SURGICAL REJUVENATION
of the
FACE

SURGICAL REJUVENATION *of the* FACE

*To my good friend and colleague —
Al Kligman
Tom Baker
2-6-96*

THOMAS J. BAKER, M.D.
Associate Clinical Professor of Surgery (Plastic)
Department of Surgery
University of Miami School of Medicine
Miami, Florida

HOWARD L. GORDON, M.D.
Associate Clinical Professor of Surgery (Plastic)
Department of Surgery
University of Miami School of Medicine
Miami, Florida

JAMES M. STUZIN, M.D.
Assistant Clinical Professor of Surgery (Plastic)
Department of Surgery
University of Miami School of Medicine
Miami, Florida

Medical Illustrator
David Peace

SECOND EDITION
with 584 illustrations

Mosby

St. Louis Baltimore Boston Carlsbad Chicago Naples New York Philadelphia Portland
London Madrid Mexico City Singapore Sydney Tokyo Toronto Wiesbaden

Mosby
Dedicated to Publishing Excellence

A Times Mirror Company

Publisher: Anne Patterson
Editor: Robert Hurley
Associate Developmental Editor: Christine Pluta
Project Manager: John Rogers
Sr. Production Editor: Kathleen L. Teal
Design: AKA Design Incorporated
Design Coordinator: Renée Duenow
Manufacturing Manager: Betty Richmond

SECOND EDITION
Copyright © 1996 by Mosby–Year Book, Inc.

Previous edition copyrighted 1986

All rights reserved. No part of this publication may be reproduced, stored in a retrieval system, or transmitted, in any form or by any means, electronic, mechanical, photocopying, recording, or otherwise, without prior written permission from the publisher.

Permission to photocopy or reproduce solely for internal or personal use is permitted for libraries or other users registered with the Copyright Clearance Center, provided that the base fee of $4.00 per chapter plus $.10 per page is paid directly to the Copyright Clearance Center, 27 Congress Street, Salem, MA 01970. This consent does not extend to other kinds of copying, such as copying for general distribution, for advertising or promotional purposes, for creating new collected works, or for resale.

Printed in the United States of America
Composition by the Clarinda Company
Printing/binding by Walsworth Publishing Co.

Mosby–Year Book, Inc.
11830 Westline Industrial Drive
St. Louis, Missouri 63146

Library of Congress Cataloging in Publication Data

Baker, Thomas J.
    Surgical rejuvenation of the face / Thomas J. Baker, Howard L. Gordon, James M. Stuzin. – 2nd ed.
      p.   cm.
    Includes bibliographical references and index.
    ISBN 0-8016-0153-3
    1. Facelift. 2. Face–Surgery. 3. Surgery, Plastic. I. Gordon, Howard L., 1927-   . II. Stuzin, James M. III. Title.
    [DNLM: 1. Face–surgery. 2. Surgery, Plastic–in old age. WE 705 B168s 1993]
RD119.5.F33B35   1993
617.5′20592–dc20
DNLM/DLC
for Library of Congress   93-42944
                                                            CIP

96 97 98 99 00 / 9 8 7 6 5 4 3 2 1

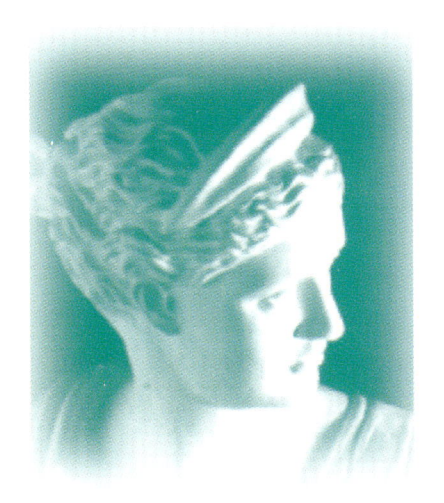

Preface

Why a second edition? Progress. Since the first edition of *Surgical Rejuvenation of the Face* was published, several advances have been made in aesthetic surgery. From what began essentially as an art form, passed down in methodology from teacher to pupil, scientific and anatomic thinking have gradually permeated into aesthetic surgery. In critically evaluating our own surgical results over the past several years, we have tried to isolate those clinical findings that by self-determination we thought needed improvement. By criticizing our own work, from both positive and negative aspects, we believe we have made alterations in the various techniques of our surgery that have led to both improved short-term and long-term results. The purpose of this book is to offer our current view of the procedures we use in rejuvenation of the aging face. Only those procedures we have personally used or have developed are described in detail. No implication is made that ours is the only, or even the best, way to achieve good results. All we mean to say is that this is how we do it now.

One of the difficulties in presenting such a simple concept—the way we do it now—is that techniques change as time goes by. When we look at videotapes of surgical procedures that we performed several years ago, we can see obvious differences between past and present techniques. How sure we often were that an apogee had been reached. And how wrong we were many times. If one compares the first and second editions of this textbook, the evolution of our surgical thinking in aesthetic surgery is apparent.

When we began the practice of the art and skill termed aesthetic surgery, we attended many conferences and meetings. We listened to long descriptions of currently used techniques, and we watched endless processions of wonderful results paraded across projection screens. We hoped that if we listened and watched long enough we too would be privy to the "secrets" of performing high-quality surgery and achieving consistently good results. The secret, of course, is that there are no secrets. Consistently good results are obtained by integrity and devotion to the pursuit of excellence, and dissatisfaction with the status quo. In our hearts, we all know when we are exerting ourselves to the utmost in this pursuit, and we know when we are not.

We present a combined aesthetic surgical experience of more than 70 years. During the first few years following our residencies, we knew we were well trained in the areas of trauma, congenital defects, and burns, but in the areas of aesthetic surgery we found our training lacking. In the early days of our practice, the mention of aesthetic surgery to our teachers was often met with a supercilious sniff of disdain. This remains somewhat true today. There are still training programs in which aesthetic surgery is looked down on. We find this somewhat hypocritical, since many of those who tend to deemphasize aesthetic surgery are guilty of performing these procedures on a regular basis but would rather those around them not know that they have placed any personal emphasis on this area of plastic and reconstructive surgery. The public today expects a plastic surgeon to be an expert in

PREFACE

aesthetic surgery first and foremost, and we believe it is the responsibility of those of us who are doing a significant volume of aesthetic surgery to pass the information along to our colleagues.

It is hard to recall the moment when pupils became teachers, but the moment has passed. In our type of practice, we are asked on a daily basis by visitors, residents, and fellows about techniques and principles. The questions sound very much like those we asked such a short time ago. It is our impression that the rising interest in aesthetic surgery has paralleled the evolution of surgical thinking in this field.

Inevitably there is change. Several areas of experience have been the source material for this second edition. First and foremost has been a better understanding of facial soft tissue anatomy and the anatomic changes that occur in the aging face. In evaluating our own cases, we decided to go back to the anatomy laboratory and undertake fresh cadaver dissections to analyze the anatomic changes that needed to be addressed in the aging face. As we began to understand the anatomic changes that occur with aging, we developed perhaps a more scientific approach to addressing these problems. For as we understand how the face ages, and know how to safely manipulate the surgical anatomy, we can approach surgical rejuvenation primarily as a reconstructive procedure, with the primary aim being to reconstruct the anatomy and reverse the changes due to aging. This is quite different from approaching these procedures as simply cosmetic techniques, lacking in scientific basis, and often introducing surgical distortion into the result. The anatomic analyzes and their clinical applications remain the core part of this current edition. We know that techniques will continue to evolve, but facial anatomy remains the constant on which these techniques must be based.

Another area of expertise that this book draws from is the shared accumulative experience of our colleagues from all over the world. One of the most savory benefits of attending meetings has been the opportunity to exchange surgical tidbits with our friends.

Still another source has been the daily association with young plastic surgeons who are nearing the completion of or who have recently completed their training. Since 1978 we have offered fellowships in aesthetic surgery. Each young surgeon has spent from 1 to several months in our offices. It has been an opportunity for them to assist in surgery on a daily basis and to participate and observe the administrative activities of private practice. We have treasured these one-on-one relationships, not only because we have come to know so many bright and engaging young surgeons but also because in teaching them what we do we have been compelled to codify and organize our own thoughts and procedures.

Finally, a large source of our experience included here has come from the teaching symposium on aesthetic surgery that we have produced since 1967.

Sometime before 1967 we observed that some of the surgical results and procedures described at meetings were not easily reproducible in the real world of our own operating rooms. In other words, it is sometimes easier said than done. We concluded that there was a need for a type of meeting where the surgeon would be called on to perform the procedure just described.

The first aesthetic surgical symposium was held at Cedars of Lebanon Hospital, Miami, in February 1967, and was attended by 100 plastic surgeons at all stages of their careers. The first faculty of our meeting included Salvador Castanares, M.D., and Thomas D. Rees, M.D. The attendees of the meeting included many old-timers as well as residents still in training. Most of the audience were newly in practice and eager to learn about aesthetic surgery from the only source available—each other. This symposium has been held annually since 1967, and has expanded to where it is overly subscribed each year. There have now been more than one hundred invited faculty members from all over the world, and the list reads like a "Who's Who" in plastic surgery. Registrants attending the Baker-Gordon-Stuzin Cosmetic Surgery Symposium have now exceeded 7,000. We, the authors, have profited greatly from the parade of visiting professors, and have personally improved our techniques as a result of these associations. The give and take of these seminars has been invaluable, not only to the registrants but to us as well.

It is an amalgamation of our close association with these visiting professors and our respected colleagues, our experience in regional and national meetings, and our return to basic science in the anatomy laboratory, combined with years of personal objective experience, that we have tried to summarize and present in this volume.

There is little doubt that the techniques we describe herein will be improved on, and indeed this is our wish. Our specialty is not static, but is forever moving forward. Aesthetic surgery is an art form that strives for perfection. That is our goal, and this is our contribution.

Acknowledgment

We gratefully acknowledge the efforts of Margaret Carapezza, without whose dedication and commitment to preparing the manuscript this textbook would not be possible.

THOMAS J. BAKER, M.D.

HOWARD L. GORDON, M.D.

JAMES M. STUZIN, M.D.

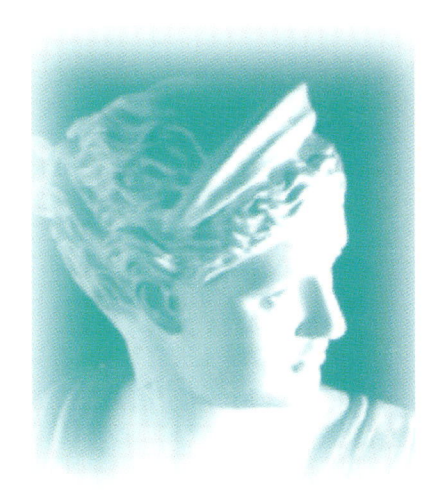

Contents

One   PATIENT-SURGEON RELATIONSHIP, *1*

Two   INTRAVENOUS SEDATION AND DRUG MANAGEMENT IN OUTPATIENT SURGERY, *11*

Three   CHEMICAL PEELING (PHENOL AND TRICHLOROACETIC ACID) AND DERMABRASION, *45*

Four   RHYTIDECTOMY, *147*

Five   BLEPHAROPLASTY, *385*

Six   CORONAL BROW LIFTING, *527*

Seven   ANCILLARY PROCEDURES, *575*

SURGICAL REJUVENATION *of the* FACE

One

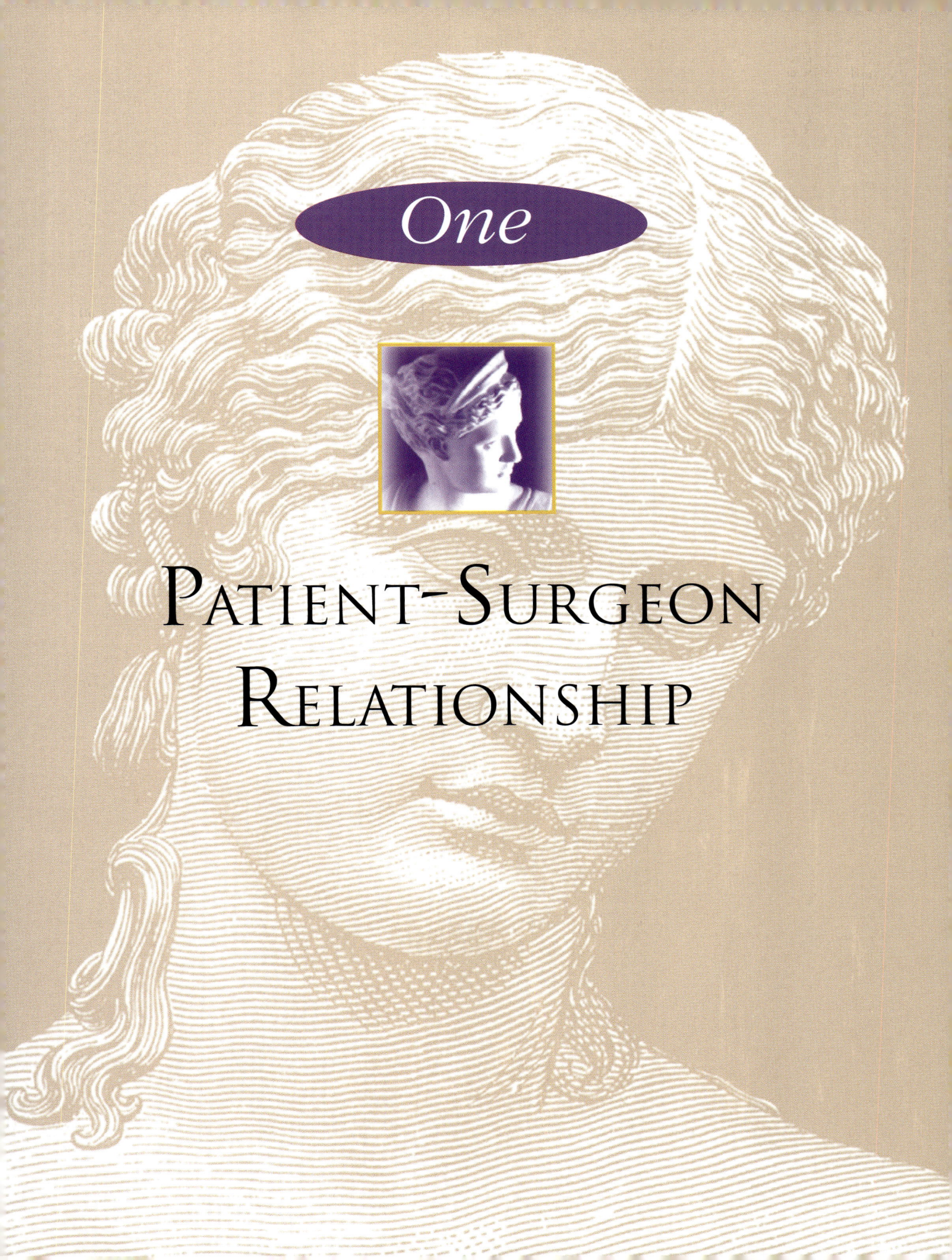

Patient-Surgeon Relationship

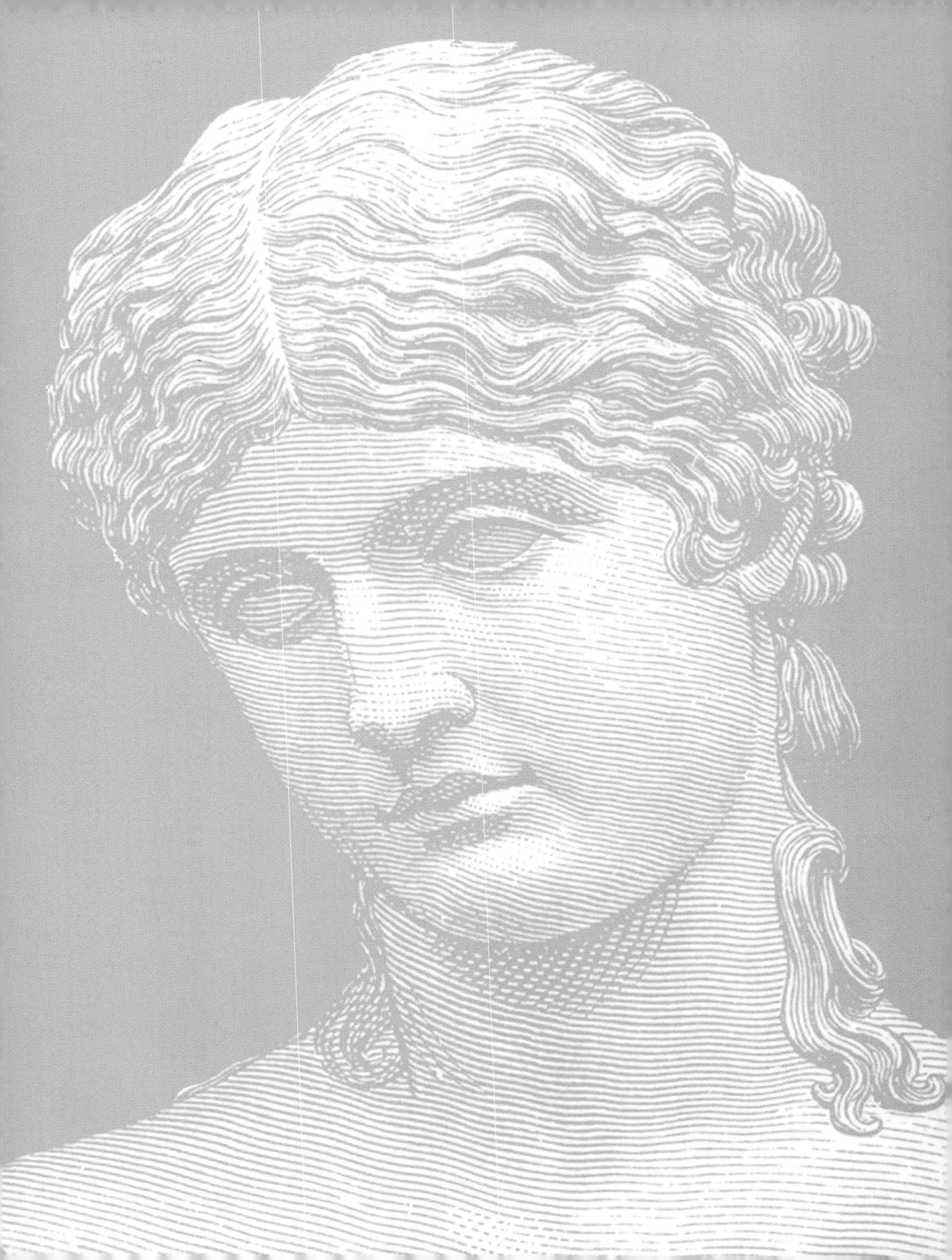

BEFORE MEETING

Our relationship with a patient often begins indirectly before we meet in person. It begins by hearing about us from former patients, friends, or colleagues and deciding to see us about a problem. Patients usually have preconceived notions about what plastic surgeons are like in general and even a specific idea of what *we* are going to be like.

INITIAL CONTACT

Because the patient's first contact with the surgeon is often made by telephone, the office personnel should be familiar with the proper technique of handling telephone conversations. The telephone manner is as important as the information conveyed. Our employees are instructed to be friendly and responsive to prospective patients and express an interest in helping them.

An experienced receptionist can often recognize a difficult patient during the initial phone contact. We have found that if the *office personnel* suspect that the new patient will be a problem, then we will probably find that the patient *will* be a problem.

Our office personnel are given specific information to supply over the telephone, such as when appointments can be scheduled, what the cost of a consultation is, and what general areas of plastic surgery we perform. They do not give medical advice or quote specific surgical fees but can give a general range of costs. We answer all medical questions.

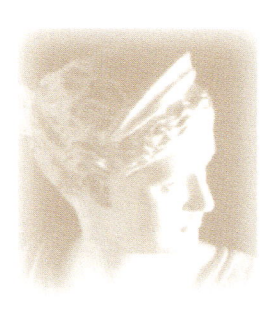

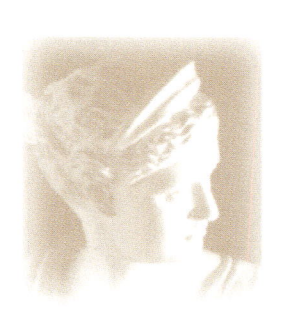

At this point the completed questionnaire can be reviewed with the patient. We ask about any previous surgery, if there are any health problems, any cigarette smoking and alcohol drinking habits, any drugs she may be taking, the presence of allergies, and if she has any current medical problems. By engaging in this conversation, the patient becomes more relaxed and the examination can proceed. If the patient's spouse or another relative accompanies her for the initial examination, this person is invited to be in the room during the interview.

We then take the patient into a brightly lit examining room and assess those changes that would improve her appearance. We combine the patient's wishes with our recommendations and develop a preoperative plan, a step-by-step description of what is to be done, and explain it to the patient. We clarify those features that can be significantly improved, those that may not be greatly improved, and those that might not be improved at all. We also explain the pros and cons of doing these various surgical procedures as well as the possible complications or undesirable results that might occur. The procedures are outlined in explicit detail so that the patient understands what is proposed, such as lines of incision, resultant scars, possible discomfort, time required for the surgery, types of medications used, the anticipated postoperative result, and the postoperative course.

We describe what will happen on the morning of the surgery. We tell the patient what she will experience in the operating room, and if there is going to be pain, we discuss it. Most people appreciate a forthright and honest physician. We inform the patient of the average length of the convalescent period and specifically when she will be able to return to work or full activity. She is told here for the first time, and it will be repeated many other times, how long it will be before she can expect to see the final result. If the patient does not inquire about risks and complications, we tell her briefly what the most common risks are and the likelihood of each occurring.

The patient is also told that this initial interview is not her last chance to talk to us. She is welcome to return as many times as she wishes for preoperative consultation, and at no extra cost. There is only an initial consultation fee. But be cautious of the patient who requests excessive preoperative visits. It is very likely that she is not hearing what is being said and it is this patient that is most likely to swear that, "He never told me!"

A week or two before the date of the surgery, the patient returns

BAKER & GORDON PLASTIC SURGERY ASSOCIATES

Name of Patient _____ Date _____

Date of Birth _____ Age _____ Married/Single/Sep./Div./Wid.

Address _____
       (permanent)   Zip Code

_____
       (local)   Zip Code

Home phone _____ Bus. phone _____ Name of Husband or wife _____

Referred by _____

Occupation _____ Employed by _____

Employer's address _____ Business phone _____

If a patient is a minor, who is legally responsible _____

1 Have you ever suffered from:
Heart disease ☐ High Blood Pressure ☐ Chest disease ☐ Recent sore throat ☐ Cold ☐ or Flu ☐ Do you have a cough ☐ Have you suffered from Bronchitis ☐ Asthma ☐ Have you had a recent chest x-ray ☐, or Electrocardiogram ☐

2 Do you suffer from Allergies ☐ or Hay Fever ☐

3 Have you ever had Diabetes ☐ Blood Disease ☐ Kidney disease ☐ Jaundice ☐ Glaucoma ☐ Cancer ☐

4 Have you ever been treated for Anemia ☐ Do you bruise easily ☐

5 Have you had any serious illness or accidents _____

6 Are you allergic to any medication; if so, which drugs _____

7 Have you ever had problems with bleeding ☐

8 Have you or any relative had a bad reaction from General or Local Anesthetic _____

9 Have you taken any of the following drugs: Aspirin ☐ Tranquilizers ☐ Water pills ☐ Blood Pressure pills ☐ Pain pills ☐ Antihistamines ☐ If so, when _____

10 Do you have any of the following habits
Smoking ☐ frequency _____
Alcoholic beverages ☐ frequency _____
Recreational drugs ☐ frequency _____

11 Have you had any previous surgery including plastic surgery ☐ What kind/When/Where
_____
_____
_____
_____

12 Have you ever consulted a professional for emotional problems ☐

13 What medications are you presently taking
_____

14 When was the last time you had a complete medical examination _____

15 Name of personal physician _____

16 Do you wear glasses? _____

17 Name of your Ophthalmologist
_____
_____

REASON FOR SEEING THE DOCTOR

Appointment with Dr. _____ SIGNATURE _____

FRONTAL   **BASAL**   **RIGHT**   **LEFT**

Patient Questionnaire.

to the office to have the laboratory work done, photographs taken, and to ask any last-minute questions.

Each patient is required to read and sign a consent form before any surgery. The consent forms are specific for each procedure. The patient also signs an additional statement to the effect that she has read and understood the particulars in the consent. Finally, all of the conditions in the written form are described verbally during the preoperative consultation.

Despite these efforts to create an informed consent, most patients do not hear or remember much of what is said or read. For this reason it is a good idea to reinforce the information by repeating it during future patient visits.

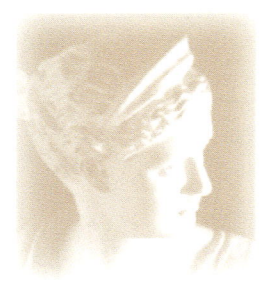

THE DAY OF SURGERY

Most of our surgery is done in our outpatient surgical unit adjacent to our office. Patients arrive early in the morning. This immediate preoperative period is critical in setting a tone for the morning. Patients are usually apprehensive before surgery. If an already jittery patient is not handled in a soothing and reassuring way, there are times when no amount of sedation and tranquilization will help.

The attitude and demeanor of the surgeon and staff affect the way the patient feels about the surgical experience and outcome. Staff members speak to the patient in quiet, reassuring tones, addressing her by name, and not using inappropriate personal terms like "honey" or "sweetie." The patient is attended while she is disrobing and being prepared for surgery. This is not a time to be alone.

We always have background music in our operating rooms; it relaxes and soothes the patient. Every effort is made to make the patient comfortable. Because operating rooms are kept notoriously cold, blankets are used to cover the patient. Arm boards are padded, heels are padded, and knees are flexed. We recently began using water-filled mattresses on the operating tables, much to the delight of our patients.

A staff member remains with the patient in the immediate hours after surgery and until the patient leaves for a recovery facility or home. If the patient's eyes are covered, it is reassuring if someone is there to talk to and provide reassurance. If the patient is somewhat drowsy and confused, someone is there to tell her that the surgery is over and all is well. Appropriate medication should be administered at the first sign of pain.

POSTOPERATIVE PERIOD

Patients require frequent and sometimes constant reassurances during the days and weeks following surgery. It is one thing to be told that there will be swelling and discoloration. It is quite another to look in the mirror in the morning and see the swelling and bruises.

We encourage our patients to return to the office any time they have questions or problems, and we are scrupulous about returning telephone calls. Our patients know that they can always reach us if necessary.

■ Postoperative Results

Why do aesthetic surgery patients seem to require more reassurance postoperatively than other surgical patients? It may be because the goals are not as clearly defined and recognized in cosmetic surgery as in general surgery. Most general surgery patients present with a specific complaint or problem. Once diagnosed the correction may be straightforward: the pain of appendicitis is gone, the bulge of the hernia is absent, or the tumor has been removed. Cosmetic surgical goals are more difficult to define. Patients want to look better—but how much better? When asked if they note improvement in the way they look, many say, "Of course, I look a lot better, but . . ."

We find that frequent reiteration of the original goals is valuable. Patients need to be reassured that everything is progressing on schedule.

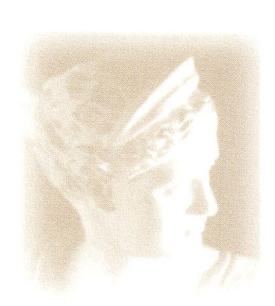

Surgeon Dissatisfaction

Sometimes we are dissatisfied with the postoperative result, whereas the patient seems perfectly satisfied. What a dilemma! Why bring up an imperfection or a less-than-optimal improvement? The tendency to keep silent is understandable. In our experience, we have almost invariably found that an open and frank appraisal of the result, pointing out a further improvement possibly as a secondary procedure, is welcomed. The patient may or may not agree to a further improvement. We always explain that this secondary procedure can be done anytime within a reasonable period, about a year in the case of a facelift that could use a little more tightening. We do not charge for the secondary procedure. The patient feels that she has been treated fairly, and the relationship has invariably been enhanced.

Patient Dissatisfaction

Patient dissatisfaction stems from several sources; a major one may be unrealistic expectations. It is important during the entire surgeon-patient relationship, beginning with the first interview, to be as specific as possible in describing obtainable goals. The patient may expect her facelift to influence her career path or solve her marital problems, both unrealistic goals, whereas the surgeon's expectations may include only tightening the neck skin and achieving a more youthful appearance. If the surgeon does not listen to the patient's desires and explain what can be realistically accomplished, he or she may be faced with a dissatisfied patient such as the one described in the following paragraph.

> A short, slightly overweight woman, about 55 years old, had undergone a facelift uneventfully. At the 6 weeks' postoperative visit the result was entirely successful in our eyes, but she looked at herself in the mirror and said half-angrily and half-wistfully, "So where's Elizabeth Taylor?"

Obviously, we had not successfully communicated our realistic expectations. We have found disparate expectations between patient and surgeon to be the major source of dissatisfaction.

Another source of patient dissatisfaction is the less-than-perfect result. Whether this is because of an unforeseen complication or a mistake in surgical judgment, we have found it far better to face the problem immediately with the patient and plan how to correct it rather than deny there is a problem. Sooner or later some correction will have to be made, either by the original surgeon or by someone else. The vast majority of people welcome and admire truthfulness and honesty.

Other sources of dissatisfaction are usually temporary. During the period of healing the patient may be afraid that the edema and discoloration of the tissues are not dissipating as quickly as she thought or as quickly as was the case with a friend of hers who was treated by another surgeon. These fears are legitimate and should be dealt with in a reassuring and supportive way. We have sometimes found the repetition of a question such as, "When will the swelling go away?" to be exasperating, but we try to remember that the patient is really saying, "Please tell me again that everything is okay."

Sometimes those relatives and friends who are sharing the experience with the patient belittle the results of the surgery or make the patient feel guilty for having had it done at all. There is nothing we can do in this circumstance except make an extra effort to be supportive and available. We try to review briefly the original goals and the timetables for achieving them on every preoperative and postoperative visit.

In the face of a less-than-optimal result and a dissatisfied patient, we have found that consultation with another physician is a valuable aid. If this suggestion comes from the operating surgeon, the patient is usually reassured that everything possible is being done to solve the problem. Almost invariably the patient returns to the original surgeon, her confidence restored by the consultant.

If the request for a consultation comes from the patient, it should be welcomed as a way of obtaining needed help and showing sincere concern for the patient's welfare. We always offer to help find a qualified consultant and often call the consultant to make the appointment.

Withheld or grudging cooperation will only make a difficult situation worse.

What if the dissatisfied patient is not your own? Here more than ever it is important to be honest and forthright with the patient. To be judgmental and condemning of what has gone before is counterproductive for all concerned. With the patient's permission, we usually contact the original surgeon, if possible, in the presence of the patient. The patient can be made to feel that all efforts are being made in a constructive direction. This is preferable to the patient's feeling that efforts are being made to cover up a mistake. We usually encourage such patients to return to the original surgeon. We also must be willing to accept these patients for treatment if it is indicated.

There is no certain way to guarantee a good relationship with a patient, but being aware of one's self as a physician and as a human being goes a long way toward establishing a satisfactory relationship. If the physician is skilled, sympathetic, and listens to the inner voice of intuition—so much the better.

Two

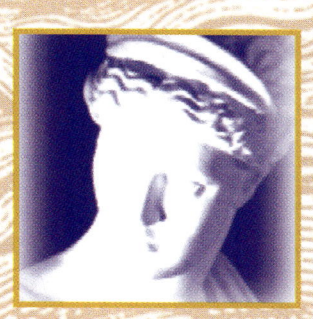

Intravenous Sedation and Drug Management in Outpatient Surgery

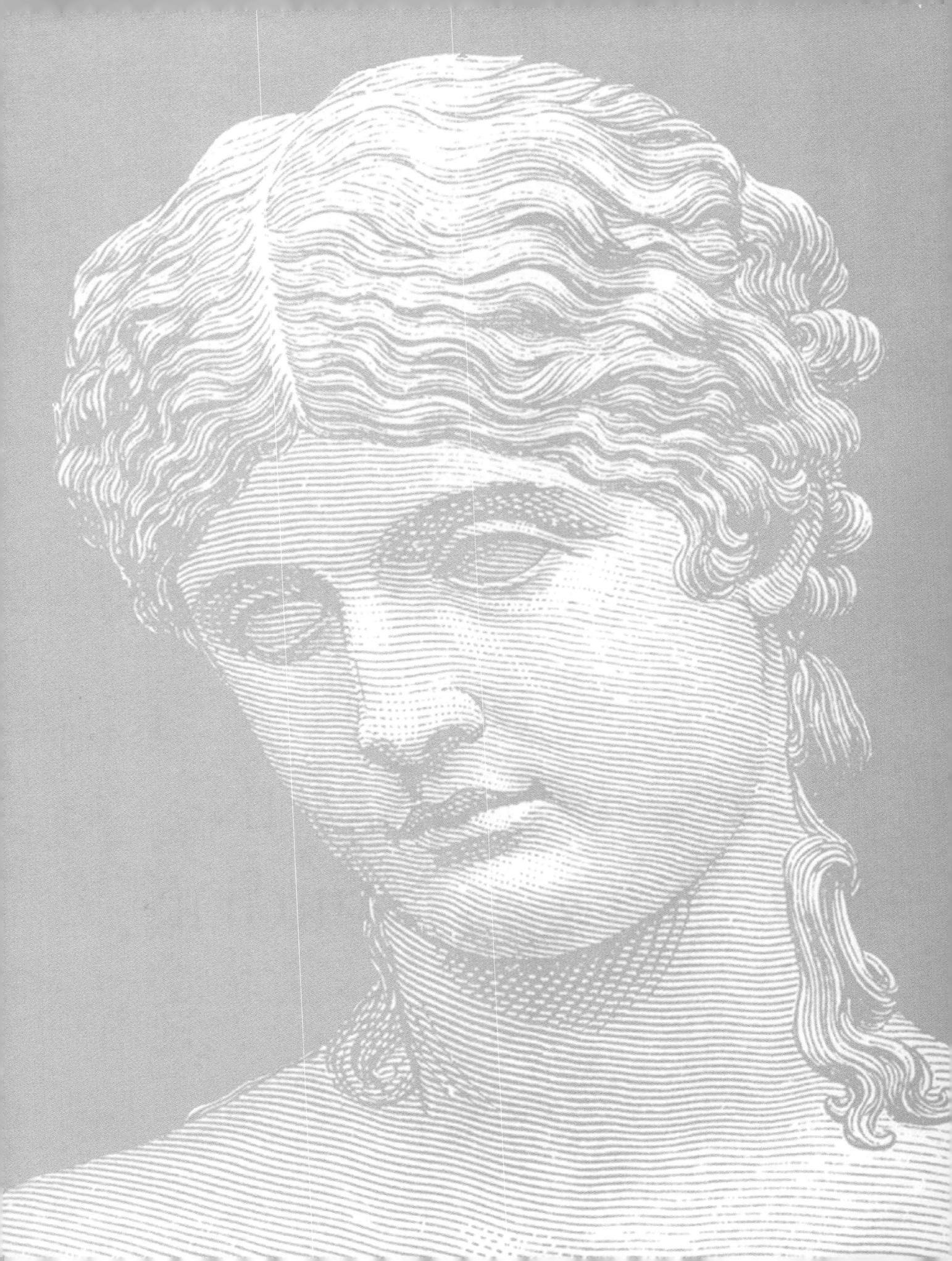

DRUG MANAGEMENT IN OUTPATIENT SURGERY

The vast majority of our aesthetic procedures are performed under local anesthesia using intravenous (IV) sedation. The prerequisite for smooth surgery is a comfortable patient who is adequately monitored and exhibits a level of sedation that is kept constant throughout the surgery. There are many choices available as to drug management in outpatient surgery, and the surgeon cannot possibly be familiar with all of the drugs available today, much less the new ones introduced almost daily. Nonetheless, a working knowledge of the basic drug groups is required, understanding their risks and benefits, deciding which medications to use, and how to manage their use in the safest and most efficient manner. This chapter provides a rationale for drug selection that will attempt to suit both the patient's and surgeon's needs during outpatient surgery.

BASIC PHARMACOLOGIC PRINCIPLES

Three pharmacologic concepts are helpful in understanding drug management in outpatient surgery: (1) the therapeutic index, (2) the dose-response curve, and (3) drug potency. These terms need to be explained before we evaluate the risks and benefits of the different drug groups. Also, a basic understanding of the pharmacokinetics of drug metabolism is required, including plasma protein binding, drug half-life, and drug elimination.

■ Therapeutic Index

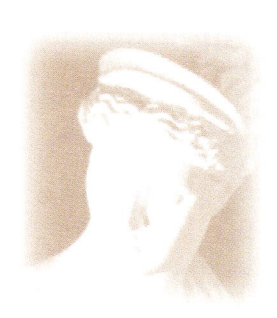

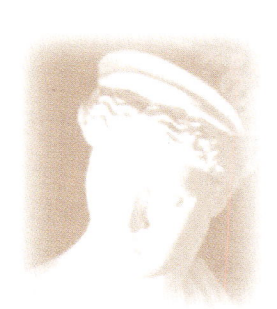

The *therapeutic index* is the ratio between the drug dose that kills 50% of the animal test subjects (LD_{50}) and the median effective drug dose (ED_{50}). The LD_{50} is insignificant in clinical application, and the therapeutic index would be better explained as the ratio between the toxic dose and the effective dose, or how far the usual therapeutic dose can be exceeded before toxicity is encountered. For example, the hypnotic dose of barbiturates in relation to the toxic dose yields a favorable therapeutic index, but since much more of the drug must be used to induce anesthesia, the therapeutic index is less favorable and there is a smaller margin of safety. The more effective a particular drug is in relation to its toxicity at any given dose, the safer and more desirable that drug is.

Dose-Response Curve

Another pharmacologic concept frequently discussed in relation to specific drugs is the *dose-response curve.* As shown in the accompanying diagram, if the dose of a drug is plotted along the horizontal coordinate of a graph and the effect of the drug, either desired or a side effect, along the vertical coordinate, it may be concluded that a drug with a steep dose-response curve has a stronger potential for toxicity or overdose than a drug with a shallow dose-response curve.

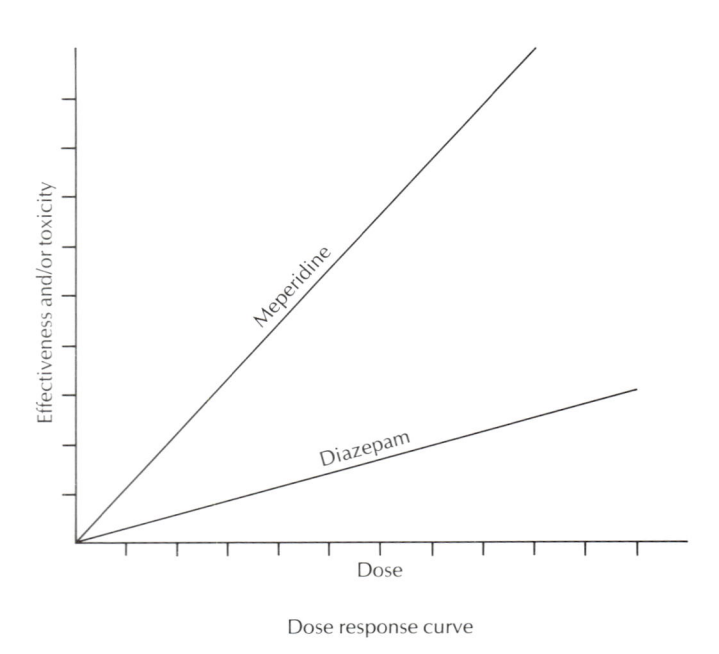

Dose response curve

For example, diazepam (Valium) has a shallow dose-response curve compared with the steep curve of meperidine (Demerol). This indicates that a therapeutic dose of diazepam can be greatly increased without reaching toxic levels. Toxic levels of meperidine can be reached more quickly with a relatively smaller increase, and so the margin of safety is smaller.

From a clinical point of view, the concept of *overdosage* is more important than dose response. All drugs have a spectrum of clinical response, and the safety of the drug depends on the person administering the agent and the adequacy of patient monitoring. The variability from patient to patient in terms of response to anesthetic agents requires that judicious incremental dosages of medications be given and that the patient be carefully evaluated regarding therapeutic response.

Potency

Drug potency also warrants consideration. *Potency* is the relationship between biologic activity and unit dose weight. Within the usual limits of drugs that are commercially available to the average practitioner, potency is generally irrelevant. If one drug is twice as potent as the next, but the efficacy is the same, all the surgeon needs to do is double the dose of the drug with the lesser potency. Efficacy is the primary concern, not potency.

Pharmacokinetics

Drugs can be given orally (e.g., diazepam for premedication) and by injection to the operative field, (e.g., lidocaine). Once in the blood, a certain fraction always binds to plasma proteins, so only the unbound portion is available to affect the receptor organ. Plasma protein binding is important in patients on chronic medication, since some of the binding sites will be occupied by the chronically ingested medication. In these situations an administered drug may be unbound and reach "overdose concentrations" sooner. It is also possible that an agent will be displaced from binding sides by administered drugs, and this can produce an overdose effect of its own (e.g., dicumarol will decrease blood clotting when displaced from its binding sites and may increase the bleeding tendency). The one agent commonly used in our outpatient surgery that is not bound to plasma proteins is ketamine.

Most drugs are metabolized by the liver and eliminated predominantly through the kidneys. The patient with impaired function of these organs will usually require lower doses of administered drugs, since these medications will be metabolized and eliminated more slowly. Some chronically taken agents will induce increased enzyme activity in the liver and increase the dosage required for clinical effectiveness. Among these enzyme inducers are barbiturates and antiepileptic drugs, as well as cigarettes and alcohol. This increased enzyme activity means that any drugs administered during surgery will tend to be metabolized and deactivated more rapidly, and anesthetic agents will therefore have to be administered more frequently or given in larger amounts.

Drug Interaction

The drug interactions of most concern in outpatient surgery involve drugs used in psychiatry for the treatment of depression: tricyclic antidepressants and monoamine oxidase (MAO) inhibitors. Patients on these agents may prove to be sensitive to epinephrine, and unpredictable or prolonged extremes of cardiovascular responses may occur. This is especially true for the MAO inhibitors, and it is advisable that patients taking these medications discontinue these drugs 2 weeks before surgery. While similar considerations are warranted regarding tricyclic antidepressants, most patients using these drugs tolerate the small doses of epinephrine administered with local anesthetic agents and show little cardiovascular response during surgery. Nonetheless, we tend to administer epinephrine incrementally in these patients and evaluate the cardiovascular response before the wide dispersal of anesthetic agents in the operative field. If possible, however, we prefer that the patient stop these medications preoperatively.

Drug Management

Many patients are on chronic medication before surgery, and most of these agents should be continued throughout the perioperative period. We believe that antihypertensive, cardiac, and hormonal agents should be continued right through the day of surgery. For patients who are on oral hypoglycemic medication or require insulin for the management of blood sugar control, consultation is always obtained with the patient's internist to ensure proper control of glucose levels perioperatively. Patients requiring the regular administration of aspirin or anti-inflammatory agents that contain prostaglandin inhibitors are taken off these medications at least 2 weeks before to surgery.

Pharmacology of Individual Agents
Local anesthetic agents

Local anesthetics prevent the generation and transmission of nerve impulses; these effects are transient and reversible. Clinical applications include local infiltration and block anesthesia, surface anesthesia, spinal anesthesia, epidural and caudal anesthesia, and IV anesthesia. For the most part, in our outpatient surgical setting, we use these agents for local infiltration and block anesthesia.

Local anesthetics usually start out as weak bases that are converted into salts and ionized in solution. Only the ionized form of the drug is available for its pharmacologic effect. A tendency toward acidity will impede, and alkalinity will enhance, the activity of these drugs.

The main site of action of local anesthetics is at the cell membrane. They block impulse conduction by interfering with the increased membrane permeability to sodium ions produced by membrane depolarization. In other words, they stabilize the cell membrane.

Nerve fibers can be classified as A, B, or C fibers. A fibers are the largest and are myelinated; B fibers are smaller and myelinated; C fibers are the smallest, are unmyelinated, and tend to transmit painful stimuli. Local anesthetic drugs depress the smallest and unmyelinated fibers first and the largest and myelinated fibers last. Therefore the order of functional loss after the administration of a local anesthetic is pain, temperature, touch, proprioception, and skeletal muscle tone.

Absorption of a local anesthetic, or any drug for that matter, depends on the injection site, its vascularity, the dose, and the presence of a vasoconstrictor, such as epinephrine, mixed with the injected solution. The more vascular the site of injection, the higher the blood level achieved, and the sooner the peak concentration in the blood. Also, the more vascular the site of injection, the more rapidly the effects of the drug wear off.

For a given site, absorption depends on the dose alone, not on the concentration of the solution injected.

Local vasoconstriction, caused by epinephrine mixed with the solution, will slow absorption and maintain the anesthetic effect for a longer time. Absorption brings the anesthetic into the bloodstream. While the anesthetic is bloodborne, a portion is bound to plasma protein fractions. This limits the amount of drug that is freely disfusable and subsequently effective.

Most local anesthetics are classified either as esters or amides. Common ester-linked local anesthetics are procaine, chloroprocaine, and tetracaine. These are hydrolyzed in the plasma and excreted in the urine. Amide-linked local anesthetics such as lidocaine, mepivacaine, prilocaine, and bupivacaine are metabolized in the liver and excreted in the urine. These metabolites are less toxic than the parent drugs, with the single exception of prilocaine, whose metabolic products are reported to cause methemoglobinemia.

As a rule, the amides are less likely to produce an allergic reaction than the esters. In fact, most allergic reactions to local anesthetics are misdiagnosed, and are probably overdoses of the anesthetic or reactions to either the preservative in the anesthetic or to the epinephrine mixed with the anesthetic.

Properties of local anesthetics that should be considered when choosing one for use include potency, duration of action, speed of onset, and toxicity. By far, the most widely used local anesthetic today is lidocaine. Its effect begins shortly after administration, its duration is satisfactory for most procedures, and there is a minimal chance of producing a true allergic reaction.

Some local anesthetics are more lipid-soluble than others. For example, etidocaine is highly lipid-soluble compared with lidocaine. For that reason it affects myelinated motor nerves for a very long time. A motor nerve block sometimes lasts for 1 or 2 days.

Drugs such as etidocaine and bupivacaine that have a high protein-binding capacity may bind to the protein in the heart muscle. If a cardiac arrest were to occur with these drugs, it would necessitate long and complicated resuscitation. One perfect anesthetic does not exist, for if it did we all would be using it.

In almost every instance, local anesthetic toxicity is purely a matter of overdose. There are maximum safe allowable doses for each local anesthetic with and without epinephrine, and these should not be exceeded. The total dose is the important consideration, not the concentration of the solution (Table 2-1).

TABLE 2-1 Suggested maximum doses of local anesthetics*

Anesthetic†	Body weight (mg/kg)	Dose for average adult (mg)‡
Procaine (Novocain)	14.0	1,000
Prilocaine (Citanest)	10.0	600
Lidocaine (Xylocaine)	7.0	500
Mepivacaine (Carbocaine)	7.0	500
Tetracaine (Pontocaine)	1.5	100
Bupivacaine (Marcaine)	4.0	250
Etidocaine (Duranest)	6.0	400

*Adapted from de Jong RH: *Local anesthetics*, ed 2, Springfield, Ill, 1977, Charles C Thomas.
†All anesthetics include epinephrine.
‡These are *suggested* maximum doses that provide optimal therapeutic effects with minimal side effects. These doses are not necessarily either "safe" or the absolute maximal dose. Severe reactions can be encountered with much smaller doses.

Headache, tinnitus, dizziness, blurred vision, a flushed or chilled feeling, confusion, slurred speech, nystagmus, shivers, muscle twitches, and convulsions are the signs and symptoms of progressive central nervous system (CNS) toxicity in the case of local anesthetic overdose. Most of the early signs of a toxic reaction relate to CNS stimulation, and a patient who is conscious enough to speak can relate these symptoms to the surgeon. In severe toxic reactions, the early CNS stimulation progresses to convulsions and to cardiovascular collapse (see first box below).

Prophylaxis for local anesthetic toxicity is primarily dose control, followed by adequate ventilation and administration of oxygen. The preferred treatment of the toxic state includes ventilation and possibly the administration of diazepam for control of seizure. *The problem is not the convulsion; the problem is hypoxia* (see second box below).

SIGNS OF CENTRAL NERVOUS SYSTEM TOXICITY

Headache	Flushed or chilled feeling
Light-headedness	Confusion
Tinnitus	Slurred speech
Drowsiness	Nystagmus
Dizziness	Shivers and muscle twitches
Blurred vision	Convulsions

MANAGEMENT OF CENTRAL NERVOUS SYSTEM TOXICITY

Prophylaxis: ventilation, oxygen administration, barbiturates, diazepam (preferred), dose control
Treatment: ventilation, airway support, oxygen administration, diazepam, Trendelenburg's position
Remember: the problem is not the convulsion; the problem is *hypoxia*

Analgesics

Analgesics are drugs that have a predominant pain-relieving action. Most analgesics used as preoperative medication are narcotics. Narcotics are given to increase the patient's pain threshold. Narcotics mainly alter the patient's response to painful stimuli. The patient may still feel the pain, but does not respond to it in the usual way.

As a risk factor, narcotics cause some degree of respiratory depression, particularly when given in combination with other respiratory depressants such as barbiturates.

Drug half-life has to be considered when administering narcotics. Half-life refers to the time required after drug administration for 50% of the drug to be eliminated. For instance, a patient with respiratory depression who receives a narcotic antagonist that has a very short half-life, such as naloxone (Narcan), may become renarcotized if the original narcotic has a longer half-life than the antagonist. For this reason, a second dose of the antagonist (naloxone) may be required 30 minutes to 1 hour after the first dose to maintain adequate reversal of the longer-acting agonist (i.e., morphine). Other problems frequently caused by narcotics include nausea and vomiting, as well as possible dysphoria (Table 2-2).

Fentanyl (Sublimaze) is the most common narcotic used by us. It is administered in incremental doses during surgery. Its undesirable side effects include respiratory depression and bradycardia. The peak de-

TABLE 2-2 Narcotics

Risks	Benefits
Respiratory depression	Sedation
Hypotension (with hypovolemia)	Analgesia (changes affect)
Nausea and vomiting	
Dysphoria	
Steep dose-response curve	

pressant effect following administration of fentanyl is usually noted between 5 and 15 minutes after injection, and the clinical effect of the drug lasts between 30 and 60 minutes. The analgesic potency of 100 µg (equal to 2 cc) of fentanyl corresponds to approximately 75 mg of meperidine, or approximately 10 mg of morphine. The limited duration of action of fentanyl makes it useful in an outpatient surgical setting, especially in short procedures in which the patient is expected to be alert at the end of the procedure. Clinically, we administer this drug in 25-µg increments and evaluate the effect before administering more medication. Fentanyl can be reversed by naloxone.

Meperidine differs from fentanyl predominantly in its clinical duration of action, which is 2 to 4 hours, and in that it may occasionally produce tachycardia after IV injection. Because of its potential for tachycardia, meperidine should be used with caution with a history of atrial flutter or other supraventricular tachycardias. Our main indication for the use of meperidine is in the treatment of postoperative pain in the recovery room and in patients undergoing phenol chemical peels. It also is useful in the patient recovering from neuroleptic analgesia who shows evidence of shivering. Administered in small IV doses (10 mg), meperidine is useful in controlling this troublesome symptom. Another indication for the use of meperidine is in long procedures requiring several hours of sedation. In this situation, incremental administration of 10-mg doses of meperidine is useful in maintaining a constant state of analgesia and requires less frequent dosing as compared with the use of IV fentanyl.

Barbiturates

Barbiturates are drugs that provide a significant sedative-hypnotic effect. Barbiturates commonly used include methohexital (Brevital), pentobarbital (Nembutal), secobarbital (Seconal), and phenobarbital.

In their favor, barbiturates are time-tested, inexpensive, and have predictable toxicity. They are also effective orally, and are associated with little nausea and vomiting. A disadvantage of barbiturates is that the sedative action is greater than the degree of anxiety relief. Furthermore, barbiturates have a steep dose-response curve and a low therapeutic index. The half-life of barbiturates varies from very short (e.g., methohexital sodium), to several hours, as with phenobarbital (Table 2-3). A barbiturate overdose usually requires some form of respiratory support.

The barbiturate that we use most commonly in our practice is methohexital. Methohexital is an ultra-short-acting barbiturate and can be used as a supplementary sedative near the end of the procedure in doses of 10 to 20 mg. We also use it in boluses of 0.5 mg/kg in unmedicated patients for very short procedures (removal of lesions) to make the patient unaware during the time the local anesthetic is administered. The 3 to 4 minutes of anesthesia gained with methohexital administration is usually sufficient to regionally block an area with local anesthetics.

Side effects of small boluses of methohexital administration are insignificant, but coughing, laryngospasm, hiccups, and muscle twitching have all been reported with larger doses. The onset of effect following methohexital administration is rapid, usually within 30 seconds (one circulation time), and its effects last for about 5 minutes. It is not bound to plasma proteins and in animals is not detected in the blood 24 hours after administration.

TABLE 2-3 Barbiturates

Risks	Benefits
Degree of sedation greater than anxiety relief	Sedation
Respiratory depressant	Antianxiety effect
Painful intramuscular injection	Inexpensive
Long half-life	Predictable toxicity
Steep dose-response curve	Effective orally
Low therapeutic index	Little nausea
	Time-tested

Benzodiazepines

Benzodiazepines are antianxiety drugs, often referred to as minor tranquilizers. They include chlordiazepoxide (Librium), diazepam (Valium), oxazepam (Serax), lorazepam (Ativan), and midazolam (Versed). The major difference between the members of this group of drugs seems to be variation in half-life, from 90 minutes in the case of oxazepam to 2 or 3 days in the case of diazepam.

These drugs seem to have more benefits than risks. They are effective anticonvulsants. Their antianxiety effect is greater than the sedative effect, and they are easily absorbed when taken orally. They are skeletal muscle relaxants and have a flat dose-response curve. Nonetheless, when used in IV sedation, these drugs should be administered incrementally and individualization of dosage is required. Respiratory sedation and even respiratory arrest have been reported with IV dosage of both diazepam and midazolam. Other risks in the use of benzodiazepines include painful IV administration, which is more common with the use of diazepam than with midazolam. These drugs show poor intramuscular absorption, and patients often complain of a hangover after drug administration. Possible addiction to these drugs when taken chronically should be considered.

Midazolam is the benzodiazepine most commonly used in our practice. It exhibits a CNS depressant effect causing sedation as well as relief of anxiety, and an increase in dose produces drowsiness and sleep. The most important beneficial effect in terms of outpatient surgical management is the amnesia that is observed in approximately 80% of patients following IV administration of this medication.

Its undesirable effects relate to its CNS confusion, as well as possible respiratory depression. Hiccups have been reported in approximately 4% of patients and if this is exhibited at the time of IV administration, midazolam should be discontinued and diazepam substituted in its place.

Overdose of benzodiazepines clinically manifests itself as snoring followed by airway obstruction. This commonly responds to jaw elevation and airway support. The respiratory depressant effects of midazolam are often not apparent immediately and usually appear approximately 2 to 3 minutes after the IV bolus has been given. For this reason, midazolam should be administered in incremental doses of 1 to 2 mg and the doses separated by at least 2 minutes. This is especially important in the older patient in whom the respiratory depressant effects appear to be more common.

We would note here that the respiratory depression seen with midazolam administration is different from the overdose observed with narcotics. Usually the patient who has shown depressant effects with midazolam will exhibit airway obstruction that responds to airway support and jaw elevation. The patient will then take a breath by herself. This is in contrast to an overdose with narcotics, in which case the patient makes no respiratory effort despite an open airway. In other words, the respiratory depression with the benzodiazepines will usually respond simply to airway support, whereas the overdose seen with narcotics requires ventilation either by an Ambu bag via mask or tube, as well as reversal with naloxone. We would emphasize this basic difference in the management of overdosage between benzodiazepines and narcotics. Benzodiazepine overdosage requires *airway support*, whereas narcotic overdosage also requires *ventilation.* The use of a benzodiazepine antagonist (flumazenil [Mazicon]) and narcotic antagonist (naloxone) should also be considered.

Midazolam is short-acting. After IV administration, sedation is achieved in 3 to 5 minutes, although it will take only 1 to 2 minutes if a narcotic premedication has been given. Peak sedation will take 30 minutes to occur and the effect usually wears off between 60 to 120 minutes. We use midazolam in 1- to 2-mg increments and frequent boluses during a longer case are required to keep a continuous level of sedation.

Diazepam is the other benzodiazepine we use. It differs from midazolam in that it is much longer-acting, and its half-life is similarly longer. It is supplied for injection in a mixture of propylene, ethanol, and water, which can produce a burning sensation when given intravenously. It is also less potent than midazolam and we give increments of 2.5 mg of diazepam for IV sedation. Our main indication for diazepam is as a premedication (10-15 mg orally), or in incremental IV boluses during longer procedures in which several hours of sedation are required.

Benzodiazepine antagonists

The benzodiazepine antagonist flumazenil is currently available. Flumazenil is indicated in those situations in which patients show respiratory depression with hypoventilation secondary to benzodiazepine overdosage. In this clinical situation, the first means of therapy should be, of course, to establish airway support and ventilation. As an adjunct, 0.4 mg of IV flumazenil has been shown to be effective in reversing the sedative and psychomotor effects of the benzodiazepines. Because the half-life of flumazenil is short, resedation can occur in patients who have received longer-acting benzodiazepines, especially in large doses (greater than 20 mg midazolam) or in procedures that have lasted longer than 60 minutes. Any patient who is treated with flumazenil should be monitored carefully for the occurrence of resedation. We would point out that our experience with flumazenil is that it does not fully reverse the ventilatory insufficiency induced by benzodiazepines and is only an adjunct in this clinical situation. Airway support and cessation of benzodiazepine administration remain the primary means of treating hypoventilation resulting from benzodiazepine overdosage.

Antihistamines

Antihistamines are included with sedative-hypnotics because of the strong sedative effect they produce. Diphenhydramine (Benadryl) and promethazine (Phenergan) are used preoperatively for their calming and antihistaminic effects. Promethazine can enhance the effects of narcotics. Diphenhydramine is particularly effective as a preoperative medication for the very young or very old who do not tolerate barbiturates.

Hydroxyzines

Hydroxyzines include drugs such as hydroxyzine pamoate (Vistaril) and hydroxyzine hydrochloride (Atarax). An advantage of hydroxyzine pamoate is its ability to potentiate the analgesic effect of narcotics. It also has antihistaminic and anticholinergic effects that may make it useful as a preoperative medication. Hydroxyzines are antiemetic and offer some degree of anxiety relief, making them particularly suitable for preoperative medication.

Risks associated with these drugs include poor intramuscular absorption and the pain of intramuscular injection. This group of drugs has a long half-life.

Phenothiazines

Phenothiazines are considered major tranquilizers, and are usually grouped into three categories: the piperidines, the aliphatics, and the piperazines. The piperidine group includes thioridazine (Mellaril) and mesoridazine (Serentil) and is the least potent. The aliphatic group includes promazine (Sparine), chlorpromazine (Thorazine), and triflupromazine (Vesprin), and is of medium potency. The piperazine group includes trifluoperazine (Stelazine), perphenazine (Trilafon), prochlorperazine (Compazine), and fluphenazine dihydrochloride (Prolixin), and is the most potent. A benefit derived from using this group of drugs is their nonaddictive nature; they are very effective in changing the mood and behavior of the patient without excessive sedation.

These drugs have many side effects (e.g., chlorpromazine has strong antiemetic and antihypertensive effects). Many phenothiazines also have some anticholinergic and antiadrenergic effects (Table 2-4).

The most common use of phenothiazines in our practice is the use of chlorpromazine as an intraoperative agent in the control of blood pressure. The IV administration of chlorpromazine causes a lowering of blood pressure due to a combination of central action and peripheral α-adrenergic blockade, which produces peripheral vasodilation and occasionally reflex tachycardia. The response in terms of blood

TABLE 2-4 Phenothiazines, butyrophenones, and thioxanthines

Risks	Benefits
Postural hypotension	Antiemetic
Dysphoria	Low risk of tolerance
Potentiates narcotics	Low risk of dependency
Blood dyscrasias	Antipruritic
Skin rashes	Antianxiety effects with little sedation
Endocrine (e.g., amenorrhea)	Antipsychotic effects

pressure to very small (1.0-2.5 mg) IV doses of chlorpromazine is often dramatic. In the patient undergoing rhytidectomy, chlorpromazine administration will lower blood pressure. Incremental dosage up to 7.5 mg over a period of time will usually control intraoperative hypertension in most patients. One must keep in mind that chlorpromazine is usually provided in solutions of 25 mg/mL and this must be diluted so that only 1.0- to 2.5-mg incremental doses of this medication are administered to prevent severe intraoperative hypotension.

Butyrophenones

Two commonly used butyrophenones are haloperidol (Haldol) and droperidol. Droperidol is available as a solitary agent (Inapsine) and in combination with fentanyl (Innovar).

Droperidol is an agent that we have begun to use more commonly in our practice for premedication and anesthesia induction. In IV doses of 2.5 to 5.0 mg, droperidol offers intraoperative sedation, is long-acting, and also offers strong antiemetic effects. The main purpose of using droperidol is as a preoperative inducing agent, which lessens the amount of preoperative midazolam or diazepam required for sedation when ketamine is used to provide dissociative anesthesia.

Anticholinergics

Anticholinergic drugs are competitive antagonists of acetylcholine or organs innervated by postganglionic cholinergic nerves. The cardiovascular system, the CNS, the gastrointestinal system, the eyes, and the urinary tract are all affected. Unpleasant clinical effects include dryness of the mouth and respiratory tract, tachycardia, blurred vision, hot and dry skin, and CNS excitement.

Anticholinergics (parasympatholytics) have historically been used as preoperative medications. The major anticholinergic drugs are atropine and, to a lesser degree, scopolamine. These drugs are administered to reduce tracheobronchial secretions. Previously, when ether was commonly used as an inhalant general anesthetic, these secretions needed to be minimized because of ether's irritation of the tracheobronchial tree.

Atropine and scopolamine easily pass the blood-brain barrier. If an anticholinergic is indicated for a specific case or even as a routine preoperative medication, a drug like glycopyrrolate (Robinul 0.2 mg) is perhaps a better choice because it does not pass the blood-brain barrier and the CNS side effects are avoided.

In our practice, the administration of atropine is usually confined to the treatment of intraoperative bradycardia that is vasovagal in origin. Atropine is administered in 0.4-mg IV increments.

Adrenergic blocking agents

The adrenergic blocking agents constitute another group of drugs the surgeon needs to be familiar with when considering preoperative and intraoperative medications. Antiadrenergics inhibit the action of catecholamines and other adrenergic agonists on their specific receptors.

Although most aesthetic surgeons do not prescribe them, many patients will come for surgery after recently taking or while still taking some form of adrenergic blocking agent. These drugs have many different uses. They are commonly used to treat angina pectoris, cardiac arrhythmias, hypertension, heart failure, and as migraine prophylaxis, as well as other conditions such as glaucoma and certain varieties of tremors.

The adrenergic blocking drugs can be classified as α- or β-adrenergic blocking agents, indicating the presence of two types of receptors. In tissues that possess both α- and β-receptors, such as most peripheral blood vessels, α-stimulation causes contraction and β-stimulation causes relaxation. α-Adrenergic blocking drugs cause vasodilation, and in organs such as the heart, whose receptors are almost entirely β-receptors, β-blockers oppose the excitatory effects of norepinephrine.

α-Adrenergic blocking agents include tolazoline (Priscoline) and phentolamine (Regitine). These drugs cause peripheral vasodilation, resulting in lower blood pressure and orthostatic hypotension.

The adrenergic blocking agents most often encountered preoperatively are β-adrenergic blocking agents. These drugs, such as propranolol (Inderal), competitively antagonize the effects of catecholamines on the β-receptors. Consequently, there is decreased heart rate, slowed atrioventricular conduction, decreased cardiac contractility, increased bronchoconstriction, lessened plasma renin activity, and possible hypoglycemia.

Intraoperatively, the administration of propranolol in 1-mg increments is occasionally required in patients who develop supraventricular tachycardia in response to administered epinephrine. If the patient is tolerating a rapid rhythm, we wait several minutes for the epinephrine response to wear off before considering the administration of an adrenergic blocking agent. Nonetheless, low doses of propranolol can be useful in these situations, as well as with patients who develop atrial flutter with a rapid ventricular response.

α-Adrenergic agonists

Clonidine represents a selective α_2-adrenergic agonist that has been used in the treatment of systemic hypertension. It exhibits both peripheral as well as central effects, and it is an activator of central α_2-receptors in the lower brainstem which is believed to be responsible for its clinical effect in lowering blood pressure.

In outpatient surgery we have found clonidine to be a useful preoperative medication in the regulation of blood pressure, specifically in patients undergoing rhytidectomy. In patients with normal blood pressure 0.1 mg of clonidine is administered preoperatively by mouth. In patients with a history of hypertension, 0.2 to 0.3 mg of clonidine is used. The effects of clonidine are usually apparent within 1 hour of administration, and because of the long duration of this drug, a systolic blood pressure in the range of 90 to 110 mm Hg is apparent for up to 12 hours following its administration. In our opinion, this represents the ideal blood pressure range in patients undergoing a long and potentially bloody procedure such as rhytidectomy, and offers blood pressure control in the early postoperative period when hematoma development is most common. The use of clonidine as a preoperative agent also appears to have a sedative effect that reduces the amount of other sedatives and analgesic agents required during the surgery.

The major side effect of clonidine is the development of a dry mouth and orthostatic hypotension, which is most evident in the recovery room as the patient is getting ready to leave the outpatient surgical facility. Orthostatic hypotension resulting from clonidine responds rapidly to IV fluid administration, as well as patient stimulation.

Dissociative anesthetic agents

Ketamine. Ketamine hydrochloride is a phencyclidine derivative that has limited usefulness because of its psychic and circulatory side effects. This drug is not new; for many years it has been used in young children who require multiple, frequent anesthesia without muscle relaxation for short procedures such as burn dressings and debridements. There are many reports of postanesthetic psychic problems related to the use of ketamine. They range from terrifying dreams during the anesthesia to flashbacks and schizophrenic-like episodes occurring later.

Our current enthusiasm for using this drug relates to its high therapeutic index; i.e., there is a very large margin of safety because the effective dose is far short of the toxic dose. This drug provides an ideal way of achieving a short pain-free period.

Elimination of the postanesthetic psychotic side effect following ketamine administration has been accomplished by dose control and the concomitant use of midazolam, diazepam, or droperidol to provide sedation before to ketamine administration. Using this low-dose ketamine regimen in combination with sedative agents, we have eliminated this unpleasant reaction in more than 10,000 cases.

Most of our patients receive 5 mg of diazepam orally about 30 minutes before going to the operating room, and in the operating room enough droperidol and midazolam is given intravenously to produce a drowsy state so that the patient's speech is slurred, but she can still be aroused. Commonly, 2.5 to 5.0 mg of droperidol is administered and 2 to 3 mg of midazolam is given to achieve the necessary degree of sedation.

Following the administration of the sedative agents, ketamine is given intravenously over 60 seconds. The usual dose is between 0.5 and 1.0 mg/kg.

Ketamine has a different mode of action than other anesthetic agents. The drug induces a cataleptic or trancelike state, during which the patient appears to be dissociated from her surroundings and does not feel any pain, but also does not appear to be asleep. The gag and cough reflexes are preserved, and the laryngeal protective reflex, used in swallowing, also remains active. As a result, airway obstruction and aspiration are less likely to occur during ketamine anesthesia than with many other agents. The patient usually reports feeling nothing and remembering nothing during this period. There is usually a transient, perhaps 5- or 10-minute, period of hypertension and tachycardia. We have also had several cases of increased tenacious secretions of the naso pharynx and mouth after using ketamine, and on rare occasions the patient required suctioning of the oropharynx. This is usually observed when using high doses of ketamine and is prevented by the preoperative administration of glycopyrrolate (0.2 mg).

When a second dose of local anesthetic needs to be given, perhaps when multiple procedures are to be done, a second dose of ketamine can be administered 1 or 2 hours later. We usually use one half to two thirds of the original dose. We have used this regimen of ketamine with midazolam or diazepam or droperidol in a variety of cases, including rhytidectomies, blepharoplasties, rhinoplasties, augmentation mammoplasties and mastopexies. Our experience and those of the patients have been so overwhelmingly favorable that we are expanding the use of this technique.

Following ketamine administration, in patients with a history of hypertension, occasionally the blood pressure will remain high longer than the arbitrarily set limit of 10 minutes. We have found that a small amount of chlorpromazine, in 1- to 2-mg increments, will usually lower the blood pressure to a normal level within several minutes. With clonidine premedication, this appears to be a less common problem.

Much of the criticism of ketamine from anesthesiologists is related to their experience with much higher doses of ketamine without the accompanying midazolam or diazepam. The key to successful use of this valuable drug is dose control and the use of sedative agents before ketamine administration.

Propofol. Propofol (Diprivan) is an IV hypnotic agent commonly used in the induction or maintenance of neuroleptic analgesia, as well as in general anesthesia. Intravenous injection of propofol produces hypnosis rapidly and smoothly, usually with minimal excitation, with a rapid induction of anesthesia usually within 1 to 3 minutes following administration of the medication. While the half-life of propofol ranges from 5 to 12 hours, the rapid redistribution from the CNS to other tissues following cessation of the drug accounts for the relatively rapid recovery from anesthesia after administration is discontinued.

Other drugs that cause CNS depression, such as sedatives and narcotics, increase the CNS depression induced by propofol and therefore lower the dose necessary for neuroleptic analgesia. Because of this, the dosage should be individualized and titrated to the desired effect according to the patient's age and clinical status. If propofol is going to be used as an inducing agent at the time of local anesthetic administration, it can be given in boluses of 2.0 to 2.5 mg/kg. More commonly, we use this medication as a maintenance infusion at a rate of 0.1 to 0.2 mg/kg/min, titrating the dosage to the patient's clinical needs. The main advantage of propofol is the relative safety of this drug in terms of cardiovascular and respiratory depression, as well as the rapid elimination of clinical effect following cessation of drug administration. The relative disadvantage of this medication is its high cost, and specifically in long procedures such as rhytidectomy, several ampules of this drug are required to maintain adequate neuroleptic analgesia.

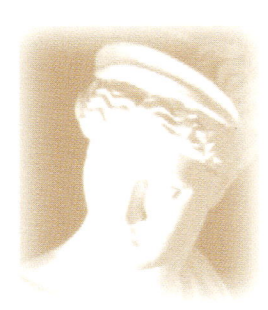

TECHNIQUE OF DRUG MANAGEMENT IN OUTPATIENT SURGERY

Neuroleptic analgesia provides sedation for patients in whom anesthesia for the operation is obtained by infiltration of the surgical field with local anesthetics. This sedation should be heavy enough to render the patient comfortable during the operation and amnesic following the procedure. It should also provide the surgeon with a steady and quiet operative field, and should be safe enough to result in only minimal interference with the patient's vital signs.

■ Monitoring Depth of Neuroleptic Analgesia

Just as in general anesthesia, the depth of neuroleptic analgesia results from a balance of depression and stimulation. The depression is produced by the IV drug administration, and the stimulation comes from touching, preparing, injecting, and rotating the head passively. In addition to the electronic monitors that must be used, the patient's face and the respiration should be directly observed.

We use several different systems for monitoring patients during sur-

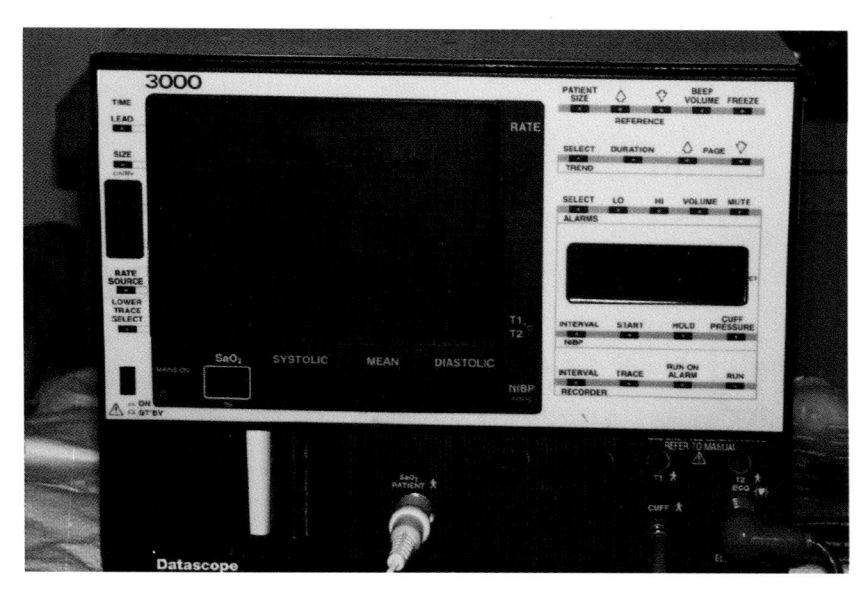

Neuroleptic anesthesia requires that the patient be monitored. An automatic digital blood pressure display is valuable for checking blood pressure and pulse during the procedure. A continuous ECG display is also required. Perhaps the most important monitor we use today is that of oxygen saturation. The device pictured here offers all of this information that is constantly updated throughout the surgical procedure.

gery. An automatic digital blood pressure display is valuable for checking blood pressure and pulse during the procedure. A continuous electrocardiographic (ECG) display is also required. Perhaps the most important monitor we use today is that of oxygen saturation. This device enables the surgeon to rapidly determine that the airway is patent and the patient is ventilating adequately. Respiratory depression is recognized at a very early stage using this monitoring device, and airway intervention is given rapidly should it be required following a drop in oxygen saturation.

Technique

Immediately upon arrival in the operating suite, all patients are premedicated with 5 mg of diazepam by mouth. In patients undergoing rhytidectomy, depending on their preoperative tendency toward hypertension, they are given between 0.1 and 0.3 mg of clonidine by mouth. The patient is then taken to the operating room where monitoring devices for blood pressure, ECG, and oxygen saturation are attached, and an IV line is started.

For the average patient (approximately 130 lb), 5 mg of droperidol (equals 2 cc), 25 μg of fentanyl (equals 0.5 cc), and 1 to 2 mg of midazolam are administered slowly. The patient is then prepared and draped, and observed for the full effect of this induction dose. It should be noted that the full effects of the IV droperidol take up to 30 minutes to occur. Additional increments of fentanyl or midazolam are given as needed until adequate sedation is obtained. Approximately 1 minute before injection of the local anesthetic agent, 30 to 40 mg of ketamine is then given over a 60-second interval. Approximately 90 seconds after the ketamine has been administered, the local anesthetic injection can be administered during this period of dissociative anesthesia.

Maintenance of the neuroleptic analgesia is achieved during the procedure by additional increments of 1 to 2 mg of midazolam as well as incremental doses of fentanyl, usually given in 25-μg doses. We use midazolam as the sedative agent and administer it when patients are awake, talking, or opening their eyes. Fentanyl is used for pain relief and is given when the patient shows signs of moving, restlessness, or in response to painful stimuli. We would emphasize that if the patient is reacting to painful stimuli, the first response should be to ensure that the anesthetic block is adequate rather than administering more sedative. A well-blocked patient will basically be pain-free, thereby requiring less supplemental analgesia.

Usually these drugs are given approximately every 20 to 35 minutes, and occasionally both drugs are given simultaneously. In procedures lasting about 2 hours, usually 10 to 15 mg of midazolam and 75 to 100 μg of fentanyl are administered during the entire operation. In longer procedures lasting up to 5 hours, we have given up to 40 mg of midazolam, 150 μg of fentanyl, and 15 mg of droperidol. Older patients (older than 60 years of age) usually require less medication administration than younger patients.

Some patients (smokers, drinkers, and drug abusers) are hard to sedate with this technique, especially in long-lasting cases. No matter how much midazolam or fentanyl these patients receive, they often show nonspecific agitation and are commonly difficult to control. In these situations we occasionally switch to pentobarbital, since it appears to have a longer duration of action and exhibits more powerful sedative effects. Pentobarbital is administered in increments of 10-20 mg. Alternatively, we have switched to continuous infusion of propofol in these difficult patients, which can be used in place of both midazolam and fentanyl administration.

During the induction phase, the best indicator of the need for additional medication is the patient's face. If 2 to 3 minutes after the induction dose the patient has her eyes open or talks and moves spontaneously, usually another 10 to 15 mg of ketamine is administered. If the patient shows no response to the injection, the eyes remain closed, or she begins to snore, then usually adequate dissociative anesthesia has been obtained. During the maintenance phase, neuroleptic analge-

SUMMARY OF TECHNIQUE OF NEUROLEPTIC ANALGESIA

Premedication	Diazepam 5–10 mg po
	Clonidine 0.1 mg-0.3 mg po
Induction	Droperidol 2.5-5.0 mg
	Fentanyl 25-50 μg
	Midazolam 1-3 mg
2 minutes before injection of local anesthetic agent	Ketamine 30-40 mg
Maintenance	Midazolam 1-2 mg for being awake, talking, opening eyes
	Fentanyl 25 μg for moving, wiggling, restlessness
	Meperidine 10 mg IV used in place of fentanyl in the early portions of long cases for moving, wiggling, restlessness

sia is judged in a similar way, and midazolam or fentanyl is administered as previously noted. Often the first sign of "getting light" is a movement of the foot. If untreated, the next movement is of the shoulder or head. In our opinion, it is best to titrate these patients early and catch the need for additional medication before the patient becomes fully awake. On the other hand, we prefer to keep the patient light rather than risk the untoward complications associated with overdosage of medication.

For longer procedures (lasting more than 2 hours), we commonly use diazepam in 2.5-mg IV increments in place of midazolam for the first half of the operation, since it has a longer half-life and requires less frequent redosing as compared with midazolam.

COMPLICATIONS AND THEIR TREATMENT

■ Airway Obstruction

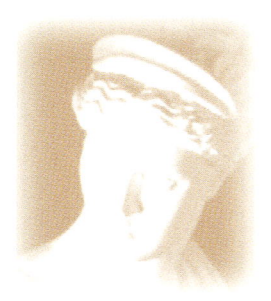

Airway obstruction is usually the result of too much medication given too suddenly, especially between the induction dose and any stimulation. The first sign of obstruction is snoring. This is usually harmless. Snoring is usually associated with adequate oxygen saturation. One must realize however, that snoring is a sign of heavy sedation and total airway obstruction is not far away. As airway obstruction progresses, the tongue falls backward, preventing air from entering the lungs. Patients will commonly attempt respiration but chest movement will appear abnormal. Instead of rising, the chest now retracts and with each chest retraction the abdominal wall bulges, often in a jerky manner. In these situations, immediate treatment is imperative. The head should be tilted backward and if this is still ineffective, the jaw needs to be supported and pulled forward. To do this, the tips of the middle fingers should be engaged behind the angle of the mandible and the jaw pulled forward until the lower teeth are in front of the upper teeth. Following jaw support, the patient will exhibit adequate respiration and commonly will require jaw elevation for only a few breaths until able to maintain the airway without external support. It is important to realize that despite airway obstruction, additional oxygen is usually not required. *These patients simply require support of the airway and once the airway is opened, there is usually adequate oxygen in the air to oxygenate the patient.* It has been our experience that only patients with chronic lung disease require supplemental oxygen during neuroleptic analgesia if proper attention is given to monitoring, titration of medication, and airway support. *Supplemental oxygen does not serve as an adequate substitute for proper airway support.*

Respiratory Depression

Respiratory depression, like airway obstruction, is usually a result of too much narcotic being given suddenly. The signs of respiratory depression are a lack of respiratory movement and a drop in oxygen saturation. The patient does not respond to encouragement "to take a big breath," and jaw elevation alone does not help. If a patient exhibits respiratory depression, immediate ventilation with a mask and Ambu bag and insertion of an oral or a nasal airway are helpful. Naloxone 0.4 mg should be given immediately and is usually effective within seconds. Repeat doses of naloxone may be required within 1 to 2 hours depending on the amount, type (i.e., short- or long-acting narcotic), and time since the last administration of the narcotic.

Hypo- or Hypertension

Blood pressure drops below 80 mm Hg systolic may be due to blood loss, carotid sinus pressure, or vasovagal response. These drops in blood pressure are often treated with fluids and Trendelenburg's position, and occasionally require administration of ephedrine given in 10-mg increments. If a patient exhibits a vasovagal response associated with a slow pulse and hypotension, the treatment of this problem is administration of 0.4 mg of atropine along with IV fluid boluses.

Systolic blood pressure almost always increases after the injection of local anesthetic containing epinephrine. If the blood pressure remains elevated above 150 mm Hg systolic for longer than 10 to 15 minutes after the injection, we tend to treat this patient with chlorpromazine, as previously discussed. For prolonged hypertension unresponsive to chlorpromazine, we occasionally use hydralazine (Apresoline) administered in 5-mg increments.

Cardiac Arrhythmias

Sinus arrhythmias and occasional atrial and ventricular extrasystoles are harmless, and are usually noticed before drugs are given and the procedure is started. If the patient exhibits frequent or multifocal premature ventricular contractions (PVCs), it is best to postpone surgery and obtain a cardiology consult.

Tachycardia (heart rate greater than 100 beats/min) is often due to nervousness or the epinephrine injection. It usually disappears with adequate sedation. Bradycardia (heart rate less than 50 beats/min) should be treated with 0.4 mg of atropine if symptomatic or associated with hypotension.

The development of intraoperative cardiac arrhythmias is fortunately rare during neuroleptic analgesia. If arrhythmias do occur, one must be sure that they are not a result of hypoxia with resultant acidosis and that the patient has adequate airway support and ventilation. Intraoperative blood loss with hypotension can similarly be associated with arrhythmias and obviously should be corrected. The development of multifocal PVCs usually responds well to IV lidocaine administration. If significant cardiac arrhythmias develop during surgery, the procedure should be terminated at the earliest possible point and the arrhythmia controlled. Cardiology consult and further monitoring of the patient should be given similar consideration.

Shivering

Shivering can be a nuisance to the patient as well as to the recovery room personnel. It also increases oxygen requirements. Factors contributing to shivering include a nervous patient, exposed skin surfaces, a cold operating room, cold preparation, and IV solutions, as well as a possible reaction to injected lidocaine. If shivering develops and persists in the recovery room, it can usually be ameliorated with 10-mg

IV boluses of meperidine. Occasionally, we have used 1- to 2-mg doses of chlorpromazine in the patient with persistent shivering.

Neuroleptic Malignant Syndrome

Neuroleptic malignant syndrome is a rare complication of neuroleptic therapy and is mainly discussed in the psychiatric literature. Approximately 500 cases, mostly young males, have been reported. It is distinct from malignant hyperthermia, which is triggered by inhalation anesthetics and certain muscle relaxants and is genetically determined.

Neuroleptic malignant syndrome may manifest at any time from a few hours to many weeks after exposure to neuroleptic drugs. Symptoms evolve gradually over a period of 2 to 4 days and consist of hyperthermia, hypertonicity of skeletal muscle, and fluctuating consciousness. It is believed to be caused by a decreased availability of dopamine in the brain. Dantrolene, amantadine, and bromocriptine have been used as treatment in addition to supportive therapy.

PATIENT MANAGEMENT IN THE RECOVERY ROOM

Following the termination of the procedure, it is important that the patient be adequately monitored in a well-staffed recovery room area. Since most of the agents used in these procedures are short-acting, the patient should be able to respond to verbal commands upon awakening on the operating table. The patient should also be able to walk the short distance from the operating room table to the recovery room with assistance. Rarely in our practice is a wheelchair required to transport a patient to the recovery room. Patients are monitored for at least 2 hours postoperatively and then discharged to the care of a responsible person. They are not allowed to drive a motor vehicle.

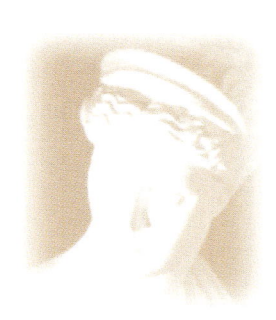

In the recovery room we treat complaints of pain with 10-mg increments of IV meperidine. If the pain occurs close to discharge time, acetaminophen-propoxyphene (Darvocet) or acetaminophen-oxycodene (Percocet) is given by mouth. Nausea and vomiting have been rare since the introduction of droperidol into the neuroleptic analgesia armamentarium. If they do occur, we prefer to give 5-mg intramuscular doses of prochlorperazine.

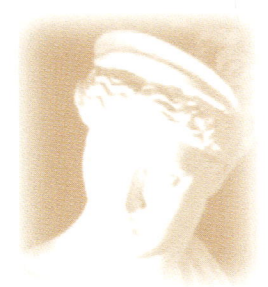

POSTOPERATIVE PATIENT NEEDS

During the period immediately following surgery, the patient may have pain and feel anxious. These symptoms can be alleviated with the appropriate analgesic or tranquilizer. If oral medication for pain is to be administered, we have found that prescribing on a regular schedule rather than on demand appears to be more effective. If the surgeon waits until the patient's pain becomes severe enough to seek medication, many times an oral analgesic such as acetaminophen (Tylenol) will not be as effective as desired. On the other hand, if pain following the surgery is anticipated and a mild analgesic is given every few hours while the patient is awake, a level of analgesia is maintained and the same drug can be used more satisfactorily. If medications are necessary for sleep for a few days after the surgery, we usually prescribe flurazepam (Dalmane).

Pain and the patient's reaction to it are difficult to evaluate. If the attitude of the surgeon and his or her assistants is that there will be little or no pain, that is frequently the experience of the patient. On the other hand, if the surgeon and assistants concentrate on the painful aspects of the postoperative period and communicate this repeatedly to the patient, then that becomes the patient's experience.

SURGEON NEEDS

The needs of the surgeon should also be considered. To do his or her work well, the surgeon needs a calm and quiet patient. Sedatives are frequently administered to alleviate patient anxiety or fear, but sedation, which does not provide relief from tension, has a questionable value and carries considerable risks. Heavy sedation should be avoided. Although some surgeons do not like to have patients awake and able to talk during surgery, or able to hear or at least remember conversations going on before or during surgery, there is a large price to pay for this degree of sedation. The patient will have depressed respiration, and the level of consciousness cannot be monitored as easily.

Nothing dismays the recovery room team as much as being unable to discharge a patient at the expected time because of oversedation. One of the benefits of using short-acting agents is a rapid return of the patient to normal. Each surgeon should evaluate his or her own philosophy in this matter and design a specific pharmacologic regimen to accommodate the needs of both surgeon and patient.

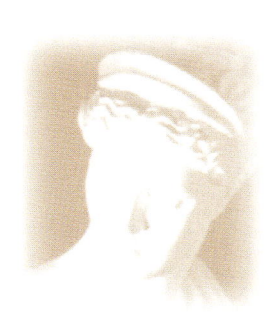

SUGGESTED READING

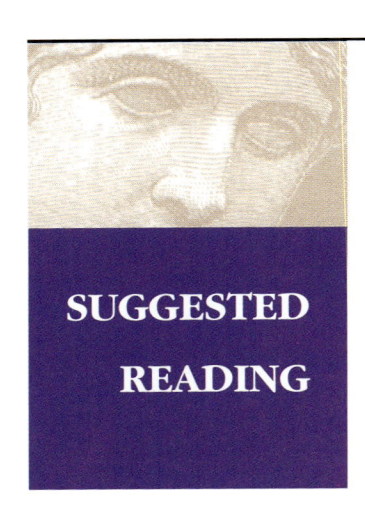

Baker TJ, Gordon HL: Midazolam (Versed) in ambulatory surgery, *Plast Reconstr Surg* 82:244, 1988.

Colon GA, Gubert N: Lorazepam (Ativan) and fentanyl (Sublimaze) for outpatient office plastic surgical anesthesia, *Plast Reconstr Surg* 78:486, 1986.

Cunningham BL, McKinney P: Patient acceptance of dissociative anesthetics, *Plast Reconstr Surg* 72:22, 1983.

de Jong RH: *Local anesthetics,* ed 2, Springfield Ill, 1977, Charles C Thomas.

Gilman AG, Rall TW, Nies AS, et al: *The pharmacological basis of therapeutics,* ed 8, New York, 1990, Pergamon Press.

Gordon HL: The selection of drugs in office surgery, *Clin Plast Surg* 10:277, 1983.

Gordon HL: Drugs for outpatient surgery. In Regnault P, Daniel RK (eds): *Aesthetic plastic surgery,* Boston, 1984, Little, Brown.

Goth A: *Medical pharmacology,* ed 10, St Louis, 1981, Mosby.

Graham WP: Anesthesia in cosmetic surgery, *Clin Plast Surg* 10:285, 1983.

MacKenzie N, Grant IS: Propofol for intravenous sedation, *J Anesthesia* 42:3, 1987.

Skelly AM, et al: A comparison of diazepam and midazolam as sedatives for minor oral surgery, *Br J Anaesth* 56:1279, 1984.

Stromberg BV: Anesthesia in plastic surgery, *Clin Plast Surg* 12:1-145, 1985.

Vinnik CA: Intravenous dissociation technique for outpatient plastic surgery: Tranquility in the office surgical facility, *Plast Reconstr Surg* 67:799, 1981.

White PF, et al: Comparison of midazolam and diazepam for sedation during plastic surgery, *Plast Reconstr Surg* 81:703, 1988.

Three

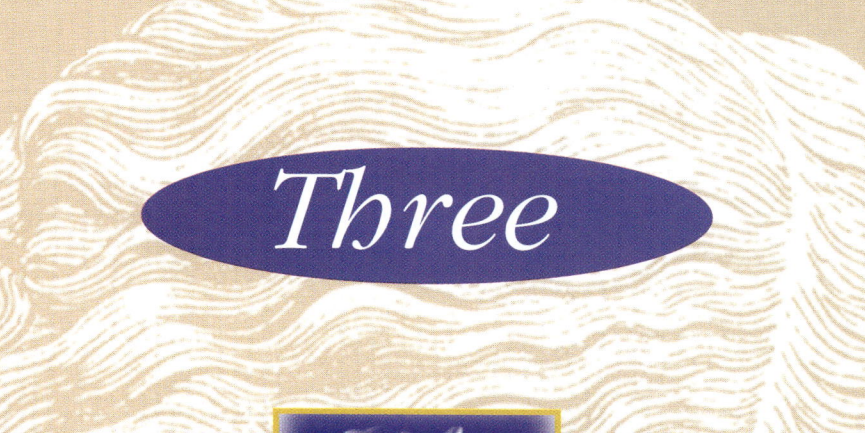

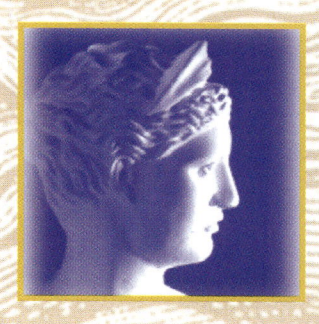

Chemical Peeling (Phenol and Trichloroacetic Acid) and Dermabrasion

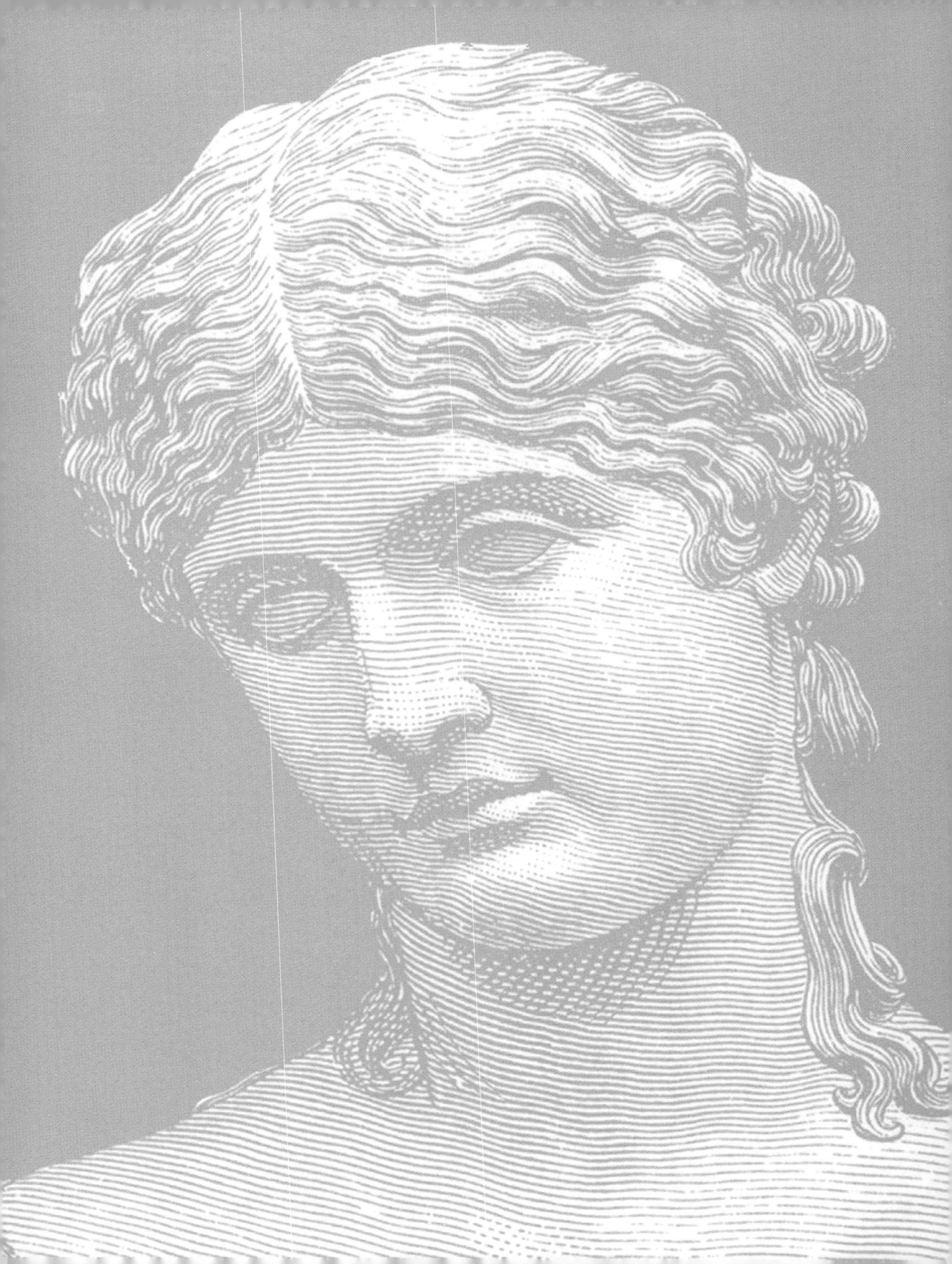

Some facial skin problems do not respond to direct surgical therapy. Specifically, multiple fine facial rhytides, uneven skin pigmentation or hyperpigmentation, and acne scars are conditions in which standard surgical techniques have limited application. Disorders localized to facial skin are often better approached through other procedures such as chemical peeling and dermabrasion.

Chemical peeling and dermabrasion are processes that affect both the epidermis and superficial dermis, producing a smoothing of surface irregularities and altering skin pigmentation. Although both treatment modalities have been used in the past to treat similar clinical problems, trial and error has given the clinician a better understanding of which process is better suited to the specific pathologic condition; they should no longer be used interchangeably.

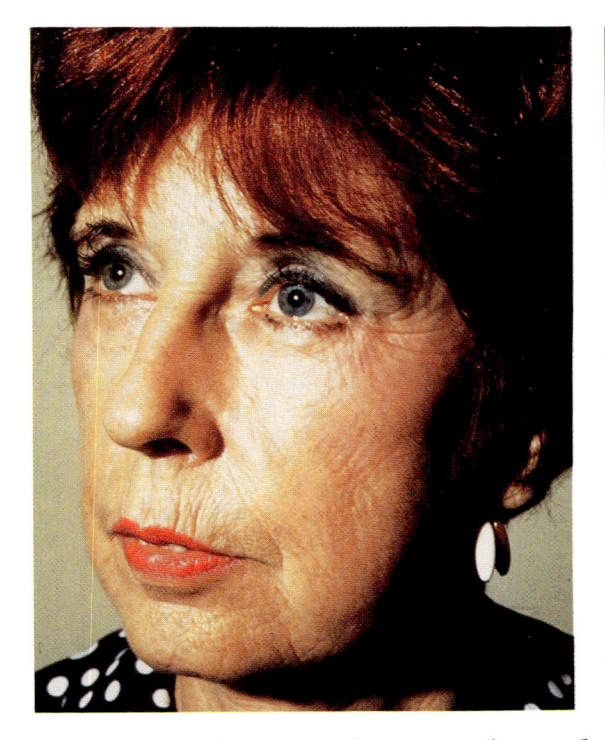

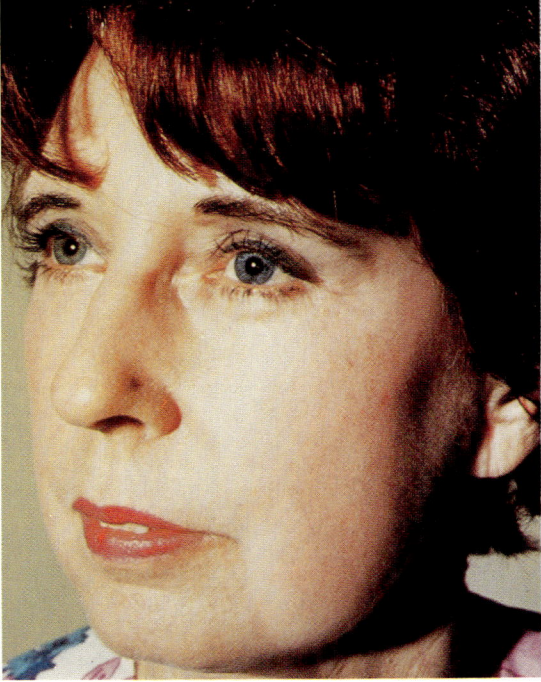

This 48-year-old woman has severely sun-damaged skin in the photograph on the **left.** *There is deep wrinkling in all areas, causing the skin to appear prematurely aged. A full-face peel was performed 1 year before the photograph on the* **right** *was taken. No surgery has been performed.*

SURGICAL REJUVENATION
OF THE FACE

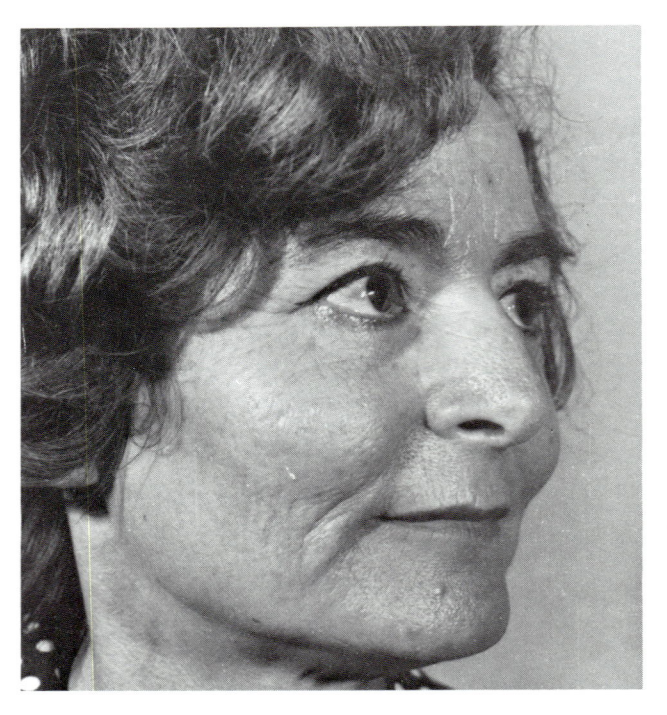

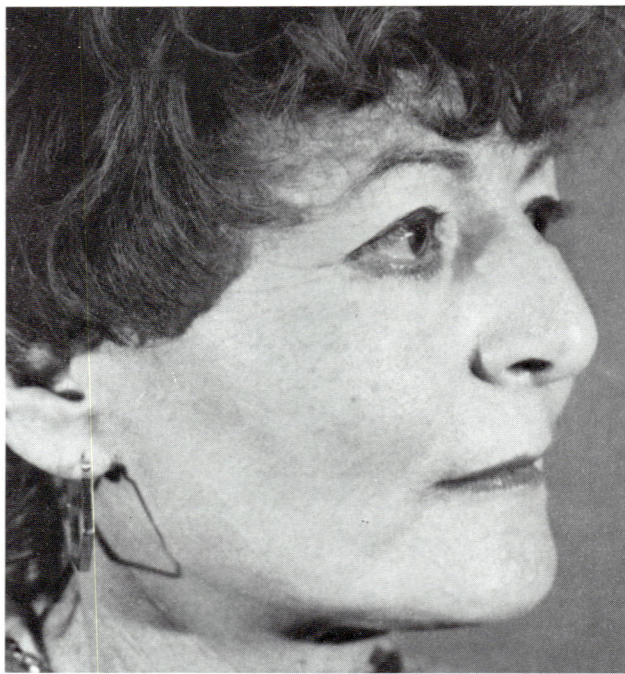

This 52-year-old woman's facial skin shows fine wrinkling. The patient is shown 6 years after a full-face peel. Most of the fine wrinkling is still gone. The face also shows a general tightening effect. No surgery has been performed.

CHEMICAL PEELING (PHENOL AND TRICHLOROACETIC ACID) AND DERMABRASION

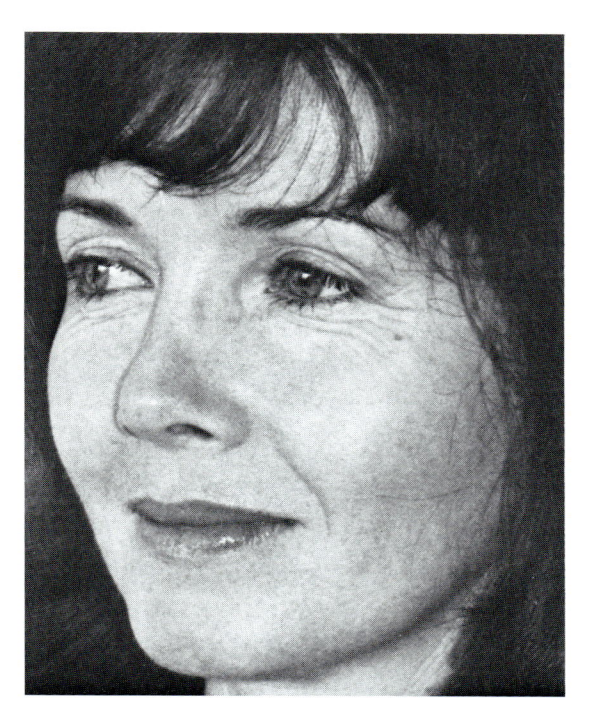

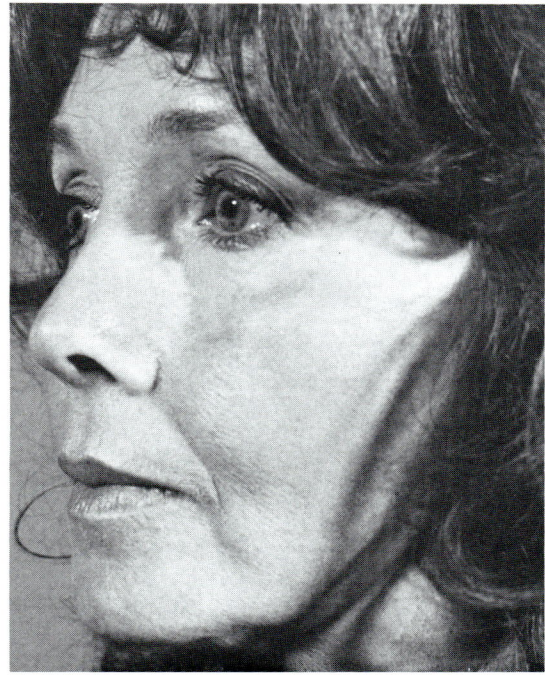

This 38-year-old woman has premature fine wrinkling, most evident around her eyes. The patient is shown 11 years after a full-face peel. The improvement in the appearance of the facial skin has persisted, although some generalized gross sagging of the soft tissues has occurred.

SURGICAL REJUVENATION OF THE FACE

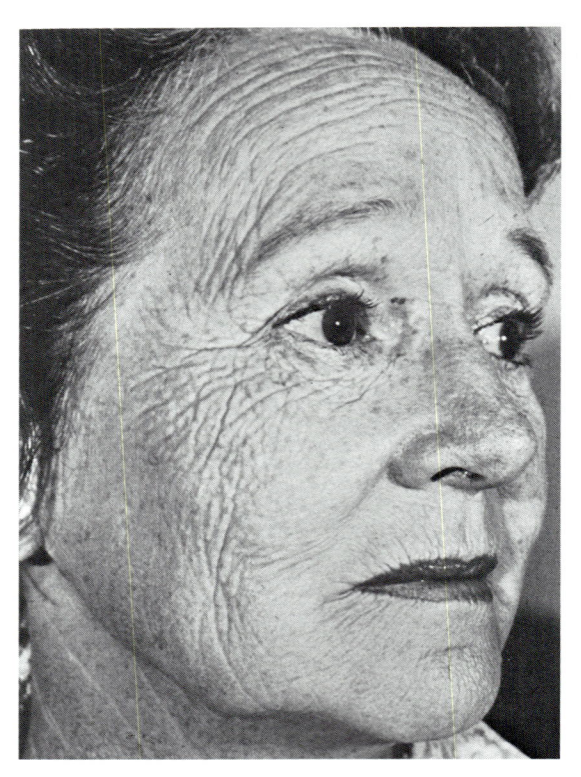

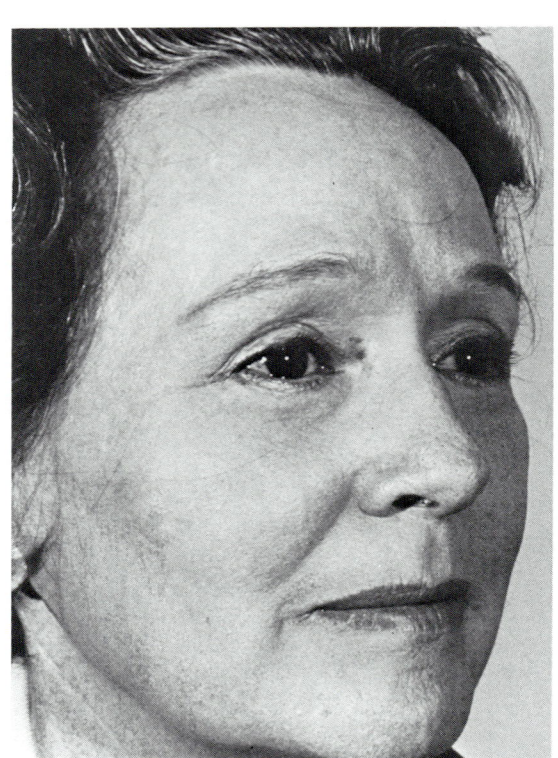

This 50-year-old woman had prematurely aged skin, partly as a result of years of exposure to the sun. The patient is shown 3 months after a full-face peel. No surgery has been performed.

CHEMICAL PEELING (PHENOL AND TRICHLOROACETIC ACID) AND DERMABRASION

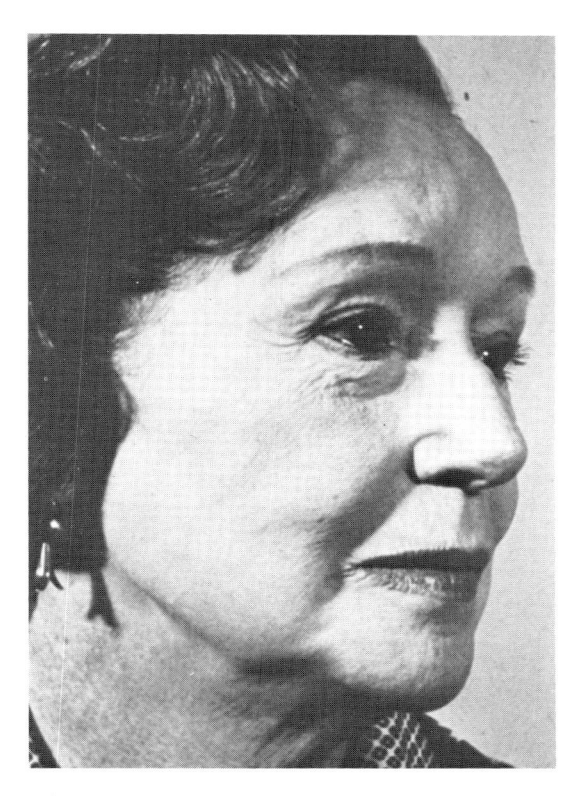

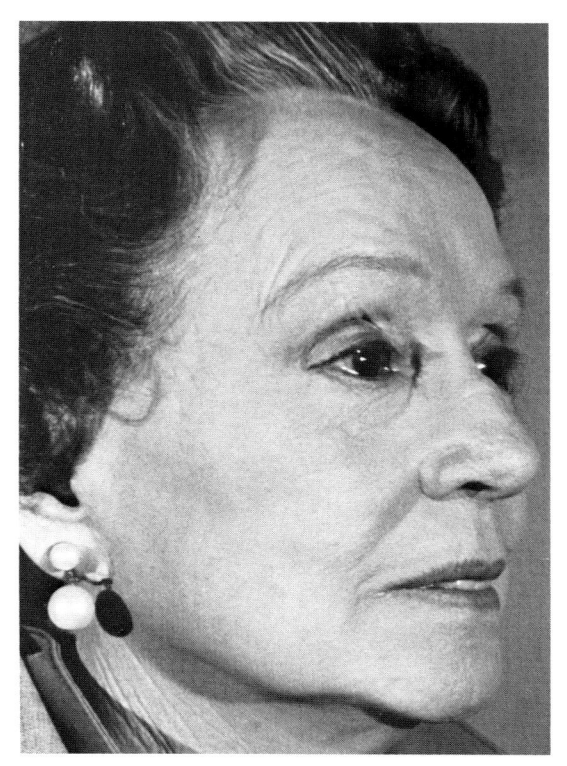

The patient is shown 7 years after a full-face peel. The soft tissues of the face are sagging, but the skin texture retains improvement from the peel. The patient is shown 14 years after the full-face peel. Note the persistence of the peeling effect.

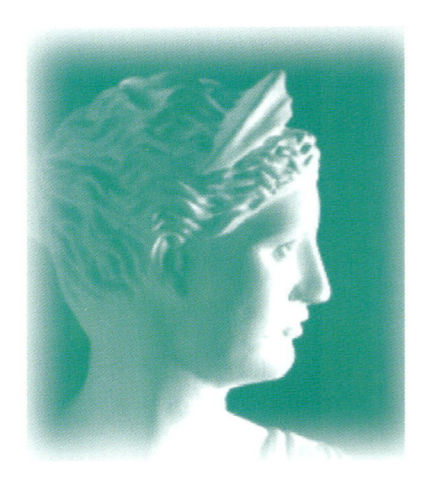

A

CHEMICAL PEELING: PHENOL

Chemical face peeling involves the application of a chemical mixture to produce a controlled and predictable chemical injury. Upon healing, the skin is smoother, firmer, appears more youthful, and is less lined. Phenol peeling is most commonly used to remove fine facial wrinkles, to treat irregular hyperpigmentation of facial skin, and to ablate precancerous lesions (actinic keratoses) following radiation (solar) exposure.

■ Historical Background

Although there is no recorded evidence, it is likely that prehistoric peoples recognized and used abrasives, oils, and simple drugs as beautification treatment for aging skin. The oldest record of cosmetic treatment by physicians is found in the Ebers Papyrus, circa 1560 B.C., which outlines methods for removing wrinkles, dyeing hair and eyebrows, and correcting squints, along with other procedures for beautifying the body. Early chemosurgery probably took the form of certain types of acid treatment. Exfoliation of the skin was accomplished by the direct application of poultices made from mineral and plant substances. Sulfur, mustard, and limestone are known to have been used.

During the early part of the twentieth century, chemical face peeling was used occasionally by lay operators, although MacKee and Karp are known to have used liquid phenol for the treatment of acne scars as early as 1903.

During the late 1940s and early 1950s, the treatment was given considerable publicity by the news media. Claims were made that the Fountain of Youth had at last been found. In 1960, a Chicago newspaper reporter underwent the treatment herself and described her experiences daily in a series of articles. There were photographs taken of her before, during, and after the treatment. The results were wonderful. Almost all her wrinkles had been removed, and the woman looked incredibly younger. Most of the medical community smiled knowingly at this obvious attempt to dupe the gullible public. Since we knew of no way to accomplish such a marvelous improvement in the texture of aging skin, we concluded that the story was a hoax and that the photographs had been skillfully retouched. As peeling became more common, results observed by physicians of patients being treated in "lay" clinics stimulated a greater interest in the scientific investigation of chemical peeling. Based on the concrete evidence we saw in patients in our practice who had undergone this treatment, we were forced to rethink our opinion of chemical peeling.

At first, we went to the local lay operator who was doing the peeling to find out what was being used. Predictably, he or she would not even discuss it with us, much less divulge the formula.

Little by little, we amassed a body of information about the treatment. Some of the data came from patients who had been treated. All of them described the smell of carbolic acid and a tan powder that smelled like iodine. They all reported that the treated areas had been covered with some type of adhesive tape. A search of the medical literature provided a few more clues as to what was being done to remove wrinkles in such a mysterious way.

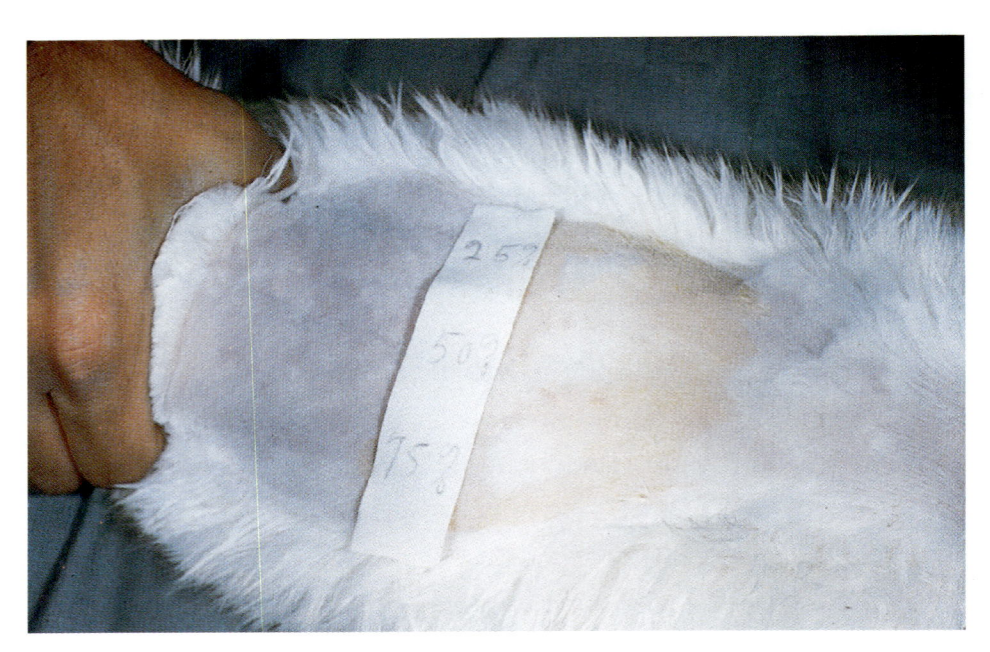

Before using phenol chemical peeling on humans, we first applied it to the underbelly of experimental rabbits in various concentrations and noted rapid healing with loss of dermal pigmentation in all concentrations used.

The first application of the diluted phenolic solutions was applied experimentally to spots on the shaved skin of rats and rabbits. Chemical burns resulted, and the skin healed. We then decided to test human skin. The first test spot was on the freckled forearm of one of us (T.J.B.), and the small white spot persists to this day. We then treated a small spot on the face of our brave secretary, and it also healed easily. Taking a deep collective breath, we decided on a clinical trial. We chose to "peel" the forehead of a very elderly woman who was to have a face-lift at the same time. We reasoned that if a catastrophic skin loss occurred, we would cover the forehead with a skin graft as a single anatomic area. The result was beautiful, and for a long time we peeled foreheads at the same time that face-lifts were performed. Most patients returned at a later date to have the rest of their face peeled. Although there were never any complications from having a fresh surgical wound so close to a contaminated chemical burn, we soon began our

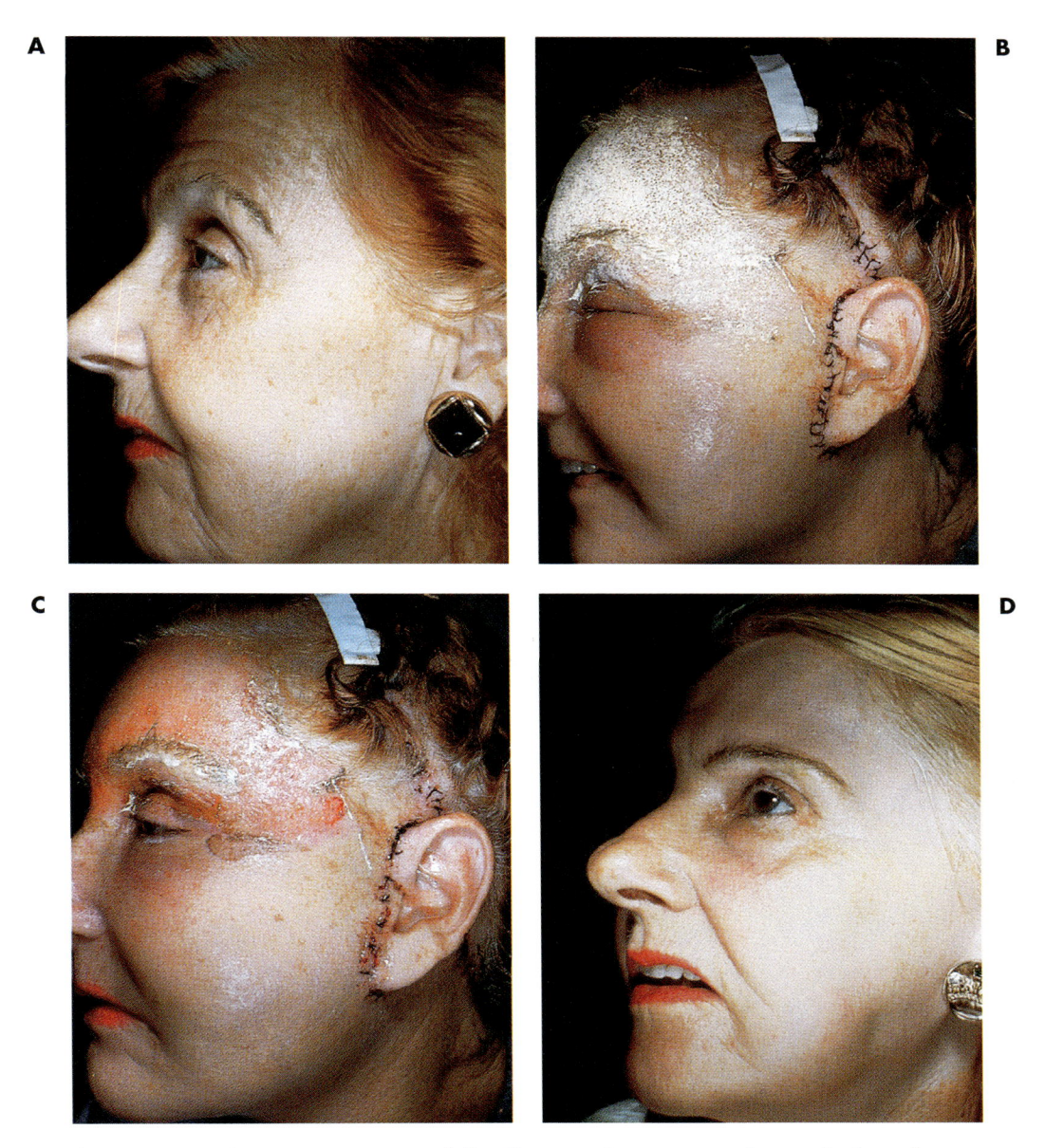

CHEMICAL PEELING (PHENOL AND TRICHLOROACETIC ACID) AND DERMABRASION

A, Preoperative appearance of the first patient we performed phenol peeling on, in 1960. In this patient, it was elected to perform a face-lift and, in conjunction with this procedure, a phenol peel of the forehead and glabella. B, Same patient immediately postoperatively following face-lift and phenol peel of the forehead C, 6 days following the procedure. D, Late postoperative result. Because of the rapid postoperative healing seen following a phenol peel in this patient, associated with a dramatic improvement in forehead rhytides, we maintained the courage to continue investigating the clinical application of phenol chemical peeling.

present procedure: except for small areas around the mouth, we do not peel major areas of the face at the same time that major areas of the face are operated on.

We were struck not only by the efficacy of this treatment but also with the rarity of troublesome complications. Our first papers on this subject were published in 1961, and we continued to publish and present material at medical conferences for many years. During the first 8 or 10 years, however, our medical colleagues were almost universally reluctant to accept or even seriously consider this new technique.

Finally we brought a patient to the American Society of Plastic and Reconstructive Surgeons (ASPRS) meeting in Las Vegas, Nevada (1972).

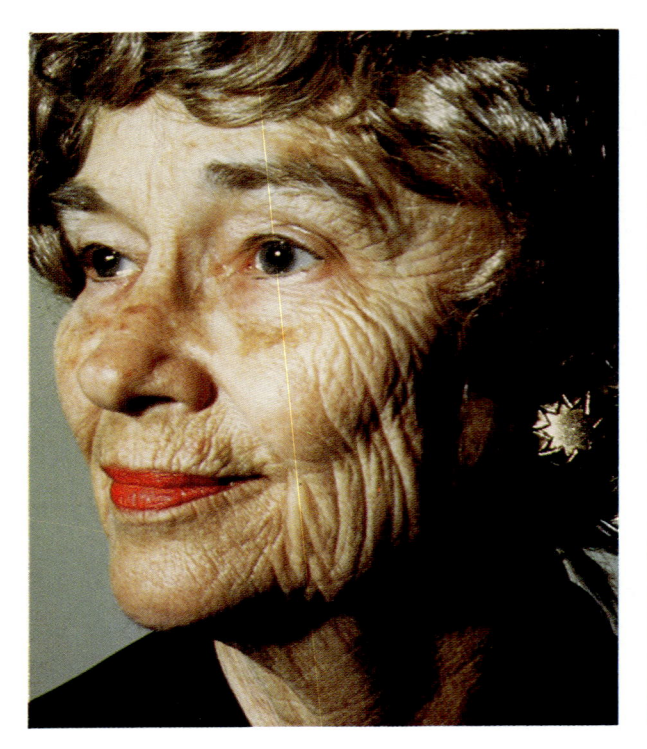

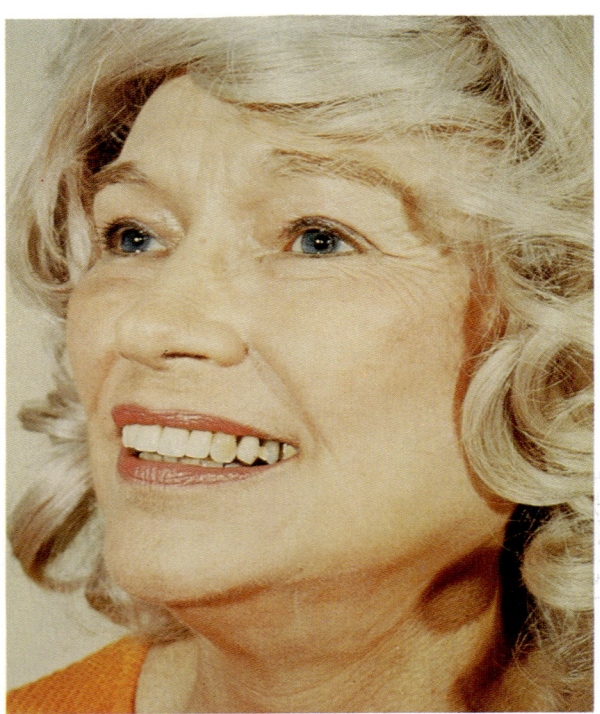

This 67-year-old woman has the common stigmata of the aging face. There is a generalized sagging of the skin and subcutaneous tissues of the face and neck. There is also an abundance of fine wrinkling, as well as blotchy hyperpigmentation. A surgical face-lift and blepharoplasty were performed and 3 months later a chemical peel was done. The photograph on the right is the patient's appearance 6 months after the combined peel and surgery.

She had had a surgical face-lift, blepharoplasty, and a full-face chemical peel. We showed slides depicting her appearance before treatment, and then turned on the houselights and displayed her in person. Since then, the peeling technique has become more widely accepted and our results have been duplicated by those colleagues who have been willing to give it a try.

Histology of Sun-Damaged and Aging Skin

Patients seeking chemical peels of the face are generally middle-aged women who have spent too much time in the sun and have suffered structural skin damage, in addition to the normal changes of aging. Degenerative changes occur both in the dermis and epidermis. The histologic changes of aging parallel those from actinic damage, the difference being perhaps more quantitative than qualitative. More accelerated and severe changes are seen after chronic sun exposure.

The histologic changes that occur with aging and following actinic exposure explain the fine wrinkling, laxity, and mottled pigmentation commonly present in these patients. Premalignant changes commonly occur in the epidermis, most often in the form of microscopic actinic keratoses. It is known from the flares produced by topical treatment with fluorouracil that the great majority of actinic keratoses are subclinical. Additionally, spotty downgrowths from the epidermis consisting of melanin-laden keratinocytes and numerous melanocytes are typically seen in sun-damaged skin. This is the histologic counterpart of the solar lentigo, commonly known as the senile freckle. Incipient basal cell cancers and microinvasive squamous cell cancers are found infrequently.

A deep chemical peel is capable of ablating most of these epithelial lesions as well as creating a new superficial dermis. It is important to appreciate the extent of the histologic damage that occurs following actinic exposure.

Dermis

Elastosis is the hallmark of sun-damaged skin. It consists of thickened, coiled, tangled, dense masses of altered elastic fibers. Routine hematoxylin-eosin (HE) staining of actinic skin reveals a basophilic degeneration of collagen and elastic fibers. Mowry staining shows an increase in ground substance in the form of acid mucopolysaccharides present within the dermis. Elastic tissue stains reveal that the dermis appears to be replaced by a solid mass of damaged elastic fibers, which in undamaged skin constitute less than 5% of the dry weight of the dermis. As the elastosis deepens, the collagen disappears proportionately. Thus the fibrous network that normally provides dermis with its viscoelastic properties is degraded and the skin shows little resistance to stretching. Other findings in sun-damaged skin include a sparsity of vessels, which are irregularly placed and variably dilated. Large, thin-walled veins account for the telangiectasia of photodamaged skin. A chronic inflammation signifying chronic injury is reflected in the patchy perivascular infiltration of lymphocytes, histiocytes, and mast cells observed in these specimens (Figure 3-1).

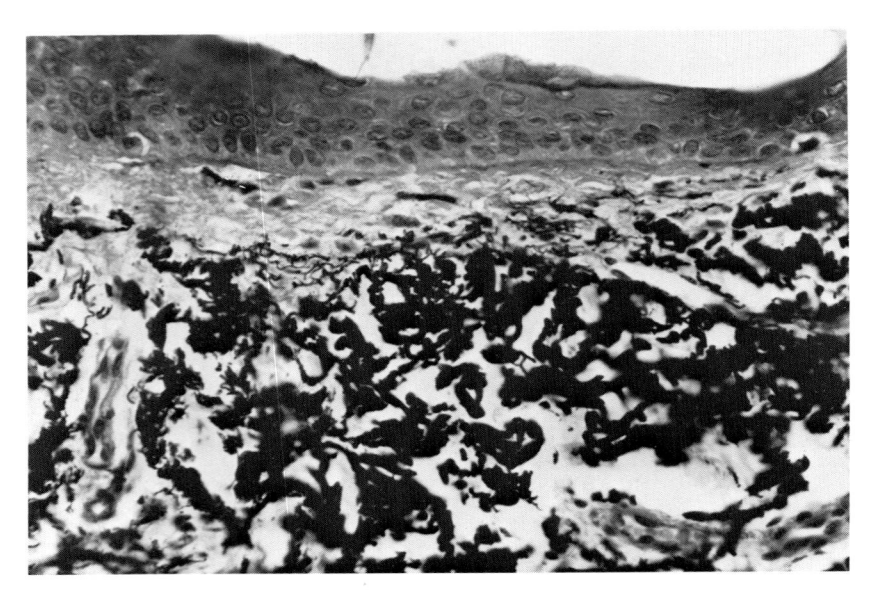

FIGURE 3-1 A portrait of sun-damaged facial skin. The epidermal cells are in disarray, showing variability in size and staining properties. Beneath the flat epidermis there is a thin, clear band of collagen, an ongoing attempt to repair dermal damage. The deep dermis is composed of thickened, tangled, abnormal elastic fibers, characteristic of actinic elastosis. (Luna stain, ×406.) (From Kligman AM, Baker TJ, Gordon HL: **Plast Reconstr Surg 75:652–659, 1985. Used by permission.)**

A thin subepidermal band of fine collagen seems to be exempt from these degenerative changes. This eosinophilic band of collagen, without elastin being present, is termed the *grenz zone* and represents the region where new collagen is generated continuously by hyperplastic fibroblasts in an attempt to repair the ravages of ultraviolet light. This region of the papillary dermis, immediately below the basal layer of the epidermis, is largely responsible for the regenerative changes seen after chemical peeling.

Epidermis

The epidermis in sun-damaged skin is variably thickened and composed of disorderly cells varying in shape, size, and staining properties. These cells are small, have pyknotic nuclei, and exhibit cellular disarray with loss of vertical polarity. The basement membrane beneath the epidermis is thickened, ragged, and often blurred (Figure 3-2).

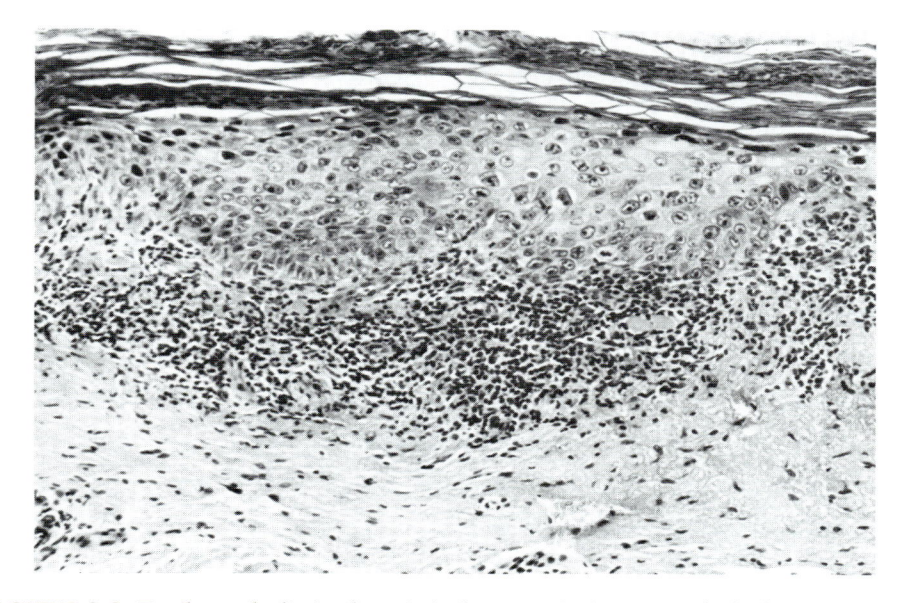

FIGURE 3-2 Early, subclinical actinic keratosis in unpeeled skin. The epidermis shows atypical cells, great cytologic variability, and a dense subepidermal lymphocytic infiltrate. (HE, ×160.) (From Kligman AM, Baker TJ, Gordon HL: **Plast Reconstr Surg** *75:652–659, 1985. Used by permission.)*

The pigment-forming melanocytes are more numerous, unevenly distributed, frequently enlarged, and misshapen. The quantity of melanin granules within keratinocytes is extremely variable. Some epidermal cells appear to be engorged with dense pigmentation, whereas others are virtually empty. This uneven distribution of melanin explains the blotchiness of photodamaged skin (Figure 3-3).

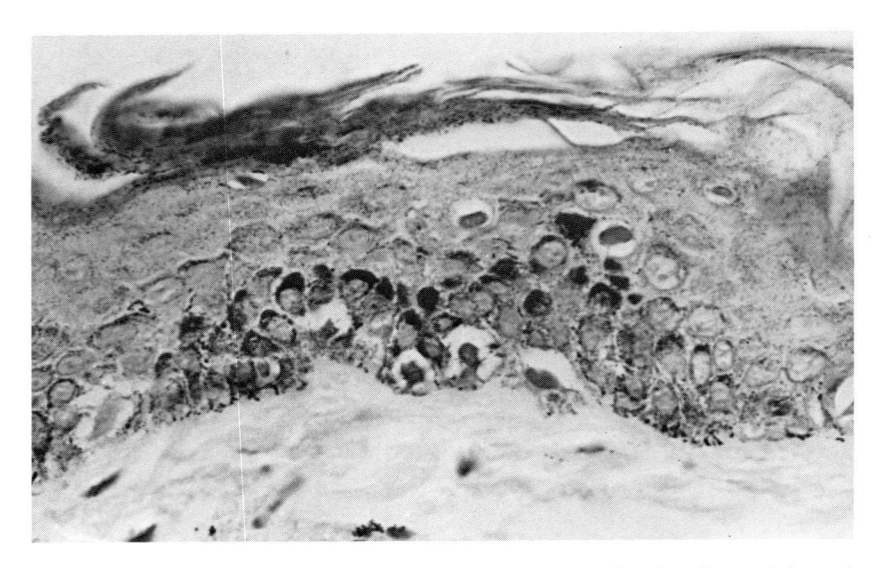

FIGURE 3-3 Uneven distribution of melanin granules in the epidermis. Some cells are engorged with melanin, whereas others contain very little pigment. In the center are three large adjacent melanocytes, probably nonfunctional. The blotchiness of sun-damaged skin is largely due to irregular pigment distribution. (Fontana's stain, ×650.) (From Kligman AM, Baker, TJ, Gordon HL: Plast Reconstr Surg *75:652–659, 1985. Used by permission.)*

CHEMICAL PEELING (PHENOL AND TRICHLOROACETIC ACID) AND DERMABRASION

In response to ultraviolet light, freckle-like, deeply pigmented macules, termed *solar lentigo* (or senile lentigo), are commonly produced. These represent a downgrowth of pigment-laden cells produced by hyperplastic melanocytes (Figure 3-4).

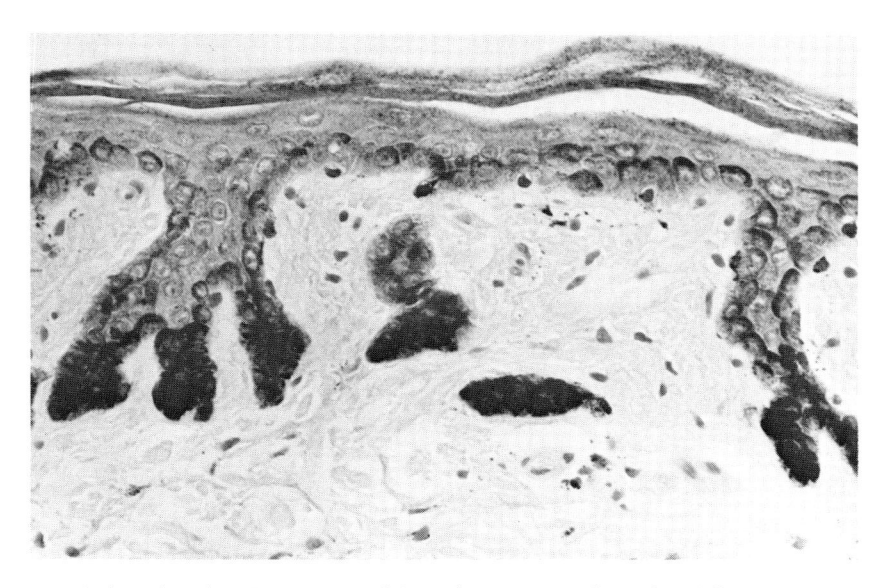

FIGURE 3-4 Solar lentigo. Branching downgrowths of epidermis contain huge amounts of pigment secreted by numerous melanocytes clustered at the tips of the rete pegs. (Fontana's stain, ×406.) (From Kligman AM, Baker TJ, Gordon HL: Plast Reconstr Surg 75:652–659, 1985. Used by permission.*)*

Histologic Changes in Peeled Skin

The application of phenol produces a controlled chemical injury. The depth of phenol penetration extends into the papillary dermis, and clinical changes are a direct result of the changes produced in the superficial dermis and epidermis: the removal of the damaged elastotic skin and the reconstruction of this layer with neocollagen following wound healing. As with other partial-thickness injuries to the skin, the healing seen after chemical peeling proceeds from the epithelial appendages.

Biopsies obtained 48 hours after phenol peeling demonstrate a keratocoagulation necrosis of the epidermis extending through the papillary dermis and surrounded by a marked inflammatory reaction. Epidermal regeneration begins at 48 hours and is usually complete within 7 days. Dermal regeneration lags behind epidermal healing, and biopsies taken 2 weeks following treatment show only a partial reconstitution of the dermis; attempts at re-formation of the rete pegs, dermal thickening, fibroblastic proliferation, and deposition of new collagen are also observed. By 3 months the most striking change apparent in dermal anatomy is the alteration of the upper dermal collagen from a wavy, disorganized form to a rigid, compact shape, replacing the disorganized collagen seen in elastosis.

It is important to note that the findings identified after complete healing within 3 to 4 months following phenol chemical peel appear to be extremely long-lasting. Although the changes noted between peeled and unpeeled skin on histologic examination are most readily apparent within the first few months following treatment, distinct differences remain even as long as 20 years following chemical peel. The aging process continues, but the histologic changes produced by peeling are permanent and their clinical appearance is similarly long-lasting.

Dermis

Even under low power magnification, the changes seen within the dermis after peeling are profound and contrast with the histologic appearance of the adjacent unpeeled skin. A new, wide band of dermis, measuring 1 to 2 mm in width, is found directly beneath the epidermis and is sharply defined from the tangled mass of elastotic fibers representing the old, unpeeled dermis. The newly formed matrix consists of compact and parallel bundles of collagen arranged horizontally. A fairly dense network of fine elastic fibers course through this zone, often disposed in a parallel pattern conforming to the configuration of the collagen fibers. Even in specimens obtained as long as 20 years after peeling, these elastic fibers remain fine and numerous (Figure 3-5).

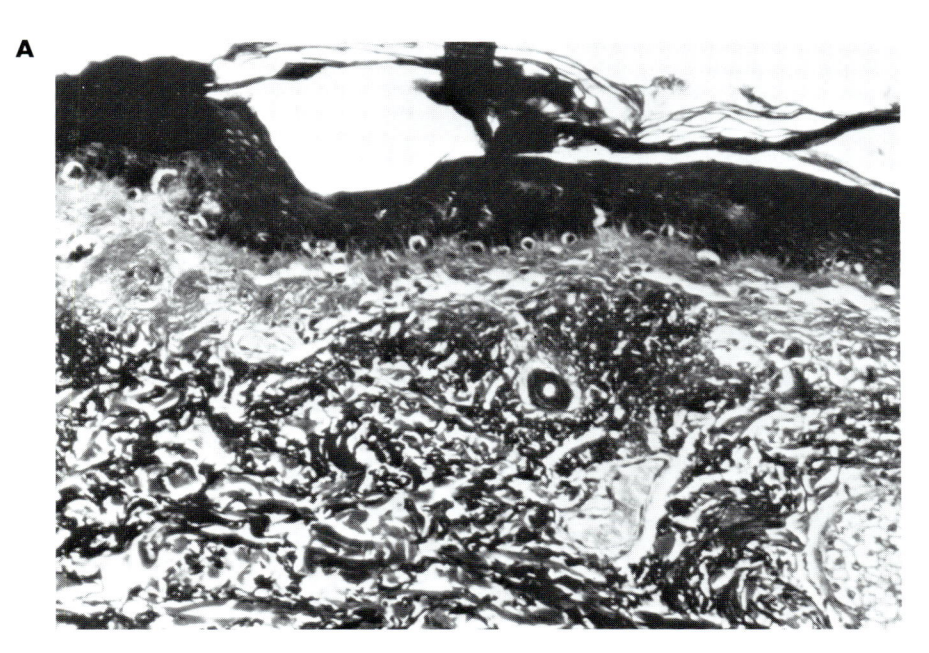

FIGURE 3-5 A, unpeeled specimen showing an eosinophilic grenz zone and marked dermal elastosis below. *Continued.*

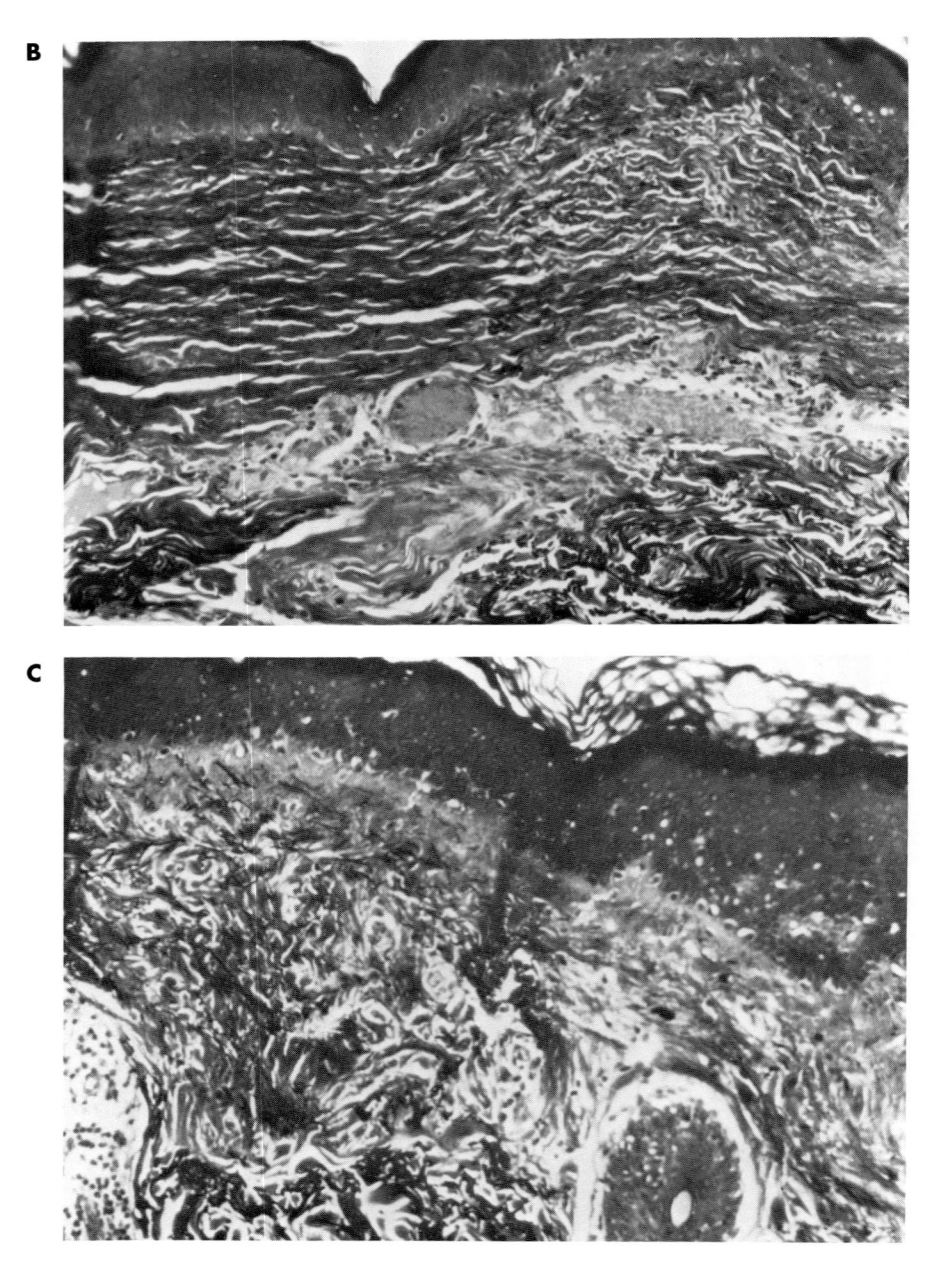

FIGURE 3-5, cont'd. B, Same patient 12 years after peel showing a wide band of new fine, parallel collagen bundles. C, another patient, 20 years after peeling. The reconstructed collagen band is about 3 mm wide. The old elastotic dermis is at the bottom. (From Kligman AM, Baker TJ, Gordon HL: Plast Reconstr Surg 75:652–659, 1985. *Used by permission.)*

Mowry staining shows a considerable diminution in the presence of ground substance within this dermal band, as compared with adjacent unpeeled skin. Small blood vessels in the reconstructed zone appear normal and are not surrounded by lymphocytic infiltrates. Inflammatory signs of chronic actinic damage are not present. Telangiectatic vessels are found only within the deep dermis, which is beyond the reach of the peeling solution. It is important to note that the newly formed collagen and elastic fibers seen within the papillary dermis explain how finely wrinkled, slack skin becomes smoother, fuller, more turgid, and more resilient after a phenol chemical peel (Figure 3-6 to 3-8).

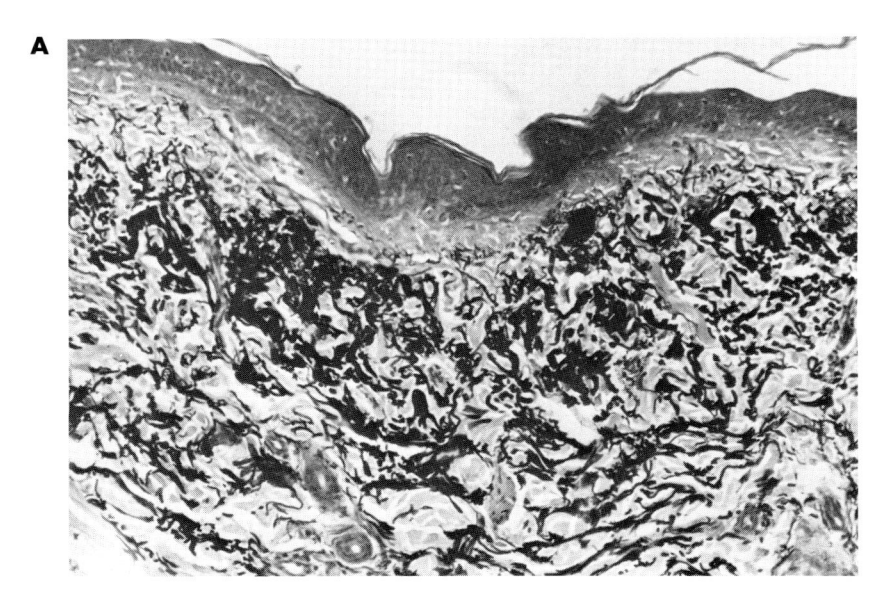

FIGURE 3-6 A, Unpeeled specimen illustrating intense elastosis. (Luna stain, ×160.)

Continued.

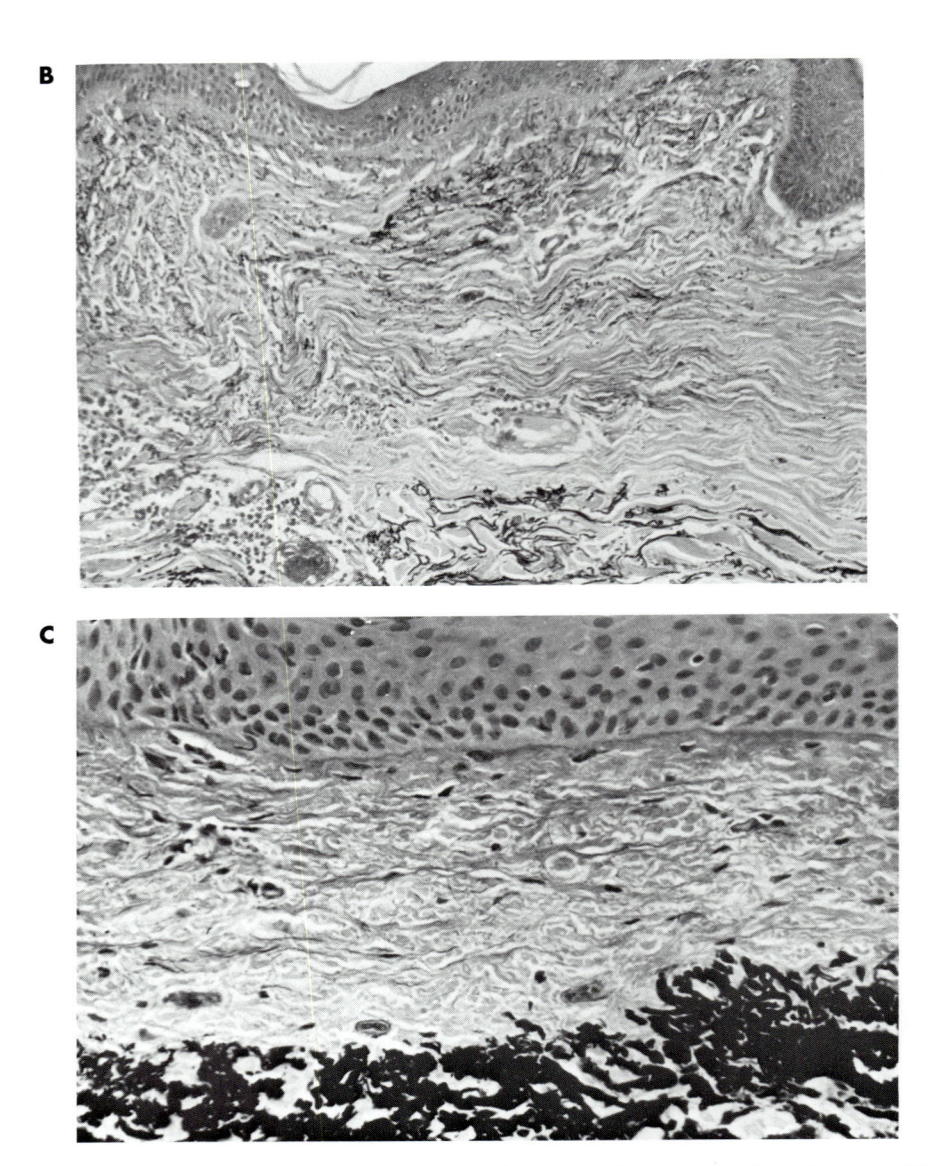

FIGURE 3-6, cont'd. B, Same patient 14 years after peel, showing a wide band of horizontally arranged collagen bundles that intertwine with fine elastic fibers. (Luna stain, ×96.) C, Another patient 4 years after peel, showing the sharp demarcation between the new collagen band and the old elastotic dermis below. (Luna stain, ×406.) (From Kligman AM, Baker TJ, Gordon HL: **Plast Reconstr Surg 75:652–659, 1985.** *Used by permission.)*

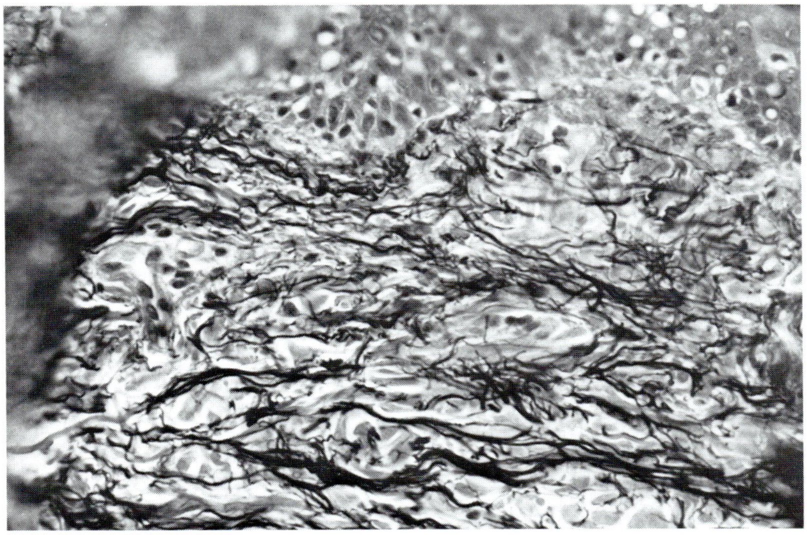

CHEMICAL PEELING (PHENOL AND TRICHLOROACETIC ACID) AND DERMABRASION

FIGURE 3-7 Specimen 20 years post peel showing redevelopment with the new collagen band of numerous relatively normal elastic fibers, mainly parallel to the surface. (From Kligman AM, Baker TJ, Gordon HL: Plast Reconstr Surg 75:652–659, 1985. Used by permission.*)*

SURGICAL REJUVENATION OF THE FACE

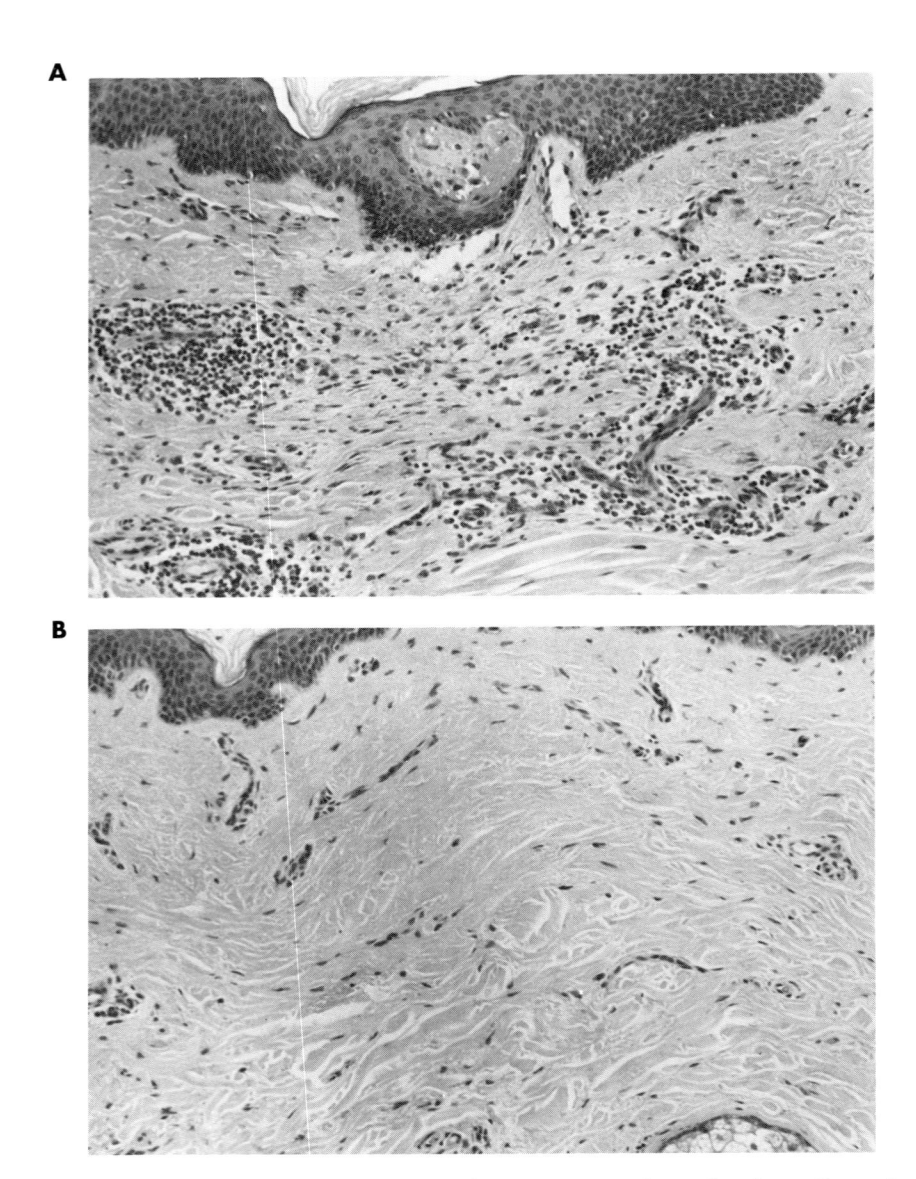

FIGURE 3-8 *A, Unpeeled specimen showing a perivenular lymphocytic infiltrate, usually present in sun-damaged skin. B, Specimen from the same patient 18 years post peel. There is no sign of inflammation. The population of dermal mesenchymal cells, including fibroblasts, is seemingly normal. (Luna stain, ×153.) (From Kligman AM, Baker TJ, Gordon HL:* **Plast Reconstr Surg** *75:652–659, 1985. Used by permission.)*

Epidermis

Following peeling, the epidermis is no longer in disarray. The cells stain evenly and have become a more uniform shape, and there is a return of vertical polarity. Lentiginous downgrowths are rarely seen.

Although peeled skin tends to be hypopigmented, the belief that this results from the destruction of melanocytes cannot be supported. Melanocytes are present and are often of increased density, as compared with those of unpeeled skin. They are, however, incapable of synthesizing normal amounts of melanin. Close inspection shows the melanocytes of the basilar layer to contain many fine pigment granules, and this pigment is evenly dispersed with no tendency to form local accumulation of pigment or lentigines. Microscopic actinic keratoses are not observed in peeled skin (Figure 3-9 and 3-10).

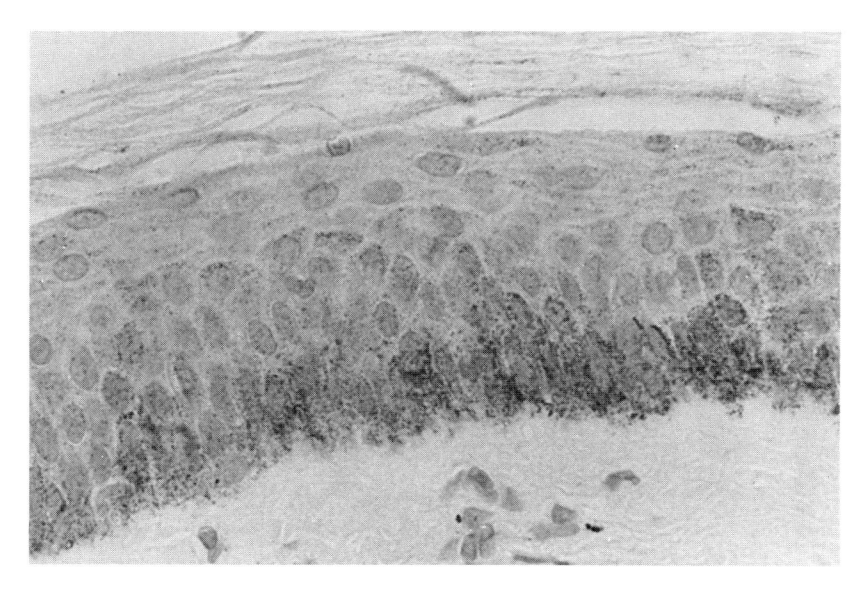

FIGURE 3-9 Even distribution of melanin granules 20 years post peel. The basilar layers contain many small melanin granules. This is the basis of clinical hypopigmentation. (Fontana's stain, ×650.) (From Kligman AM, Baker TJ, Gordon HL: **Plast Reconstr Surg** *75:652–659, 1985. Used by permission.)*

SURGICAL REJUVENATION OF THE FACE

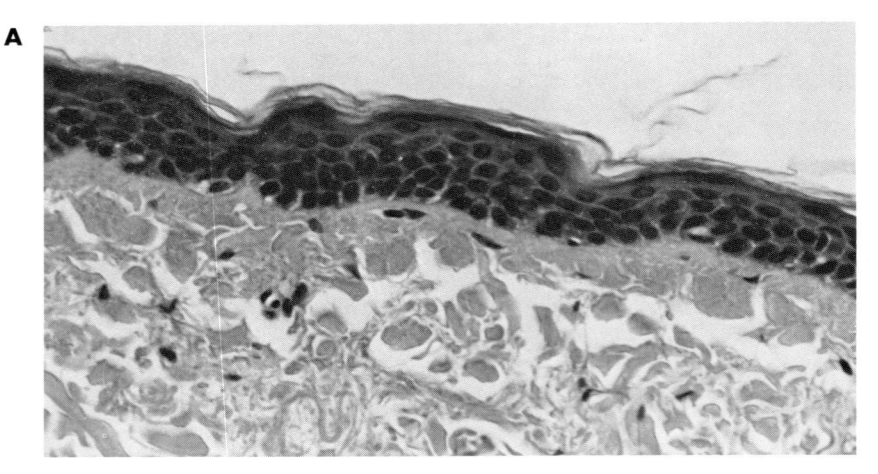

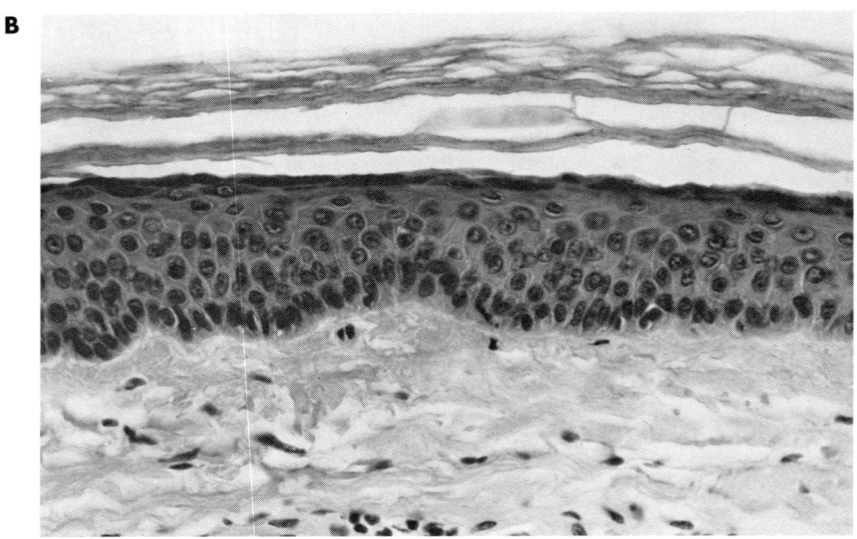

FIGURE 3-10 A, Unpeeled specimen showing cytologic irregularities of the epidermis and loss of polarity. The dermal matrix shows large spaces, reflecting increased ground substance, and abnormal fibrous architecture. (HE, ×406.) B, Peeled specimen from same patient 12 years later. There is a return of orderly differentiation, accompanied by elimination of cellular variability. This is essentially a normal epidermis. The dermal matrix has a normal appearance. (HE, ×406.) (From Kligman AM, Baker TJ, Gordon HL: Plast Reconstr Surg *75:652–659, 1985. Used by permission.)*

Conclusion

The clinical and histologic effects of deep phenol peeling are extraordinarily long-lasting. Even after 10 to 15 years, the contrast with unpeeled skin is striking. The immediate effect of phenol is to destroy the epidermis and the upper elastotic dermis to a depth of 2 to 3 mm. This is considerably deeper than that obtained by dermabrasion, and by contrast, 25% trichloroacetic acid (TCA) barely reaches the upper dermis. The probable reason for the long-lasting effect of the phenol peel is the greater depth of tissue damage and resultant formation of the new stratified collagen layer.

The epidermis regenerates to a markedly normal degree from the epithelial appendages, primarily from the numerous facial follicles. In the deeper dermis, surviving fibroblasts proliferate to construct an entirely new dermal matrix made up of fine, compact collagen bundles in a neat, parallel array. This fibroplasia should not be confused with scarring. As in normal wound healing, collagen deposits precede the re-forming of elastic tissue. In peeled skin, new elastic fibers do not become abundant until years later. This arrangement parallels that of the collagen bundles. The regenerated elastic fibers seem structurally normal and apparently can fulfill the chief function of elastic tissue—keeping the skin under tension and enabling it to snap back to its original state after a deforming force. Peeled skin shows this property to a remarkable degree.

The chief purpose of a peel is cosmetic—to restore aged and sun-damaged skin to a more youthful appearance. However, this understates the full medical impact of the phenol peel. Premalignant epithelial transformations, such as small actinic keratoses, and incipient basal and squamous cell carcinomas are also eliminated. Thus the peel has a significant prophylactic effect on skin cancers, the majority of which occur on facial skin. It has been established by half-face planing that the reappearance of actinic keratoses is markedly slowed after dermabrasion. This must hold true even more so for the deeper phenol peel. In our practice, we have rarely noted facial skin malignancies in patients who have undergone previous chemical face peeling where phenol was the active agent.

Indications

Proper patient selection is the most important aspect of obtaining satisfactory results following treatment. In the beginning, we used chemical peeling to treat many conditions until, by trial and error, we discovered what the chemical peel was suited for. For example, little benefit was seen after chemical peeling for the treatment of acne scarring. Nor did chemical peeling improve the appearance of capillary hemangioma and telangiectasia, and it has little effect in reducing the hyperpigmentation seen in some split-thickness skin grafts.

Two clinical conditions have responded well to chemical peeling. Peeling is effective in the treatment of facial wrinkling and is also helpful for the patient with blotchy skin pigmentation caused by pregnancy, chloasma, birth control pills, chronic sun exposure, and various dermatitides.

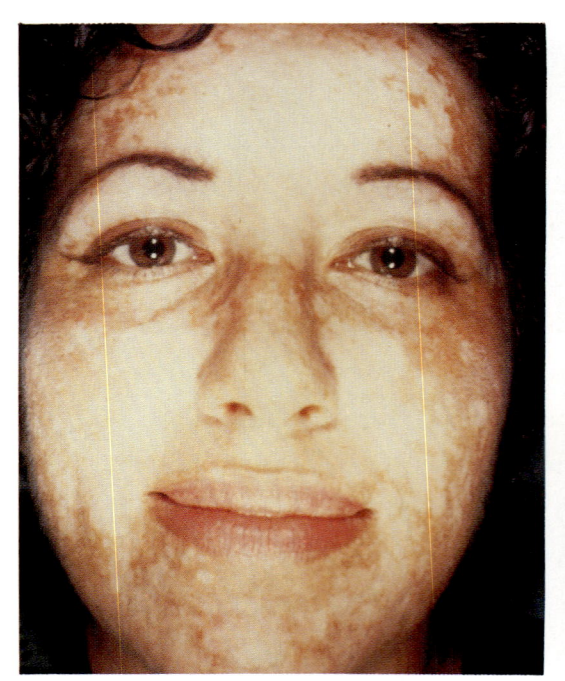

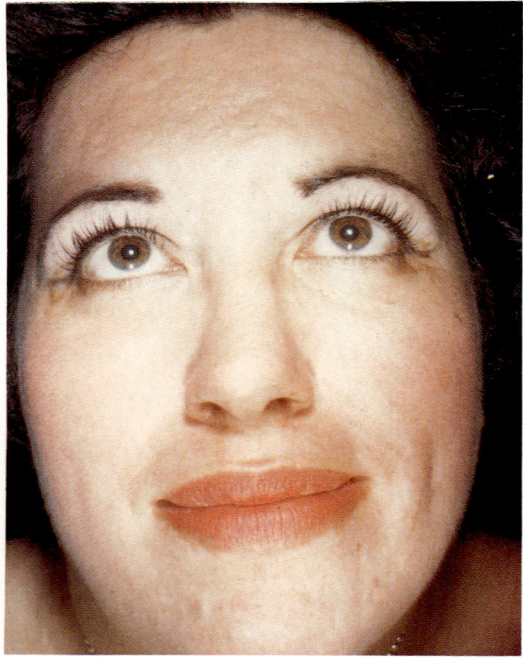

This 28-year-old woman had a generalized allergic drug reaction of the facial skin, and hyperpigmentation of the skin followed. The patient is shown 7 months after full-face peel to remove hyperpigmentation.

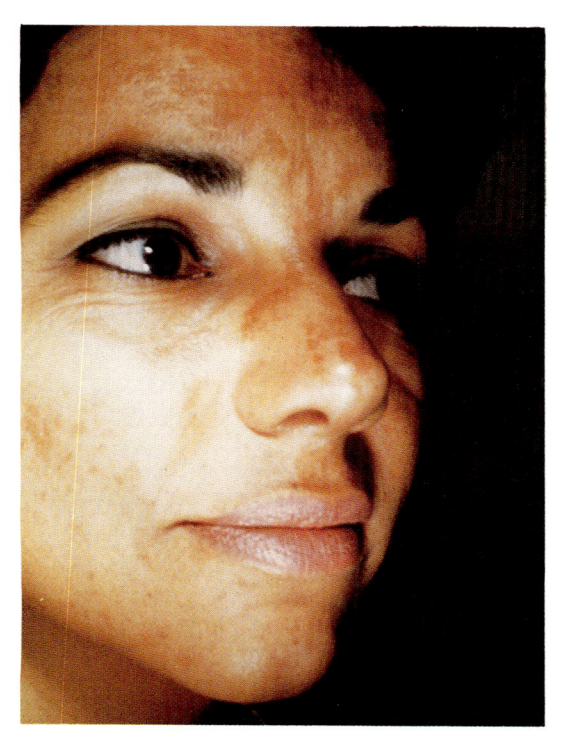

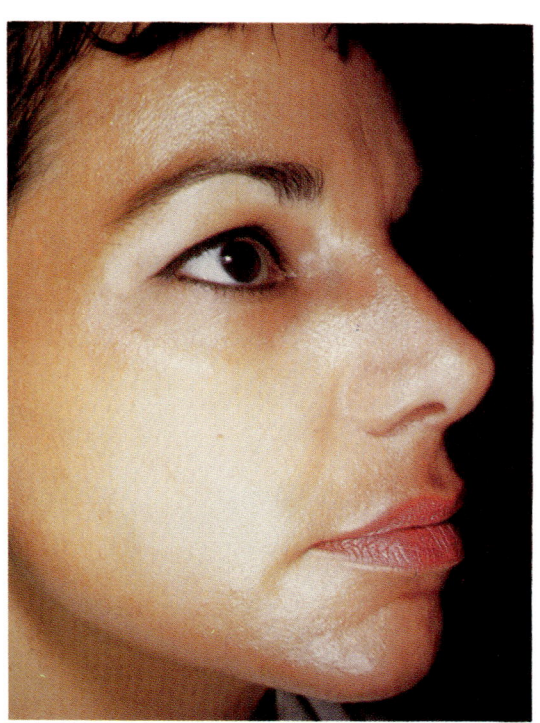

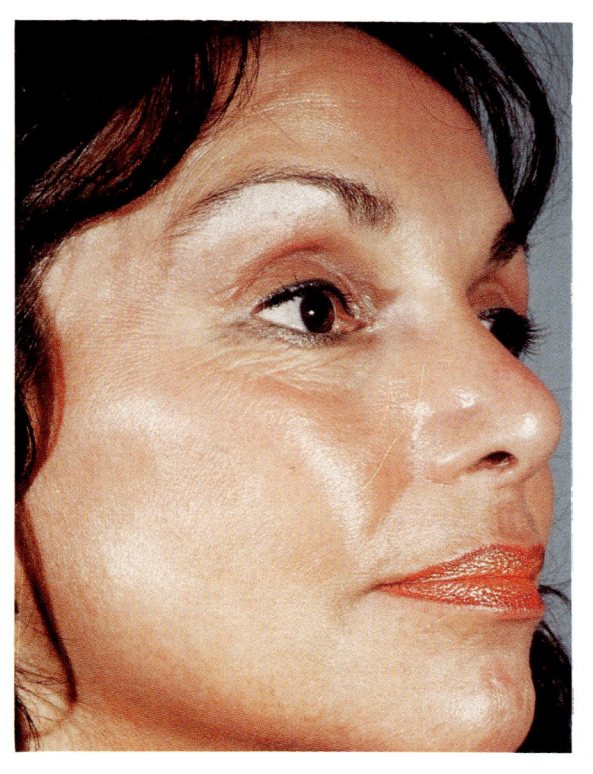

CHEMICAL PEELING (PHENOL AND TRICHLOROACETIC ACID) AND DERMABRASION

This hyperpigmentation of facial skin, primarily in the areas of the nose and the forehead, is the result of birth control pill use and exposure to sunlight. The patient has an olive Mediterranean complexion. The patient is shown 1 year after a full-face peel. Essentially all of the pigmented areas have been removed without excessive bleaching of the skin. The patient is shown 10 years after full-face peel to remove the pigmented blotches.

SURGICAL REJUVENATION OF THE FACE

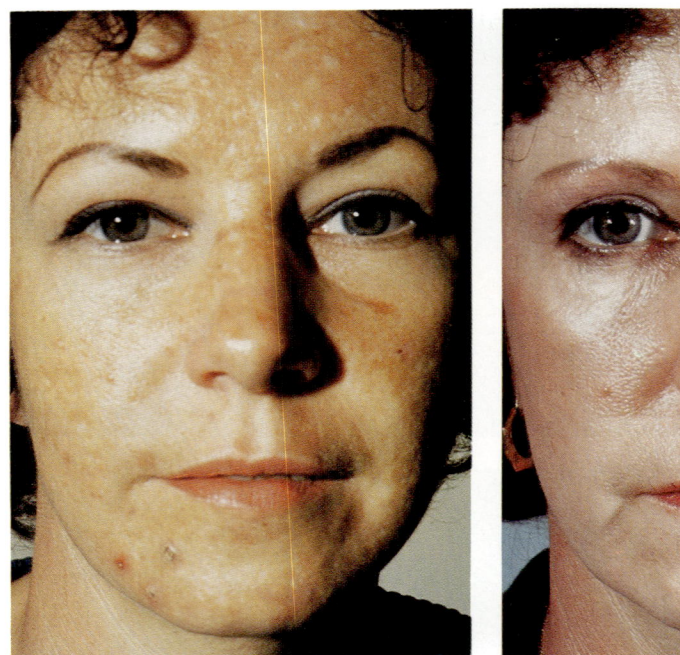

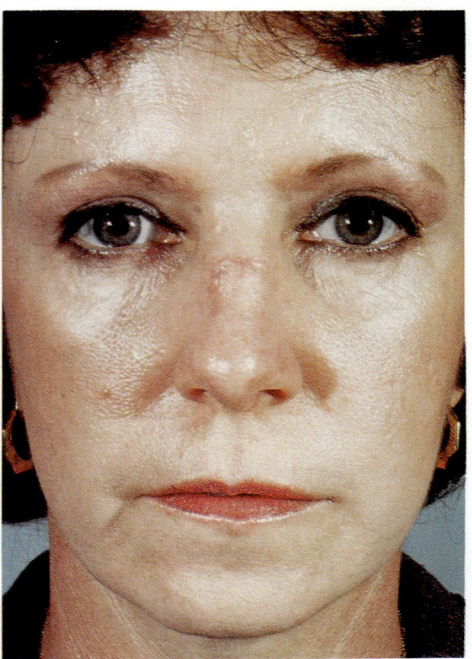

Blotchy facial hyperpigmentation in a 25-year-old woman after repeated bouts of adolescent acne. The patient is shown 10 years after full-face peel that removed facial blotches. The scar on her nose is not related to the peel.

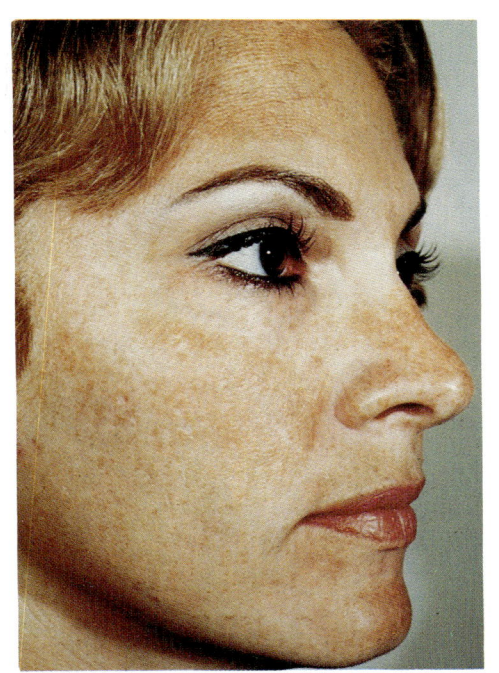

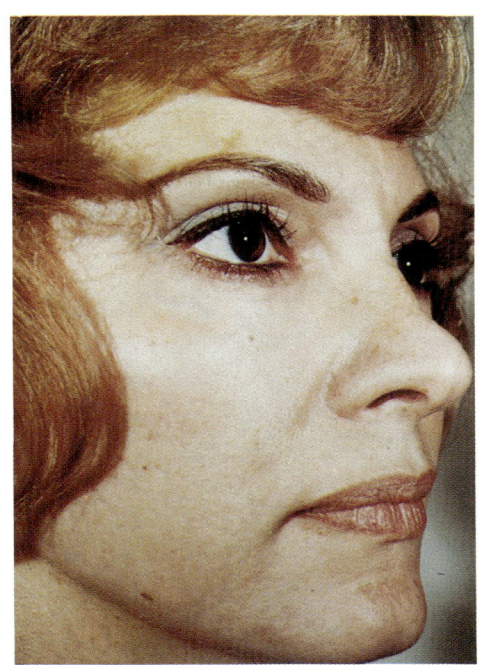

CHEMICAL PEELING (PHENOL AND TRICHLOROACETIC ACID) AND DERMABRASION

Uniform distribution of hyperpigmentation after prolonged exposure to sunlight. The patient is shown 2 years after a full-face peel with no recurrence of blotchy pigmentation.

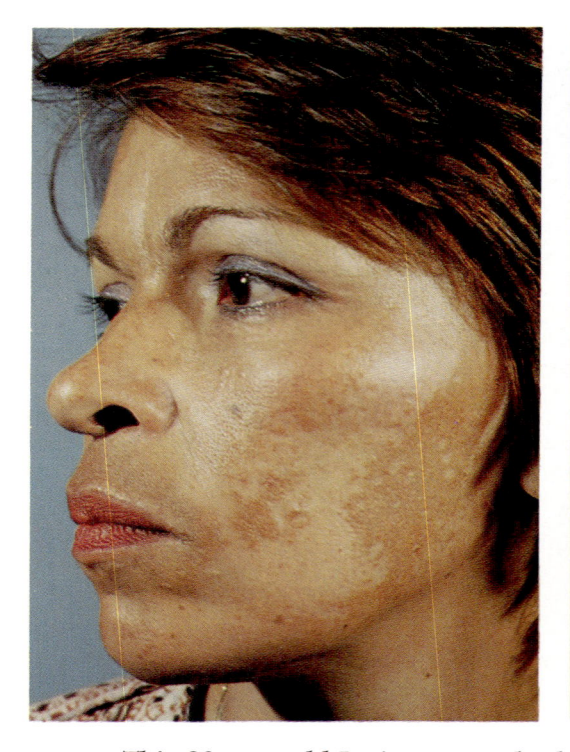

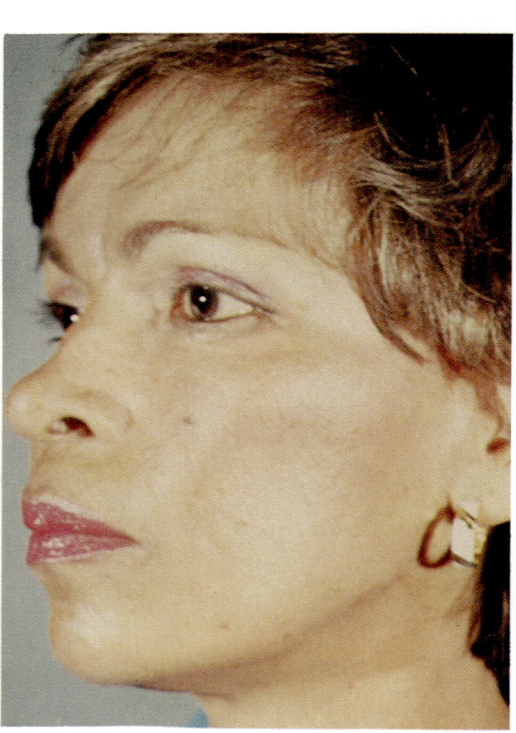

SURGICAL REJUVENATION OF THE FACE

This 30-year-old Latin woman had a full-face peel done elsewhere that left irregular blotching; the cause was unknown. The patient is shown 2 years after repeat full-face peel to remove blotching.

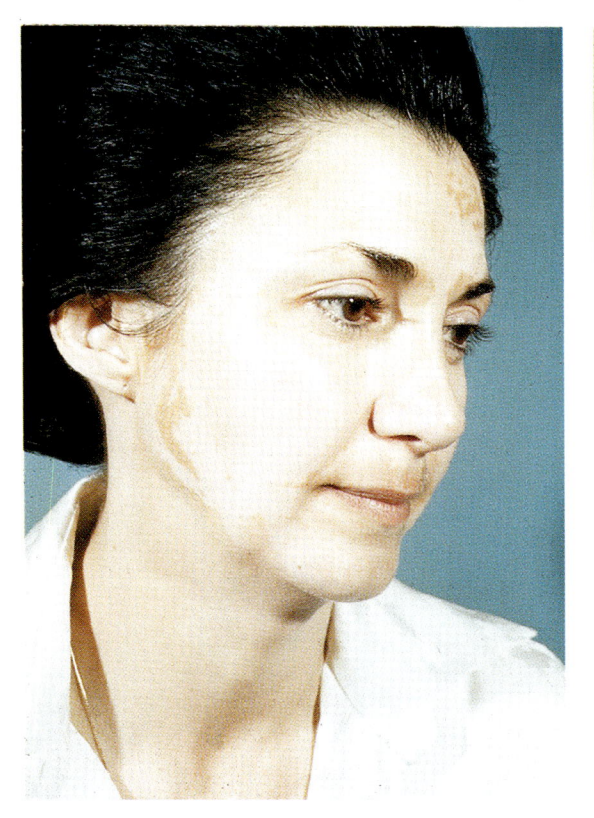

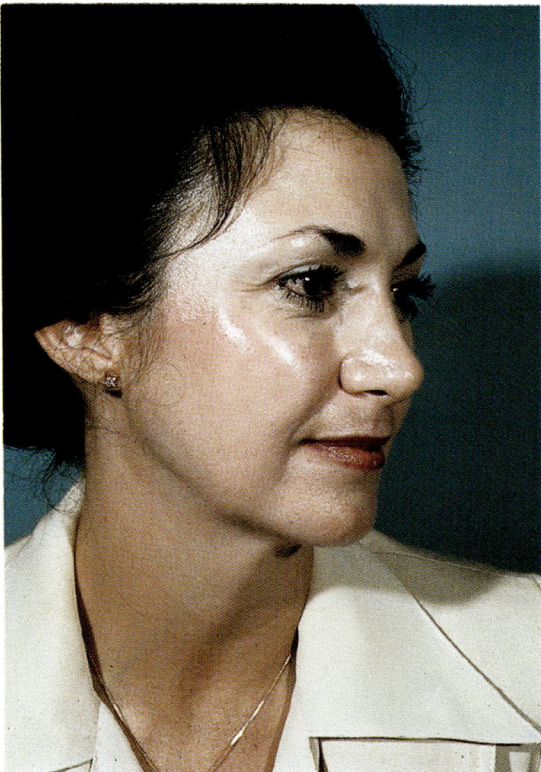

CHEMICAL PEELING (PHENOL AND TRICHLOROACETIC ACID) AND DERMABRASION

Preoperative appearance of peel done for blotchy facial hyperpigmentation. Appearance following full-face phenol chemical peel.

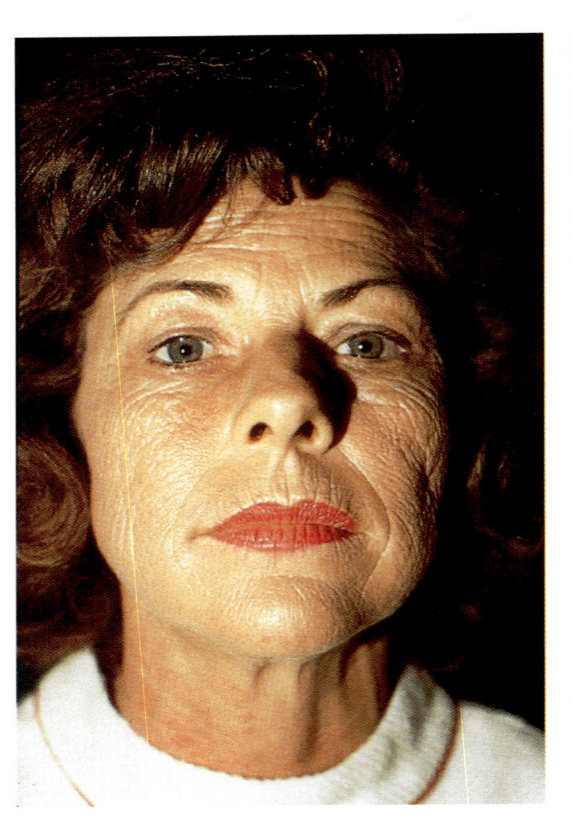

SURGICAL REJUVENATION
OF THE FACE

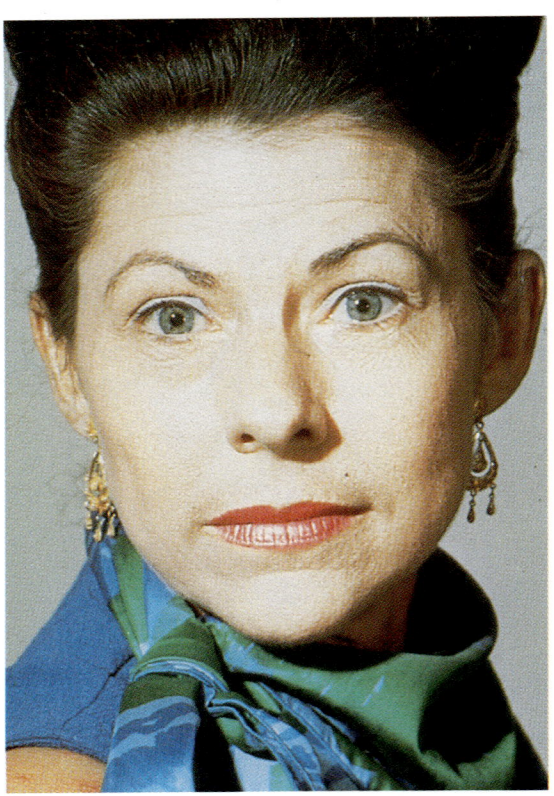

Preoperative appearance of patient with multiple fine and coarse facial rhytides. Patient seen 15 months following full-face phenol chemical peel.

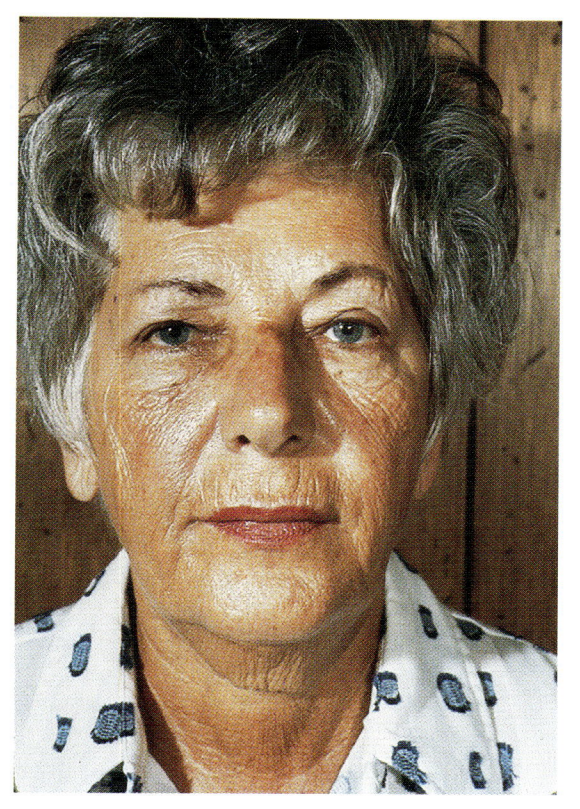

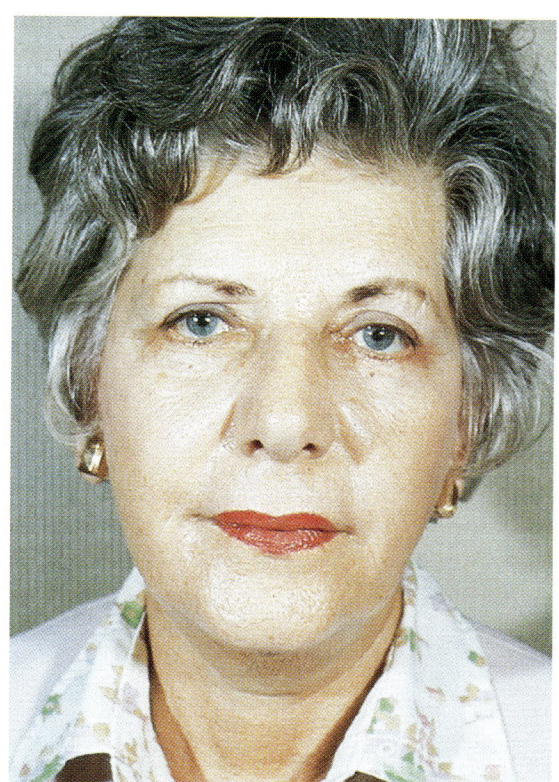

CHEMICAL PEELING (PHENOL AND TRICHLOROACETIC ACID) AND DERMABRASION

Preoperative appearance of patient with blepharochalasis, facial laxity, and coarse and fine facial rhytides. Patient seen following upper and lower blepharoplasty, and rhytidectomy. Three months following the surgical procedure, the patient underwent a full-face phenol peel. She is seen here 6 months following the chemical peel.

SURGICAL REJUVENATION OF THE FACE

Precancerous lesions following sun exposure can also be treated by facial peeling. While 5-fluorouracil (5-FU) has largely replaced chemical peeling in the treatment of actinic keratoses, we occasionally see patients with severe epithelial dysplasia following actinic exposure, which responds extremely well to a deep facial peel. The restoration of dysplastic epithelium following chemical peeling is an added benefit in patients who present with sun-damaged skin and actinic keratoses who undergo peeling for facial wrinkles.

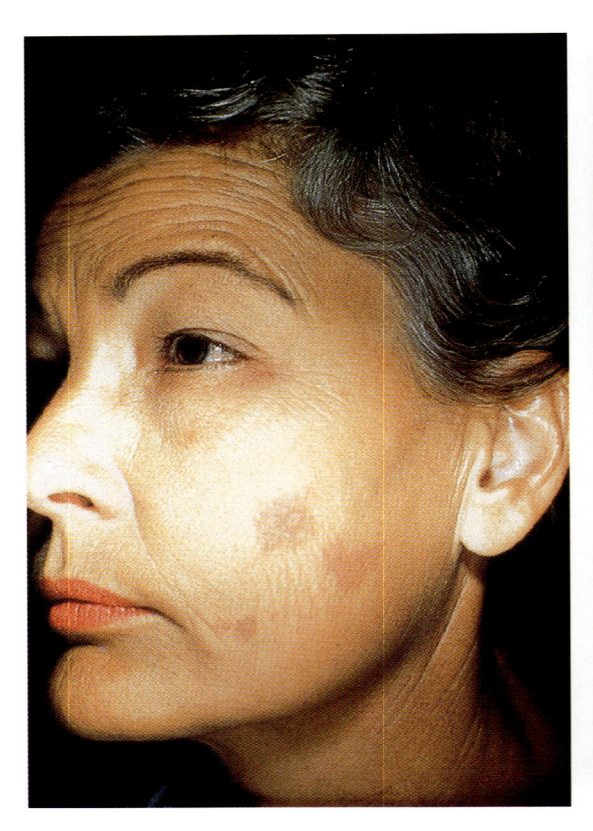

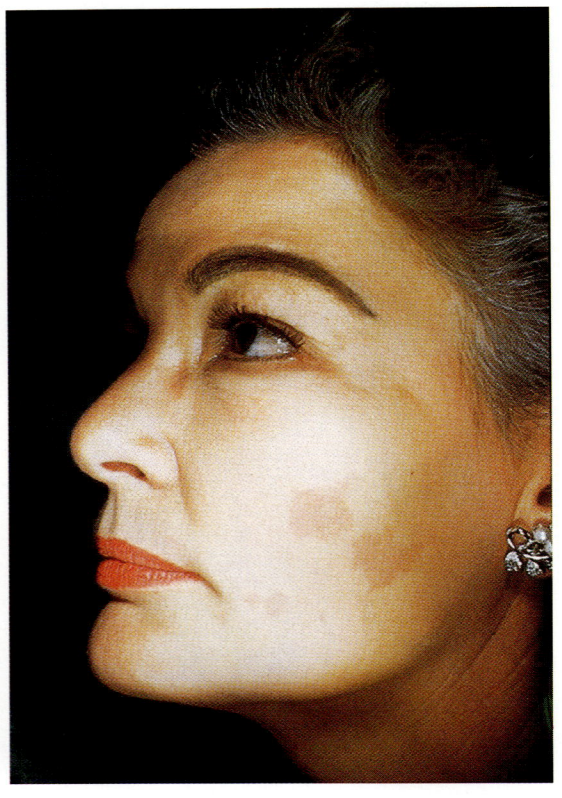

Preoperative appearance of patient seen with predominantly fine facial rhytides as well as port-wine stains of the left cheek. Patient's appearance following full-face phenol peel. Note the improvement of the facial rhytides as well as the general bleaching of her facial pigmentation. We would also point out that there has been no change in the appearance of the port-wine stains present preoperatively. While phenol peeling will produce a bleaching of facial pigmentation, it has no effect on the appearance of vascular malformations or hemangiomas.

We emphasize that chemical peeling is not indicated for treatment of port-wine stains, telangiectasias, hypertrophic scars, and scars resulting from burns. Little benefit is seen in these conditions following chemical peeling. Similarly, scars resulting from acne show little improvement following phenol chemical peel. Acne scars are usually more effectively treated by dermabrasion, and a peel treatment should be reserved for patients whose scars are very superficial.

■ Toxicology

Phenol is a keratocoagulant. It was originally used in carbolic acid as a disinfectant. Because of the extreme keratocoagulation that phenol produces, its use and depth of penetration are quite different from those of TCA. Phenol produces an all-or-none response; that is, low concentrations of phenol do not necessarily produce a light peel, nor do higher concentrations produce a deeper peel. In fact, the opposite appears to be true. When one uses high concentrations of phenol, more rapid and complete coagulation of the keratin in the epidermis occurs and the coagulant layer produces a barrier to further penetration of the acid, lessening its effect on the dermis. We find it interesting that histologic studies have shown that 100% phenol produces 35% to 50% less penetration than a 50% solution. Raising the concentration of phenol may increase the risk of systemic toxicity without producing improved clinical results.

Systemic absorption of phenol occurs through the skin following chemical peeling. Phenol is detoxified in the liver and eliminated in the urine. A toxic dose produces injury to both liver and kidney and can depress the respiratory centers and myocardium. Nonetheless, despite systemic absorption, the blood levels observed following full facial application are low and appear to show that the small volumes of phenol used during facial peeling pose little risk of toxicity.

Perhaps more important to a physician performing a phenol chemical peel is the possibility of rapid absorption. Truppman and Ellenby noted a high incidence of cardiac arrhythmias when greater than 50% of the face was treated with phenol in less than 30 minutes. When the same area was treated over 60 minutes or more, arrhythmias did not occur. Presumably, high levels of phenol absorption can produce myocardial irritability. The arrhythmias observed range from atrial tachycardia to premature ventricular contractions. Because of this possibility, all patients undergoing phenol facial peel should be monitored electrocardiographically and have an intravenous line in place should antiarrhythmic medication prove necessary. We would note that in the thousands of phenol chemical peels that we have performed, electrocardiographic changes following have been rare, especially if the phenol is applied regionally over a period of 1 or 2 hours. In our practice, we have never had to administer antiarrhythmic medications in the treatment of electrocardiographic abnormalities following phenol peeling.

Patient Selection and Contraindications

Patient selection is perhaps the most important factor in obtaining satisfactory results with phenol chemical peel. Unlike TCA, which at least in light peels can be applied to most persons, phenol facial peels require a greater patient selectivity. This is largely secondary to the bleaching effect seen following phenol peeling. Patients with fair complexions are obviously better candidates than those with olive-toned skin. Patients with a dark complexion tend to show an obvious line of demarcation between the treated and untreated areas. Caution should also be exercised when peeling black and Asian patients. In general, regional peeling can be performed in patients who are fair, whereas olive complexions usually require full-face peeling to minimize the contrasting hypopigmentation observed between treated and untreated skin. Thick and oily skin seems to respond less favorably to peeling and has a greater tendency to develop areas of spotty hyperpigmentation.

We have learned to avoid the red-haired, freckle-faced person, who, on discovering fine wrinkles around the eyes and mouth, goes to the office of the nearest plastic surgeon and implores, "Do something!" The peeling would definitely remove the wrinkles, but it would also remove all those little pale freckles. And it would remove them right down to

CHEMICAL PEELING (PHENOL AND TRICHLOROACETIC ACID) AND DERMABRASION

the line where the treatment stopped, leaving a permanent and obvious sharp line of demarcation between the skin that was treated and the untreated skin. Worst of all, once done, nothing can be done to remedy it. We know of no way to feather this edge or line of demarcation to make it less apparent.

Even if a small area of the face, such as the upper lip, is peeled on this type of patient, there is always such a disparity in color between the freckle-free lip and the rest of the face that more problems are created than solved. We strongly discourage persons with this type of skin from having the treatment unless they are willing to accept the consequences.

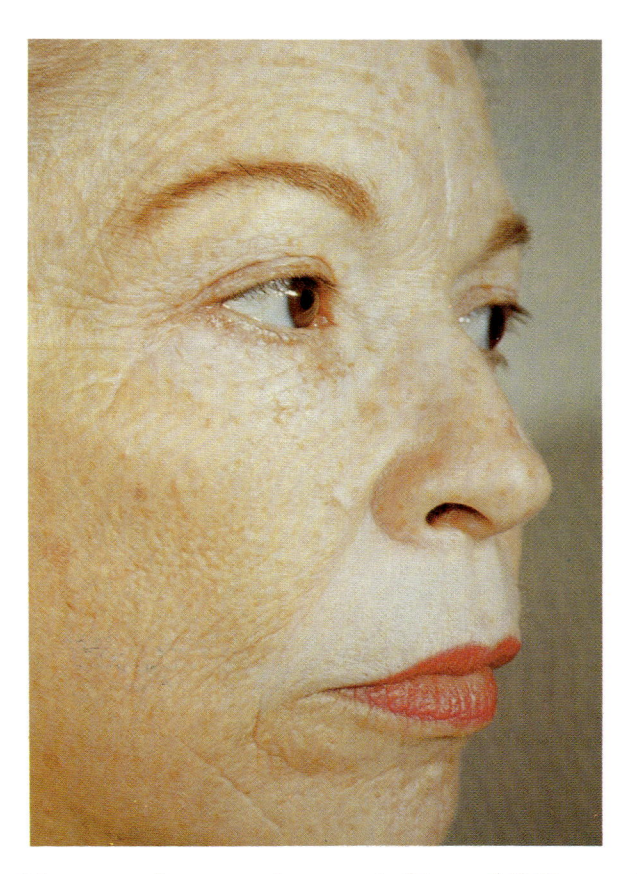

This 46-year-old woman has sun-damaged skin, exhibiting wrinkling and freckling. She has red hair and very fair skin. Peeling her upper lip removed wrinkles and freckles but left a sharp contrast between the treated and the untreated areas.

Likewise, in the case of a patient with severely sun-damaged skin, we believe that regional peeling tends to produce a conspicuous line of demarcation and that the procedure may be contraindicated. This type of skin has many fine wrinkles, which, to be sure, will be removed. The problem is the permanent lightening of skin color caused by the treatment.

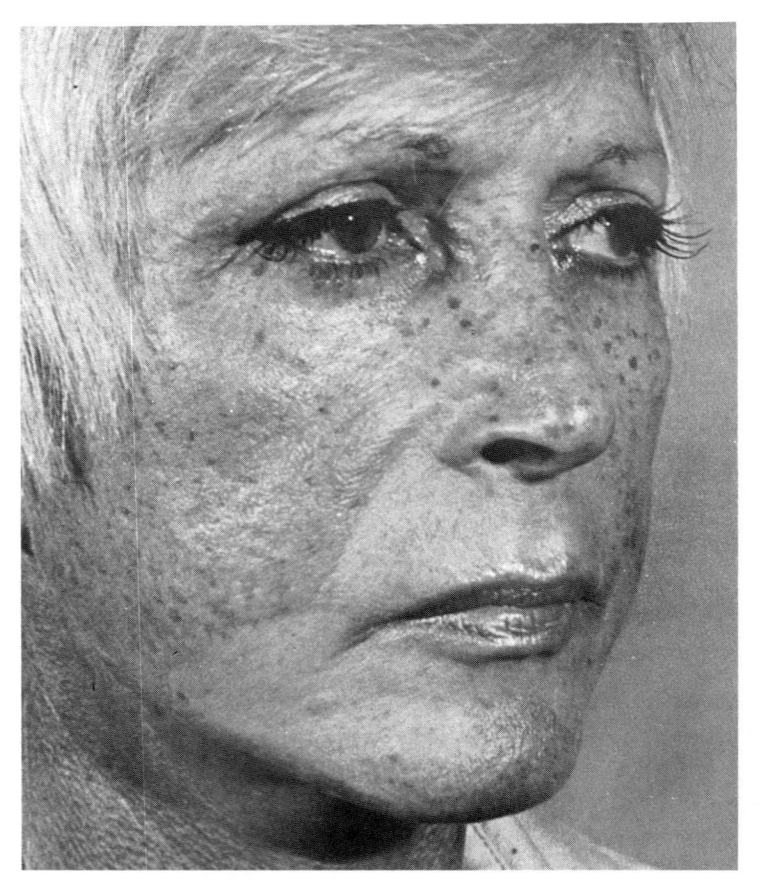

This 44-year-old tennis player has severely sun-damaged skin. A perioral peel was performed that was extended onto the lower cheek. The obvious line of demarcation is unsightly and difficult to conceal with makeup. The only solution now is to peel the rest of the face, although there will then be a sharp line of demarcation below the mandibular border.

Males, with few exceptions, are not good candidates, because the use of covering cosmetics is not appropriate and thick male skin in most instances does not respond as well as the thinner skin of females.

Phenol chemical peeling should not be used in the treatment of rhytides or hyperpigmentation of the neck, thorax, or extremities. Attempts at peeling these areas have occasionally resulted in hypertrophic scarring, which may relate to the paucity of skin appendages in these areas, as compared with facial skin. Because of the large areas to be treated, there is also the danger of systemic phenol toxicity.

Spot peeling can be performed on individual lentigines on the dorsum of the hands and fingers. Judicious, direct application of pure phenol on these pigmented lesions is particularly effective in eliminating these common signs of aging. On patients requesting a more generalized treatment for lentigines of the forearm and hands, we have limited experience with the use of light- to medium-depth TCA to improve the so-called age spots that are commonly seen in the elderly patient.

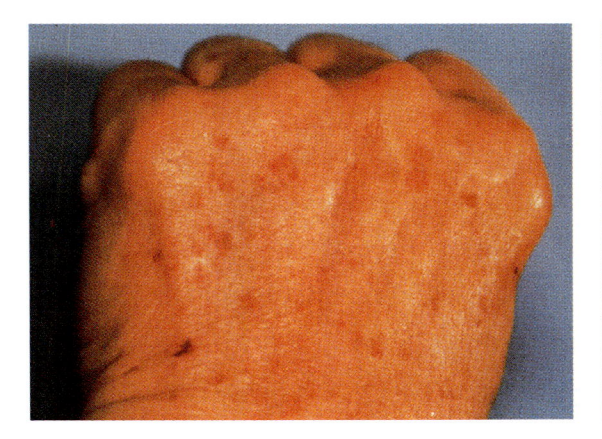

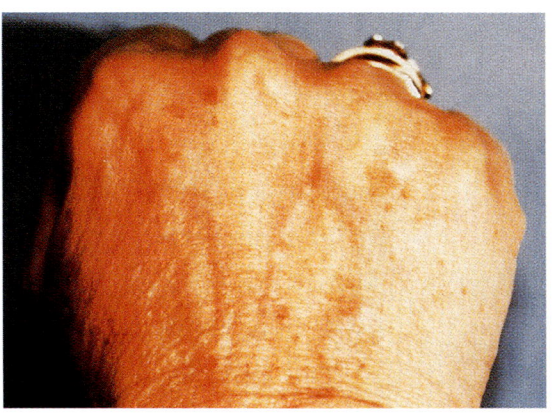

Spot peeling of phenol for individual lentigines present along the dorsum of the hand is quite effective. In this patient, spot peeling was performed on lentigines of the right hand, whereas no treatment was performed on the left hand. Note the substantial difference in appearance between the treated and untreated hands of this patient.

Preoperative Visit

Most patients who come for consultation about the aging of their face have some kind of surgical face-lifting procedure in mind. The clinician has many questions to answer during this initial interview. The most common public misconception about the treatment of the aging face is that surgical face-lifting removes *all* wrinkles. When patients say "wrinkles," they usually mean not only the generalized sagging of the skin and the subcutaneous soft tissues of the face but also the fine lines. We spend much time with prospective patients explaining that surgery removes the excess skin caused by gravitational pull, but peeling removes the lines on the remaining skin. An analogy used in this explanation goes as follows:

Suppose that you had a favorite and expensive garment that no longer fit because of recent weight loss. You might take the garment to a tailor and have him reduce the size of the garment by removing the excess fabric. The garment now fits perfectly. This tailoring corresponds to the surgery contemplated. However, you notice that the tailor did not press the garment, so that while you now have a garment that fits, it is still wrinkled. The steam pressing that the tailor now does to remove the wrinkles corresponds to the peeling.

Frequently, patients who come to our office requesting face-lifts leave wanting facial peels instead. After the explanation of what each procedure does, they realize that peeling fits their expectations more than surgery does. The reverse is less often true—that someone comes in for a peel who really needs a surgical procedure. Patients who are sophisticated or educated enough to ask about peeling usually know something about the procedure.

The benefits of peeling as opposed to rhytidectomy must be explained thoroughly to the patient before chemical peel is undertaken. If the patient is likely to benefit from both procedures, it is preferable to perform the face-lift first and follow with the chemical peeling 3 months later. *Under no circumstances should chemical peeling be performed on undermined skin at the time of rhytidectomy. This is an invitation to the catastrophic possibility of full-thickness skin loss.* Eyelid peeling and blepharoplasty should *never* be performed at the same time. Regional perioral peeling is commonly performed at the time of rhytidectomy, but we emphasize that the *skin undermining must stop a few centimeters short of where the peeling solution is applied* to minimize the possibility of hypertrophic scarring.

Patient Education

When a patient comes to us for an initial consultation, we try to be as specific as possible in telling her what to expect. Our experience has been that the more the patient knows before the procedure, the smoother the course will be. We all tend to fear the unknown. Many surgeons use a printed information sheet, and others use various audiovisual devices. Time spent informing the patient is well invested. The following is an example of what we say to the patient during an initial interview.

You want to know if the fine lines and wrinkles on your face can be removed? The answer is yes, they can be removed, but instead of an operation, a chemical skin treatment called peeling is needed. This treatment is designed to remove fine wrinkles and brown blotches, but is not a substitute for surgical face-lifting.

> Your skin will be treated in our clinic. We will make every effort to make you as comfortable as possible, but I must tell you that some phases of the treatment will be painful. We put chemicals on your face, and you will experience a burning sensation that lasts for several minutes. Then we fashion an adhesive-tape mask, leaving holes for your eyes, nose, and mouth. After a time the burning sensation will return and last longer than before. We will give you medication to relieve your pain, but you must expect some unavoidable discomfort during the first day. A few hours after the mask is applied you will be moved to a recovery center where experienced people will take care of you. By the second day you will have little or no discomfort. You will return to our office 48 hours after your treatment, and the mask will be removed; this is somewhat painful but only lasts a moment.
>
> During the rest of the first week you will wash and lubricate your face

yourself. We will tell you what to do on a daily basis. At the end of the first week, your skin will be quite red, but smooth and clean. By the end of the second or third week the redness will have faded to resemble a sunburn, and you will be able to wear makeup. You probably will be able to return to work at this time. Complete healing, that is, when the redness has totally faded, will usually occur in 10 to 12 weeks. When your skin has healed, it is our expectation that your wrinkles or blotches will be gone and your face will be a little lighter in color than before. You will notice a line of demarcation between the treated and the untreated skin. If you decide to have cosmetic surgery in addition to the full facial peel, it can be done before or after this procedure, but not at the same time—the minimum interval is 3 months.

There are a few important instructions to the patient about skin care after the healing process is complete.

Following a peel, the skin does not react in the usual manner to sunlight exposure; instead, the skin pigment is distributed unevenly, producing an unpleasant blotchy discoloration. For this reason, patients are to avoid exposure to sunlight as much as possible.

Another reason to avoid exposure to the sun is to minimize the line of demarcation between the area that was treated and the surrounding skin. The untreated skin will tan as before, but the treated skin will not, thus producing a difference in color and therefore a more obvious line of demarcation. If sun exposure is unavoidable, the skin should be covered with a maximum-protection sunscreen.

Sometimes the skin is drier than usual after a peel. A regular regimen of daily lubrication is advised. Any lubricant will do, and the choice is usually left to the patient.

Procedure

Ingredients

The chemical mixture used to perform a peel is composed of the following ingredients:

3 mL *USP* liquid phenol

2 mL tap water

8 drops liquid soap

3 drops croton oil

The phenol, *USP* liquid phenol, is a prepared solution of approximately 88% phenol concentration. It is readily available from most chemical supply houses. We have always mixed tap water with this solution, but if the available water contains contaminants, distilled water should be used. The liquid soap we use most often is Septisol, but any liquid soap will do. Its purpose is to help emulsify the mixture. Croton oil is extracted from the seeds of *Croton tiglium,* an Asiatic plant. This ingredient may be difficult to find. Some pharmaceutical houses in large cities still stock this archaic medication that was used years ago as a purgative and vesicant. If croton oil cannot be found, the peel can be done without it. We use it because it enhances the keratolytic and penetrating action of the mixture.

Technique

Phenol peeling should be performed in a hospital or ambulatory surgical facility. Full-face peeling requires sedation before and during the procedure. An intravenous catheter should be in place, and the patient should be monitored with electrocardiographic and pulse oximetry equipment. Because eyelid edema is anticipated for 2 to 3 days after full-face peeling, experienced personnel must be available if the procedure is performed on an outpatient basis. For regional perioral or spot peeling of the face, the need for sedation, monitoring, and postoperative care is minimized.

The night before the procedure, the patient washes her face thoroughly to remove all traces of makeup, and this is repeated the next morning. Upon arrival at the hospital or clinic, the patient is premedicated, the authors' preference being oral diazepam. Before application, intravenous meperidine (50 mg) is effective in alleviating the discomfort of the peel, and this can be supplemented as needed. Local anesthetic agents are not used.

The skin is again cleaned with liquid soap and water, thoroughly dried, and washed with diethyl ether to remove all surface oils that might interfere with the peeling.

SURGICAL REJUVENATION OF THE FACE

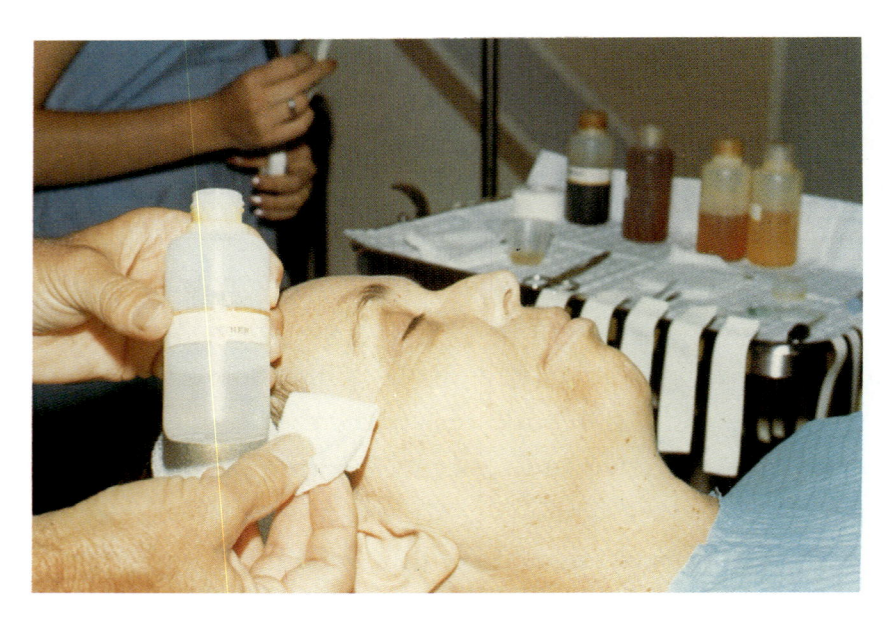

The sedated patient has had her face cleaned with diethyl ether to remove superficial skin oils. The phenol mixture has been freshly made and is on the tray in the background.

The chemical mixture for peeling is freshly prepared before each case. The ingredients do not mix readily and need to be stirred vigorously before each application.

The peeling mixture is applied to the face with a cotton-tipped applicator. The mixture is applied evenly and uniformly over the entire area and into each wrinkle. The skin becomes pearly white on contact with the chemicals, and the patient experiences a mild burning sensation, which gradually subsides as the local anesthetic property of phenol takes effect. The application is carried slightly into the hairline to minimize the line of demarcation where the peeling stops. The peeling process does not affect the hair follicles and therefore does not cause alopecia. The applicator is semimoist rather than saturated to prevent the solution from dripping onto areas where it is not wanted. Any site that the solution touches will be affected. Lightly rolling the applicator onto a piece of gauze absorbs excess liquid and helps to avoid this problem.

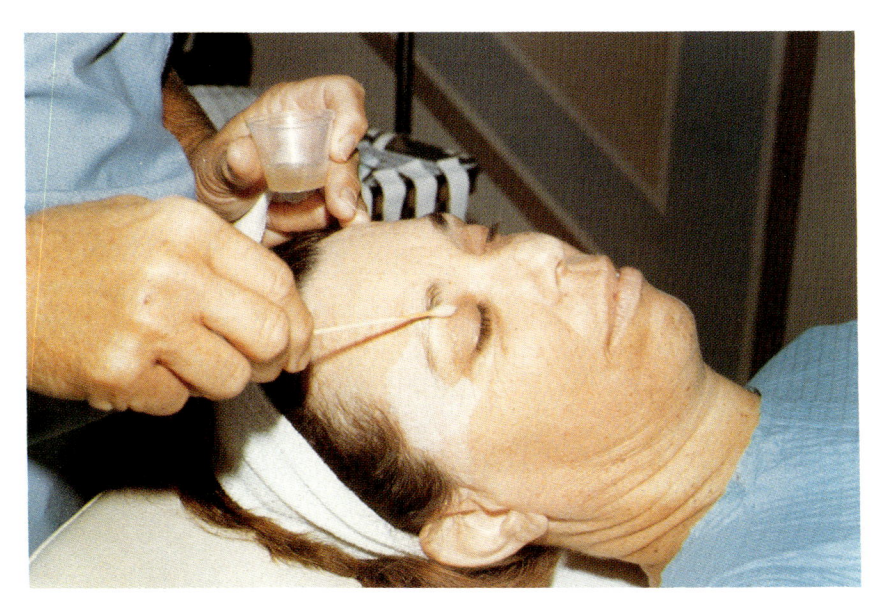

CHEMICAL PEELING (PHENOL AND TRICHLOROACETIC ACID) AND DERMABRASION

The phenol mixture is applied to the facial skin with a cotton-tipped applicator. Note that the skin immediately turns a distinctive grayish-white color. The patient experiences a burning sensation.

The phenol is applied slowly to lessen patient discomfort and minimize the possibility of too rapid absorption. The solution is applied to the forehead first. The painting is carried close to and into the eyebrows. If the upper eyelids are to be treated, the applicator must be almost dry to prevent the phenol from coming into contact with the cornea and conjunctiva. The mixture is applied to the skin between the brow and the upper tarsal fold, but the skin overlying the tarsal plate is left untreated. Peeling in this region leads to enormous eyelid edema, which can be slow to resolve. The upper eyelid skin can be taped, but no tape is applied directly over the eyebrows.

After the first area is treated, it is covered with an occlusive dressing, usually waterproof tape, and 20 to 30 minutes are allowed to elapse before proceeding to the next area. The malar region and cheeks, including the lower eyelids, are then treated. When chemical peeling of the lower eyelids is performed, the skin is moistened to within 2 mm of the ciliary margin. An assistant holds the upper eyelids open to pre-

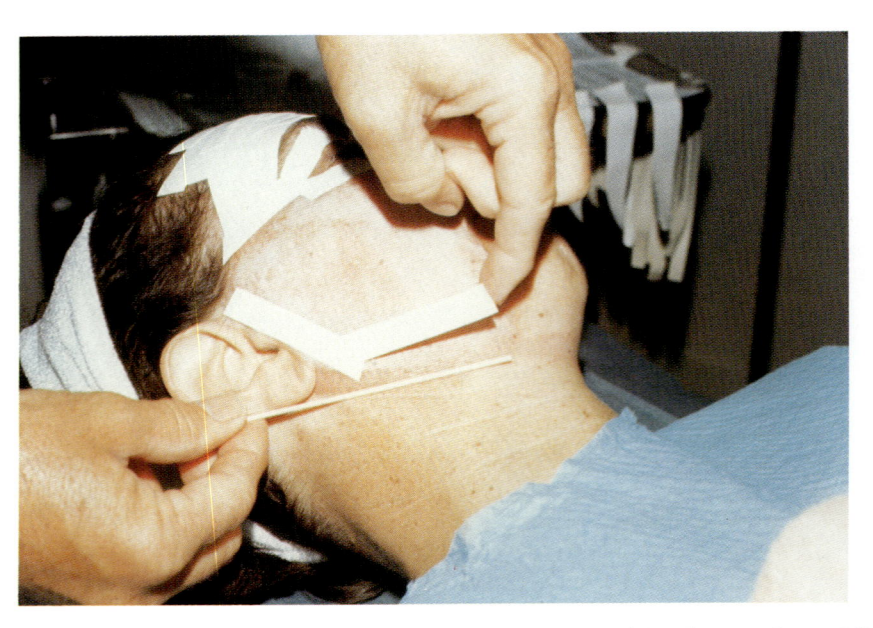

The forehead, cheeks, and perioral area are painted in that order with the phenol mixture, and each area is immediately covered with waterproof adhesive tape before proceeding to the next area.

vent blinking until each of the lower lids has been treated, blotted, and allowed to air-dry. A supply of water to irrigate the eye in case of mishap is an important safeguard. This will minimize the possibility of corneal injury.

The mixture is applied regionally to the entire face down to a line 2 to 3 cm below the inferior margin of the mandible. The mixture should extend onto the neck only far enough to camouflage the treated area as much as possible. Around the mouth, care should be taken to apply the chemicals at least to the vermilion border and preferably slightly into it. Application along the vermilion removes the vertical wrinkles of the upper lip, especially the smaller ones that radiate from the vermilion border. The ear lobes are commonly wrinkled, and these fine wrinkles can be treated if the patient wishes.

CHEMICAL PEELING (PHENOL AND TRICHLOROACETIC ACID) AND DERMABRASION

Application of the Waterproof Mask

After the skin has been completely covered with the chemical mixture, a mask of waterproof adhesive tape is applied directly to the skin, leaving only the eyes, eyebrows, nostrils, and mouth exposed. Short pieces of tape are easier to apply than long ones and seem to conform to the curves of the face better. When the tape is first applied, it may not adhere well, but as the body heat warms the adhesive and early edema occurs, adherence improves. The short strips should not be applied tightly; if they are applied improperly, the skin beneath can become folded or pleated and the skin in the depth of the fold will not be in contact with the tape. This produces streaking and unevenness in the final texture and color of the skin.

After the area to be treated is covered with strips of half-inch tape, a second layer is placed over the first, using strips of 1-in. tape. This second layer reinforces the mask and ensures that all areas are covered.

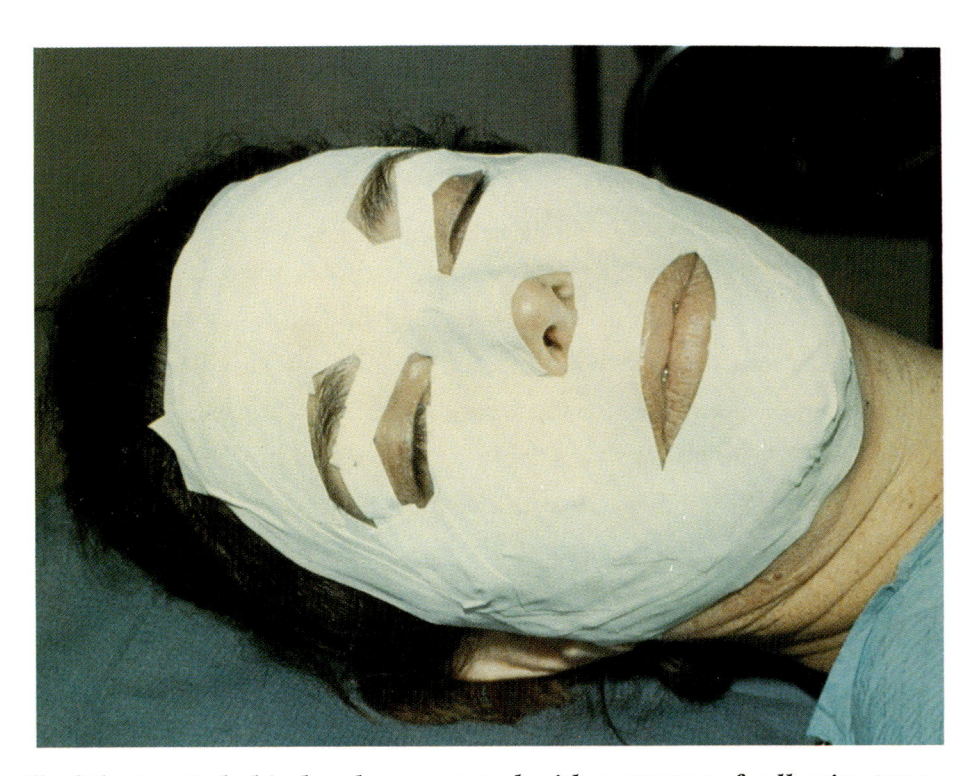

All of the treated skin has been covered with waterproof adhesive tape.

Alternative to Tape Mask: Petroleum Jelly

It has long been our impression that occlusive taping maintains the concentration of phenol at the skin surface and produces a more complete and longer-lasting peel. Numerous studies have confirmed this observation. The occlusive dressing prevents evaporation of the phenol solution as well as promoting tissue maceration, both factors leading to increased penetration of the phenol solution. It should be noted that if a lesser result is desired with phenol peeling, the way to produce this is to perform peeling without an occlusive dressing.

The disadvantages of taping include increased patient discomfort and the inability to evaluate what is going on beneath the mask. Mask removal is uncomfortable. Drying of the skin after application of thymol iodide at the time of tape removal is unpleasant, and separation of the crusts from the face after desquamation and healing may be painful.

Over the last several years we have found ourselves less frequently using a tape occlusive dressing following phenol peel. In its place we have substituted an occlusive dressing using a thick layer of petroleum jelly (Vaseline). The occlusiveness provided by the petroleum jelly has proved to be almost as effective as the standard tape mask, and the results parallel those obtained with occlusive tape. The advantages of petroleum jelly include greater patient comfort, the ability to evaluate the wound beneath the petroleum jelly, and the prevention of streaking, which can occur from uneven tape application. Eschar formation and crust separation are avoided after the peel by the constant use of facial lubricants, our preference being A & D ointment.

The technique of applying petroleum jelly is quite simple. As the phenol mixture is regionally applied and allowed to dry, each treated area is then covered with a thick layer of petroleum jelly.

The dressing is applied only once, immediately following the phenol peel, lubricating the wound and serving as the occlusive dressing.

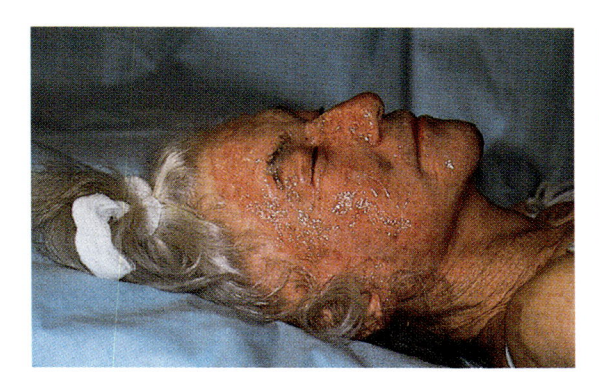

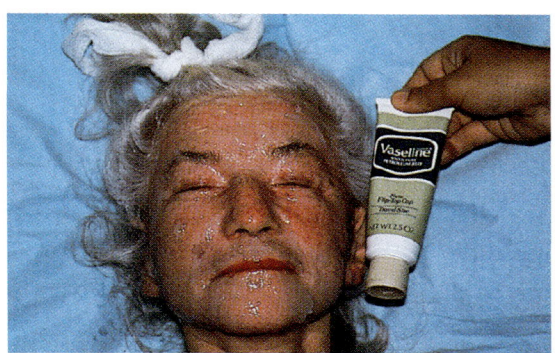

As an alternative to a tape occlusive dressing, we have achieved comparable results with the use of a petroleum jelly (Vaseline) occlusive dressing. The patient is seen here following a full-face phenol peel with the subsequent application of a thick layer of petroleum jelly that serves as the immediate postpeel occlusive dressing.

Wound lubrication is continued throughout the early postpeel period with a greasy petroleum-based ointment, such as A & D ointment. Gentle washing of the peeled area with cool tap water is begun on the first postpeel day, and this routine of washing followed by ointment application is continued until wound healing is complete (5–7 days). At no time is the wound allowed to desiccate, and by the constant use of moisturizers, eschar formation and crust separation are prevented.

Having used petroleum jelly in this way for several years, it is our opinion that the occlusive dressing is most important in the hours immediately following phenol application and that it is during this period that a mechanical barrier enhances the results of the chemical peel. While covering the peeled areas for a shorter time, as compared with the tape mask, petroleum jelly provides effective occlusion immediately following the chemical peel.

SURGICAL REJUVENATION
OF THE FACE

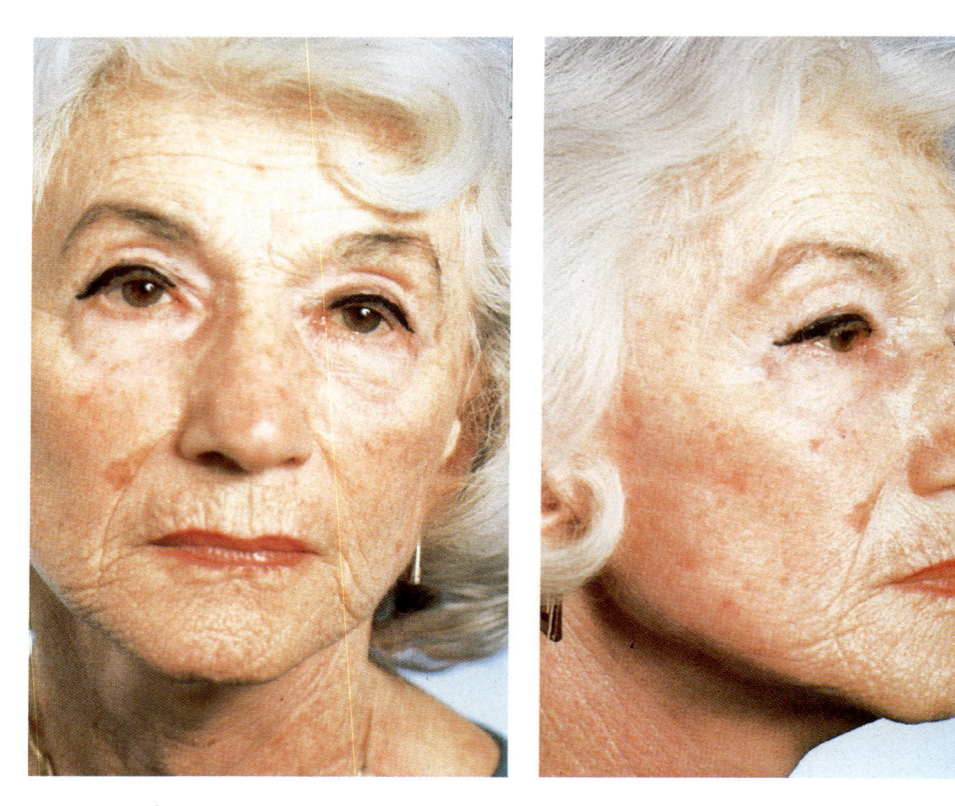

Prepeel appearance. Prepeel appearance.

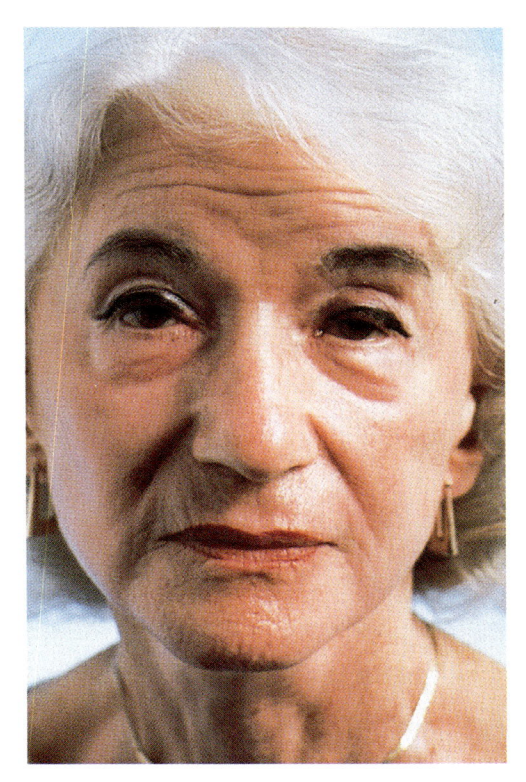

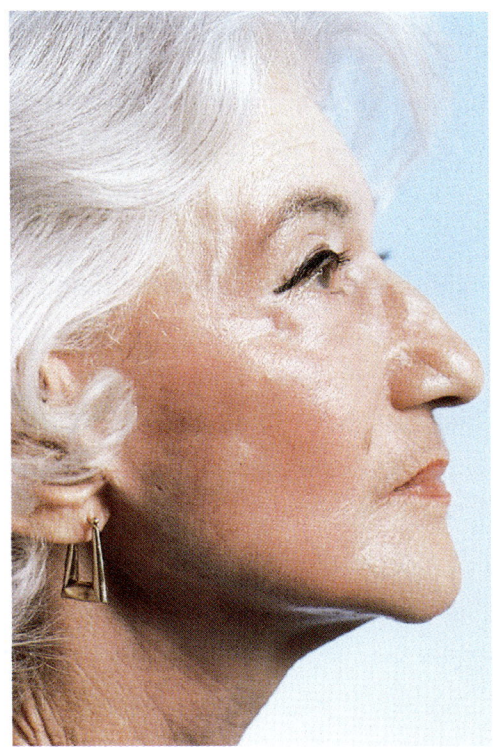

CHEMICAL PEELING (PHENOL AND TRICHLOROACETIC ACID) AND DERMABRASION

Appearance following a full-face phenol peel performed with the use of petroleum jelly. Appearance following a full-face phenol peel performed with the use of petroleum jelly.

We currently use petroleum jelly in all our peels done for problems of facial pigmentation as well as peels done for fine facial wrinkling. Petroleum jelly does not achieve quite the penetration seen with the use of a tape mask, and in patients presenting with coarse facial wrinkling, the so-called weather-beaten look, it is our impression that tape occlusion produces a more profound result. In contrast to fine facial wrinkling, patients with coarse wrinkles following chemical peel show a more improved appearance when tape is used. We reserve tape occlusion for these difficult clinical problems.

In summary, the use of phenol remains either an all-or-none phenomenon and varying the concentrations of phenol will not produce a lighter or deeper peel. The way to control the depth of phenol penetration is not by varying the concentration, but rather by the use or nonuse of an occlusive dressing. The lightest phenol peel is produced without an occlusive dressing. The use of petroleum jelly produces a peel of intermediate depth, and is useful for most clinical problems. Finally, a tape mask produces the deepest phenol penetration and should be reserved for problem patients presenting with coarse facial rhytides and severe actinic damage.

Postpeel Care

Within 1 to 2 minutes after the phenol mixture is applied, the initial burning sensation subsides because of the local anesthetic action of the phenol. Approximately 20 to 30 minutes after the tape mask is applied, the burning sensation returns, this time to a greater degree and for a longer period. Analgesia is helpful in keeping the patient comfortable during this time, and narcotics are usually necessary. Facial edema reaches a maximum during the first 6 to 12 hours after treatment. The eyelids are often swelled shut and the patient may not be able to open her eyes for 48 hours.

The patient is instructed to talk and chew as little as possible to ensure that the tape remains adherent to the skin. Liquids are encour-

CHEMICAL PEELING (PHENOL AND TRICHLOROACETIC ACID) AND DERMABRASION

aged and should be taken with a straw. The head of the bed is elevated, and the patient is allowed out of bed with assistance.

Most of the burning sensation subsides after the first 12 to 24 hours and so does the necessity for medication. Patients may ambulate during the second 24 hours; their mobility is limited only by their ability to see between the edematous lids.

If a mask is used, it is removed after 48 hours. The removal may be somewhat painful and may require medication. At 48 hours, many areas of taping begin to separate spontaneously. The tape mask is split

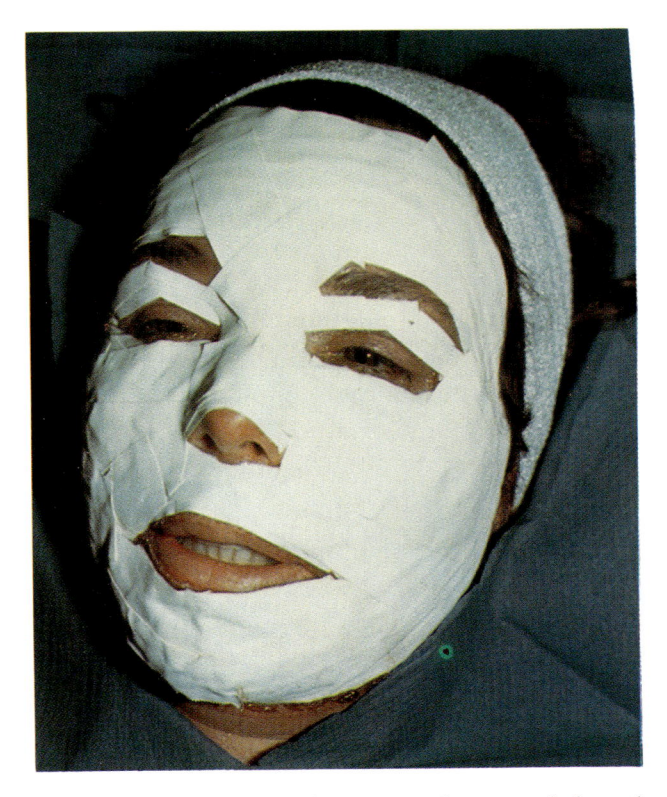

The mask has been in place for 48 hours, and most of the edema of the face has subsided. Note some seepage of the serous exudate from under the edges of the mask.

in several places to facilitate removal. A superficial layer of epithelium, adherent to the undersurface of the dressing, is usually removed with the tape. The appearance of the newly uncovered skin, resembling a uniform second-degree burn, can be alarming to the uninitiated. The skin is edematous and moist. It is covered with a thin layer of loose necrotic epithelium and coagulated exudate. Any loose material or crusts can be lightly washed away at this time.

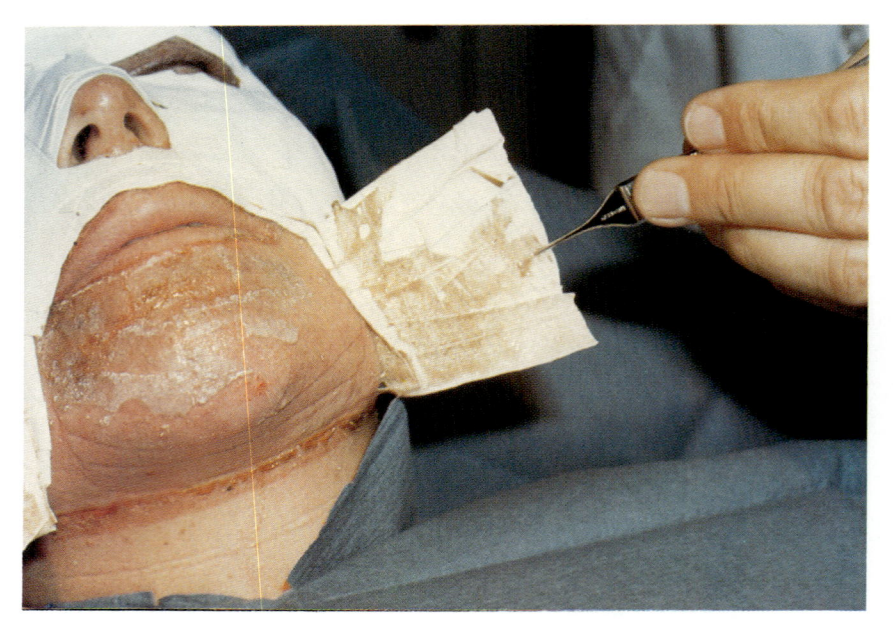

The tape mask is split in several places to facilitate removal. There is necrotic epithelial debris stuck to the underside of the tape.

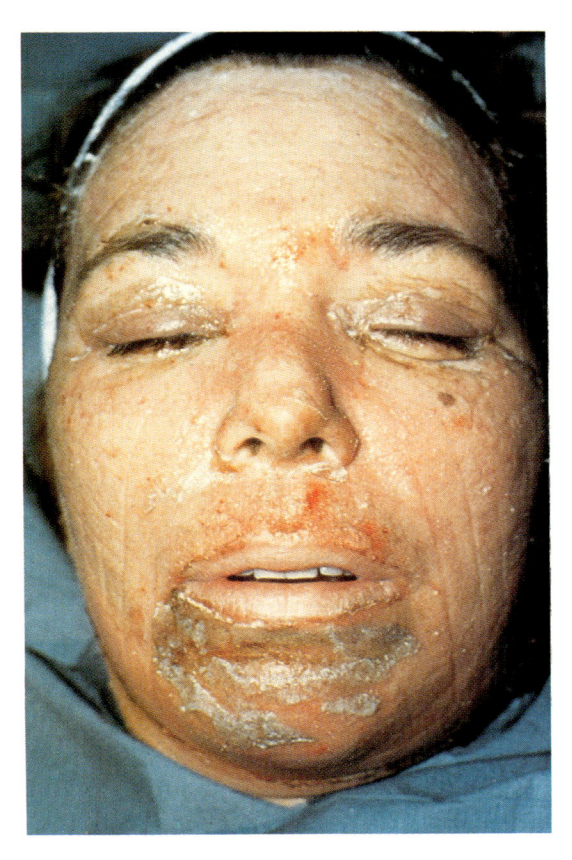

CHEMICAL PEELING (PHENOL AND TRICHLOROACETIC ACID) AND DERMABRASION

The tape mask has just been removed. The skin surface shows some necrotic debris still adherent in the area of the chin. Many areas of punctate hemorrhage and moderate edema are seen.

SURGICAL REJUVENATION OF THE FACE

After the mask has been completely removed, the skin is covered with thymol iodide powder, for its drying and bacteriostatic effects. A large cotton ball twisted around the end of an applicator stick can be used as a powder puff.

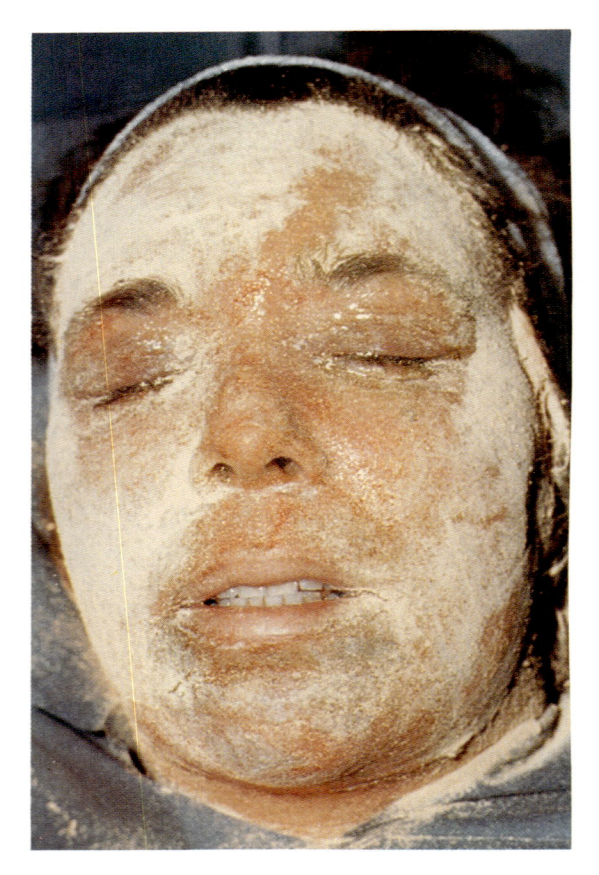

The face has been dusted with thymol iodide powder immediately after removal of the tape.

The powdered surface is left open and allowed to dry for 24 hours, while a thin, yellow-brown crust forms. Twenty-four hours after mask removal the face is covered, powder and all, with A & D ointment to soften and loosen the crusts. The face is washed with warm water and ointment is applied several times daily until the crust separates, usually 1 week after peeling.

After crust separation the skin appears erythematous, but the edema usually subsides rapidly. The patient is instructed to continue washing her face several times daily and to lubricate the skin between washings with a moisturizer. Pain is rare during this period, but itching can be a problem. Ice water compresses are useful in controlling this symptom, but rarely sedatives or topical steroids may be necessary.

The patient can begin to use cosmetics over the treated areas at the end of 2 weeks if healing is proceeding in a normal fashion. The erythematous color usually persists for 10 to 12 weeks, but in rare cases may last up to 6 months.

Since chemical peeling removes a significant amount of pigment from the basal layer of the epidermis, the process eventually lightens the skin and reduces natural protection against the sun. Patients who undergo peeling should be warned to avoid direct or reflected sunlight for extended periods until healing is complete. This precaution is especially important in the postoperative period when the skin remains erythematous and has not yet faded in color. Most cases of blotchy pigmentation following chemical peel arise in patients who have disregarded the advice to avoid exposure to the sun.

Specific recommendations with regard to the sun include the following:

1. Peeled skin will never tan normally, and precautions for lifetime use of sunscreens need to be followed.

2. Patients should avoid direct sunlight for 3 to 6 months, especially during the middle of the day. If they must be in the sun, they should wear a wide-brimmed hat and apply a maximum-protection sunscreen.

3. Reflected sunlight should be avoided. This is a particular problem when driving automobiles. Makeup bases with sunscreen and a sunscreen with a high sun protection factor must be worn at all times.

Regional Peeling

There are instances in which only an isolated area of the face needs to be treated, most commonly the upper lip alone or the entire peri-

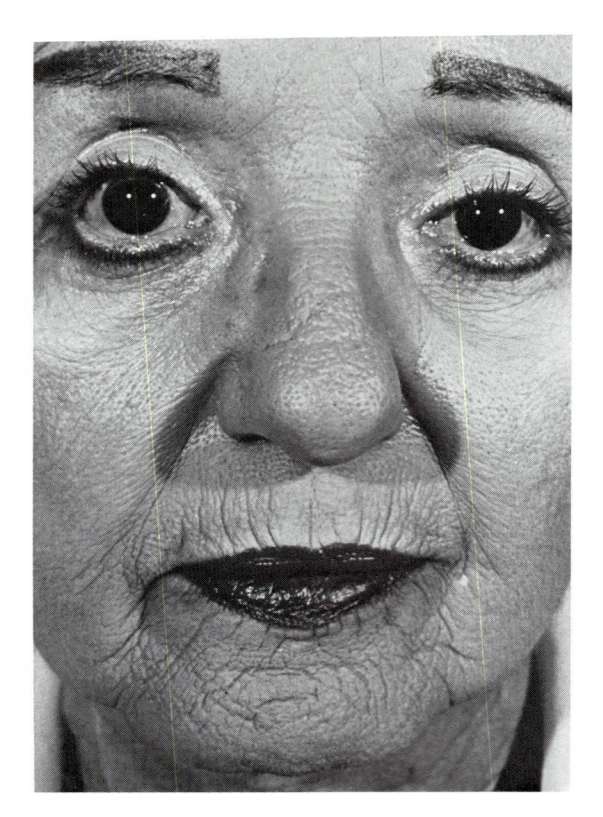

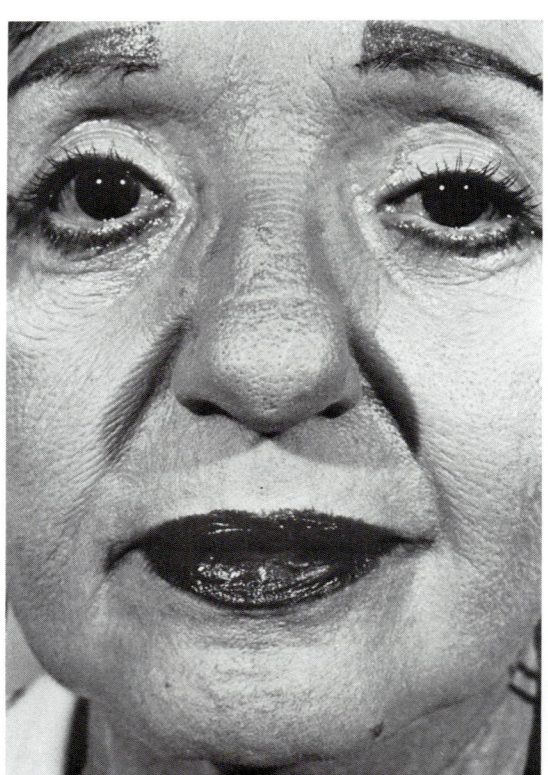

This 62-year-old woman has generalized wrinkling and sagging of the facial skin. The most severe wrinkling is in the perioral area. Her general complexion is fair and without freckles. The patient is shown in the photograph on the right 1 year after chemical peel of the perioral area only. No surgery has been performed.

CHEMICAL PEELING (PHENOL AND TRICHLOROACETIC ACID) AND DERMABRASION

oral region. The same formula as in full-face peeling is used in regional peeling, and care is taken to apply the mixture slightly onto the vermilion border and to include not only the nasolabial folds but an area extending 2 to 3 mm beyond it. If the peel stops at the nasolabial fold, it will merely accentuate the line rather than partially eliminate it.

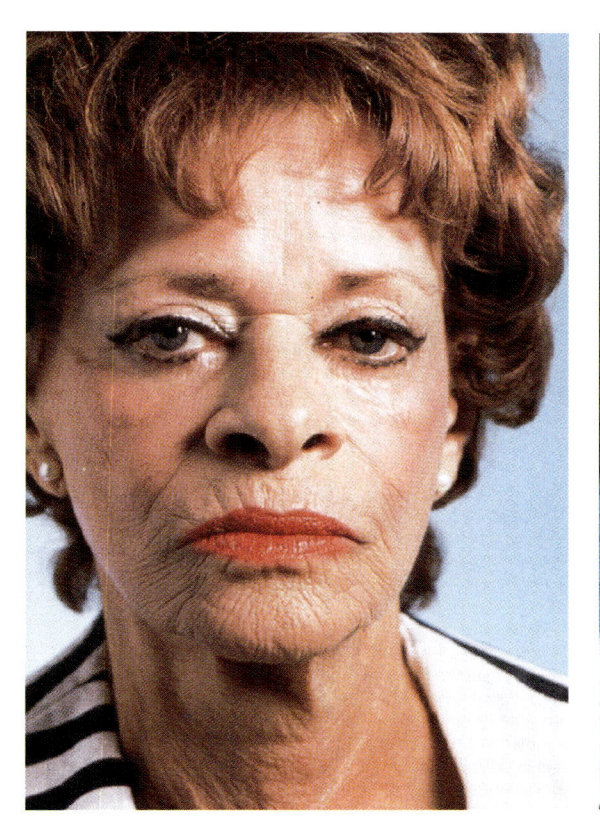

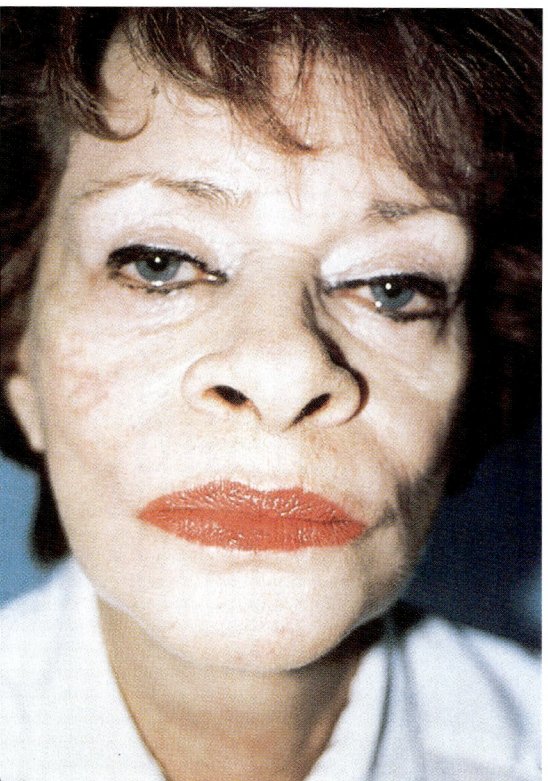

Preoperative appearance. Postoperative appearance following regional perioral peel performed with the use of petroleum jelly occlusive dressing.

SURGICAL REJUVENATION OF THE FACE

Regional peeling is an excellent treatment for the fine upper lip wrinkles and the lines radiating from the vermilion into which lipstick tends to run. Deep lines beneath the lower lip, especially those below the commissure of the mouth and paralleling the mentalis muscle, are perhaps the most difficult lines in the face to eliminate, and only modest improvement is seen in this region after peeling.

Regional peeling of the periorbital region and glabella can also be performed in properly selected patients, usually those of light complexion.

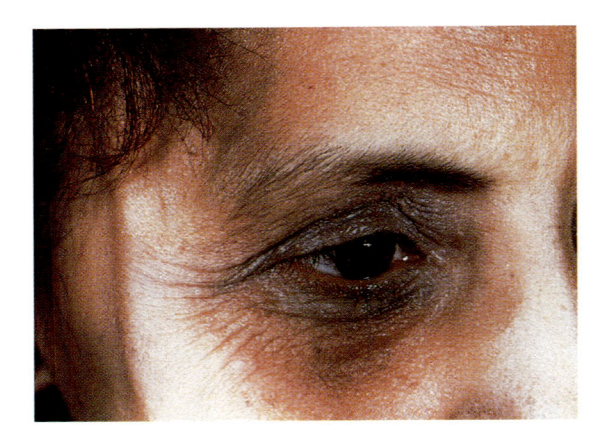

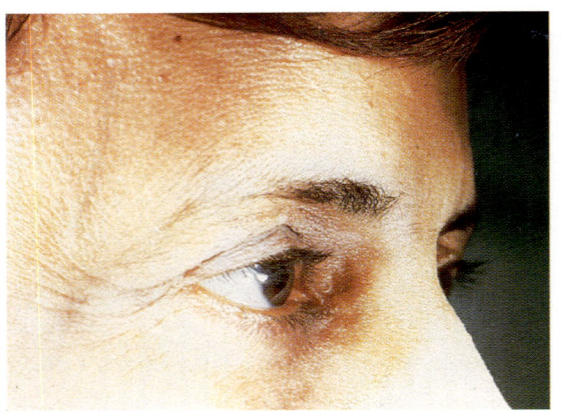

Prepeel appearance. Appearance following phenol peel to the periorbital region. Note the improvement not only in facial rhytides but also of the dark pigmentation noted before the peel in the lower eyelid.

Regional perioral peeling is commonly performed on an outpatient basis, often as an isolated procedure without sedation or monitoring. The use of regional blocks can prove useful in these situations.

Complications and Undesirable Results

We have found the complication rate from chemical peeling to be extremely low if we define *complications* as only those reactions that are unexpected and serious. On the other hand, there are some undesirable results that are so common that one could consider them to be natural consequences rather than complications.

Skin Depigmentation

Depigmentation of the skin after peeling is almost unavoidable except in the fairest of fair-skinned persons. In those whose skin is not homogeneously tanned but rather colored by a confluence of freckles and other sun-induced blotches, the bleaching effect is the most pronounced. Many people with red hair have this type of skin. We usually recommend that patients with this type of skin forego the treatment.

We always stop the peel at a point just under the jawline in order to hide the line of demarcation as much as possible. Some patients have little or no contour definition at the jawline, and these patients must be told that the line will be conspicuous. Often we apply the adhesive tape so that the last quarter-inch of treated skin is not covered. We do this in an attempt to have the last little edge of peeled skin not show the bleaching effect as profoundly, and thereby feather, or blend, the edge.

Milia

Another undesirable result of treatment, so common that it might be called a natural consequence, is the appearance of milia. These small, superficial, epidermal inclusion cysts may occur anytime during the first 6 or 8 weeks after treatment. They may be few and scattered, or they may be numerous and confluent. They may be present for only a few days, or they may persist for many weeks. In most instances frequent vigorous washing, even scrubbing later on, solves the problem. In those few cases of persistent cysts, it will be necessary to puncture and evacuate each one.

Erythema

Prolonged erythema following the peel can be defined as marked reddened inflammation that persists past the predicted 10 to 12 weeks. We have seen cases in which the skin was significantly red for 4 or 5 months. We have never seen the erythema persist permanently. We treat prolonged redness with topical steroids, but we are unconvinced of the efficacy of such treatment. Tincture of time along with reassurance and support seems to be the best therapys.

Sensitivity to Sunlight

Increased sensitivity to sunlight occurs after peeling. This may result from the reduced number of melanin-producing cells in the basal layer of the epidermis that is always seen after peeling. All patients are advised that the skin will never tan as it did before the procedure and that they should wear a protective sunscreen during exposure to the sun.

Infection

Infections following peeling have been rare in our experience. The few we have seen were bacterial and responded to conventional antibiotic therapy.

Scarring

Scarring has been the rarest but most catastrophic complication of peeling. We have seen scarring of the facial skin in only four cases, but have seen others in consultation. Most of the scars showed some degree of hypertrophy. The majority of the problems occurred around the mouth, some as a transverse band of hypertrophic scar tissue across the middle of the upper lip, others as a thick welt of scar tissue along the side of the chin. But they can occur anywhere. The worst we have seen were on the anterior surface of the neck. Scar contractures in this area were sometimes so extreme that extension of the head was limited, and contracture release was necessary. We never peel neck skin for this reason. If neck skin is peeled, the line of demarcation along the supraclavicular area is very conspicuous. We have used various

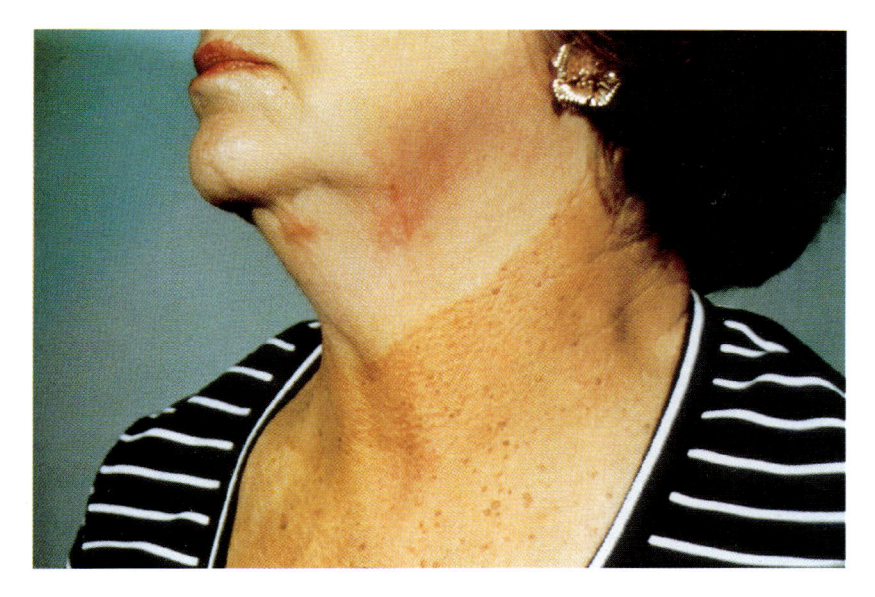

The importance of hiding the line of demarcation below the mandibular border is seen in this type of patient. When the peel is carried down to the neck, the distinction between peeled and unpeeled skin becomes obvious. Note also the scarring of the submental region following phenol peel of this area. Because of the lack of adnexal structures present within cervical skin, we avoid the application of phenol to this region.

SURGICAL REJUVENATION OF THE FACE

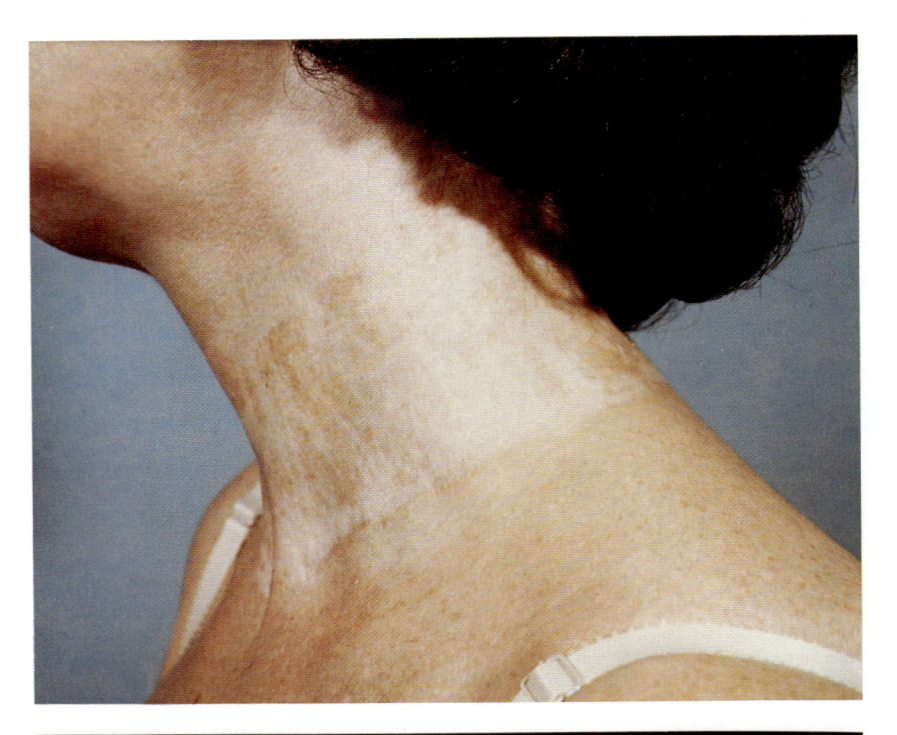

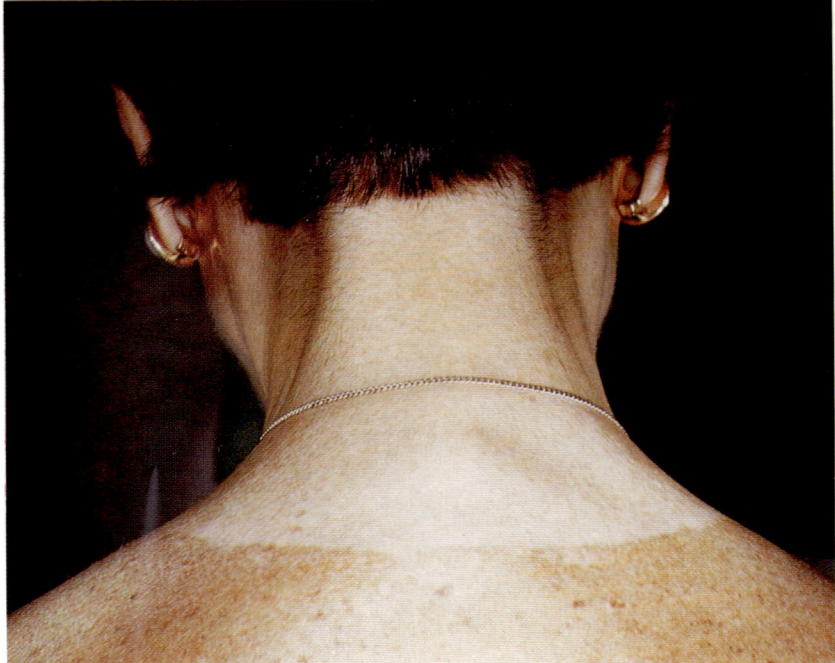

A full-face peel was carried to the obvious line of demarcation at the base of the neck. Note the uneven blotchiness of the neck often seen in peels of this area. Note the obvious line of demarcation between the treated area above and the untreated area below. This is predictable because of the deeply freckled and basically fair skin.

methods to treat hypertrophic scars, including steroids injected or applied topically, surgical excision, and x-ray therapy. Most small scars respond to treatment reasonably well, but only after a long and trying course for the patient and her physician. We have reached no conclusion as to the cause of these scars, other than that they may be due to secondary infections.

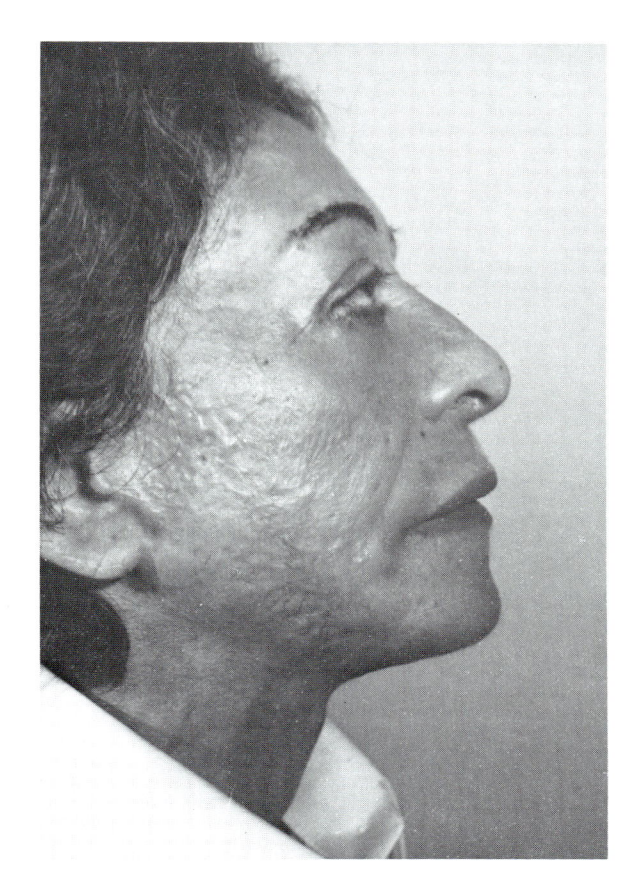

Hypertrophic scarring of the cheeks has occurred after a face peel was done by a nonprofessional.

SURGICAL REJUVENATION OF THE FACE

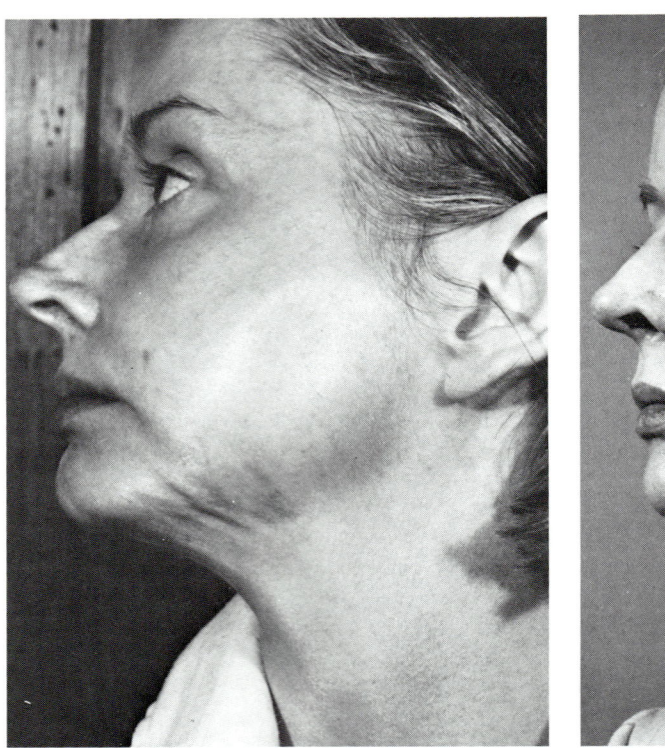

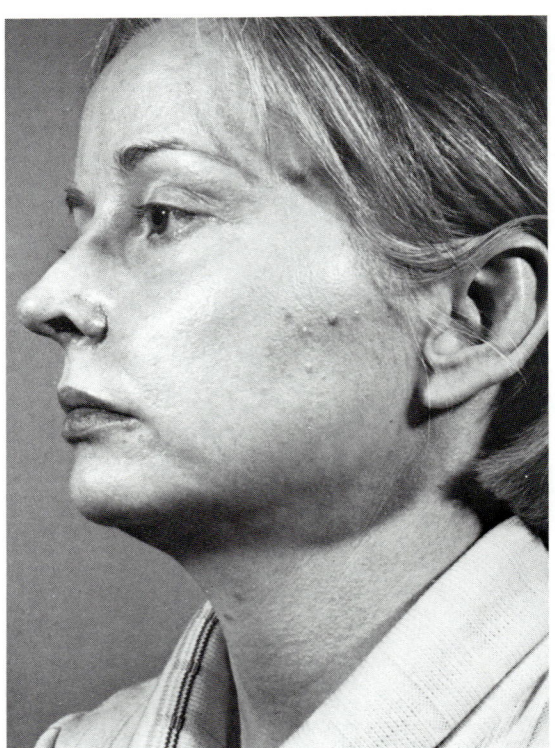

Hypertrophic scarring in the submental area has occurred after a full-face peel; the cause is unknown. The patient is shown 6 years after peeling. Marked improvement is seen in the areas of scar hypertrophy. Treatment consisted of topical steroids given over a period of several months during the first year.

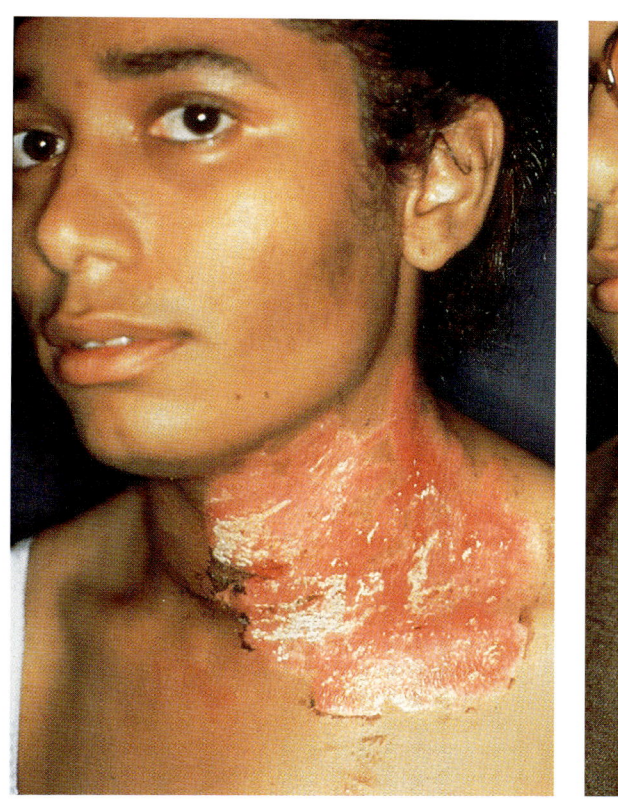

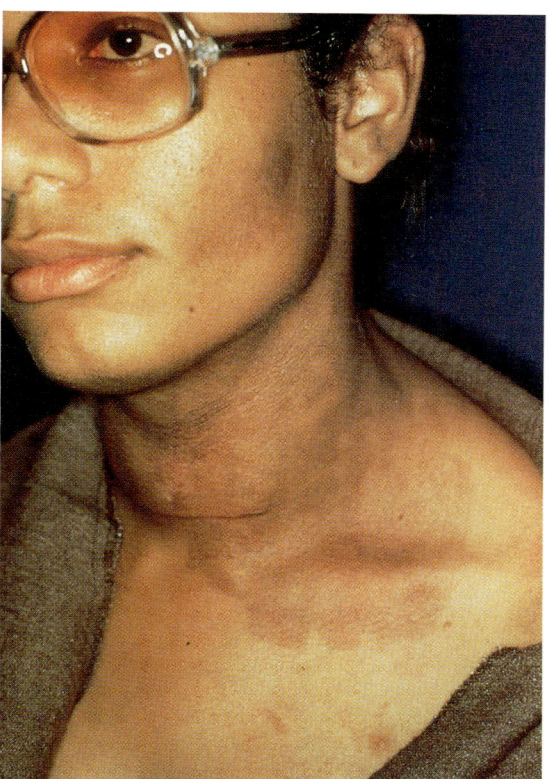

CHEMICAL PEELING (PHENOL AND TRICHLOROACETIC ACID) AND DERMABRASION

This patient was seen following an accidental spill of phenol onto cervical skin in a workplace accident. The patient eventually went on to heal from this chemical injury though she developed significant hyperpigmentation of the cervical skin.

SURGICAL REJUVENATION OF THE FACE

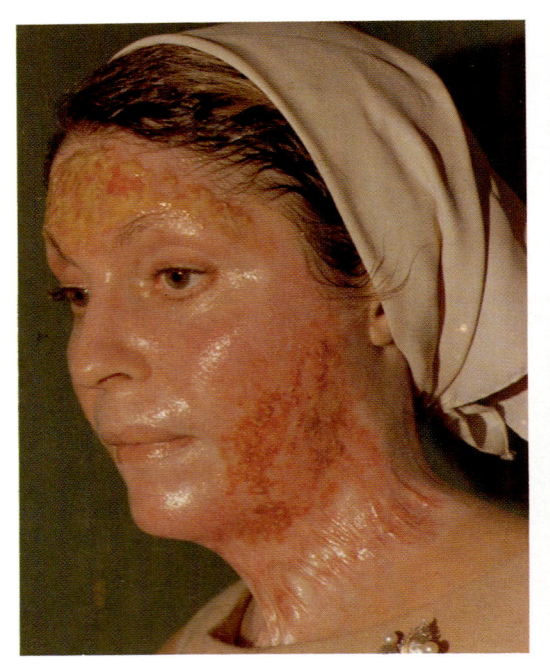

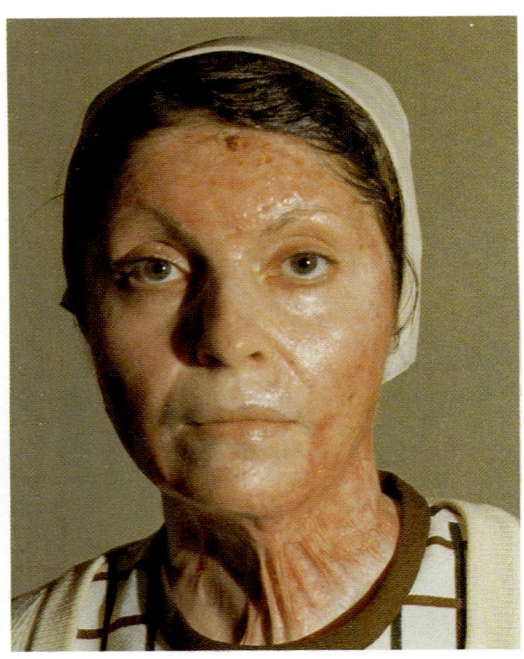

This 38-year-old woman had a chemical peel of the face and neck performed in a lay clinic. Deep second-degree and scattered third-degree burns resulted. The cause is unknown. Contractions are seen developing in the neck. This photograph was taken about 4 weeks after the peel was performed. After 7 weeks the burn scar contractures are well developed and the areas of deep second-degree and scattered third-degree burns are reepithelializing. The patient is shown 1 year after her peel and after surgical release of the scar contractures of the neck with split skin grafts.

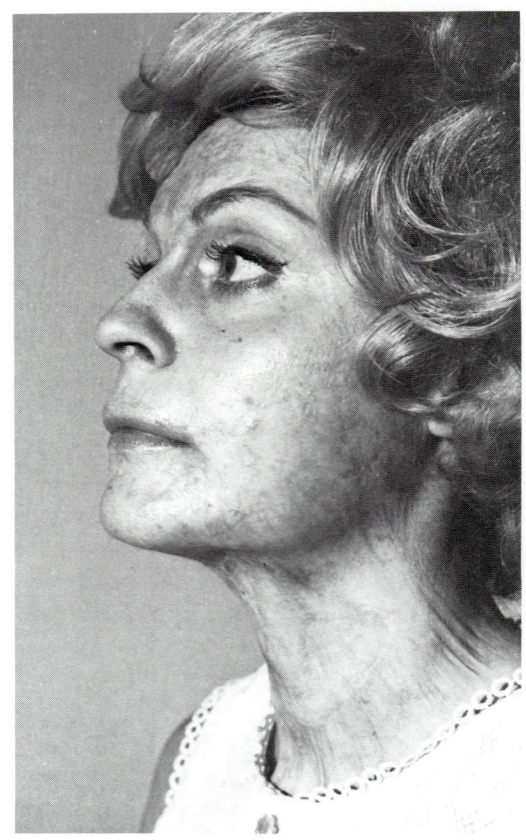

Ectropion of the Lower Eyelid

Ectropion of the lower eyelid has been seen in patients who have had previous blepharoplasty. We hesitate to perform a full-face peel on a patient who has had a lower blepharoplasty, particularly when the operation was done by another surgeon. We never know just how much lid skin has been removed when someone else has done it. Unrecognized incipient senile ectropion contributes to the danger. Only one of our patients has required full-thickness skin grafting to correct ectropion.

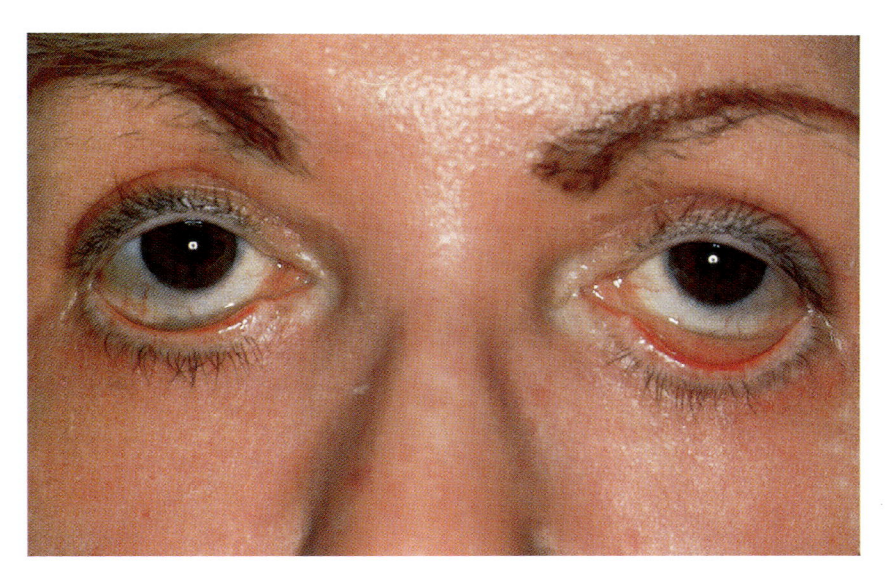

This patient is seen following a full-face phenol peel performed in another office that resulted in bilateral ectropions. Of note, this patient had a blepharoplasty before the phenol peel. It is our opinion that the combination of lower eyelid laxity and a previous blepharoplasty, in conjunction with a deep phenol peel, resulted in this unfortunate postpeel complication.

Changes of Preexisting Skin Conditions

Frequently, preexisting skin conditions show changes after peeling. These changes should be pointed out to the patient before treatment. If there is any change in the appearance of a nevus, and sometimes there is none after a peel, it is that it becomes darker, not only in contrast to the now lighter skin but also in actuality. Hyperkeratoses are completely and cleanly removed from the skin by the peeling process; in fact, on rare occasions we have used the presence of recurrent multiple hyperkeratoses as the reason for doing the procedure. This probably reduces, rather than increases, the likelihood of treated skin developing malignancies. Those patients who have multiple spider telangiectasias should be told that the process will make them more visible. On many occasions, after the erythema has faded, we have then removed each telangiectatic area with the electric cautery. We have many requests from patients who want to reduce the size of their pores. Peeling usually leaves the pores unchanged, or, if there is any effect, makes them appear somewhat larger.

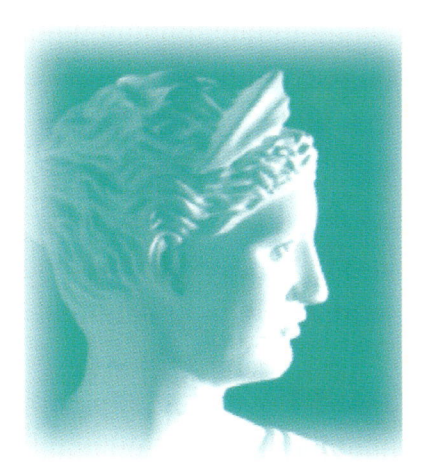

B

TRICHLOROACETIC ACID PEELS

Trichloroacetic acid has been used extensively for many years, primarily by dermatologists. Unlike phenol, which produces an all-or-none response, the concentration of TCA can be varied according to the degree of peeling desired. A 10% to 30% solution is used for light peeling, a 35% to 40% solution for intermediate peeling, and a 50% to 60% solution for deep peeling. There is reported to be greater safety with TCA, as its potential for systemic toxicity is significantly less than that of phenol.

In our opinion, there are two advantages to TCA. First, since the concentration of the peeling solution can be varied, it is possible to produce a spectrum of peeling response—from a light peel, analogous to a sunburn, to a deep peel, comparable to what is obtained using phenol. This allows the clinician to taper the results to the individual patient's needs and wishes. Also, since there is greater ability to control the depth of the peel, light- to medium-depth TCA is perhaps more suitable to the peeling of the neck, thorax, and extremities compared with phenol, which is noted to have a tendency to produce hypertrophic scarring in areas where adnexal structures are sparse.

The second difference between TCA and phenol is that TCA appears to have a lesser effect on melanocyte metabolism, producing less of the characteristic bleaching of facial skin that is seen following phenol use. For this reason TCA is perhaps more applicable in patients with dark-complected skin, as well as being perhaps better suited for regional peeling.

Trichloroacetic acid peels have their limitations. Histologic studies have shown that even with high concentrations of TCA, with and without taping, a deep TCA peel has approximately half the extent of penetration into the dermis and half the amount of neocollagen formation within the grenz zone compared with the penetration seen with phenol. In these studies, 25% TCA barely penetrated beyond the epidermis. Because of this lack of penetration and the subsequent neocollagen formation, even deep TCA peels do not seem to have the profound effect on coarse facial wrinkles that is obtained following phenol peels. This is especially true in the treatment of coarse perioral wrinkles. In general, patients presenting with coarse rhytides, severely sun-damaged skin, and significant pigmentary problems are, in our opinion, more efficaciously treated with phenol. Again, the specific needs of the patient must be tailored to the type of peel performed.

Pretreatment Routine

In all patients undergoing TCA peels, we treat their skin with tretinoin (Retin-A), as well as 4% hydroquinone, for 4 to 6 weeks before treatment. Pretreatment with retinoic acid produces significant epidermal effects, decreasing the thickness of the stratum corneum, thereby increasing the permeability of the epidermis to chemical treatment. Patients who have been pretreated with tretinoin show a greater and more uniform response following application of the peeling agent. They also appear to heal more quickly. The use of hydroquinone, which suppresses melanocyte activity, helps in preventing the tendency toward postpeel pigmentation that can occur following epidermal injury from peeling agents. Patients who show difficulty in tolerating tretinoin are treated with glycolic acid facial creams for 4 to 6 weeks before peeling. The results are comparable.

Judging the Depth of the Peel

Trichloroacetic acid, unlike phenol, does not produce an all-or-none response. Low concentrations of TCA produce a light peel, whereas higher concentrations produce a deeper peel. Other methods of increasing TCA penetration include: (1) applying more coats of the peeling solution, (2) pretreating the skin with a keratolytic agent such as Jesner's solution (salicylic acid, lactic acid, and resorcinol), and (3) mechanically abrading the skin with a gauze pad that is simultaneously used to apply the TCA solution.

The depth of the peel is judged by: (1) the appearance of the skin after the peel solution is applied, (2) the turgor of the skin as judged by light palpation, and (3) the time the skin requires to return to its normal color following TCA application.

When TCA is applied in very light concentrations, it produces an erythematous appearance. As the concentration of the peel solution increases, corresponding to a deeper penetration of the peel solution, the skin takes on a white frosting. With light peeling solutions, this frosting will be sparse and irregular, and only a light, pinkish-white frosting is seen. With an increase in the concentration of the peeling solution, the frosting tends to become uniform, and of a denser white color. The greater the degree of frosting, the greater the penetration of the peeling solution into the facial skin. If the peeling solution penetrates into the deep dermis or subcutaneous layer, rather than a dense white, the peeled skin appears gray-white, which is an indication of late healing and possible hypertrophic scarring.

SURGICAL REJUVENATION OF THE FACE

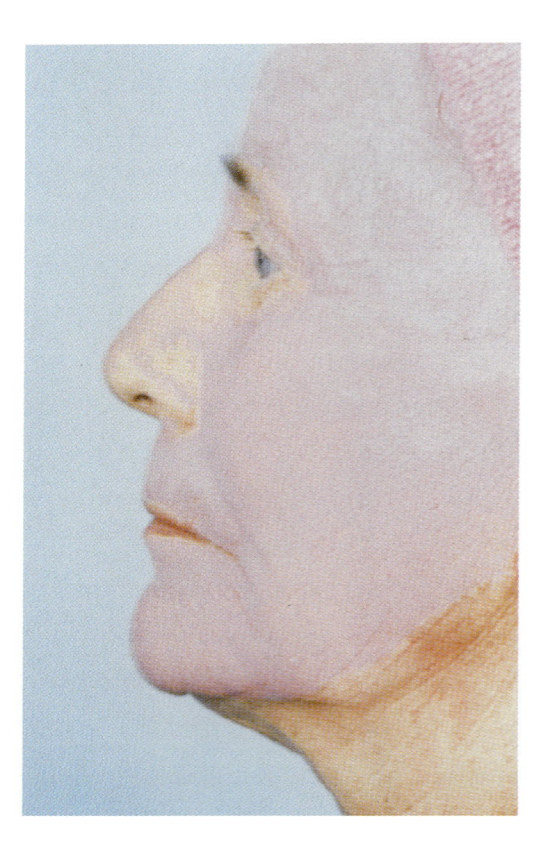

Patient is seen immediately following a 30% TCA peel. Note the pinkish-white frosting that is evident following an intermediate-depth TCA peel.

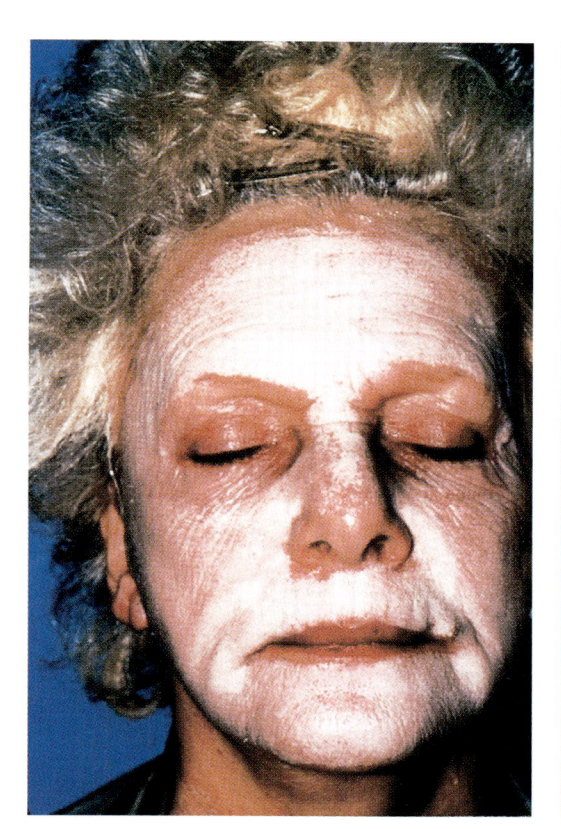

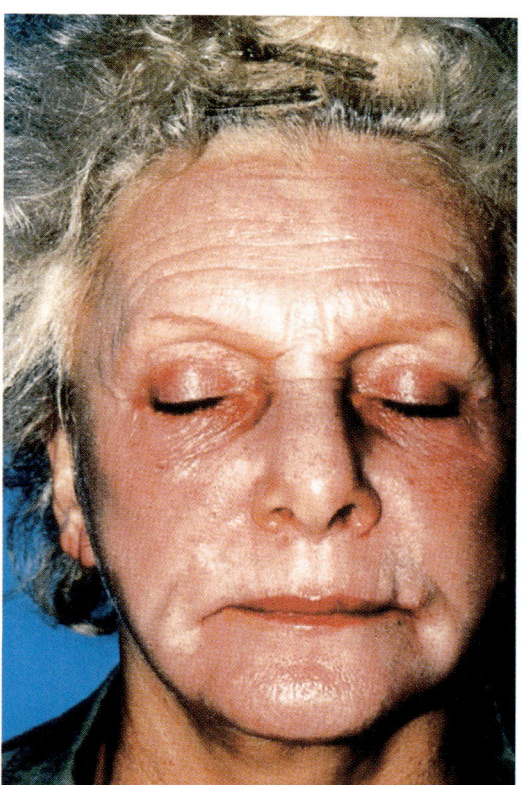

CHEMICAL PEELING (PHENOL AND TRICHLOROACETIC ACID) AND DERMABRASION

Patient is seen following heavy application of 35% TCA. Note the dense white frosting associated with deeper penetration of TCA. Patient is seen 1 hour following a 35% TCA peel. Note that the frosting has now faded and at this point the skin appears to be erythematous, similar to the appearance of a sunburn.

As the peel solution penetrates facial skin, the skin obtains a different turgor or feel by palpation. Unpeeled skin is quite soft and mobile to palpation. In lighter peels, the skin turgor increases and the smooth, sliding facial skin becomes palpably indurated. Turgor and induration increase with the concentration of TCA used and the depth of penetration of the peeling solution. As one gains experience with TCA peeling, the palpation of peeled skin and the smoothness or induration that is present following the peel serve as a useful guide to the peel's end point.

Return of color is an important factor, though it is a bit after the fact since it can be assessed only following completion of the peel. Superficial peels, which typically produce a pinkish-white frosting, will usually fade to an erythema within a 15-minute period. Intermediate peels, associated with a uniform white frosting, can take up to 30 minutes before the frosting resolves and the skin appears red. A deep peel is associated with dense, white frosting and can take up to 60 minutes to resolve. Peels that perhaps have penetrated to the deep dermis or subcutaneous layer are associated with a gray-frosted appearance and exhibit an incomplete return of color, even after a full hour has elapsed following the peel.

Technique—Light Peeling

The patient washes her face thoroughly before undergoing a chemical peel followed by degreasing the skin with either acetone or ether. Light peeling is performed with the use of a 20% to 30% TCA solution applied regionally, as with our phenol peels. We use gauze pads to apply the TCA solution uniformly. The peeling solution is usually left in place for 30 to 120 seconds, depending on the amount of frosting desired. Following this, the peel is diluted by washing the skin thoroughly with ice water. This alleviates the burning sensation that the patient experiences during the active process of peeling. At the end of the procedure the face is coated generously with 1% hydrocortisone ointment or similar petroleum-based ointment (e.g., A & D).

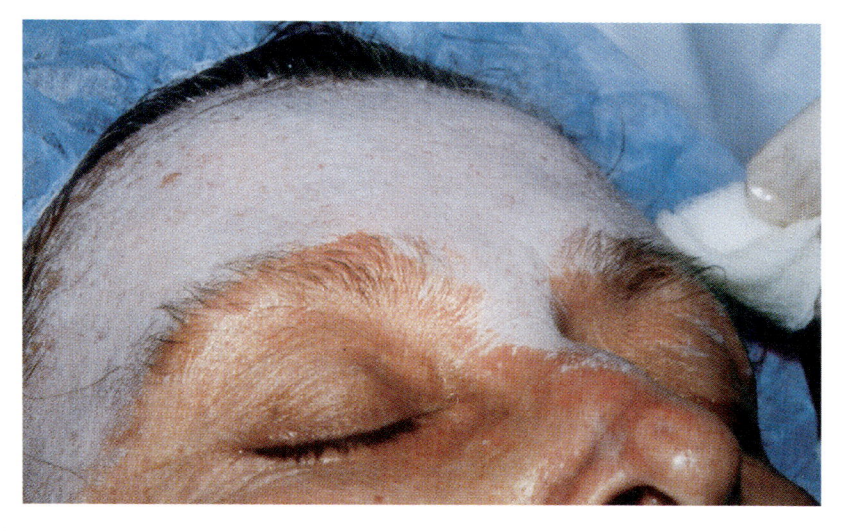

Trichloroacetic acid is applied in a regional fashion that is similar to how we perform phenol peels. We use a gauze sponge to apply the solution and gently abrade the peeling agent into facial skin. As the desired depth of peeling is obtained, as noted by frosting and induration of the tissues, the peel is then diluted with water, which alleviates the burning sensation and minimizes patient discomfort.

Postpeel Care

In patients undergoing very light peeling (to the erythema stage only), there is little associated morbidity and these patients can return to full activity with the use of a light covering makeup. In patients in whom greater frosting has been obtained, it is common to experience initial erythema of the skin, followed within 48 hours by superficial desquamation, producing a brown appearance to the keratocoagulated epithelium. We prefer not to use covering makeup during this period of desquamation, but rather to treat the skin with some sort of facial moisturizer or with a hydrocortisone-based ointment (1% Hytone). During this period, patients will commonly have to limit their social activities. In most patients undergoing peels of this depth, the desquamation usually peaks within 72 hours. This is followed by peeling of the desquamated skin for a period of 4 to 7 days as healing progresses. It is important to instruct patients not to pick at the peeling skin during this period since this can produce a mottled appearance. Patients are instructed to wash their face several times daily, and then to reapply the ointment, which serves to mechanically remove the desquamating epithelium in a gentler, more uniform fashion.

A full return to active social life without covering makeup is usually possible in 5 to 7 days following the peel. Covering makeup can be applied after most of the peeling has subsided.

Once the patient stops peeling, usually within a week to 10 days following the peel, we recommend that she restart nightly application of both tretinoin and hydroquinone. We impress upon the patient the importance of wearing sunscreens on a daily basis to prevent postpeel hyperpigmentation.

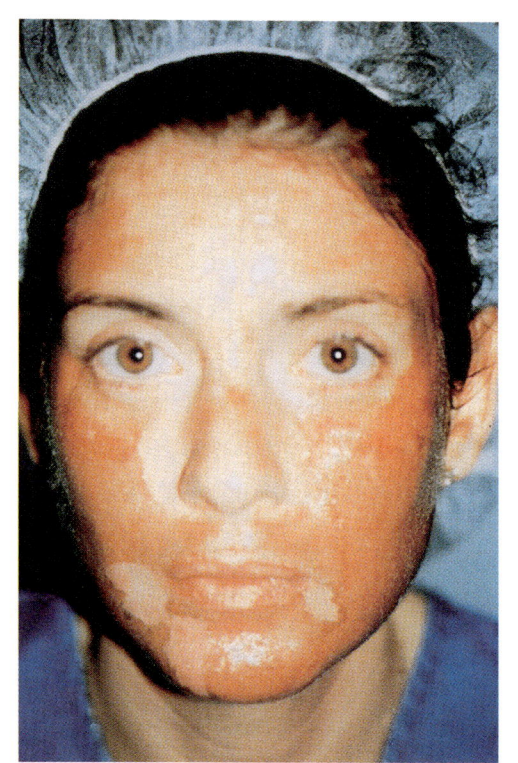

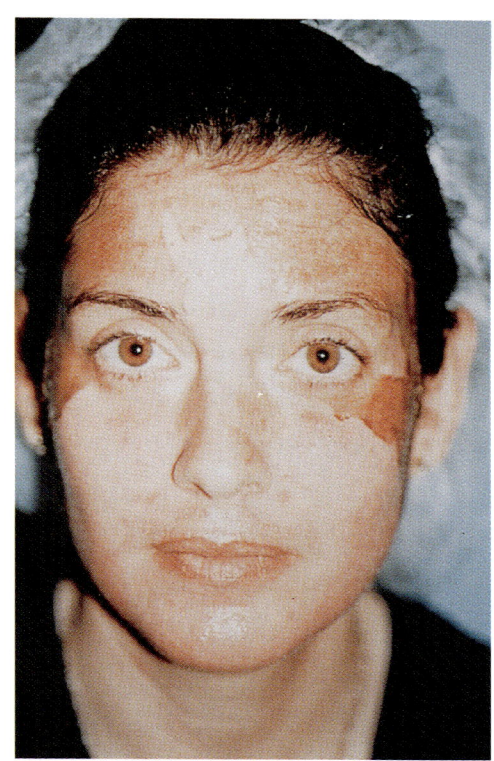

CHEMICAL PEELING (PHENOL AND TRICHLOROACETIC ACID) AND DERMABRASION

Patient is seen 72 hours following a 35% TCA peel. At this point, the desquamation appears most severe and the skin appears to be densely brown in appearance. Patient seen 4 days following a 35% TCA peel. At this point much of the desquamated skin has peeled, revealing newly healed, fresh-appearing skin.

Intermediate-Depth Peeling

Patients with multiple, coarse facial rhytides will show little improvement after light TCA peeling. In these more difficult clinical situations, deeper peeling with higher concentrations of TCA should be considered.

Intermediate to deep peeling is done with 35% to 50% TCA. These patients are treated as above with tretinoin and 4% hydroquinone, and prepared by degreasing the skin with acetone or ether. The peel solution is then applied lightly in a uniform fashion. When using higher concentrations of TCA, the frosting usually occurs quickly and is much denser than that obtained with light peeling. For this reason, one must be careful as to how many coats are reapplied to the same region as the peeling procedure is performed. For most of our intermediate peels, we prefer a 35% TCA solution. This seems to produce uniform penetration and consistent results, with a low probability of deep dermal penetration. Peeling with 50% TCA appears to leave less margin for error. Multiple applications of 50% TCA to the same area are an invitation to deep penetration followed by healing with hypertrophic scarring.

As with all our peels, we prefer to peel in a regional fashion, concentrating on the forehead, followed by each cheek, and finishing in the perioral region. Having an assistant fan the patient during TCA application helps diminish pain during the procedure, and patients appear to be able to tolerate regional application better than if the entire face is peeled at one time. Neutralizing each region with ice water after the desired frosting has been obtained quickly alleviates patient discomfort. A petroleum-based ointment, our preference being 1% hydrocortisone, is then applied to the facial skin.

The key to safety in intermediate depth peeling is not just in the concentration of the TCA which is used, but also in judging the depth of penetration as the peeling procedure proceeds. We would stress that there is a good deal of variability in terms of frosting response from patient to patient. Specifically, patients who are well prepared with retinoic acid tend to have a more rapid response to TCA application as compared to those patients who have used Retin-A sporadically. Also,

CHEMICAL PEELING (PHENOL AND TRICHLOROACETIC ACID) AND DERMABRASION

patients with thin, dry skin tend to respond more rapidly in terms of obtaining a deeper penetration of the peeling agent, as compared to patients with thick, oily skin. Finally, we would stress that there is a lag period between the time the peeling solution is applied to the skin, and the time when the maximum degree of frosting is obtained. This lag period will vary between *30 and 60 seconds*, and in performing intermediate to deep peels, it is important that the surgeon be patient in judging the maximum degree of frosting obtained prior to performing an additional application of the peeling solution.

Postpeel recovery is prolonged following deeper peeling. These patients have a significant amount of desquamation that is commonly followed by erythema. They are initially instructed to wash their face at least four times a day with water followed by ointment application. Reepithelization usually occurs within 4 to 7 days, though the skin commonly remains erythematous for several days and up to a few weeks in individual patients. In general, the deeper the peel, the more intense the desquamation and the more prolonged the postpeel erythema. Once healing is complete, reapplication of daily tretinoin and hydroquinone is useful in preventing postpeel hyperpigmentation. If a repeat peel is needed, we prefer to wait 2 to 3 months following the original procedure.

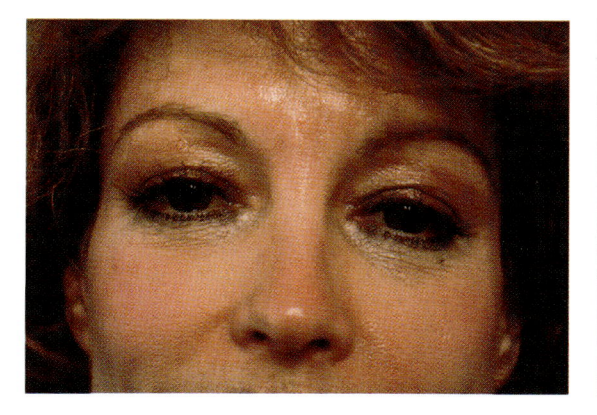

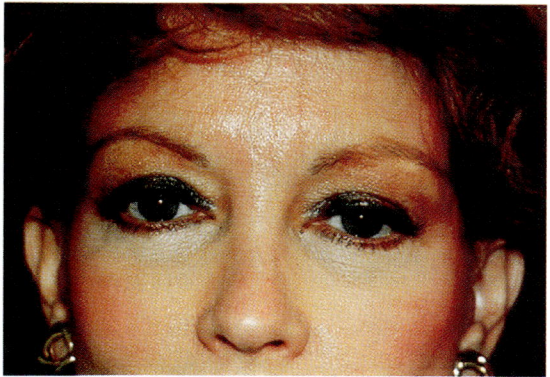

Prepeel appearance. Patient seen 5 months following a 35% TCA peel. Note the improvement in her fine facial wrinkles, most marked in the periorbital region.

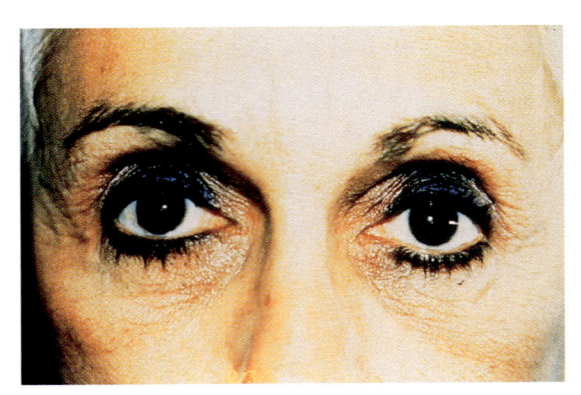

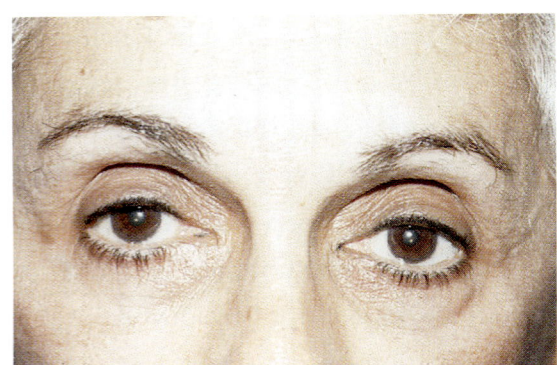

SURGICAL REJUVENATION
OF THE FACE

Prepeel appearance. Following a 35% TCA peel, note the improvement present in the periorbital rhytides and crow's feet in this patient.

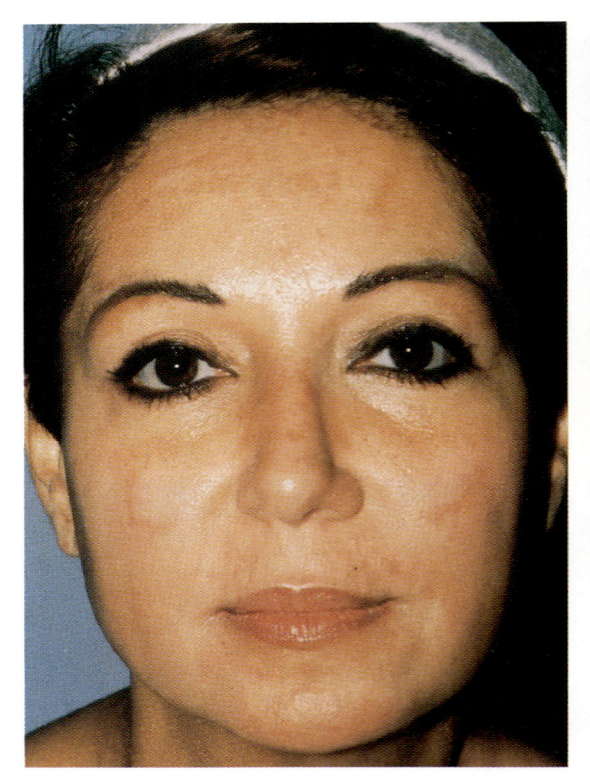

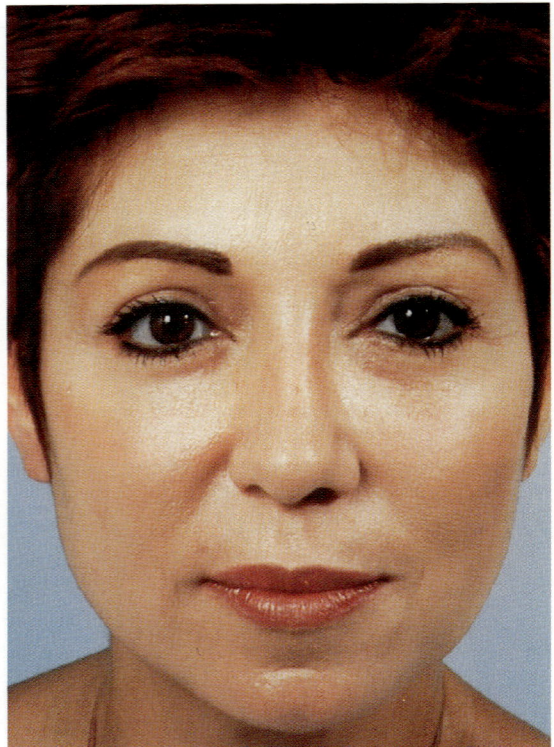

Prepeel appearance. Note the presence of blotchy facial pigmentation. Following a 35% TCA peel, note the evening of the facial pigmentation.

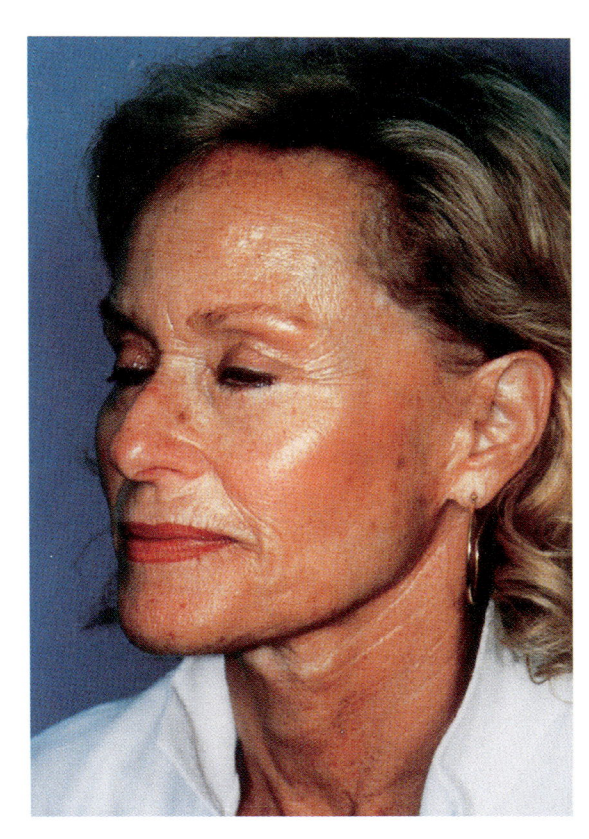

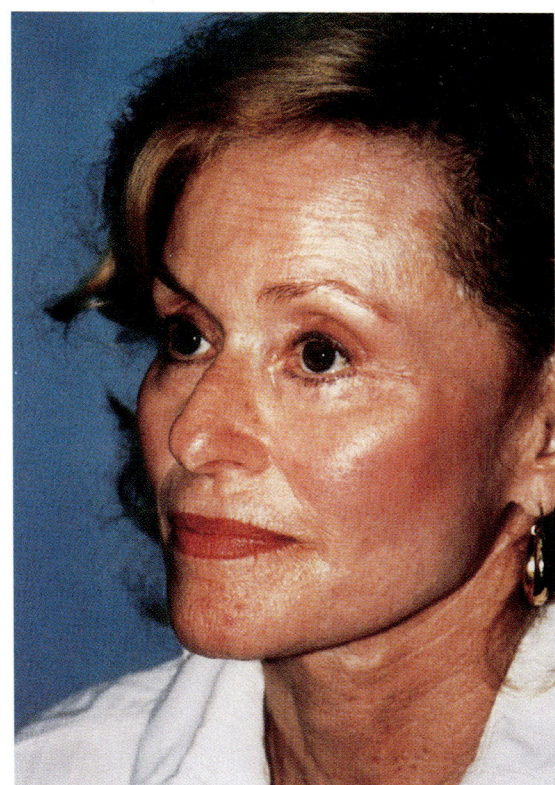

CHEMICAL PEELING (PHENOL AND TRICHLOROACETIC ACID) AND DERMABRASION

Prepeel appearance. Note the presence of discoloration of facial skin secondary to actinic exposure, as well as fine facial rhytides. Appearance following two 35% TCA peels. These peels were separated by a 3-month interval.

SURGICAL REJUVENATION OF THE FACE

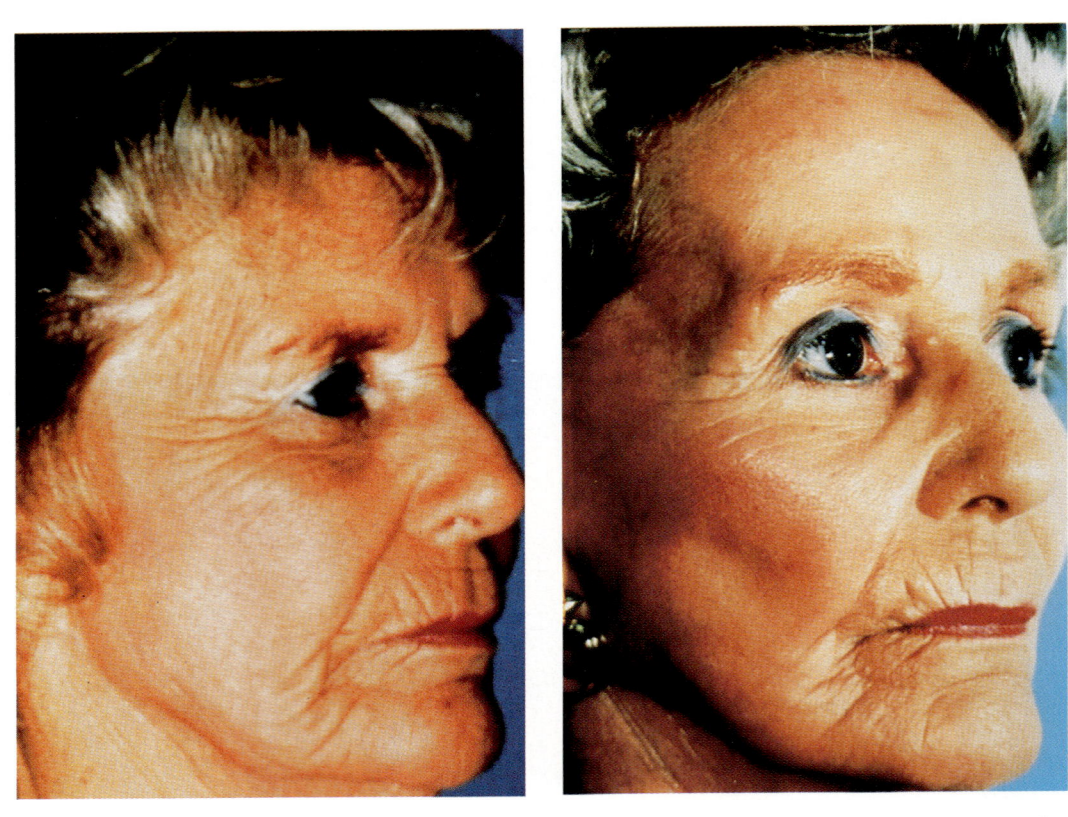

This patient is seen before undergoing a secondary face-lift. The patient's appearance following rhytidectomy and a subsequent 35% TCA peel. Note that there has been little improvement in her perioral rhytides.

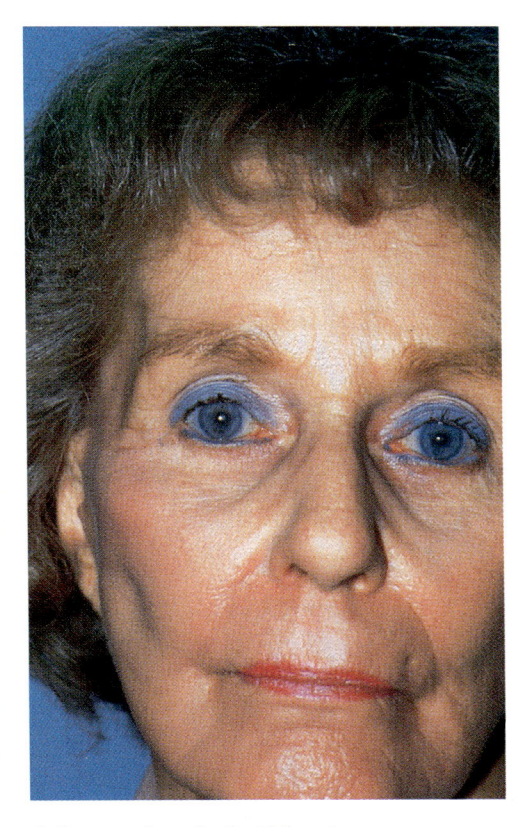

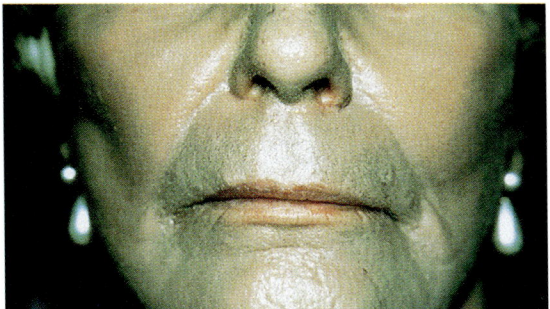

CHEMICAL PEELING (PHENOL AND TRICHLOROACETIC ACID) AND DERMABRASION

The patient then underwent phenol peeling of the perioral rhytides in conjunction with a second 35% TCA peel to the rest of the face. The final result following combination perioral phenol application in conjunction with facial TCA peeling. It must be emphasized that phenol and TCA peeling are not exclusive of each other but rather can be used in combination to improve the overall result for the patient.

■ Complications

We have noted few problems associated with TCA peeling. We advise the surgeon who is learning this technique to begin performing TCA peels with 20% to 25% solutions, and then to gradually increase the concentrations as the surgeon gains more experience. In more than one-thousand TCA peels performed in our practice, we have not seen hypertrophic scarring in any of our patients. We should note here that we rarely perform TCA peels with concentrations greater than 40% and that this concentration appears to be safe, especially if the solution is diluted with ice water once the desired frosting has been obtained. We caution physicians against using TCA in 50% solutions, since the margin for safety appears to be less. We have seen several patients present to our office following TCA peels with the development of hypertrophic scarring, presumably the result of high concentrations.

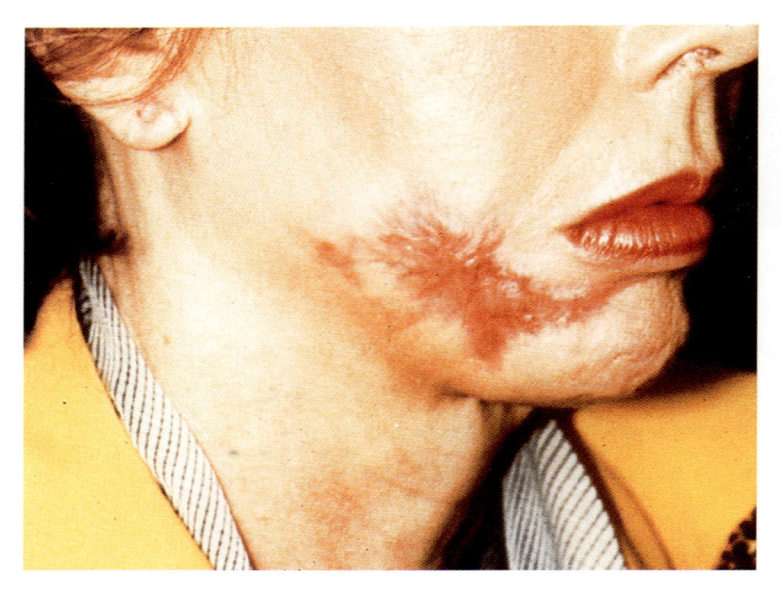

This patient is seen following a 50% TCA peel performed in an outlying office. The procedure was associated with the development of a hypertrophic perioral scar. We emphasize that 50% TCA has less margin of safety than 35% TCA solutions and that deep penetration can result in postpeel hypertrophic scarring.

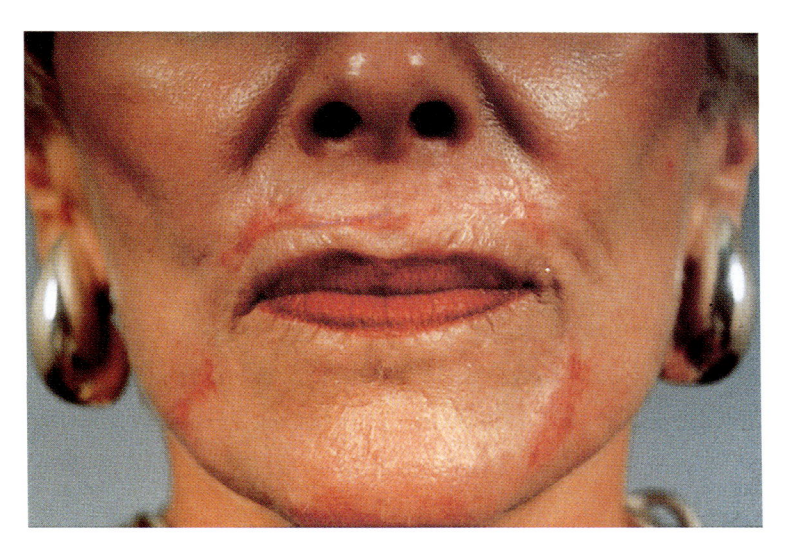

CHEMICAL PEELING (PHENOL AND TRICHLOROACETIC ACID) AND DERMABRASION

A patient seen following a 50% TCA peel performed in another office. Note the hypertrophic scarring present in the perioral region as well as the continued presence of perioral rhytides despite the deep penetration of the TCA. We have consistently been disappointed with an improvement in coarse perioral rhytides with TCA peeling and favor phenol peeling or dermabrasion to treat this difficult problem.

The most common problem we have seen with TCA peeling is postpeel hyperpigmentation. It is essential that the skin of patients undergoing TCA peeling, especially if they are of olive skin complexion, is adequately pretreated with both retinoic acid and hydroquinone to suppress melanocyte activity. Once the healing from the peel has been completed, it is again extremely important to restart these topical agents to prevent blotchy postpeel hyperpigmentation. In patients with dark complexions who are undergoing TCA peeling, we commonly perform light peeling early on and then gradually increase the concentration of the peeling agents during successive peels. Proper pre-peel preparation along with judging the patient's response to light peeling agents has proved to be very helpful in decreasing incidents of postpeel hyperpigmentation. Similarly, the patient must be told emphatically to avoid direct and reflected sunlight as well as to use covering cosmetics and sunscreens with high protection factors to prevent postpeel hyperpigmentation.

Trichloroacetic Acid vs. Phenol

The major advantage in using TCA is its versatility. It allows the clinician to individualize the depth of peeling for a particular patient's needs. While light peeling tends to be a slow road to improvement, there is little associated morbidity with this procedure and we have never seen any scarring with 20% TCA. As one moves into the deeper peels, the advantages of deep TCA peel vs. phenol need to be weighed.

The greatest advantage of TCA over phenol is the decreased tendency for bleaching of facial skin. This would make us favor TCA use in patients who are dark-complected in whom the line of demarcation between treated and untreated skin will be quite obvious post peel. Similar considerations are warranted in regional peeling of the perioral, periorbital, or glabellar regions.

In our opinion, the big disadvantage with the use of deep TCA peels is the less predictable improvement of coarse facial rhytides. Specifically, we have been disappointed with the use of TCA to treat perioral rhytides. In general, phenol is much more effective in patients with coarse facial wrinkling and significant perioral rhytides. Similarly, in patients who have severe facial hyperpigmentation localized to the dermis, we have found the uniform lightening that is obtained with phenol peeling to produce more consistent results.

Summary

In treating the patient with photoaged skin, a complete armamentarium of peeling techniques, using both phenol and TCA, allows the physician to treat a variety of difficult problems successfully and consistently. Patient evaluation and selection given the specific indications of each technique are key to a successful outcome. It is important to realize that phenol and TCA peeling are not exclusive of each other, but may be combined to improve the overall result. With experience and attention to technical detail, the physician can tailor these procedures to obtain consistent results according to the needs and desires of the patient.

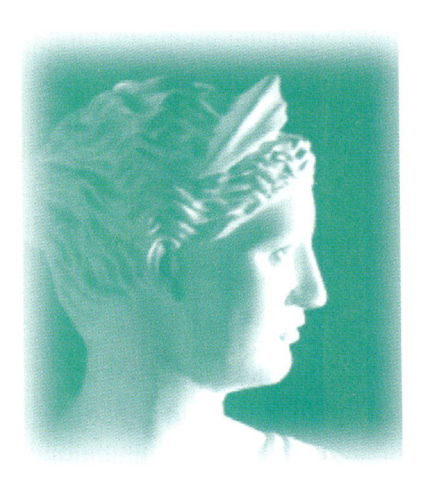

Dermabrasion

Dermabrasion is a procedure that uses abrasives to remove the epidermis and superficial dermis. The result is a smoothing of contour irregularities. It is most commonly employed in facial rejuvenation to correct facial wrinkling, specifically wrinkling in the perioral region.

Dermabrasion in the treatment of perioral rhytides has advantages over the use of phenol. Dermabrasion is a mechanical process, so the depth of treatment is more controllable and presumably lighter than phenol chemical peeling, producing faster healing and less discomfort. We know that the period of erythema following abrasion is shorter than that usually seen following phenol. For the dark-complected patient, the bleaching effect of dermabrasion is less and the contrast in color between treated and untreated skin is therefore minimized.

■ Indications

Dermabrasion is most commonly used in our practice in the treatment of perioral rhytides. While not as efficacious in the correction of wrinkling as phenol, dermabrasion usually produces significant improvement without the bleaching of perioral pigment commonly seen with phenol peels. We have found dermabrasion to be quite predictable in removing most of the rhytides present within the upper lip and reasonably effective in treating rhytides along the lower lip and chin. In patients with extremely coarse perioral rhytides, phenol is a better choice if the patient is of light complexion.

Dermabrasion is more effective than phenol peeling in the treatment of acne scarring. While patients are usually improved following a single treatment, most patients will require a second or even a third session to optimize their improvement. Despite our best efforts, most patients will retain perceptible acne scars following treatment and this eventuality must be explained to the patient preoperatively.

■ Technique

Dermabrasion is usually performed with a motor-driven instrument attached to either wire brushes, cylinders of sandpaper, or stainless steel burrs. We prefer to use a relatively low-speed, motor-driven hand piece (12,000–15,000 rpm) with various-sized, diamond-tipped fraises. These diamond-impregnated burrs produce a fine, easily controllable depth of abrasion and, when driven at relatively low speeds, yield a superficial to medium depth of surgical planing. The control provided with this equipment has essentially eliminated postoperative hypertrophic scarring. A 5-mm wheel-shaped burr is useful for abrading around the vermilion border. On the flat surface of the upper lip or cheeks, a larger, cylindrical burr is usually preferable. The dermabrasion is performed following infiltration with local anesthesia. The abrader is moved slowly and with even pressure across the skin surface, removing the epidermis and superficial dermis down to the desired level. The abrading drum should parallel the surface of the skin, the sanding process consisting of light brushing strokes carried out at right angles to the plane of rotation of the instrument. In performing the abrasion, it is important to use an even pressure and let the machine do the work. The hand piece is kept moving, rather than remaining stationary over an abraded area. This maneuver minimizes the possibility of deep planing secondary to a combination of pressure, heat, and friction. Frequent inspection of the skin surface, with the appearance of fine punctate bleeding, offers a useful guideline to the proper depth of abrasion.

Placing the skin on stretch is useful for obtaining a proper tension against which to dermabrade, and helps to produce a smooth, even planing. The depth of the abrasion should be confined to a superficial or, at most, intermediate thickness of dermis. The proper level is apparent from the multiple fine bleeding points that are seen as the abrasion is carried into the vessels that lie within the dermal papillae. It can be risky to abrade skin aggressively in the treatment of deeply placed, coarse rhytides. It is preferable to reabrade at an additional session or even consider an adjunct TCA peel following healing, rather than risk hypertrophic scarring by abrading too deeply.

SURGICAL REJUVENATION OF THE FACE

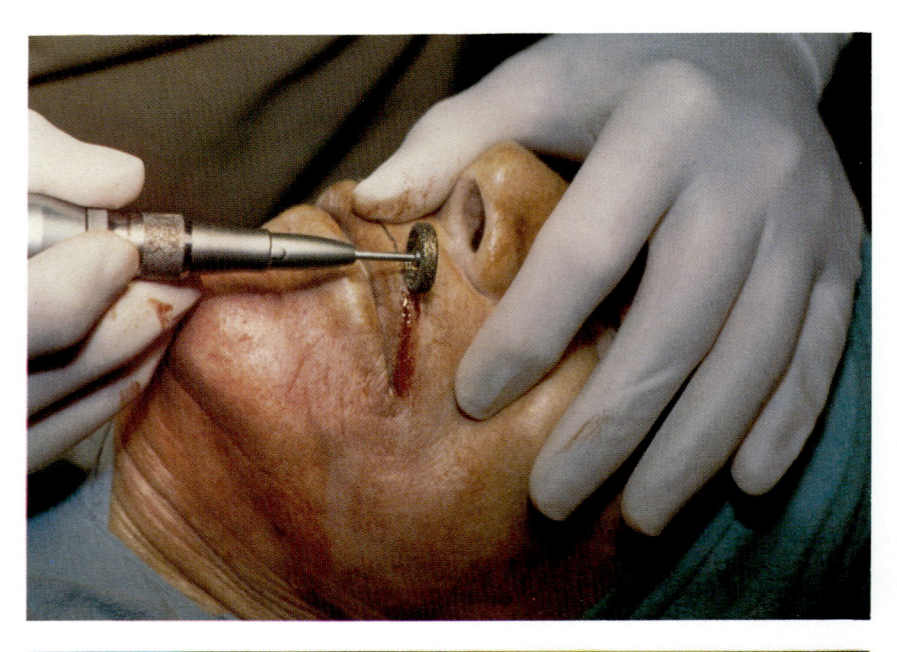

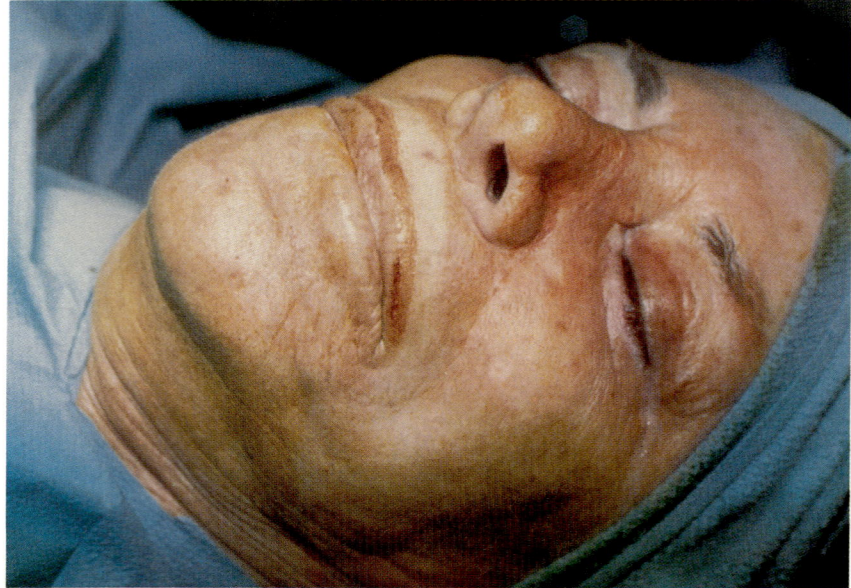

The vermilion-skin junction is abraded with a narrow fraise to outline the border. The skin adjacent to the vermilion border of the upper lip has been abraded, and the procedure is carried out on the lower lip line.

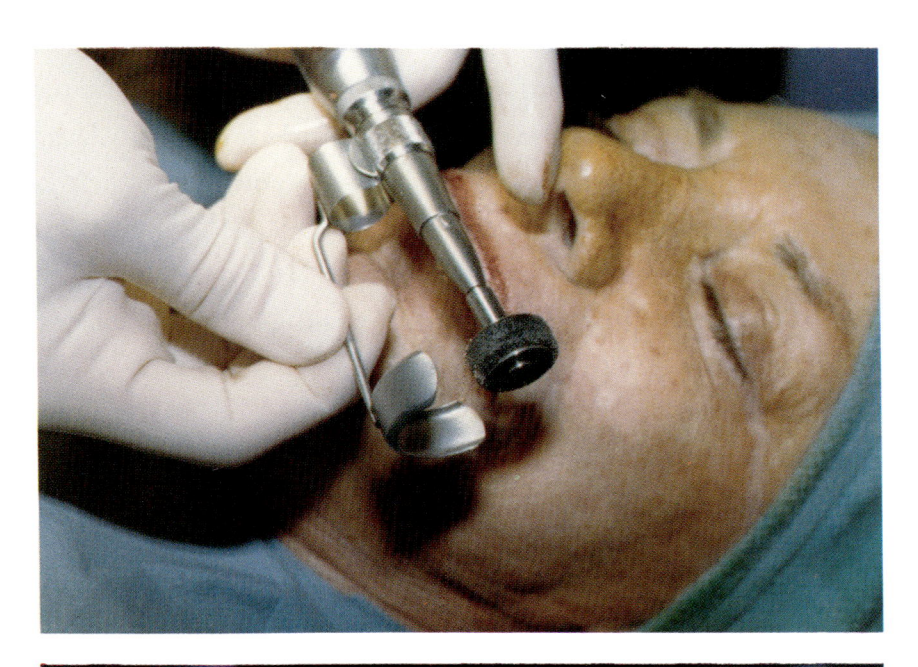

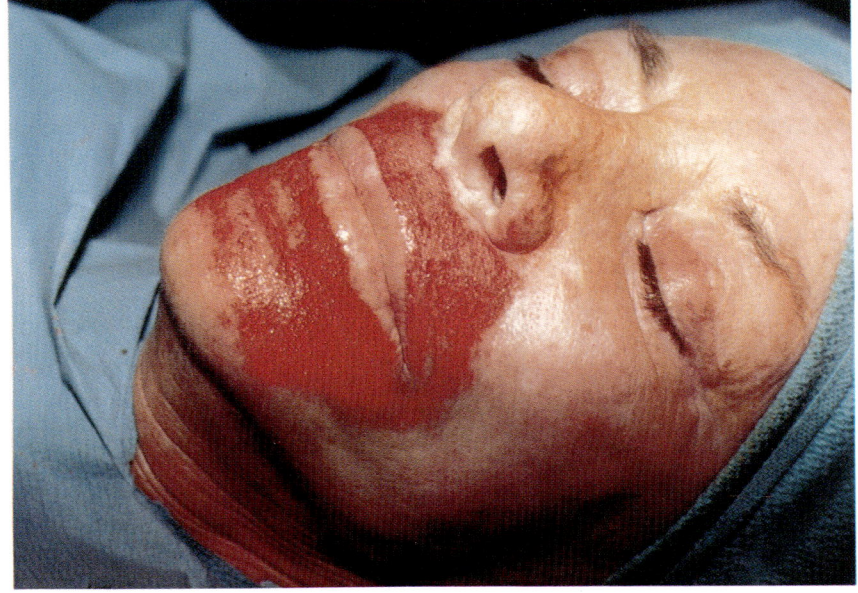

CHEMICAL PEELING (PHENOL AND TRICHLOROACETIC ACID) AND DERMABRASION

Using a large abrasive disk (in this case, a wire brush and a guard), the remainder of the perioral abrasion will now be done. The appearance of the perioral area when the dermabrasion has been completed.

Postoperative Care

After abrasion, the area is irrigated with normal saline solution and a moist gauze pad is placed on top of the abrasion. Following hemostasis, the area is covered with a greasy ointment (A & D). The patient is then instructed to wash the area several times a day with clear water and then to reapply the petroleum-based ointment, which keeps the wound lubricated and prevents eschar formation. Reepithelization is usually complete within 5 to 7 days.

The postoperative appearance of the healing surface parallels that of chemical peeling, although the erythema tends to resolve more quickly. Usually within 10 days the patient can wear covering cosmetics and return to social activity. Moisturizers are necessary until the skin returns to its normal appearance, to prevent dryness and cracking. Avoidance of sunlight and the use of sunblocks and covering makeup bases are critical to protect the skin from pigmentary changes during the period of wound healing.

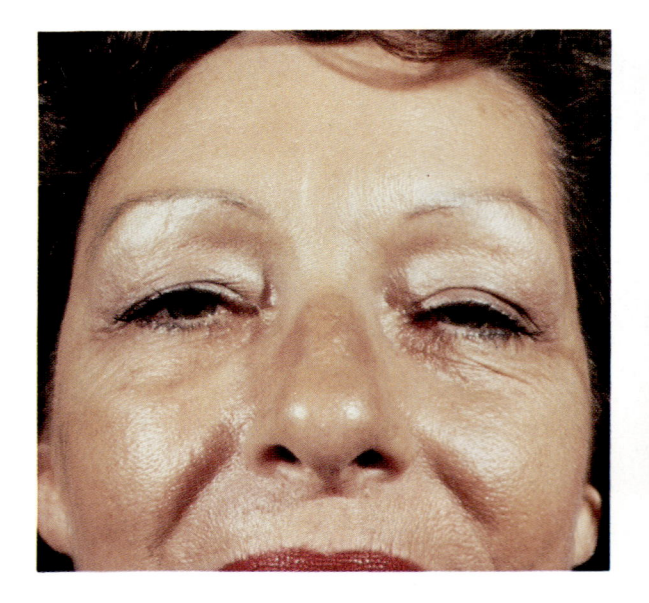

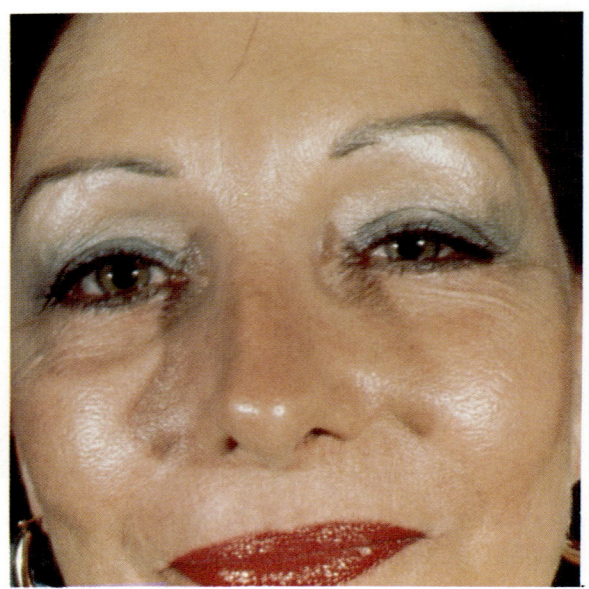

This patient requested that the lines be removed from her upper lip, by dermabrasion if possible. The appearance of the patient's lip 1 year after dermabrasion.

Q&A: FREQUENTLY ASKED QUESTIONS

Is the croton oil necessary?
The peel can be done without croton oil with comparable long-term results, although the initial erythema is deeper with croton oil. We always use a mixture containing croton oil.

Is adhesive tape necessary?
The tape acts as an occlusive dressing. The results are definitely more profound and longer-lasting when tape is used. If a lesser degree or depth of peeling is desired, the peel can be performed without tape, using a petroleum jelly occlusive dressing.

Can the thymol iodide powder be eliminated in cases of allergy to iodine?
We apply ointment directly to the face upon removal of the mask, and the results seem to be comparable to peels that follow our standard procedure.

Can peeling be done simultaneously with surgery?
We do not apply the peeling solution to any areas that have been undermined during a surgical face-lift. The only areas that we would consider peeling are those around the mouth that have not been surgically altered. We believe that the simultaneous disruption of the blood supply by undermining, and the chemical burn produced by the application of the phenol solution, are likely to produce irreversible skin changes, perhaps even necrosis.

Which should be done first, facial surgery or facial peeling?
If both procedures are planned, we prefer to do the surgery first and the peeling 2 to 3 months later. If the peeling is done first, somewhat more time must elapse before the surgery can be safely performed because of the slower healing following peeling. The choice as to which procedure to do first depends on whether the sagging of the face or the fine lines of the face are the primary concern of the patient.

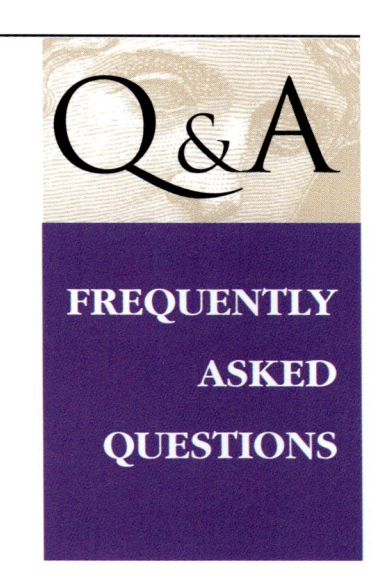

How long does peeling last?
The effect of chemical peeling is permanent and may be noted over the patient's lifetime. Some wrinkling will eventually occur, but the patient will always be less wrinkled than if she had not had the treatment. We have seen patients 15 years after peeling who still looked less wrinkled than before the treatment.

Can the peel be repeated?
In rare instances we have repeated the treatment as soon as all of the erythema and edema in the skin has subsided. This has been as soon as 3 to 4 months after the original treatment, but we usually wait 6 months to 1 year before reapplying phenol. TCA peels can be repeated more frequently. We have repeated 20% TCA peels as frequently as every 2 weeks while we usually wait 2 to 3 months before repeating a 35% TCA peel.

What is the effect on skin lesions?
Superficial lesions such as keratoses and freckles are eliminated. Lesions that occupy more depth in the thickness of the skin, such as nevi and telangiectasias, are usually more prominent after peeling. The nevi may become darker or may appear darker because of the lightening of the skin. Skin lesions such as capillary hemangiomas are unaffected.

Will peeling reduce enlarged pores?
Peeling will not reduce enlarged pores and in some instances even makes the pores appear to be more prominent.

What is the effect of peeling on the growth of facial hair?
Peeling has no long-lasting effect on the growth of facial hair. For the first few weeks, the hair may not be prominent, but eventually hair growth will be the same.

When can makeup be used?
Makeup can be safely used within 10 days to 2 weeks after peeling. This is the time when erythema is present. If the makeup causes the patient discomfort, the makeup can be removed without damage to the healing skin.

When can the skin be exposed to the sun?
Our experience has been that skin that is still erythematous, even faintly, may become blotchy when exposed to the sun, and we recommend no exposure to sun during the healing phase. After the permanent skin color has stabilized, usually within 8 to 12 weeks, we recommend shielding the skin from the sun as much as possible, using sunscreens, hats, or parasols.

SUGGESTED READING

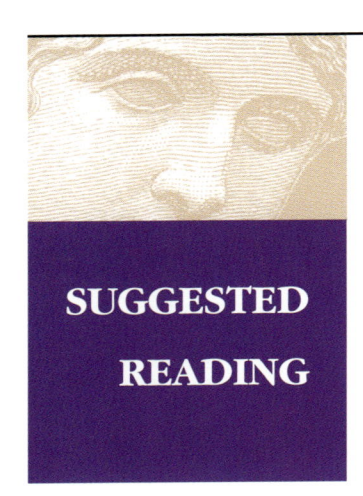

Baker, TJ and Stuzin, JM: Chemical Peeling and Dermabrasion, McCarthy, JG (Ed.) *Plastic Surgery.* Philadelphia, WB Saunders Company, 1990, p. 748.

Brody, HJ: *Chemical Peeling,* Mosby-Year Book, Inc., St. Louis, 1992.

Rubin, MG: *Manual of Chemical Peels,* Lippincott, Philadelphia, 1995.

Stuzin, JM, Baker, TJ, and Gordon, HL: Treatment of photoaging. Facial chemical peeling (phenol and trichloroacetic acid) and dermabrasion. *Clin. Plast. Surg.* 20:9, 1993.

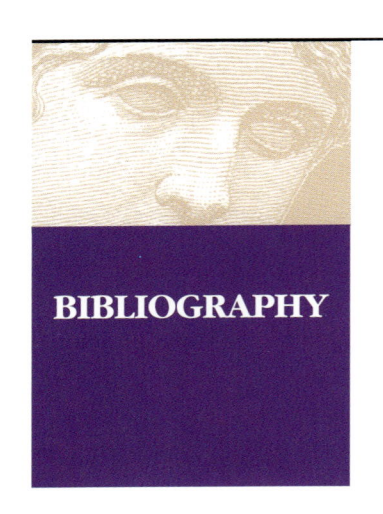

BIBLIOGRAPHY

Baker, TJ, and Gordon, HL: The ablation of rhytides by chemical means, a preliminary report, *J. Fla. Med. Assoc.* 47:451, 1961.

Baker, TJ: Chemical face peeling and rhytidectomy. A combined approach for face rejuvenation. *Plast. Reconstr. Surg.* 29:199, 1962.

Baker, TJ, and Gordon, HL: Chemical face peeling, an adjunct to surgical face lifting. *South. Med. J.* 56:412, 1963.

Baker, TJ, Gordon, HL, and Seckinger, DL: A second look at chemical face peeling. *Plast. Reconstr. Surg.* 37:487, 1966.

Baker, TJ, and Gordon, HL: Chemical face peeling and dermabrasion. *Surg. Clin. North Am.* 51(2):387, 1971.

Baker, TJ, Gordon, HL, Moisienko, P, and Seckinger, DL: Long-term histological study of skin after chemical face peeling, *Plast. Reconstr. Surg.* 53:522, 1974.

Baker, TJ, and Gordon, HL: Chemical peeling as a practical method for removing rhytides of the upper lip. *Ann. Plast. Surg.* 2(3):209-212, March, 1979.

Brody, HJ, and Hailey, CW: Medium depth chemical peeling of the skin: a variation of superficial chemosurgery. *J. Dermatol. Surg. Oncol.* 12:1268, 1986.

Brody, HJ: Variations and comparisons in medium-depth chemical peeling. *J. Dermatol. Surg. Oncol.* 15:953, 1989.

Brody, HJ: Complications of chemical peeling. *J. Dermatol. Surg. Oncol.* 15:1010, 1989.

Brown, AM, Kaplan, LM, and Brown, ME: Phenol-induced histological skin changes: hazards, techniques, and uses. *Br. J. Plast. Surg.* 13:158, 1960.

Brown, AM, Kaplan, LM, and Brown, ME: Cutaneous alterations induced by phenol: a histologic bioassay. *Int. Surg.* 34:602, 1960.

Collins, PS: Trichloroacetic acid peels revisited. *J. Dermatol. Surg. Oncol.* 15:933, 1989.

Converse, JM, and Robb-Smith, AHT: The healing of surface cutaneous wounds: its analogy with the healing of superficial burns. *Ann. Surg.* 120:873, 1944.

Deichmann, W, and Witherup, S: Phenol studies. VI. The acute and comparative toxicity of phenol and o-, m-, and p-cresols for experimental animals. *J. Pharmacol. Exp. Ther.* 80:233, 1944.

Gross, BG: Cardiac arrhythmias during phenol face peeling. *Plast. Reconstr. Surg.* 73-590, 1984.

Kligman, AM: Early destructive effects of sunlight on human skin. *J.A.M.A.* 210:2377, 1969.

Kligman, AM, Baker, TJ, and Gordon, HL: Long-term histologic follow-up of phenol face peels. *Plast. Reconstr. Surg.* 75:652, 1985.

Kurtin, A: Corrective surgical planing of skin: new technique for treatment of acne scars and other skin defects. *Arch. Dermatol. Syph.* 68:389, 1953.

Litton, C: Chemical face lifting. *Plast. Reconstr. Surg.* 29:371, 1962.

Orentreich, N, and Dunn, NP: Dermabrasion. In Goldwyn, RM (Ed.): *The Unfavorable Result in Plastic Surgery.* 2nd Ed. Boston, Little, Brown & Company, 1984, p. 919.

Rees, TD: Chemabrasion and dermabrasion. In Rees, TD (Ed.): *Aesthetic Plastic Surgery.* Philadelphia, W.B. Saunders Company, 1980, p. 749.

Resnik, SS: Chemical peeling with trichloroacetic acid. *J. Dermatol. Surg. Oncol.* 10:549, 1984.

Spira, M, Dahl, G, Freeman, R, Gerow, FJ, and Hardy, SB: Chemosurgery—a histological study. *Plast. Reconstr. Surg.* 45:247, 1970.

Spira, M, Freeman, RF, Arfai, P, Gerow, FJ, and Hardy, SB: A comparison of chemical peeling, dermabrasion and 5-fluorouracil in cancer prophylaxis. *J. Surg. Oncol.* 3:367, 1971.

Stagnone, JJ: Superficial peeling. *J. Dermatol. Surg. Oncol.* 15:924, 1989.

Stegman, SJ: a study of dermabrasion and chemical peels in an animal model. *J. Dermatol. Surg. Oncol.* 6:490, 1980.

Stegman, SJ: A comparative histologic study of the effects of three peeling agents and dermabrasion on normal and sun-damaged skin. *Aesthetic. Plast. Surg.* 6:123, 1982.

Stuzin, JM, Baker, TJ, and Gordon, HL: Chemical peel—a change in routine. *Ann. Plast. Surg.* 22:301, 1989.

Truppman, ES, and Ellenby, JD: Major electrocardiographic changes during chemical face peeling. *Plast. Reconstr. Surg.* 63:44, 1979.

Four

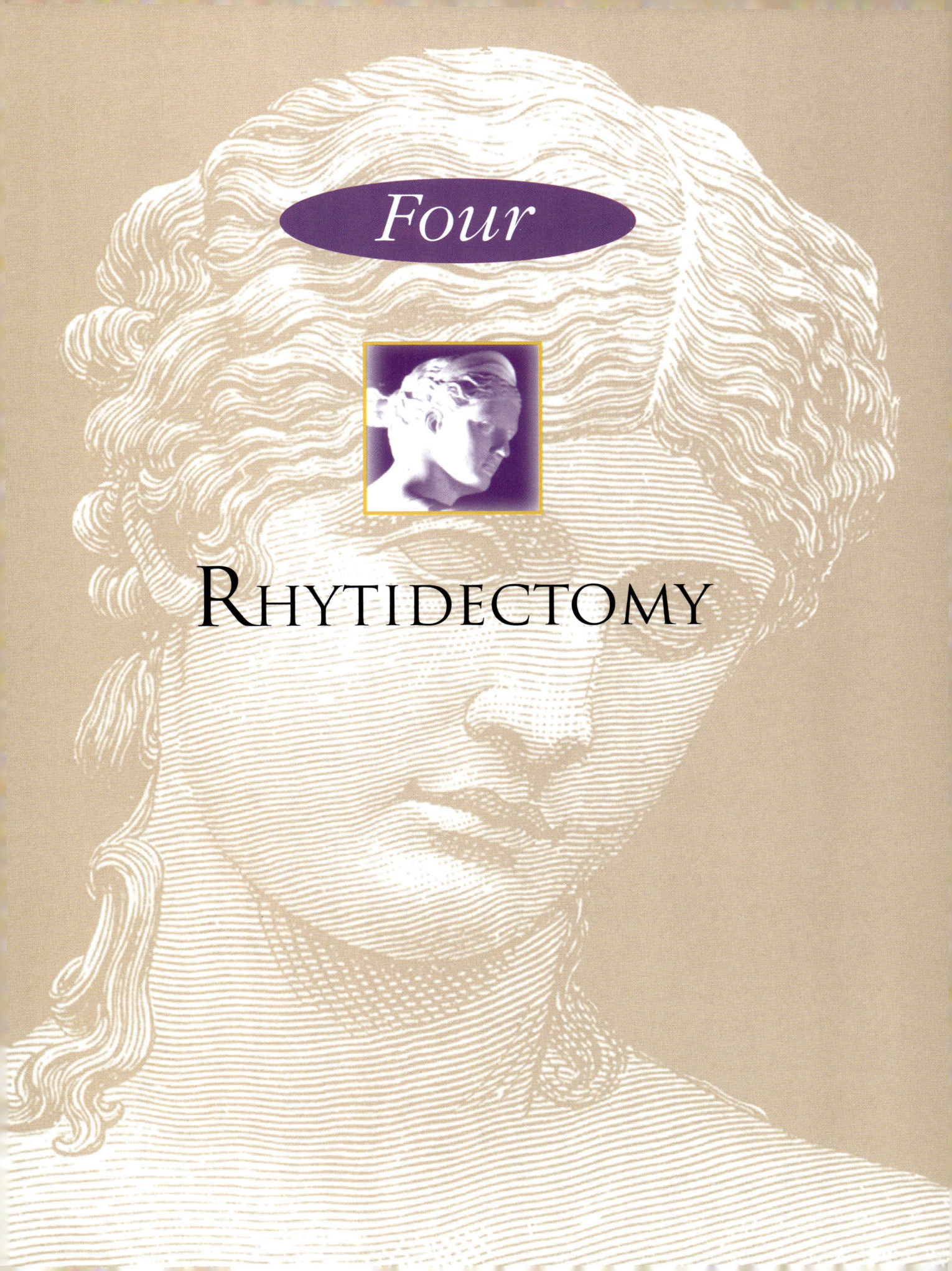

RHYTIDECTOMY

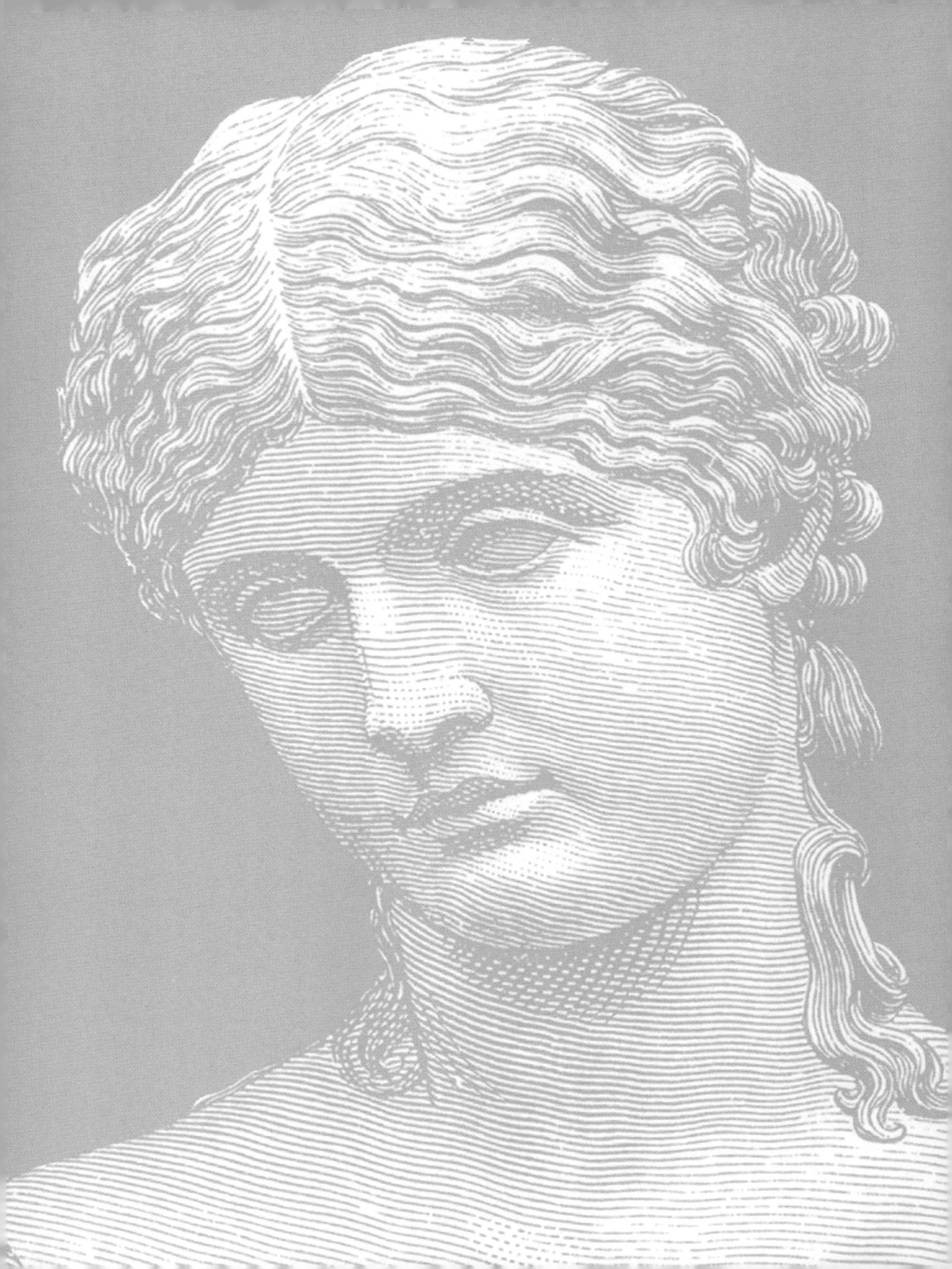

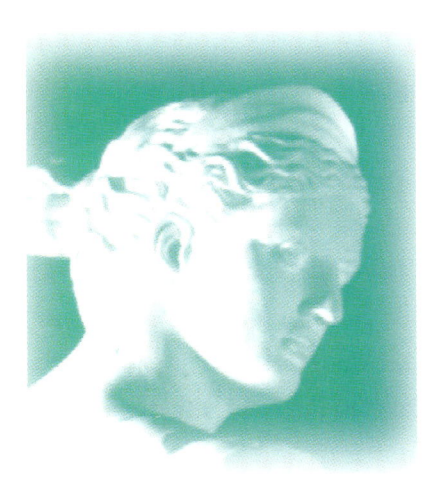

FACIAL SOFT TISSUE ANATOMY AND RHYTIDECTOMY

With the media's emphasis on youth and fitness, the topics of aging, exercise, and diet have become the issues of the day and the concerns of many. In response to these concerns, a person wanting to improve his or her self-image by looking younger may request a rhytidectomy, or facelift.

The majority of patients seeking facelifts are middle-class people seeking physical self-improvement through surgery. For many, the incentive is to remain active in the workplace. Many patients' business and social activities require daily contact with the public and they want to look good. Most patients, however, simply want to improve what they see in the mirror.

A rhytidectomy alleviates some of the damages of aging by partially eliminating folds, creases, and wrinkles caused by gravity and degeneration of the face and neck tissues. Simply stated, the operation requires the creation of two large cervicofacial flaps, which, after suspension and trimming, produce an overall tightening of the skin and fascial envelope of the face and neck. It is a challenging procedure because each patient presents a different anatomic and geometric situation.

Rhytidectomy, the so-called facelift, is a reconstructive procedure producing facial rejuvenation by correcting anatomic changes that have occurred with aging. There are certain anatomic considerations in planning and performing rhytidectomy. A thorough understanding of facial soft tissue anatomy and the effects of aging is mandatory to obtain consistent results in facelifting.

Rhytidectomy can be performed safely because facial soft tissue is arranged in a series of concentric layers. This concentric arrangement allows dissection within one anatomic plane without disturbing structures lying within another anatomic layer. The layers of the face are:

1. Skin.
2. Subcutaneous layer.
3. Superficial facial fascia (SMAS).
4. Mimetic muscles.
5. Parotid-masseteric fascia, or deep facial fascia.
6. Plane of facial nerve, parotid duct, buccal fat pad, facial artery, and vein.

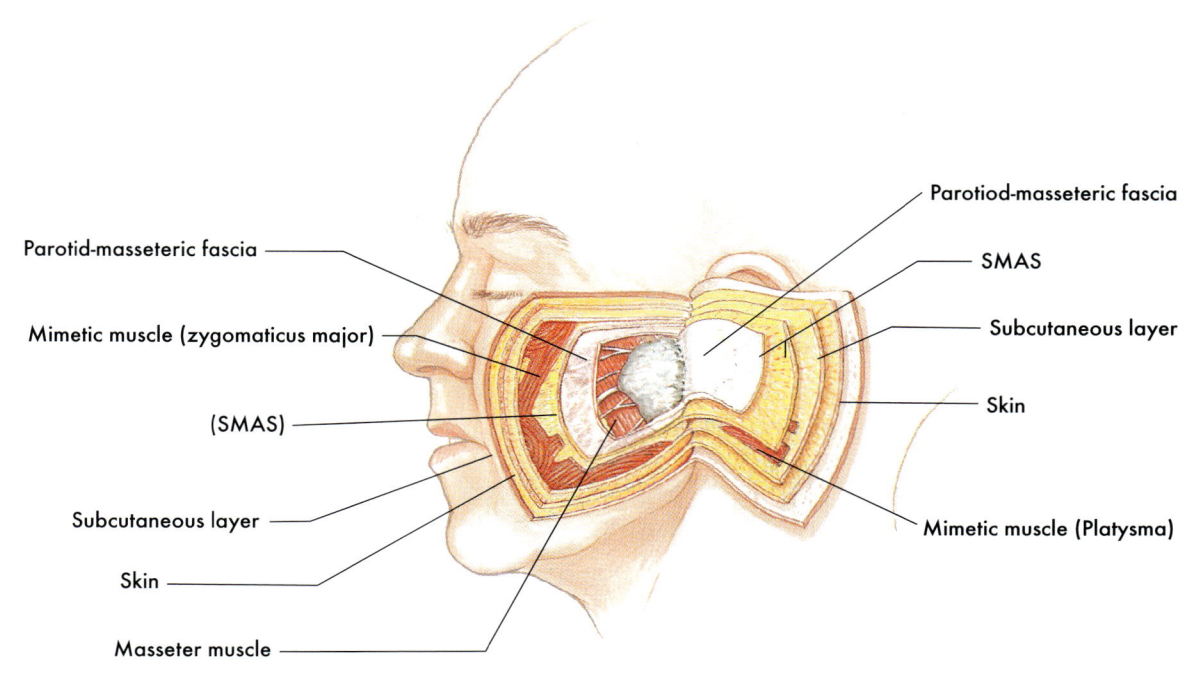

RHYTIDECTOMY

Labels (left side):
- Parotid-masseteric fascia
- Mimetic muscle (zygomaticus major)
- (SMAS)
- Subcutaneous layer
- Skin
- Masseter muscle

Labels (right side):
- Parotiod-masseteric fascia
- SMAS
- Subcutaneous layer
- Skin
- Mimetic muscle (Platysma)

The facial soft tissue is arranged in a series of concentric layers. While there is a great deal of variation in the thickness of the individual layers, the structures present within each of these layers remain anatomically constant. From superficial to deep, the layers of the face are the skin, subcutaneous layer, superficial facial fascia (SMAS), mimetic muscles, parotid-masseteric fascia (deep facial fascia), and the plane of the facial nerve, parotid duct, and buccal fat pad.

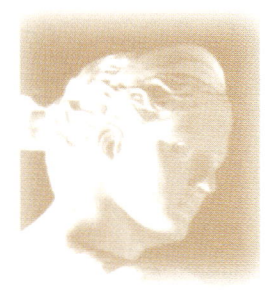

SKIN

The outermost layer of the face is skin. The aging of facial skin is influenced by actinic damage, as well as by genetic, intrinsic factors. The result of intrinsic and extrinsic aging on facial skin is termed *elastosis,* a degeneration of dermal collagen and elastic fibers. Gravitational forces affecting inelastic skin produce many of the stigmata of the aging face. Much of the improvement following rhytidectomy is secondary to a tightening of facial skin. The quality of the patient's skin greatly influences the final outcome of the procedure. Patients with poor skin elasticity, severe sun damage, and heavy facial rhytides commonly have a more disappointing result with a shorter longevity, than the younger patient with good-quality skin.

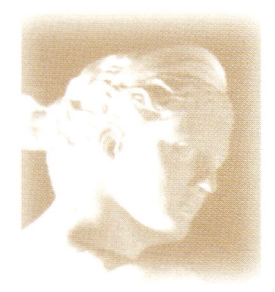

SUBCUTANEOUS LAYER

Directly deep to the skin lies a variable amount of subcutaneous fat. This fat sits directly above the superficial facial fascia (SMAS) and is the primary anatomic plane of dissection in rhytidectomy. The thickness of this layer of fat varies from patient to patient. It tends to be thicker in obese patients and thinner in patients that have previously undergone rhytidectomy. It is important to assess preoperatively the amount of subcutaneous fat within this layer since this will determine the thickness of the skin flap when undermining facial skin.

Though the subcutaneous layer is fairly homogeneous, the malar pad represents a specialized subcutaneous structure, similar to the soft tissue chin pad. The malar pad is responsible for imparting fullness over the zygomatic eminence. This pad is firmly attached to the underlying malar bone by ligaments that run from the periosteum of the zygoma through the subcutaneous portion of the malar pad and insert directly into the overlying dermis. Subcutaneous undermining in this region (McGregor's patch) tends to be fibrous as the dissection encounters and divides the numerous fibrous bands that suspend the malar pad over the underlying zygomatic eminence.

The subcutaneous layer also tends to be more fibrous overlying the parotid gland as well as directly overlying the sternocleidomastoid muscle.

SUPERFICIAL FACIAL FASCIA (SMAS)

The superficial muscular aponeurosis (SMAS) represents a discrete fascial layer that separates the overlying subcutaneous fat from the underlying parotid-masseteric fascia and facial nerve branches. When performing rhytidectomy, recognition of the SMAS is of paramount importance. As long as the integrity of this layer is maintained, facial nerve injury will not result from the dissection. An understanding of the anatomy of the SMAS and its relationship to the mimetic musculature and deep facial fascia allows extensive mobilization of the SMAS with little risk to the facial nerve branches.

The SMAS represents an extension of the superficial cervical fascia cephalad into the face. This superficial fascia forms a continuous sheath throughout the face and neck, extending into the temporal region, forehead, scalp, malar areas, nose, and upper lip. The thickness of the superficial fascia varies greatly from patient to patient, as well as from one region of the face to another. The superficial fascia is dense and thick overlying the parotid gland, and it is this anatomic component that many physicians clinically refer to when utilizing the term *SMAS*. As this fascial layer is traced superiorly cephalad to the zygomatic arch, it is termed the *temporoparietal fascia* (within the temporal region) and the *galea* (within the scalp), both of which are substantial in terms of thickness.

As the SMAS is traced medially into the cheek, overlying the masseter and buccal fat pad, this layer tends to become thinner and less distinct. Within the malar region, the SMAS is quite thin, essentially comprising the epimysium of the elevators of the upper lip.

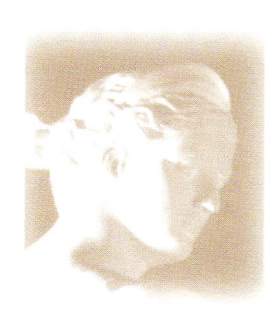

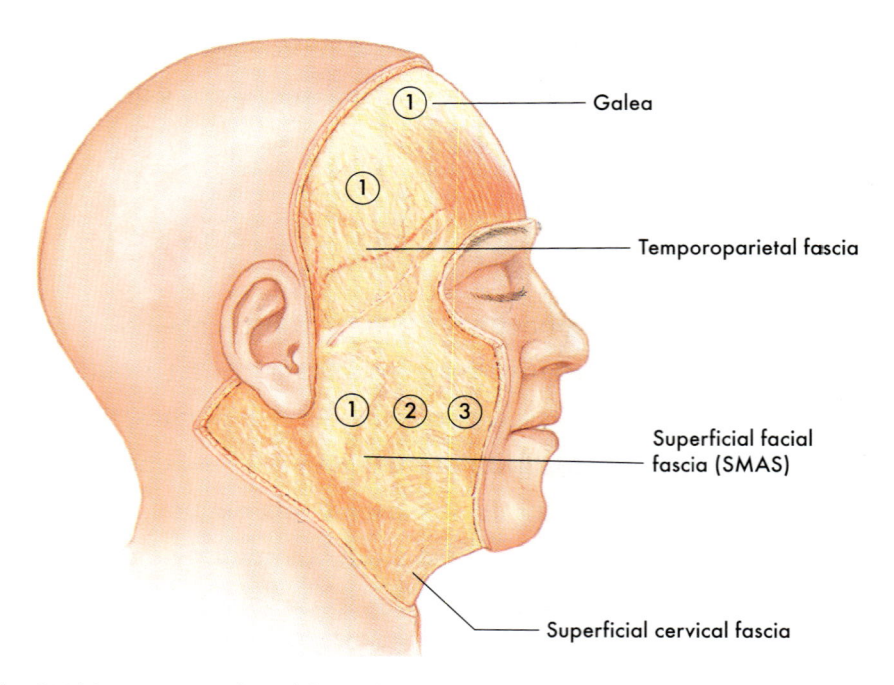

SURGICAL REJUVENATION OF THE FACE

Figure labels:
- ① Galea
- Temporoparietal fascia
- Superficial facial fascia (SMAS)
- Superficial cervical fascia

The SMAS, or superficial facial fascia, is continuous throughout the head and neck. The thickness of this layer varies from patient to patient, as well as from one region of the face to another. In some areas, the SMAS is a thick, substantial layer (1) overlying the parotid gland in the temporal region (temporoparietal fascia), and in the forehead and scalp (galea). As the SMAS is traced anteriorly in the face, it becomes thinner and less distinct (2). As the SMAS is traced into the malar region, it is quite thin, essentially comprising the epimysium of the elevators of the upper lip (3).

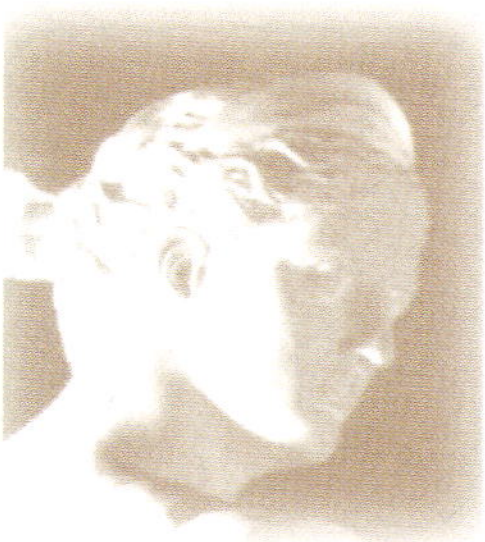

MIMETIC MUSCLES

The mimetic musculature is comprised of individual muscles that receive their innervation from the facial nerve and are responsible for facial movement. Unlike most other muscles in the body, which have origin and insertion into bones and produce movements of limbs or joints, the muscles of facial expression send fibrous insertions directly into dermis and their contraction produces movement of facial skin. The SMAS represents the aponeurotic connection between the mimetic musculature and the overlying skin.

The muscles of facial expression are situated at different depths within the facial soft tissue architecture. Some muscles are superficial, whereas others are deep. The mimetic muscles commonly overlap one another and have been described as being arranged in four anatomic layers. The muscles encountered in rhytidectomy, such as the platysma, orbicularis oculi, zygomaticus major and minor, and risorius, are examples of superficial mimetic muscles. The buccinator and mentalis muscles are examples of deep mimetic muscles.

The platysma is the mimetic muscle most involved with facial aging, and various techniques have evolved using flaps of the platysma to contour both the neck and the face.

The platysma takes its origin from within the SMAS itself, originating more superiorly in the face than is generally recognized. Its fibers can be traced in some individuals as cephalad as the zygomatic arch and as far forward as the malar prominence. As the platysma descends into the neck, it tends to become more prominent and muscular. When raising the SMAS within the cheek, usually only wispy fibers of the platysma are visualized superiorly because the muscle is poorly developed in this area in most people. As the dissection proceeds inferiorly, the platysma becomes more obvious.

Anatomically, the platysma forms a continuous muscular sheet, lending muscular support for the lower two thirds of the face as well as the anterior neck. Many of the anatomic changes seen with aging, such as platysmal bands and the formation of facial jowls, represent an attenuation of platysma support. Much of the rejuvenation obtained by rhytidectomy involves techniques to contour the aging platysma.

Dissection within the malar region exposes fibers of the zygomaticus major and minor. These muscles function as elevators of the upper lip and descend inferiorly from the malar region, past the nasolabial fold, to mingle with fibers of the orbicularis oris. Anatomically, the elevators of the upper lip are situated superficially within the facial soft tissue architecture, at a depth comparable with the adjacent platysma.

SURGICAL REJUVENATION OF THE FACE

A

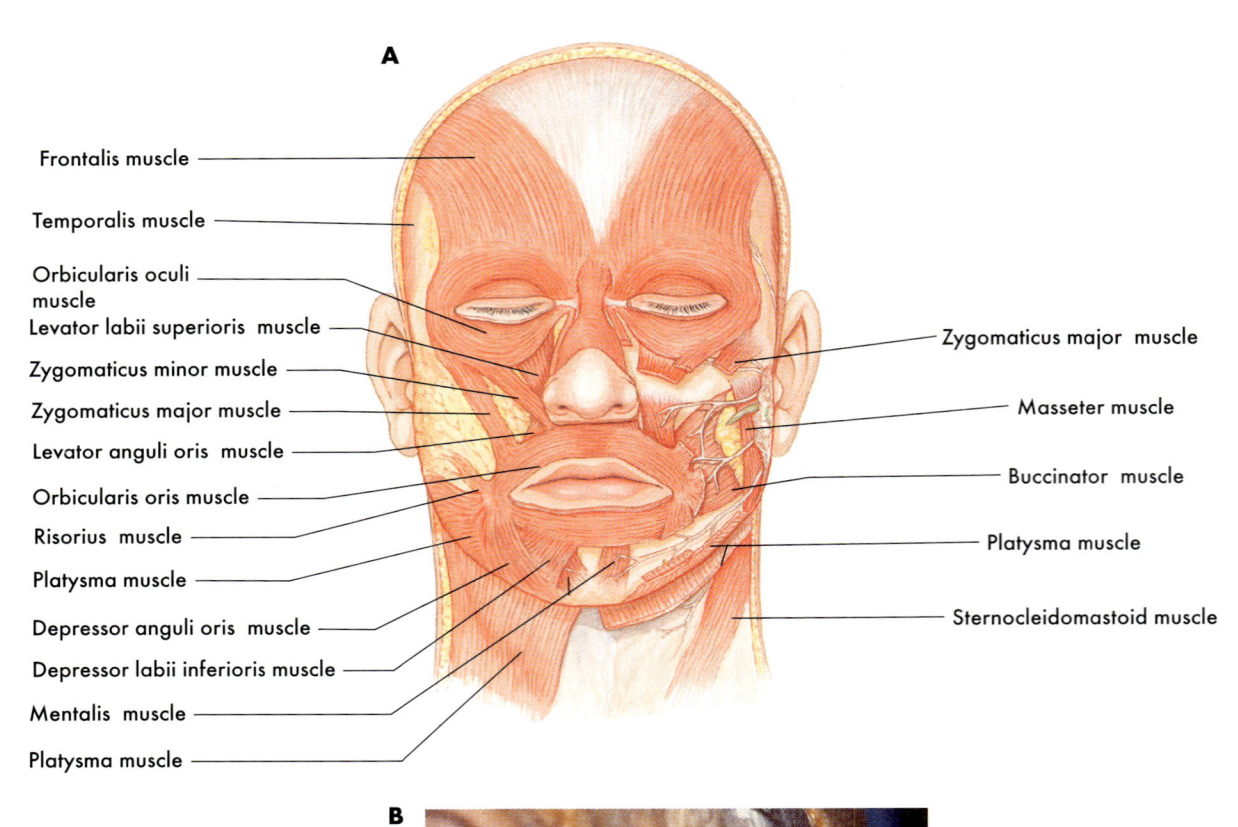

- Frontalis muscle
- Temporalis muscle
- Orbicularis oculi muscle
- Levator labii superioris muscle
- Zygomaticus minor muscle
- Zygomaticus major muscle
- Levator anguli oris muscle
- Orbicularis oris muscle
- Risorius muscle
- Platysma muscle
- Depressor anguli oris muscle
- Depressor labii inferioris muscle
- Mentalis muscle
- Platysma muscle

- Zygomaticus major muscle
- Masseter muscle
- Buccinator muscle
- Platysma muscle
- Sternocleidomastoid muscle

B

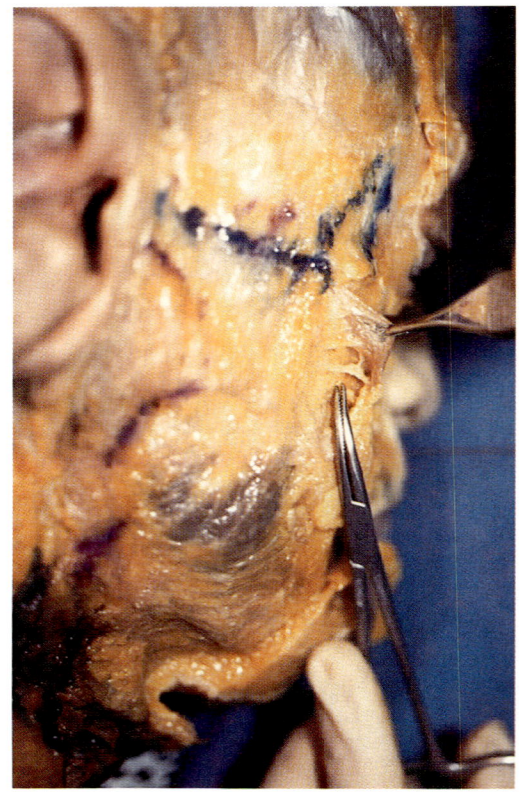

A, The muscles of facial expression are arranged in four anatomic layers that overlap one another. Since most of the mimetic muscles lie superficial to the plane of the facial nerve, they receive their innervation from their deep surfaces. Only the buccinator, the levator anguli oris, and the mentalis muscle, which lie deep to the plane of the facial nerve, receive their innervation along their superficial surfaces. B, Cadaver dissection illustrating the segmental innervation of the zygomaticus major muscle along its deep surface.

Most of the mimetic muscles lie superficial to the plane of the facial nerve and for this reason receive their innervation along their deep surfaces. Only the buccinator, mentalis, and levator anguli oris muscles, which are deep within the face, lie deep to the plane of the facial nerve, and are therefore innervated along their superficial surfaces. The surgical importance of this anatomic fact is that when performing SMAS elevation, as long as the dissection is carried along the superficial surface of the facial muscles, injury to muscular innervation will not occur. Elevation of the SMAS within the malar region will expose fibers of the underlying zygomaticus major and minor, but will not injure their innervation as long as the integrity of these muscles is not violated.

The question arises as to how it is possible to elevate the platysma in continuity with SMAS dissection and not injure its innervation. The anatomic basis for this is that the platysma usually receives two to three cervical branches in the cleft between the anterior border of the sternocleidomastoid and the angle of the mandible. As the platysma is elevated medial and inferior to the tail of the parotid, these nerve branches will commonly be encountered. Recognition of these branches, followed by preservation using blunt dissection in the region of these fibers, will allow adequate platysma mobilization while protecting its innervation.

Relationship of the Superficial Facial Fascia (SMAS) to the Mimetic Muscles

The mimetic muscles and SMAS function as a single anatomic unit in producing movement of facial skin. The superficial facial fascia is intimately associated with the mimetic muscles, and muscle contracture is translated into movement of overlying facial skin through the vertical fibrous septa extending from the SMAS into the dermis.

Anatomically, the superficial facial fascia invests the superficial mimetic muscles (platysma, orbicularis oculi, zygomaticus major and minor, and risorius). When we use the term *investiture,* we mean that not only is the superficial fascia identified along the superficial surface of these muscles but that it also lines their deep surfaces. The investiture of the mimetic muscles by the SMAS forms essentially a single anatomic layer with fascia and muscle working in continuity to produce movement of facial skin.

To understand the concept of investiture of mimetic muscles by the SMAS, it is helpful to compare dissection of the SMAS-platysma complex to dissection of a flap of temporoparietal fascia. As the thickness of the temporoparietal fascia within the temporal region invests the superficial temporal vessels and the frontal branch of the facial nerve, the thickness of the SMAS within the cheek and neck invests the platysma. Both flaps are mobilized by separating subcutaneous fat from the superficial surface of the SMAS followed by dissecting the deep surface of the flap from the underlying deep facial fascia (or deep temporal fascia). The only difference anatomically between dissection of temporoparietal fascia and dissection of SMAS-platysma is the lack of mimetic muscle within the temporal region.

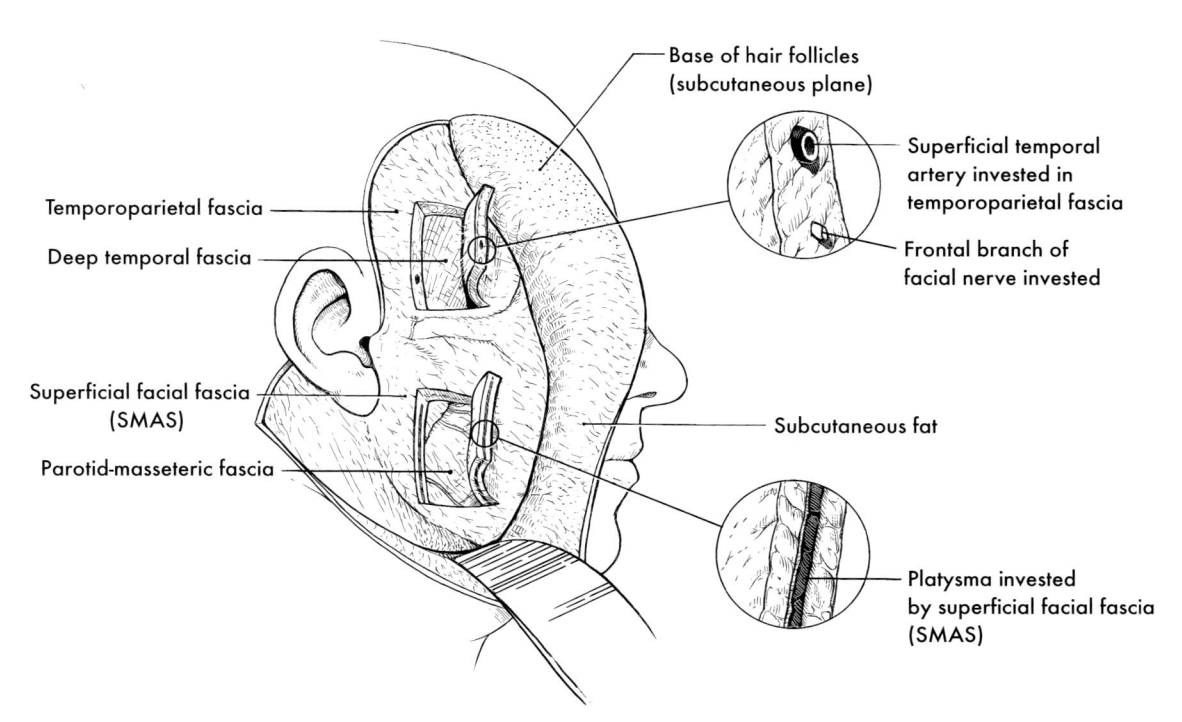

Following dissection within the subcutaneous plane, the underlying SMAS with its continuation as temporoparietal fascia is evident. The SMAS forms an investing fascial layer. In the temporal region, the thickness of the temporoparietal fascia invests the superficial temporal artery and frontal branch of the facial nerve. Similarly, within the cheek, the thickness of the SMAS invests the platysma. Dissection of a flap of temporoparietal fascia is anatomically similar to dissection of the SMAS-platysma complex, except for the absence of mimetic muscle within the temporal region. (From Stuzin JM, Baker HL, Gordon TJ: **Plast Reconstr Surg 89:441, 1992.** *Used by permission.)*

Clinically, it is possible to dissect the superficial fascia overlying the platysma, but raising fascia without platysma produces a less substantial flap than when the platysma is raised in continuity with the SMAS. Dissection along the undersurface of the platysma elevates both platysma and the fascia investing this muscle in continuity, producing a substantial myofascial flap.

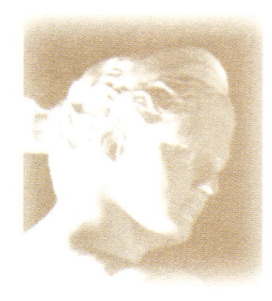

DEEP FACIAL FASCIA (PAROTID-MASSETERIC FASCIA)

Since the face and neck are contiguous, it follows that the cervical fascial layers continue cephalad, forming the facial fasciae. Since the SMAS represents a continuation of the superficial cervical fascia into the face, the corresponding deeper layer of cervical fascia (the superficial layer of the deep cervical fascia) continues into the face and has been termed the *parotid-masseteric fascia.* Its relevance to facial anatomy is infrequently discussed, but is extremely important. The significance of this anatomic layer lies in the fact that within the cheek, *the facial nerve branches, as well as the parotid duct, always lie deep to this deep fascial layer.*

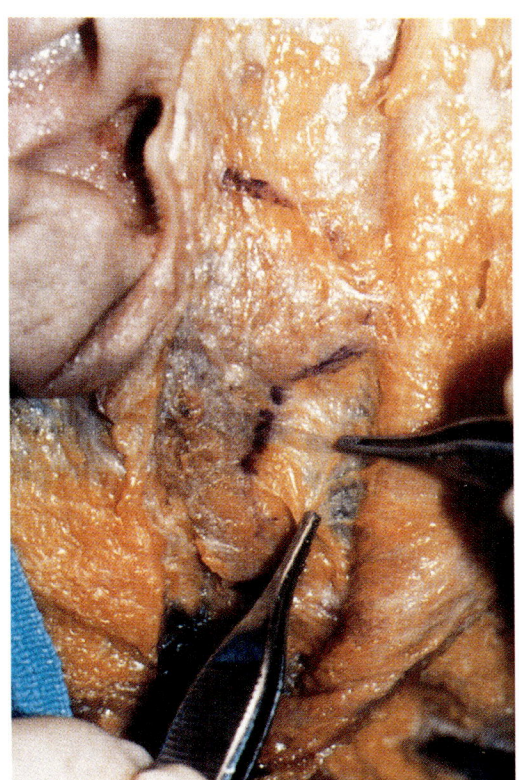

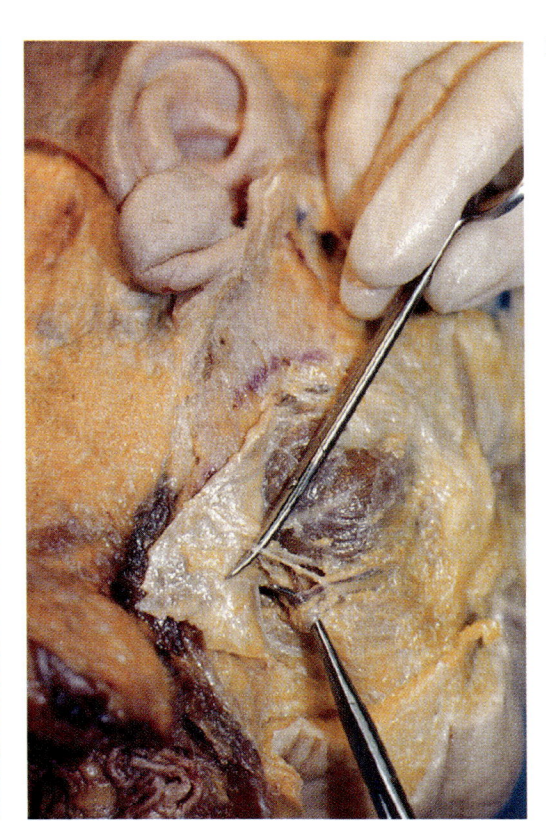

A, Cadaver dissection following SMAS-platysma elevation within the cheek exposing the underlying parotid gland, the anterior border of the parotid (marked in ink), and the parotid-masseteric fascia (held in forceps). The surgical significance of the parotid-masseteric fascia is that the facial nerve branches within the cheek are always deep to this anatomic layer. *B,* Cadaver dissection following elevation of the parotid-masseteric fascia exposing the underlying masseter muscle and the marginal mandibular nerve as it crosses the facial artery and vein. (A and B from Stuzin JM, Baker HL, Gordon TJ: **Plast Reconstr Surg 89:441, 1992. Used by permission.**)

Within the neck, the superficial layer of the deep cervical fascia is identified along the superficial surface of the strap muscles. Superior to the hyoid, this fascial layer is observed overlying the mylohyoid and can be traced superiorly over the mandibular body.

Ascending into the face, overlying the parotid, this deep fascia has been termed the *parotid capsule,* or *investing parotid fascia.* More anteriorly within the face, the deep fascia overlies the masseter muscle itself and is termed *masseteric fascia.* Medial to the masseter, the deep fascia lines the superficial surface of the buccal fat pad and parotid duct. The deep fascia extends into the malar region, lying deep to the elevators of the upper lip. An extension of deep fascia superior to the zygomatic arch, within the temporal region, has been termed *deep temporal fascia.*

RHYTIDECTOMY

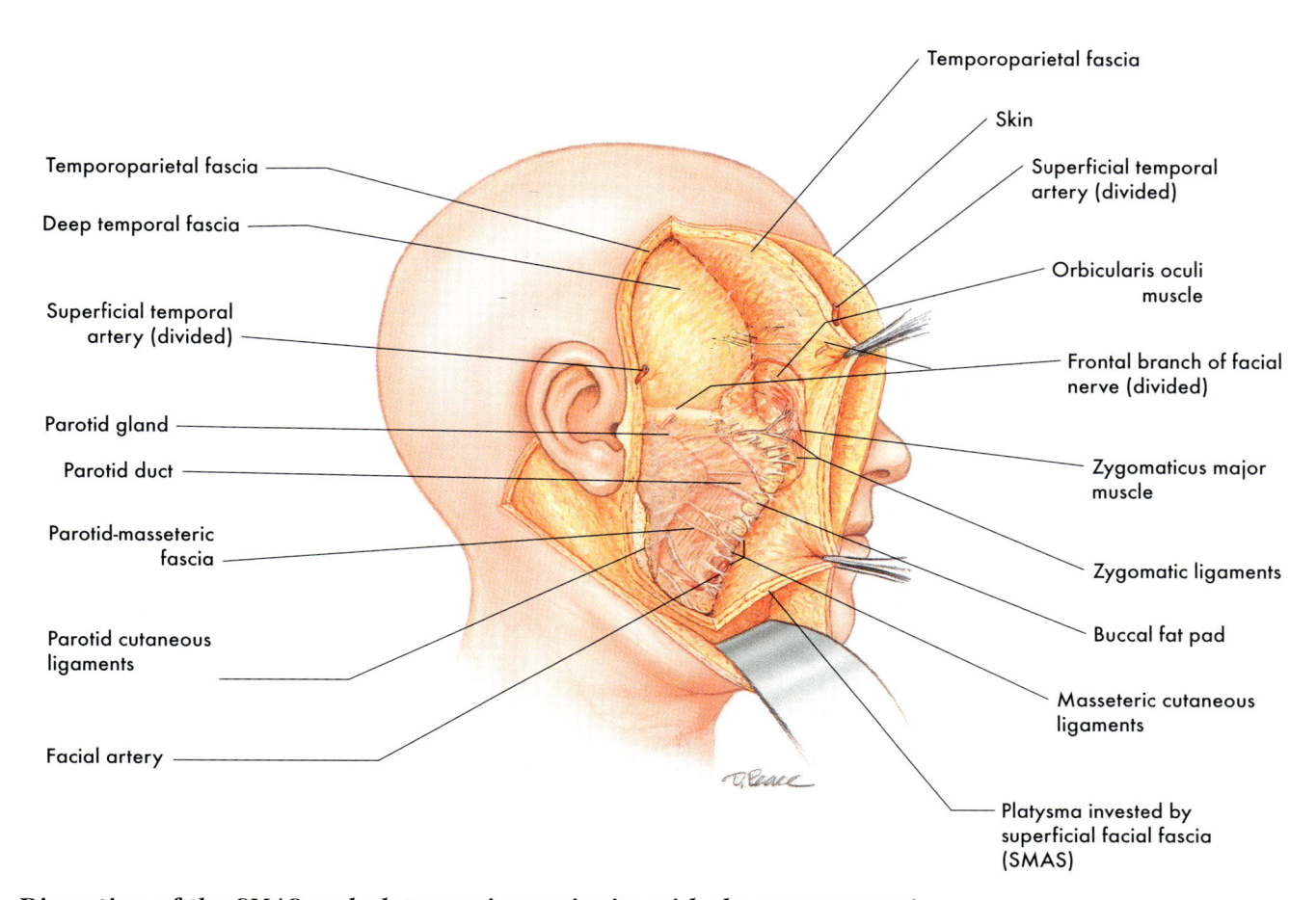

Dissection of the SMAS and platysma in continuity with the temporoparietal fascia exposes the deep facial fascia (parotid-masseteric fascia). This fascia represents a continuation of the deep cervical fascia cephalad into the face. Where this fascia is identified, it is given different names. Overlying the parotid gland, the deep fascia is termed the **parotid capsule.** *Overlying the masseter muscle, it is termed the* **masseteric fascia,** *and in the temporal region it is termed the* **deep temporal fascia.** *The significance of the deep facial fascia is that in the cheek, the facial nerve branches lie deep to the deep facial fascia. Upon reaching the mimetic muscles, the nerves penetrate the deep fascia to innervate these muscles along their deep surfaces.*

Relationship Between the Superficial and Deep Facial Fasciae

In general, two types of relationships exist between the superficial and deep facial fasciae. The more typical relationship is the separation of these fasciae by an areolar plane, which is similar to the separation of fascial planes elsewhere in the body. Areolar planes exist in specific locations including: (a) between the temporoparietal and deep temporal fascia within the temporal region, (b) within the cheek, between the SMAS and the parotid-masseteric fascia directly overlying the masseter muscle, and (c) between the platysma and underlying strap muscles within the neck.

In other regions of the face, rather than being separated by an areolar plane, the superficial and deep fasciae are intimately adherent to one another through dense fibrous attachments. Dense attachments between superficial and deep fasciae exist: (a) along the zygomatic arch, (b) overlying the parotid gland, and (c) along the anterior border of the masseter muscle.

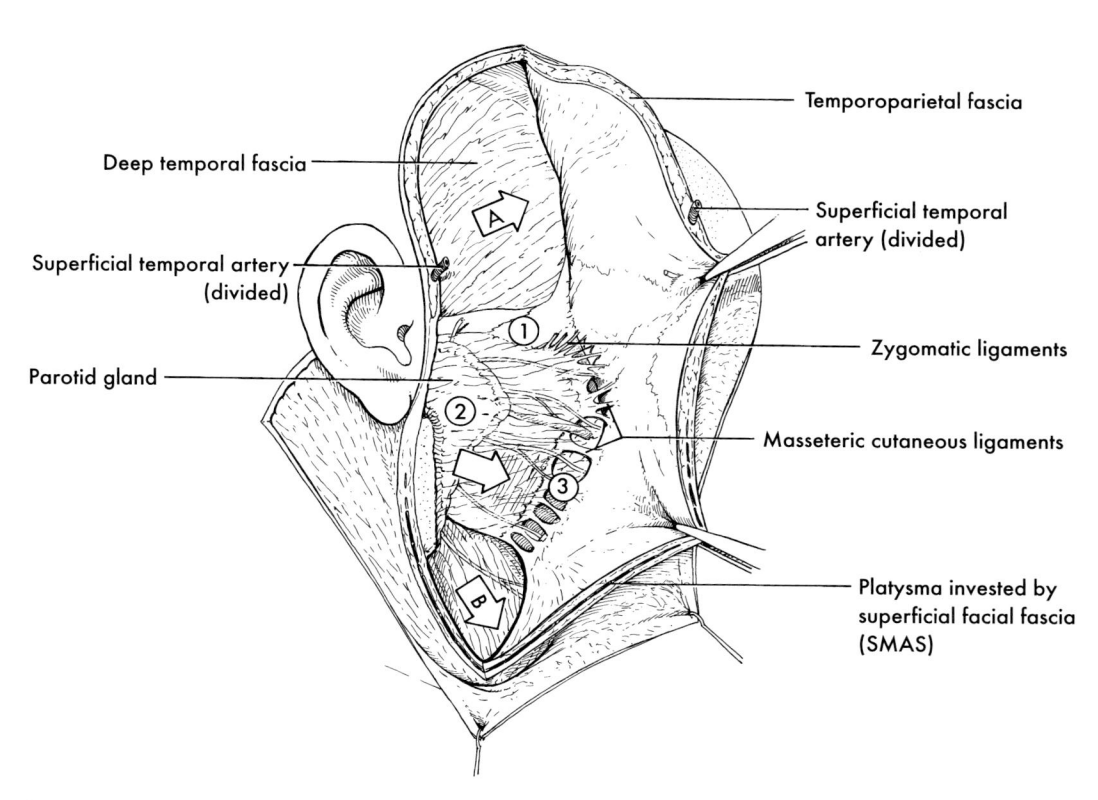

Two types of relationships exist between the superficial and deep facial fasciae. In some areas of the face, the superficial and deep fasciae are separated by an areolar plane: (A) in the temporal region between the temporoparietal and deep temporal fascias, (B) directly overlying the masseter muscle, and (C) deep to the platysma within the neck. In other locations within the face, the superficial and deep facial fasciae are densely adherent to one another. Examples of this fibrous adherence exist: (1) along the zygomatic arch, (2) overlying the parotid gland, and (3) along the anterior border of the masseter muscle. (From Stuzin JM, Baker HL, Gordon TJ: **Plast Reconstr Surg 89:441, 1992.** *Used by permission.)*

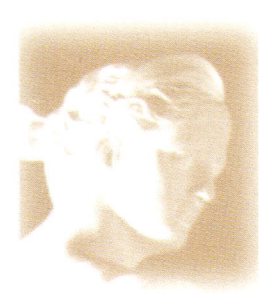

FACIAL NERVE

Facial nerve injury is the most feared complication of rhytidectomy. By understanding facial anatomy and proceeding with a careful anatomic dissection, the chance of facial nerve injury is greatly lessened.

The facial nerve is encompassed by the parotid gland in the lateral aspect of the face. Medially, it leaves the parotid to traverse along the superficial surface of the masseter muscle, lying immediately deep to the parotid-masseteric fascia, often covered by sub-SMAS fat. Medial to the masseter, the facial nerve overlies the buccal fat pad. The buccal fat pad, parotid duct, facial artery and vein, and facial nerve lie within the same anatomic plane within the cheek. As the facial nerve proceeds peripherally, it sends branches to the overlying mimetic muscles.

The frontal branch of the facial nerve is an anomaly. Unlike other nerve branches that lie deep to the deep facial fascia, *once the frontal branch crosses the zygomatic arch, it traverses the temporal region along the undersurface of the temporoparietal fascia and then peripherally penetrates this layer to innervate the frontalis muscle along its deep surface.* The temporal region, therefore, represents one area of facial anatomy where a complete violation of the SMAS layer can produce direct injury to a motor branch. For a motor branch injury to occur during undermining within the cheek during rhytidec-

RHYTIDECTOMY

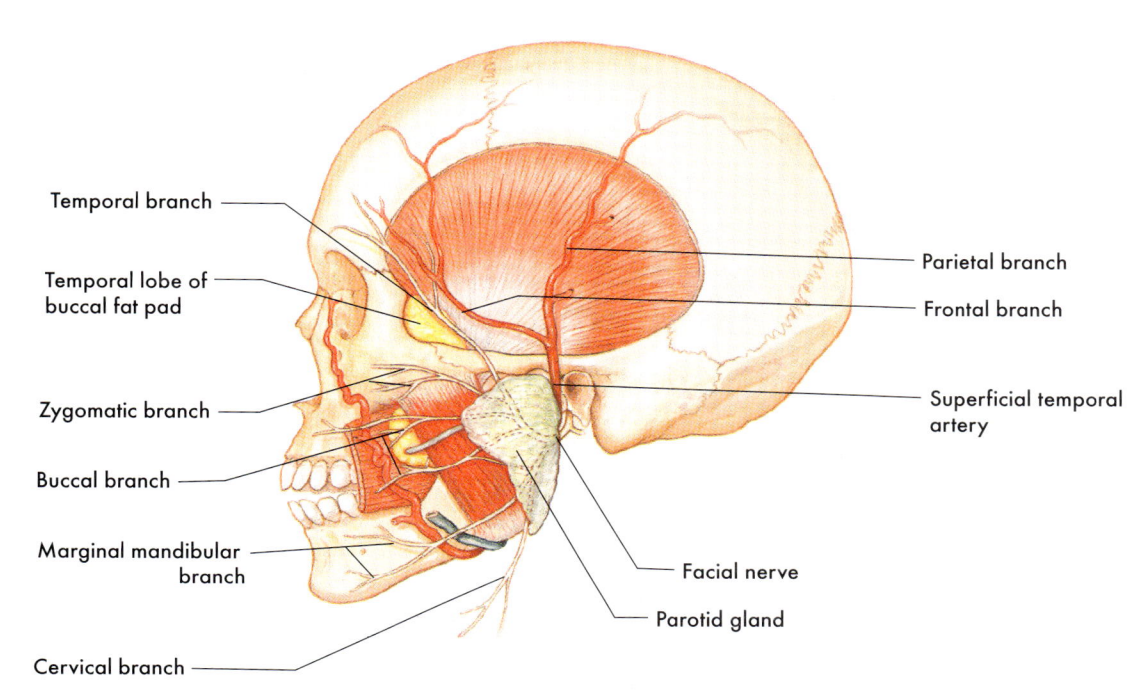

Laterally within the face, the facial nerve is encompassed by the parotid gland. After the facial nerve exits the parotid, it travels directly along the superficial surface of the masseter muscle. Anterior to the masseter, the facial nerve branches travel directly along the superficial surface of the buccal fat pad. The facial nerve, parotid duct, buccal fat pad, and facial artery and vein all lie within the same anatomic plane within the cheek.

tomy, the dissection must penetrate not only the SMAS but also the deep facial fascia. This is not the case when undermining within the temporal region. The more superficial location of the frontal branch as it traverses the temporal region places this motor nerve in a more precarious position for injury if the temporoparietal fascia is violated during dissection.

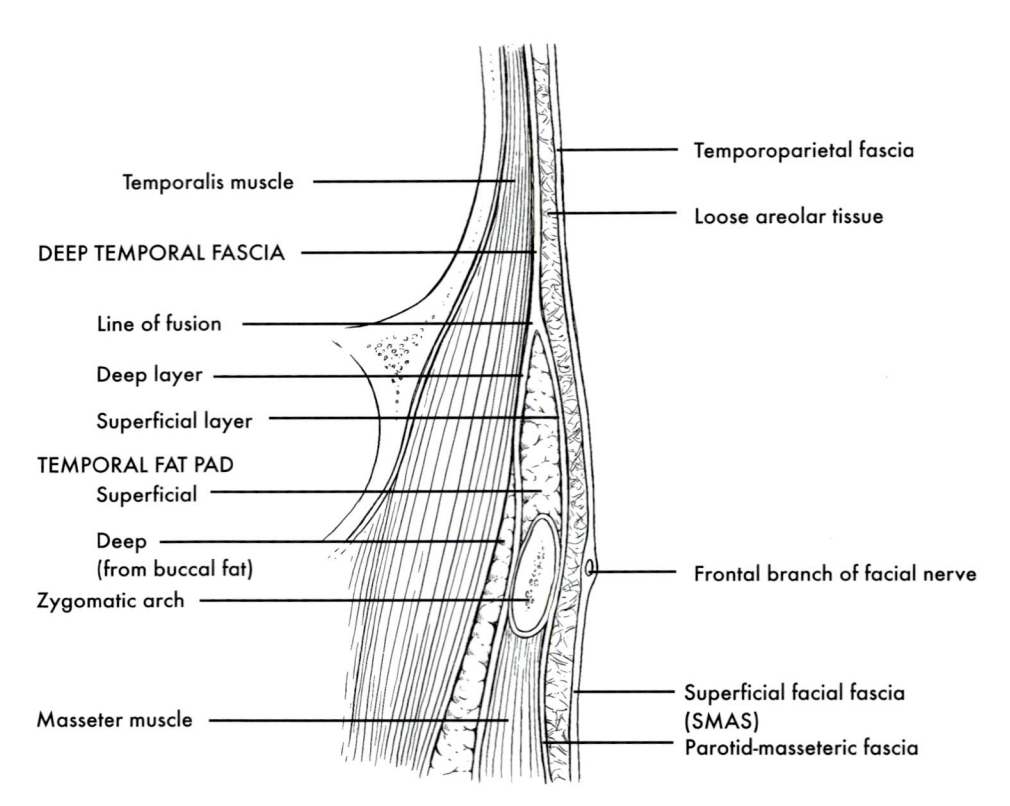

A cross-section of the temporal region demonstrates the continuation of the SMAS cephalad to the zygomatic arch where it is termed the temporoparietal fascia. Once the frontal branch of the facial nerve crosses the zygomatic arch, it runs along the undersurface of the temporoparietal fascia as it traverses the temporal region. In the region from the superior orbital rim to the zygomatic arch, the deep temporal fascia is separated into a superficial and deep layer by the superficial temporal fat pad, a structure that is separate and distinct from the underlying temporal extension of the buccal fat pad. (From Stuzin JM, et al: Plast Reconstr Surg 83:265, 1989. Used by permission.)

As an anatomic landmark, the frontal branch can be considered to travel along a line connecting the base of the tragus to a point 1.5 cm above the eyebrow. While single branching patterns exist, in some dissections as many as six nerve branches can be traced crossing the zygomatic arch. Despite the variety of branching patterns, these nerve fibers are always medial and inferior to the frontal branch of the superficial temporal artery. The frontal branch of the superficial temporal artery is easily palpated and therefore serves as a useful landmark in identifying the general path of the frontal branch during rhytidectomy.

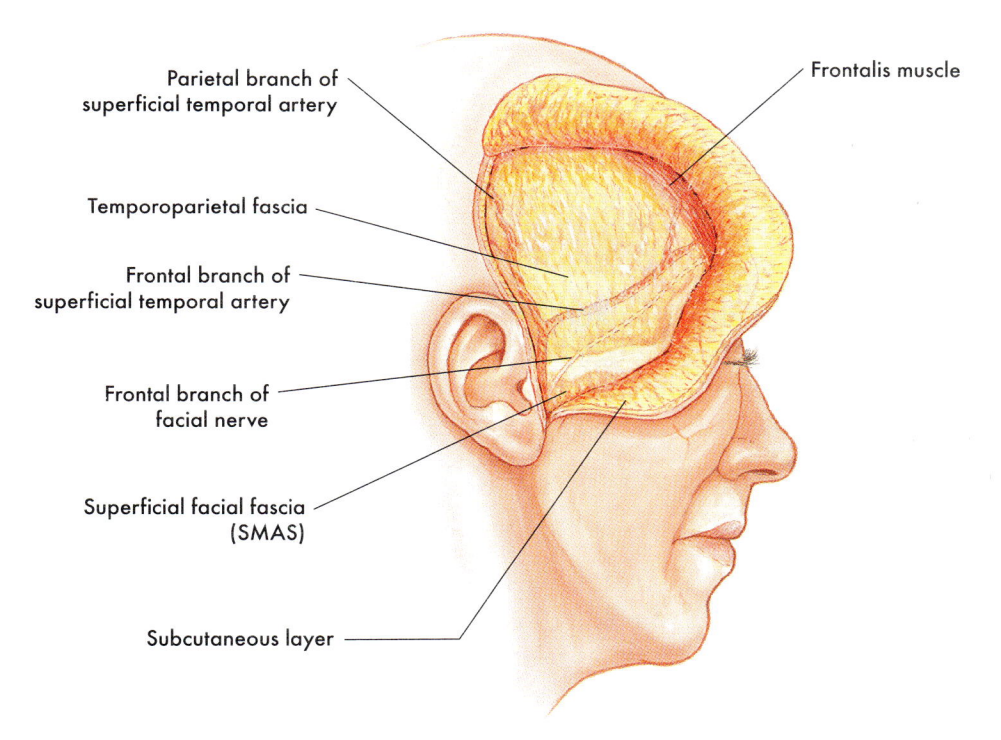

After the frontal branch crosses cephalad to the zygomatic arch, it lies directly along the undersurface of the temporoparietal fascia, usually invested by sub-SMAS fat. Peripherally, the frontal branch penetrates the investiture of the temporoparietal fascia and then innervates the frontalis muscle along its deep surface. The frontal branch of the superficial temporal artery is a useful landmark in facelifting. It is easily palpated and always lies superior and lateral to the frontal branch of the facial nerve. In general, the course of the frontal branch of the facial nerve traverses a line extending from the base of the tragus to a point 1.5 cm superior to the eyebrow.

The marginal mandibular nerve exits the parotid approximately 4 cm beneath the base of the earlobe near the angle of the mandible. In 81% of patients, this nerve will lie above the mandibular border. In 19% of patients, it will lie inferior to the mandibular border, though only in the region posterior to the facial vessels. The marginal mandibular nerve then crosses the facial artery and vein, and from this point anteriorly it runs superior to the mandibular border. Where the facial artery and vein cross the mandibular border is therefore a very useful landmark. These vessels can be palpated just anterior to the angle of the mandible, along the anterior masseter border, and serve as a quick method for localizing the marginal mandibular nerve. In this location, the nerve is superficial as it crosses over the facial vessels, and it is perhaps at this point that the marginal mandibular nerve is in greatest jeopardy. The important point to remember is that as long as subcutaneous dissection remains superficial to the SMAS and platysma, motor nerve injury will be prevented.

Although some regions of rhytidectomy dissection are danger areas, such as the area overlying the frontal branch or marginal mandibular nerve, dissection proceeds in other regions where no facial nerve branches exist. The lateral malar region overlying the zygomatic eminence is an example. The only nerve branches present within this area of the face are sensory branches. Anatomically, the lateral malar area represents a watershed between the frontal and zygomatic branches of the facial nerve and thus forms a safe region for surgical dissection.

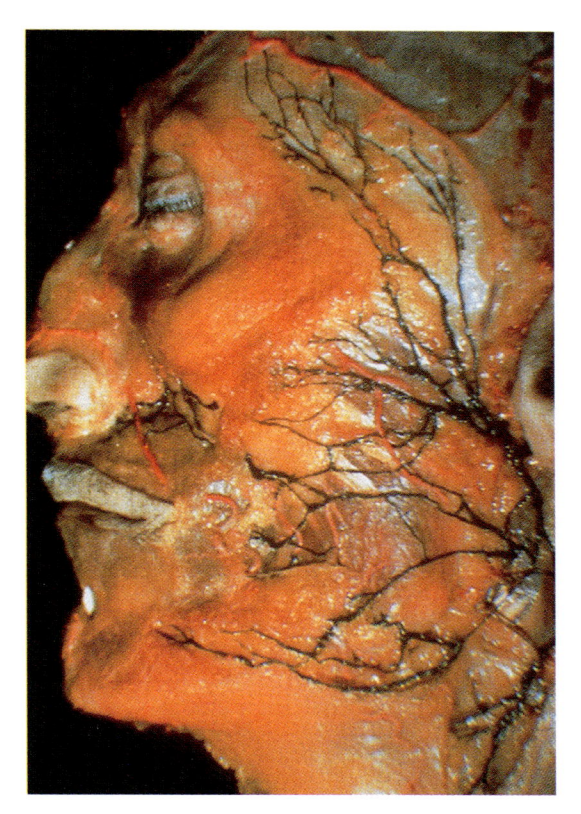

A photograph of a cadaver dissection of the facial nerve performed by Dr. Julia Terzis. Note that the area directly overlying the zygomatic buttress is devoid of motor branches and the only nerves present in this region of the face are sensory branches. For this reason, dissection in the malar area is quite safe, since the malar eminence represents a watershed between the frontal branches of the facial nerve lying superiorly and the zygomatic branches of the facial nerve that lie just inferior to the zygomatic buttress. (Courtesy of Dr. Julia Terzis, From Terzis JK, Daigle JP: Facial Nerve Reconstruction In Granick M, Hanna D, eds. Management of Salivary Gland Lesions, Baltimore, 1992, p. 251, Williams & Wilkins.

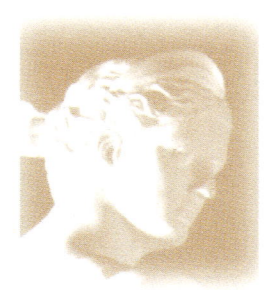

RETAINING LIGAMENTS

Facial skin is held over bony prominences by retaining ligaments, which run from deep, fixed facial structures to the overlying dermis. In performing cadaver dissection, it appears that two types of retaining ligaments exist. First, the true osteocutaneous ligaments are a series of fibrous bands that run from periosteum to dermis. The zygomatic and mandibular ligaments are examples of these structures.

A second system of supporting ligaments is formed by the coalescences between the superficial and deep facial fasciae in certain regions of the face (parotid cutaneous ligaments, masseteric cutaneous ligaments). These fascial connections, which fixate both superficial and deep fascia to underlying fixed structures such as the parotid gland and masseter muscle, similarly lend support against gravitational forces through fibrous septa that extend into dermis.

The zygomatic ligaments originate from the periosteum of the malar region. These ligaments exist as a series of fibrous septa that begin laterally in the region where the zygomatic arch joins the body of the zygoma. Similar fibers are observed overlying the malar eminence. particularly stout ligament is noted to originate along the most medial portion of the zygoma, medial to the zygomaticus minor muscle. The fibers making up the zygomatic ligaments extend through the malar pad (McGregor's patch) and insert into the overlying malar skin. The zygomatic ligaments fixate the malar pad to the underlying zygomatic eminence.

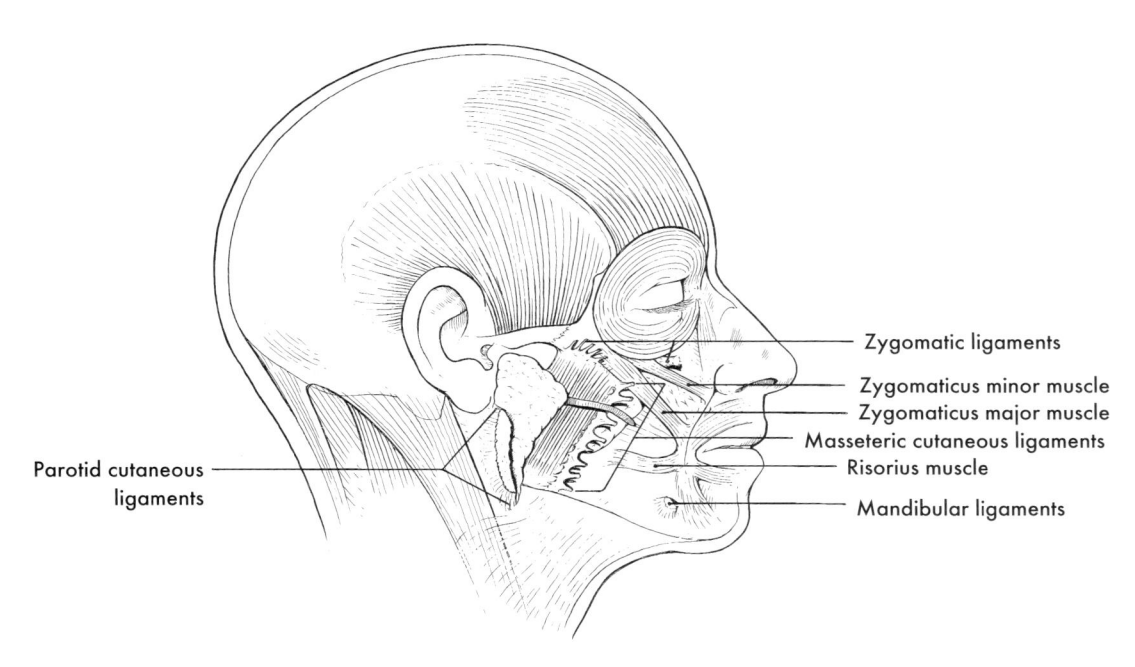

Facial soft tissue is maintained in a normal anatomic location by a series of supporting ligaments. The zygomatic and mandibular ligaments are examples of osteocutaneous ligaments that originate from periosteum and insert directly into dermis. The masseteric cutaneous and parotid cutaneous ligaments are formed as a coalescence between the superficial and deep facial fasciae. Rather than originating from periosteum, these ligaments originate from relatively fixed facial structures such as the parotid gland and the anterior border of the masseter muscle. Attenuation of support from the retaining ligaments is responsible for many of the stigmata seen in the aging face. (From Stuzin JM, Baker HL, Gordon TJ: **Plast Reconstr Surg** *89:441, 1992. Used by permission.)*

The mandibular ligaments are identified in the parasymphysial region of the mandible and extend from bone into the overlying skin. The mandibular ligaments tend to be the most discrete of the retaining ligaments, forming a series of stout fibrous bands that securely fixate the parasymphysial dermis to the underlying mandible. These ligaments also percolate through the chin pad to help support the chin superiorly to the underlying mandibular symphysis.

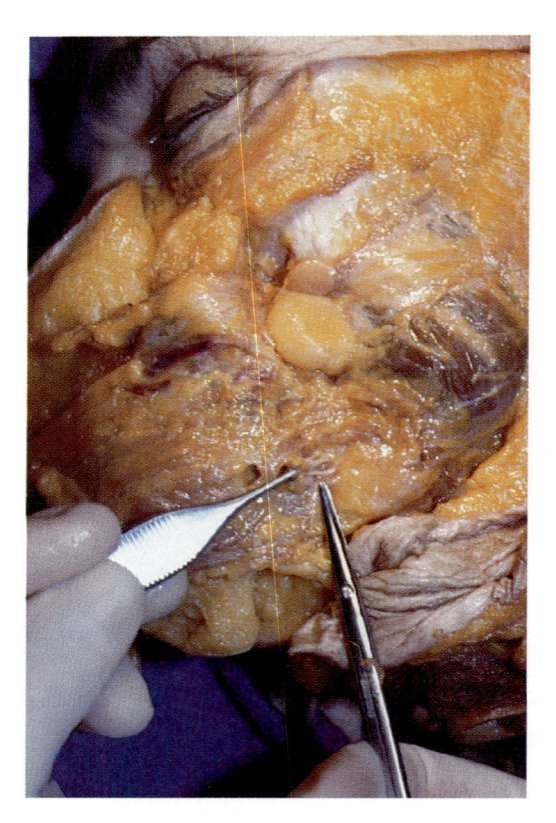

Cadaver dissection illustrating the mandibular ligaments that lie in the parasymphysial region of the mandible just lateral to the chin pad. The mandibular ligaments are the thickest and most discrete fibers identified among the retaining ligaments of the face. The mandibular ligaments firmly bind the parasymphysial skin to the underlying mandibular border.

RHYTIDECTOMY

Support of the soft tissues of the medial cheek is provided by a series of fibrous that extend along the entire anterior border of the masseter. These fibers are easily demonstrated in sub-SMAS dissection. Once the SMAS is elevated anterior to the parotid, an areolar plane exists between the superficial and deep facial fascia extending from the anterior border of the parotid to the anterior border of the masseter. On reaching the anterior border of the masseter, a series of fibrous

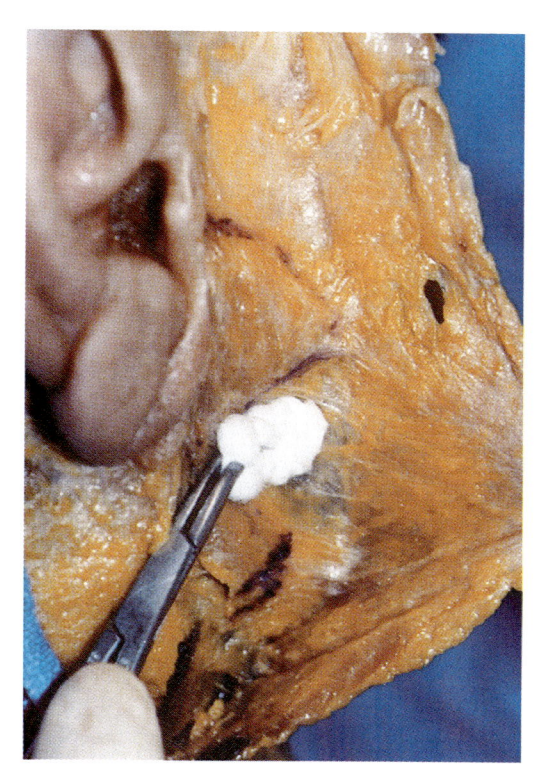

Cadaver dissection following SMAS and platysma elevation in the cheek that exposes the underlying parotid gland (the anterior border of which is marked in ink). Anterior to the parotid, an areolar relationship is encountered directly overlying the masseter muscle between the superficial and deep facial fascia. The surgical significance of this relationship is that a large portion of sub-SMAS dissection can be performed in the cheek using blunt dissection, in an area where there is little protection for the underlying facial nerve branches. This areolar plane extends from the anterior border of the parotid all the way to the anterior border of the masseter muscle, where the fibers of the masseteric cutaneous ligament are identified.

bands are identified along the entire length of the masseter beginning in the malar region and extending inferiorly to the mandibular border. These fibers represent a coalescence between superficial and deep fascia, extending from the masseter muscle vertically to insert into the overlying dermis. The fibers of the so-called masseteric cutaneous ligaments support the soft tissue of the medial cheek superiorly over the mandibular body.

In summary, there appear to be two systems of retaining ligaments supporting facial soft tissue in a superior position. The first are the true osteocutaneous ligaments, which are fibrous structures running from bone through the facial soft tissue to insert into the overlying dermis. The second system is formed by a coalescence between the superficial and deeper facial fasciae, fixating facial skin to underlying structures such as the parotid gland and masseter muscle. These ligaments tend to be finer than the osteocutaneous ligaments, and they function similarly to support facial soft tissues in their normal anatomic position.

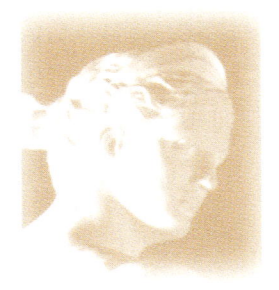

PAROTID DUCT AND BUCCAL FAT PAD

The parotid duct leaves the parotid gland on the upper third of the gland along a line extending from the tragus to the oral commissure. The parotid duct always lies deep to the parotid-masseteric fascia. After leaving the parotid, the duct travels over the superficial surface of the masseter muscle, then penetrates the buccal fat pad, buccinator, and buccal mucosa opposite the second maxillary molar. A large buccal branch of the facial nerve is commonly seen paralleling the course of the parotid duct.

The buccal fat pad can be visualized during rhytidectomy dissection anterior to the masseter muscle. A large structure, the buccal fat pad is commonly described as consisting of four segments: (1) the buccal portion, (2) the body of the fat pad, (3) the pterygoid portion, and (4) the temporal portion. During rhytidectomy, it is the buccal portion of the fat pad that is encountered within the cheek. It is important to remember that the buccal fat pad, along with the parotid duct and facial nerve branches, lie within the same anatomic plane, deep to the parotid-masseteric fascia. The buccal branches of the facial nerve travel along the superficial surface of the buccal fat pad as they course toward the mimetic muscles.

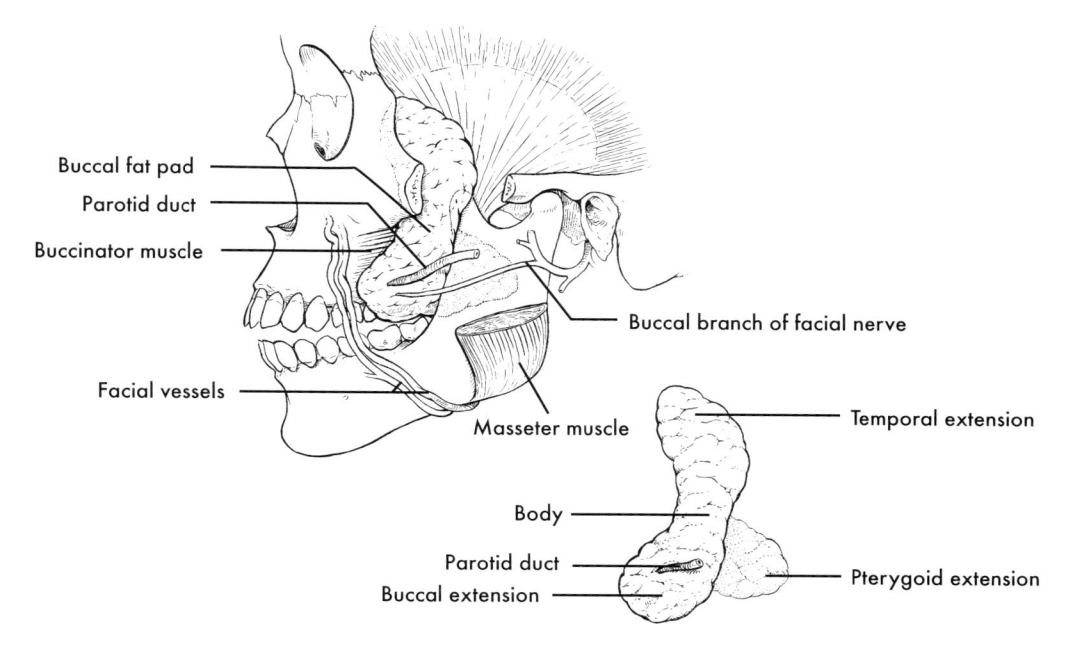

The buccal fat pad represents a specialized form of facial fat that lines the masticatory space and is similar to orbital fat in appearance and consistency. The buccal fat pad has been described as consisting of four portions: (1) the body, (2) buccal extension, (3) pterygoid extension, and (4) temporal extension. To expose the buccal fat pad in sub-SMAS dissection requires division of the masseteric cutaneous ligaments that run along the entire anterior border of the masseter muscle. If these ligaments are divided superiorly, in the region where the masseteric cutaneous ligaments join the zygomatic ligaments of the malar region, this will expose the body of the buccal fat pad (which lies superior to the parotid duct). If the masseteric cutaneous ligaments are divided more inferiorly, inferior to the parotid duct, this will expose the buccal extension of the fat pad. It is important to remember that the facial nerve branches always lie along the superficial surface of the buccal fat pad within the cheek. (From Stuzin JM, et al: **Plast Reconstr Surg 85:29, 1990.** *Used by permission.)*

If buccal fat is to be removed during sub-SMAS dissection, it can be approached by continuing the dissection to the anterior masseter border and then bluntly spreading through the fibers of the masseteric cutaneous ligament until buccal fat is encountered. Since the facial nerve overlies buccal fat within the cheek, a blunt spreading technique is preferable when harvesting buccal fat through a sub-SMAS approach.

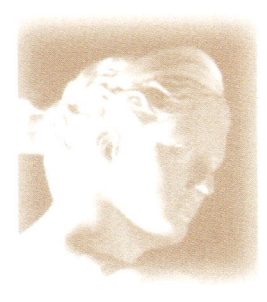

GREAT AURICULAR NERVE

The great auricular nerve is a superficial structure commonly encountered during undermining of the cervicofacial flap. A sensory nerve derived from the cervical plexus, it provides sensation to the earlobe and lateral portion of the cheek.

The great auricular nerve runs obliquely from the posterior belly of the sternocleidomastoid to the earlobe. The classic landmark for this structure is that it can be found crossing the midbelly of the sternocleidomastoid muscle 6.5 cm inferior to the external auditory canal.

To prevent injury to the great auricular nerve during undermining, it is not necessary to actually identify this structure. Rather, the key to prevention of injury is to identify the proper fascial plane of undermining, similar to what was discussed in prevention of facial nerve injury. Although it is customary to think of the superficial cervical fascia (SMAS) as being intimately associated with the platysma in the neck, this superficial fascial layer also continues laterally within the neck to overlie both the sternocleidomastoid and trapezius. The great auricular nerve traverses the lateral neck deep to this lateral extension of the superficial cervical fascia. As long as the subcutaneous undermining is continued within the lateral neck above the superficial cervical fascia, that is within the subcutaneous plane, the great auricular nerve

RHYTIDECTOMY

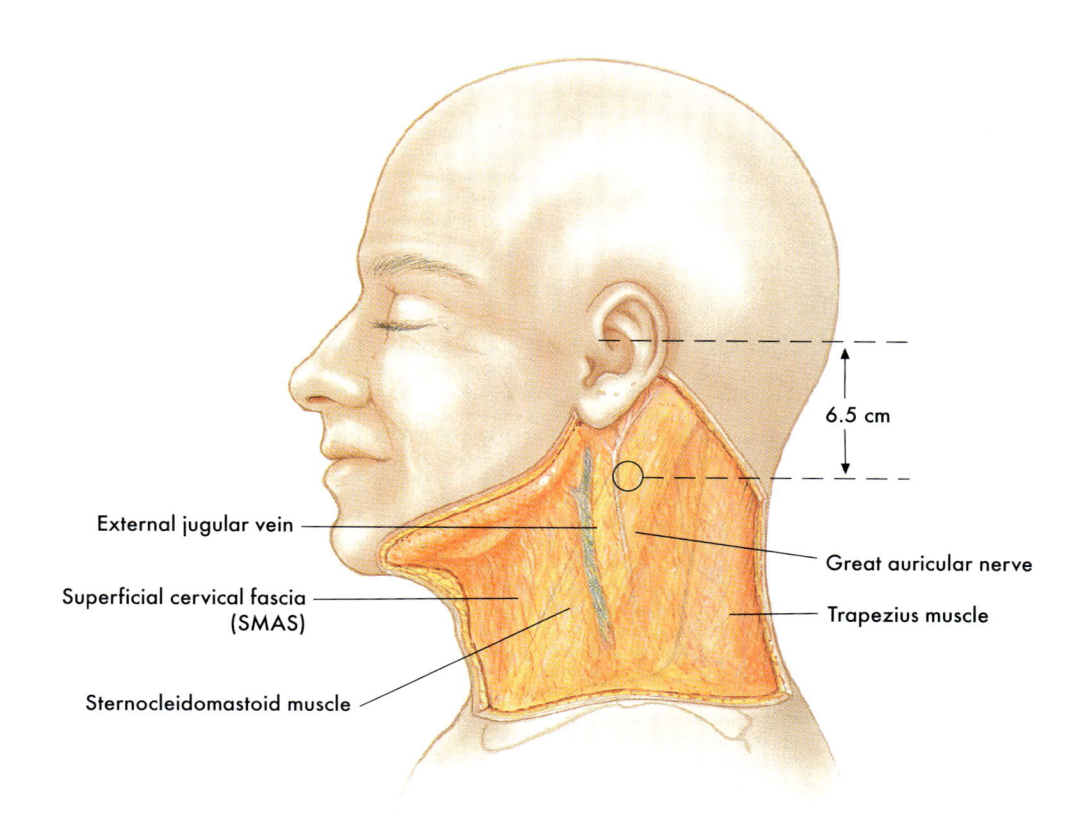

The great auricular nerve can be identified crossing the midbelly of the sternocleidomastoid muscle 6.5 cm inferior to the external auditory canal. As it traverses the cervical region, the great auricular nerve always lies deep to the superficial cervical fascia (SMAS). As long as the dissection is carried subcutaneously in the region overlying the sternocleidomastoid muscle, injury to this sensory nerve will be prevented.

will not be injured. The most common area of injury is at the most peripheral aspect of the subcutaneous undermining where the nerve crosses the posterior border of the sternocleidomastoid muscle. Attention to the proper depth of undermining, ensuring that no muscle fibers of the sternocleidomastoid are being exposed in this portion of the dissection, is important in preventing nerve injury.

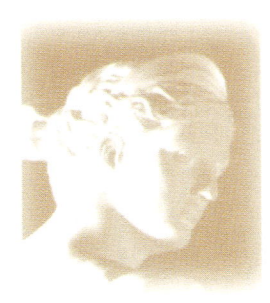

ANATOMIC CHANGES OCCURRING WITH AGING

The structures composing facial soft tissue may be arranged in layers, but they relate to one another anatomically to form a cohesive working structure, producing facial movement while providing resistance to gravitational change. Precise knowledge of the anatomic relationships between these layers is prerequisite to understanding the changes of the aging face and planning for their correction through rhytidectomy.

The retaining ligaments of the face support the facial soft tissue in normal anatomic location. As stated earlier, two types of ligamentous support exist. The attenuation of this ligamentous system, accompanied by dermal elastosis, results in the stigmata of the aging face.

The importance of the zygomatic ligaments lies in their ability to suspend malar soft tissue over the zygomatic eminence. With aging, attenuation of malar support is commonly seen, leading to the inferior migration of malar soft tissue. This soft tissue ptosis occurs adjacent to the line of muscular fixation along the nasolabial fold. It is not that the fold deepens with aging, but rather malar soft tissue lateral to the nasolabial line accumulates, accounting for fold prominence in the aging face. Attempts at diminishing the prominent nasolabial fold therefore should be directed at a restoration of malar support and repositioning of malar soft tissue in its previous position.

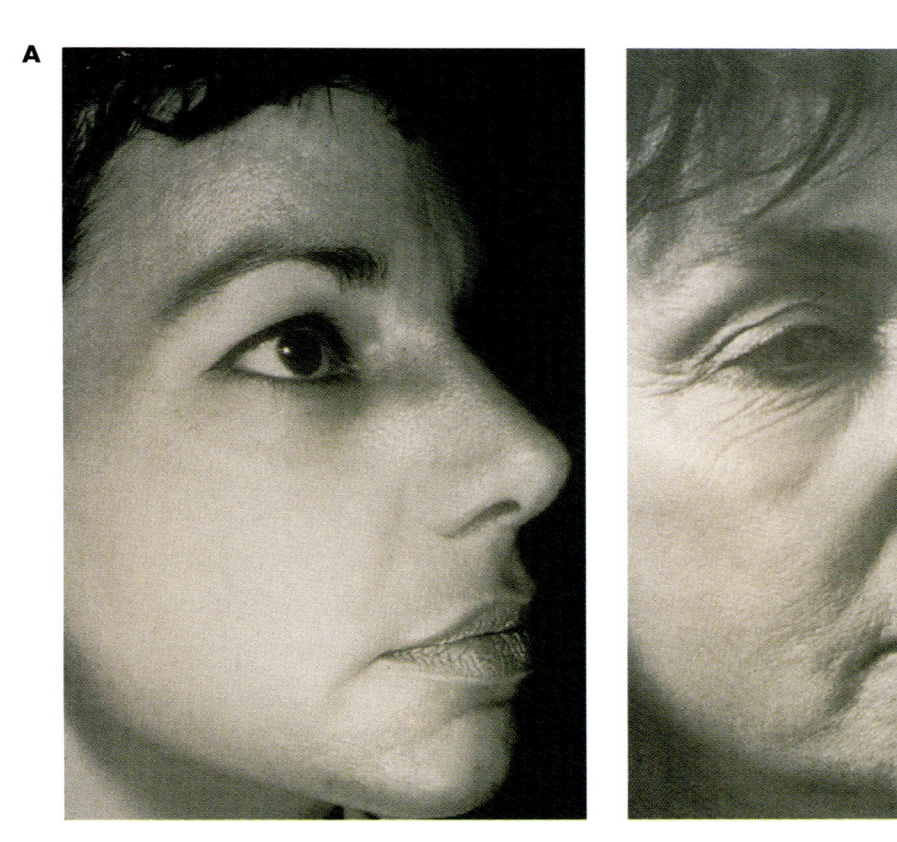

A, Patient seen at age 26, following full-face chemical peel. B, Same patient at age 57. Attenuation of the zygomatic ligamentous support suspending the malar pad and medial cheek has led to an inferior migration of these soft tissues adjacent to the line of muscular fixation of the nasolabial fold. It is not that the fold deepens with aging, but rather that an accumulation of malar soft tissue lateral to the nasolabial line accounts for fold prominence in the aging face. (A and B from Stuzin JM, Baker HL, Gordon TJ: **Plast Reconstr Surg** *89:441, 1992. Used by permission.)*

The fibers of the masseteric cutaneous ligament originate along the anterior border of the masseter, extend vertically through the platysma and subcutaneous fat, and insert into the dermis of the cheek. The importance of these fibers lies in their supporting the soft tissue of the cheek superiorly above the mandibular border. In our opinion, attenuation of support from the masseteric cutaneous ligament leads to migration of cheek soft tissue to below the mandibular border, and is largely responsible for the formation of jowls in the elderly person. If one examines the patient with prominent jowling, it is apparent that the jowl complex has anatomically constant borders. Anteriorly, the jowl is bordered by the tethering mandibular ligaments, while posteriorly the jowl complex is located along the anterior border of the masseter. Attempts at diminishing the prominent jowl should therefore be directed at restoring cheek support and repositioning the soft tissue forming the jowl complex superiorly above the mandibular border.

A and B, Attenuation of support from the masseter cutaneous ligaments allows the soft tissues of the medial cheek to descend inferiorly in the aging face, leading to the formation of the facial jowl. Because of the anatomic relationships of the retaining ligaments, the jowl has anatomically constant borders. Anteriorly, the jowl is bordered by the tethering mandibular ligaments, while posteriorly the jowl complex is positioned along the anterior border of the masseter. (From Stuzin JM, Baker HL, Gordon TJ: **Plast Reconstr Surg 89:441, 1992. Used by permission.***)*

RHYTIDECTOMY

183

A

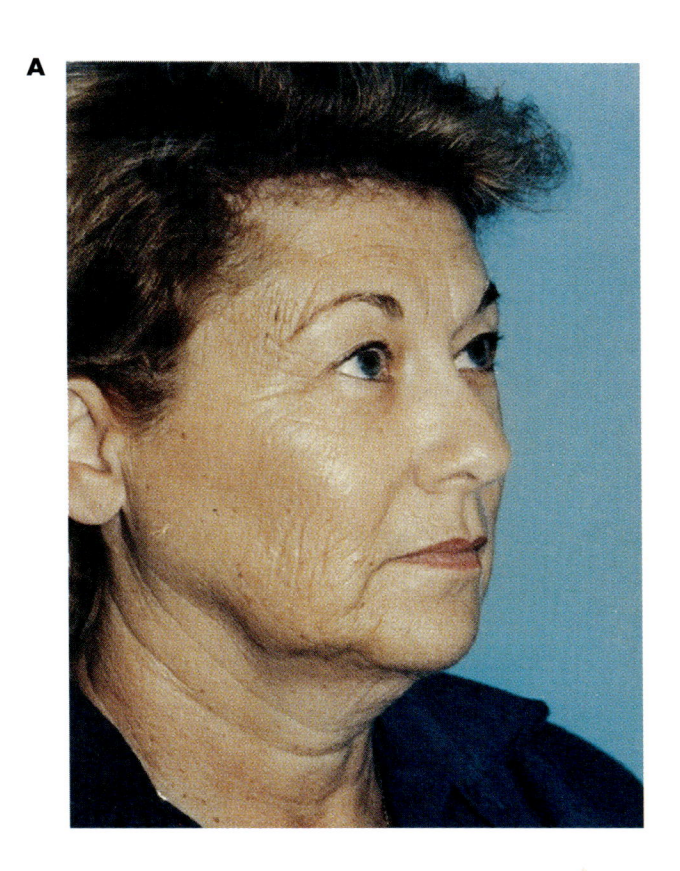

B

Masseteric cutaneous ligaments

Mandibular ligaments

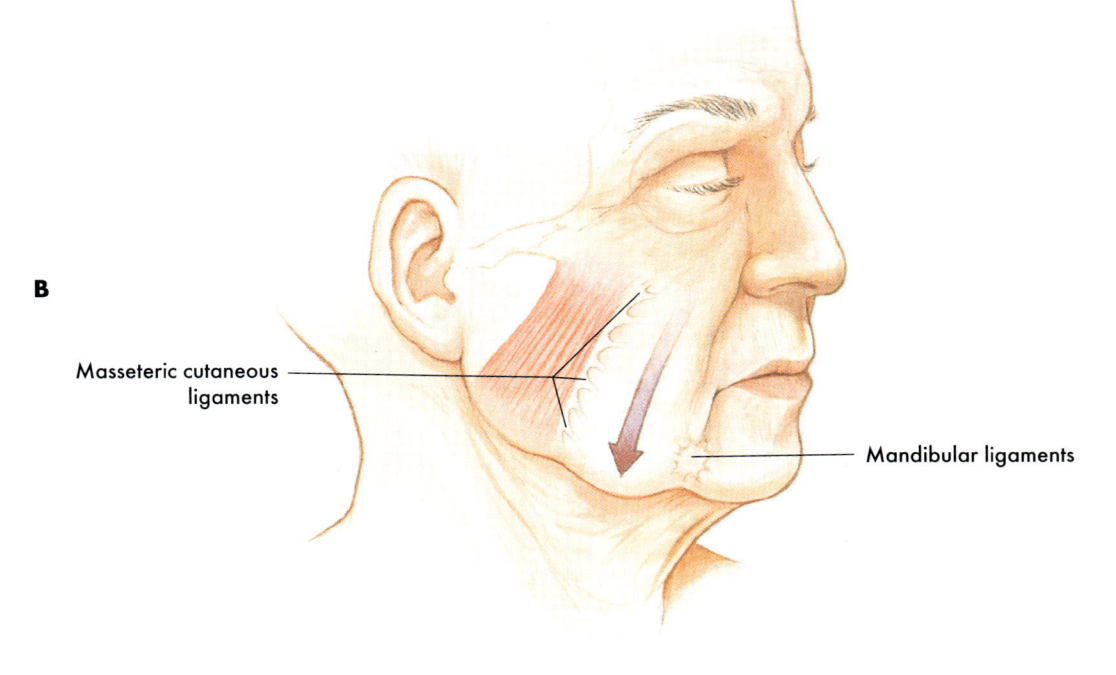

To summarize, aging is not only "skin-deep"; it also involves the deeper facial soft tissues. Attenuation of support from retaining ligaments, dermal elastosis, and facial lipodystrophy are the three main components that must be addressed to reconstruct the changes seen with aging. In general, the dermal aspects of aging are addressed through redraping of the skin flap in rhytidectomy. Obviously, lipodystrophy, which commonly occurs in the submental and cervical regions of the face and can also involve the jowls and nasolabial folds, must also be addressed through the contouring of fat. To address the problems of attenuation of support from the retaining ligaments, some form of deep layer support is mandated, usually involving SMAS-platysma contouring.

Cervical Obliquity and Platysma Bands

Similar to the retaining ligaments within the face, retaining ligaments exist within the neck and tightly hold the platysma to the underlying floor of the mouth and thyroid cartilage. These fibers are apparent along the caudal mandibular border, run throughout the fibrous subplatysmal fat that lines the submental triangle, and extend from the hyoid and superior aspect of the thyroid cartilage into the overlying platysma. This arrangement serves to hold the platysma tightly to the underlying deep cervical fascia and accounts for the acute cervicomental angle commonly associated with a youthful appearance.

As aging proceeds, cervical support for the platysma becomes attenuated. The anterior edges of the muscle descend inferiorly, accounting for the prominence of platysma bands in the aging face. As the muscle slips from its cervical support and descends inferiorly, the obliquity imparted to the neck blunts the normally acute cervicomental angle. Muscular hypertrophy, as well as shortening of the bowstringed platysma, also adds to band prominence in the aging face. Attempts at improving platysma banding and cervical obliquity must therefore cen-

Retaining ligaments

Subplatysmal fat

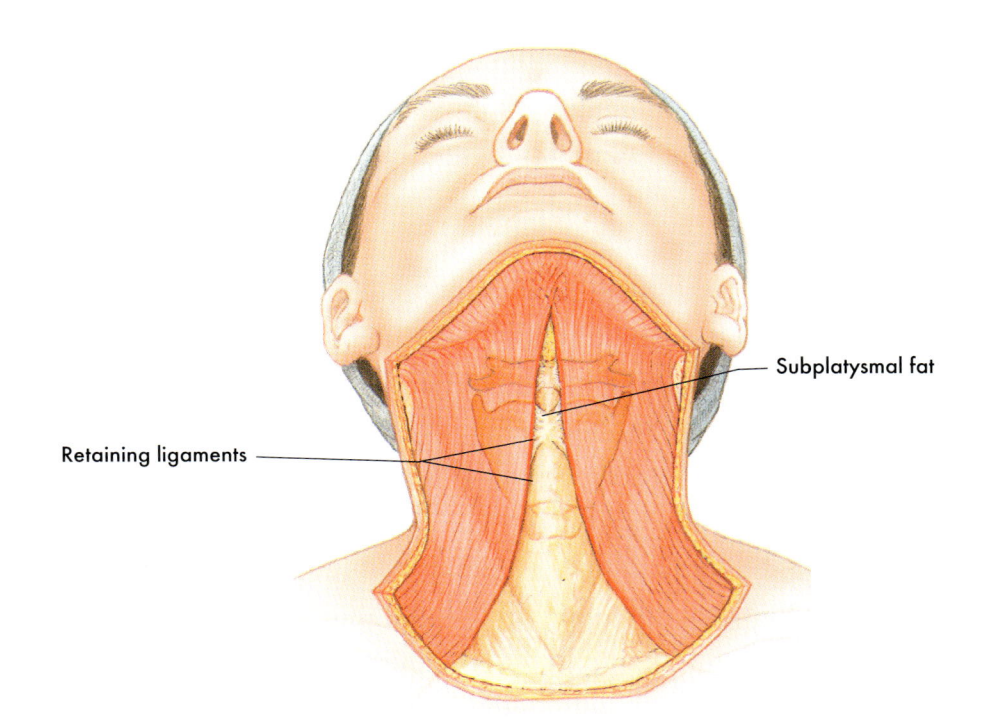

The platysma in the neck is supported in its normal anatomic position against the deep cervical fascia by a series of retaining ligaments. These fibrous bands can be identified running from the caudal border of the mandibular symphysis and extending through the fibrous submental fat as far inferiorly as the hyoid and superior surface of the thyroid cartilage. These retaining ligaments hold the young platysma tight against the floor of the mouth and adherent to the underlying thyroid cartilage. As this retaining ligament system becomes attenuated in the aging person, it allows the platysma to descend inferiorly into the neck, accounting for what is visualized as cervical obliquity and platysma banding.

ter around restoring the platysma to its normal anatomic location and contour. Any tethering within the platysma that has occurred from the muscle residing in a bowstringed position over time must also be dealt with through some form of transection myotomy to release and lengthen the muscle.

Anatomic Basis of SMAS Dissection

The anatomic relationship between the SMAS, platysma, and parotid-masseteric fascia is a subject of controversy. Much of the variation in findings can be resolved with an understanding of the investiture of the superficial mimetic muscles by the SMAS. Instead of descriptions of the SMAS lying either superficial or deep to the platysma, we believe that the superficial fascia is present along both surfaces of this muscle. The investiture of the platysma by the SMAS forms a single anatomic unit that can be dissected in continuity to form a substantial myofascial flap, which is the keystone of SMAS technique in rhytidectomy.

The anatomic relationship that exists between the superficial and deep fascia allows for extensive SMAS mobilization with little jeopardy to the facial nerve as long as this relationship is understood and maintained during the dissection. Laterally, the SMAS is densely adherent to the underlying investing parotid fascia and requires sharp dissection for elevation in this region. These attachments must be completely divided during SMAS elevation to obtain adequate flap mobility.

Once the SMAS is mobilized anterior to the gland, an areolar plane exists overlying the masseter muscle. The SMAS can be rapidly elevated using blunt technique from the anterior border of the parotid as far forward as the anterior border of the masseter, where the fibrous septa of the masseteric cutaneous ligament are encountered. As long as the underlying parotid-masseteric fascia is not violated during this dissection, facial nerve injury remains an impossibility.

Continuing the SMAS dissection into the malar region must involve a change of dissection plane to preserve the facial nerve. Since the zygomaticus major and minor are innervated segmentally along their deep surfaces, carrying the dissection deep to the elevators of the upper lip might result in motor nerve injury. For this reason, on reaching the zygomatic major, the preferred dissection plane is along the superficial surface of the muscle. Elevation of the thin fascia investing the superficial surface of the zygomaticus muscles, along with the overlying fibrous malar fat, produces a substantial flap that can be used in restoring contour to the malar region and improving the nasolabial fold. As long as malar dissection remains superficial to the elevators of the upper lip, motor nerve injury will not occur.

The degree of required SMAS mobilization will vary from patient to patient. Traction on this layer as it is mobilized, while observing the effect of contouring on various regions of the face, serves as a useful guide to the amount of SMAS dissection required.

SUMMARY

The goals in rhytidectomy are to rejuvenate and improve facial appearance. To obtain consistent results, facelifting should be approached not just as a tightening or lifting procedure but as a reconstructive procedure. The primary goal in rhytidectomy is reconstructing the anatomic changes that occur with aging. It is axiomatic that understanding facial soft tissue anatomy and the anatomic changes of aging is prerequisite to successful rhytidectomy.

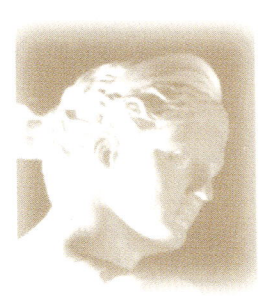

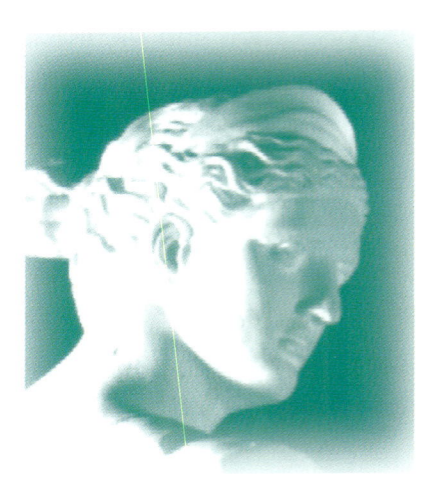

B

Preoperative Evaluation and Surgical Planning

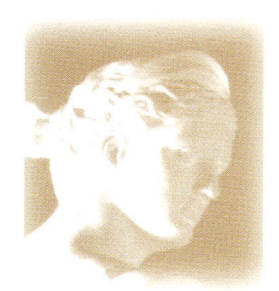

PATIENT EVALUATION

A suitable candidate for rhytidectomy should have some of the following physical characteristics: slack facial and eyelid skin, ptosis of the eyebrow, platysmal bands, jowls, or relaxed nasolabial folds. All patients undergoing this elective procedure should be in good health to minimize surgical risk. The preoperative psychological screening of candidates for rhytidectomy is covered in Chapter 1. Physical considerations include the following:

1. Preexisting scars as a result of trauma or surgery.
2. Systemic diseases such as diabetes, angina, hypertension, or Raynaud's phenomenon.

3. Actinic skin damage from repeated exposure to the elements or to radiation.

In addition, the patient should have realistic expectations about the possible results of surgery.

Patient selection is probably the most critical factor when determining the success of a proposed aesthetic procedure. The plastic surgeon must be extremely alert to any indications that the patient has *unrealistic expectations*. Disappointment is almost certain if the patient expects the surgery to correct her personal problems. A patient who expects to look 20 or 25 years younger is not being realistic. Other warning signs include the following:

1. The patient brings in a photograph of himself/herself taken 20 to 25 years ago.
2. The patient is convinced that the surgical procedure will ensure a job promotion.
3. The patient believes that his/her marital problems will be solved.
4. A widow or widower that believes the operation will lead to finding a new mate.
5. The patient is obese or careless of his/her appearance and expects that the new face will make him/her chic.
6. The patient wants to undergo the procedure to please another person, such as a lover or a family member.
7. The patient really does not need the surgery but thinks he/she does.
8. The patient requires repeated preoperative visits; this indicates that he/she does not comprehend what is to take place or what is expected.

The essential point is that if the patient's goals and expectations are realistic, they are most likely psychologically prepared for the procedure. If not, the best decision is to not proceed with the surgery.

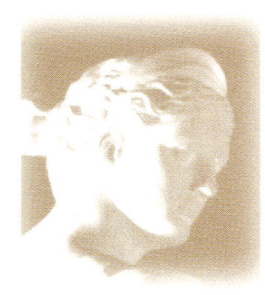

PREOPERATIVE VISIT

In addition to the initial consultation, the prospective facelift patient should be seen a few days before surgery. At that time the surgeon can review the entire operative plan and the patient can specifically outline her desires and expectations for the operative results. The patient who requests several preoperative visits should be carefully screened; this patient may not be listening to the explanations being given and may be difficult to manage postoperatively. It is our policy to ask the patient to state her specific expectations for surgery in order of priority. For example, if the neck is the patient's primary concern, that is noted. The same is true for the nasolabial folds, upper and lower eyelids, or jowls. The overall plan is discussed in complete detail for clarification of all the patient's questions.

Because the term *facelift* is familiar to the public and commonly used, it is helpful to use this term when speaking of the operation with prospective patients. The initial discussion about the facelifting procedure should cover the following issues:

- Any preoperative procedures desired, specifically upper eyelids, lower eyelids, face, neck.
- The necessity for preoperative shampoo.
- Events to expect on arrival at the hospital or clinic.
- What the patient will experience in the operating room with reference to monitoring equipment, intravenous (IV) solutions, and so on.
- Whether the sedation level will be light or heavy.

- Additional medications that may be given.
- Length of time in the operating room.
- Type of bandage to be used.
- Length of time in the recovery room.
- Anticipated amount of postoperative discomfort.
- Postoperative position in bed.
- Time of the first postoperative shampoo.
- Expected amount of swelling.
- Time of suture removal.
- Length of convalescence.
- Possible problems experienced during the first 5 days after surgery.

We emphasize during the preoperative consultation that it will be approximately 10 days after the facelift before the patient is "socially acceptable." Following this period, the patient may return to work or resume other social activities, but will usually require covering makeup for a period of several days until all ecchymoses resolve. We emphasize to the patient that it takes about 3 weeks from surgery until covering makeup is no longer required, and that he/she will continue to see changes in the appearance of the result for approximately 3 months following surgery. We tell the patient that it is common for patients to become frustrated in the early postoperative period, because the events of wound healing do not always proceed as rapidly as the patient might desire. Recovery following a facelift requires time and patience, and it is our impression that the patient who is well informed of this preoperatively has a smoother course postoperatively.

SURGICAL REJUVENATION OF THE FACE

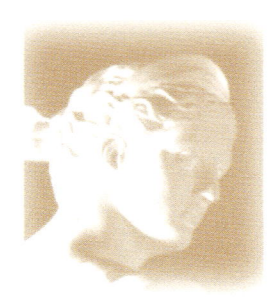

PREOPERATIVE EVALUATION

The specific problems the surgeon faces in performing a facelift can be divided into two categories: gravitational and intrinsic changes.

GRAVITATIONAL CHANGES	
Jowls	Ptosis
Nasolabial folds	Forehead lines
Sagging neck	Blepharochalasis
Drooping brows	Droopy nasal tip

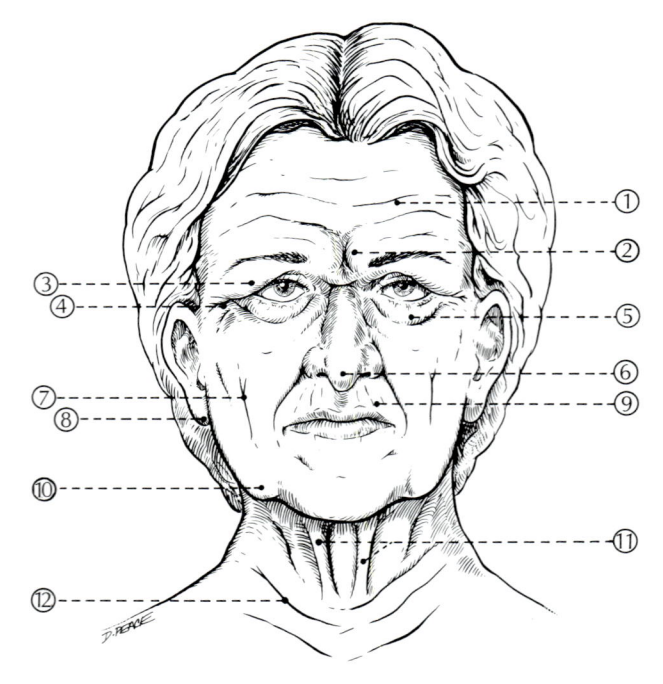

The stigmata of aging. Common findings include the following: (1) ptotic and wrinkled brow, (2) glabellar laxity and frown lines, (3) ptotic eyebrows, (4) periorbital folds and lids, (5) redundant lower eyelid skin, (6) droopy nasal tip, (7) laxity of cheeks, (8) ptotic earlobes, (9) perioral wrinkling, (10) jowls, (11) platysma bands, and (12) laxity of cervical skin. The possible combinations are infinite, and each patient must be carefully analyzed to formulate a treatment plan.

RHYTIDECTOMY

INTRINSIC CHANGES	
Loss of skin elasticity	Abnormal pigmentation
Fine epidermal lines	Epitheliomas and other associated lesions
Ultraviolet changes	Fat atrophy
Hyperkeratosis	

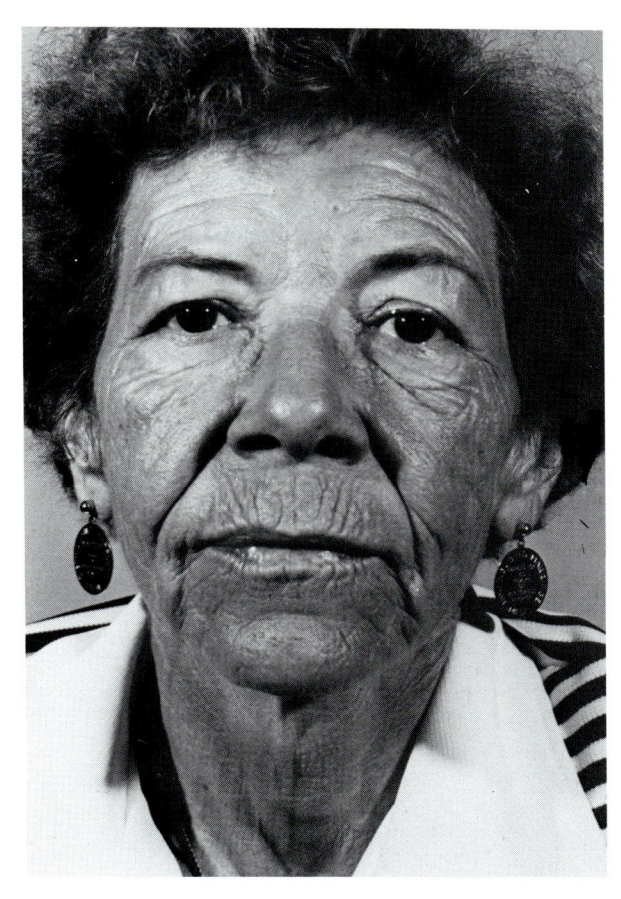

This patient demonstrates the advanced gravitational and degenerative changes shown in the artist's drawing.

We look at rhytidectomy as a reconstructive procedure, restoring facial soft tissue anatomy to a state before the degenerative effects of aging. To achieve a successful outcome, one must recognize the deformity that exists preoperatively and understand how to successfully correct the problem. Certain anatomic features bear special consideration at the time of preoperative evaluation.

Skin Quality and Elasticity

More than any other factors, skin quality and elasticity have perhaps the greatest influence on the outcome following rhytidectomy. Skin quality is influenced by the patient's heredity, age, extrinsic degeneration from actinic exposure, history of smoking, and previous weight gain and loss.

The quality of facial skin significantly influences postoperative results. Patients with severe elastosis secondary to aging and actinic damage simply do not maintain the results of rhytidectomy as long as patients with good-quality skin. Similarly, though improved following rhytidectomy, facial rhytides present preoperatively will usually remain following surgery and this must be emphasized to the patient during the preliminary consultation.

RHYTIDECTOMY

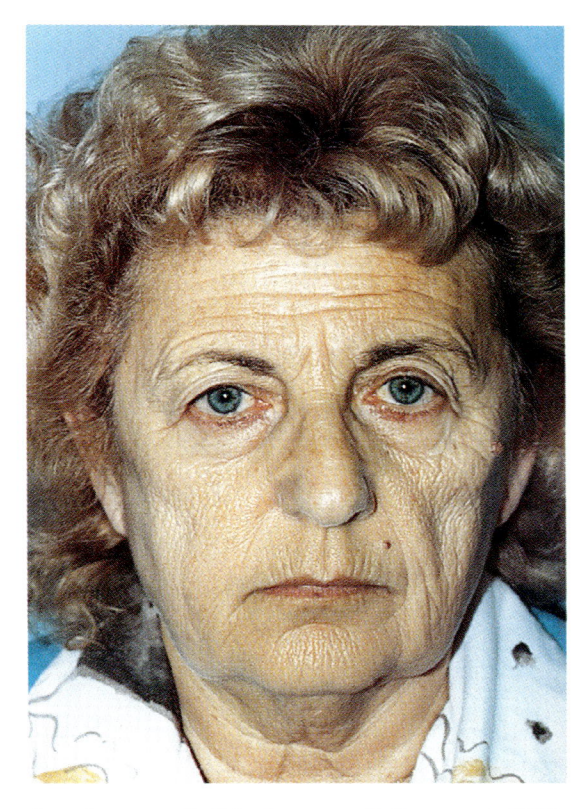

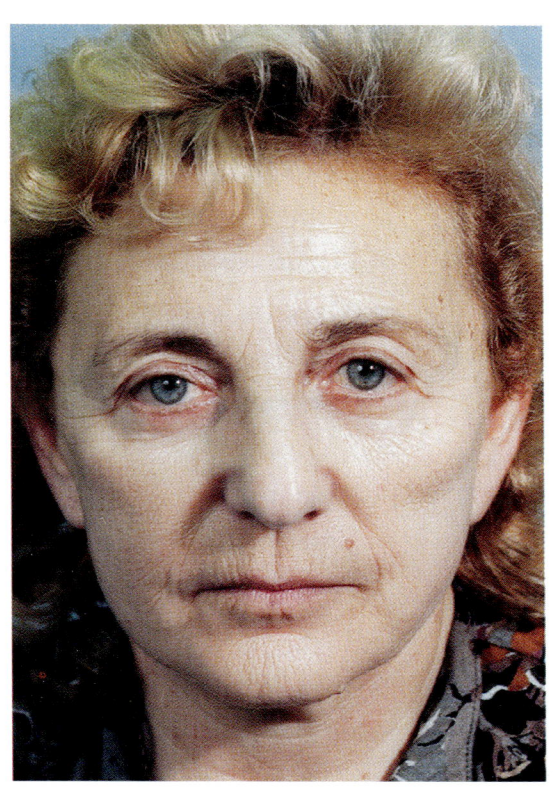

Sundamaged skin is one of the most difficult problems confronting the surgeon performing rhytidectomy. This patient is seen approximately 3 years following a primary facelift. Although wrinkles under stretch and tension are less apparent, inspection reveals that the dermal rhytides remain. Also, because of the significant degeneration of dermal collagen and elastic fibers following actinic exposure, the longevity of results in this type of patient is not as good as in the patient who presents without sun damage. A series of trichloroacetic acid peelings or a single phenol peel, done at a later date, will improve the results obtainable in patients with significant actinic damage.

Age

There is no doubt that it is easier to achieve superior results in younger facelift patients and the facelift is longer-lived compared with older patients. In general, the degenerative changes in the younger patient are less marked and skin elasticity is usually quite good. With less anatomic deformity present and better-quality soft tissue to work with, younger patients present less surgical challenge.

Patients presenting in their early forties often show only the first signs of aging (mild nasolabial folds, slight jowls, and slight fullness in the submental region). Nonetheless, these patients are usually delighted at their appearance following a fairly conservative facelift. We tell these patients that the change following rhytidectomy will not be dramatic, but will tend to produce a longer-lasting result. A facelift in the younger patient can be thought of as essentially maintenance: maintaining the current appearance while preventing the more accelerated changes of aging that commonly occur as the patient approaches the fifties.

The results in the older patient with severe degenerative changes are often dramatic. This patient requires a more aggressive approach and presents a greater surgical challenge. Interestingly, patient satisfaction is often less than that seen in younger patients despite a more dramatic improvement over the preoperative state. Although rhytidectomy will make these patients look better and more youthful, it is often impossible to make an older patient appear "young," and this is perhaps the source of discontent for some of these patients. Again, a thorough preoperative consultation is mandatory to inculcate realistic expectations in these patients. The longevity of the result is shorter in older patients and the time interval to secondary rhytidectomy is less.

Subcutaneous Fat Accumulation

Preoperative evaluation should focus on the presence of subcutaneous fat accumulation present within the face and neck. Frequently, the submental, submandibular, and occasionally the jowl areas of the face will have some degree of fatty accumulation that can be contoured to produce a more pleasing result. The presence of subplatysmal fat should also be evaluated preoperatively and can be carefully contoured during rhytidectomy if required. Much of the definition obtained along the jawline is secondary to proper contouring of the fat in the submental and submandibular region of the neck.

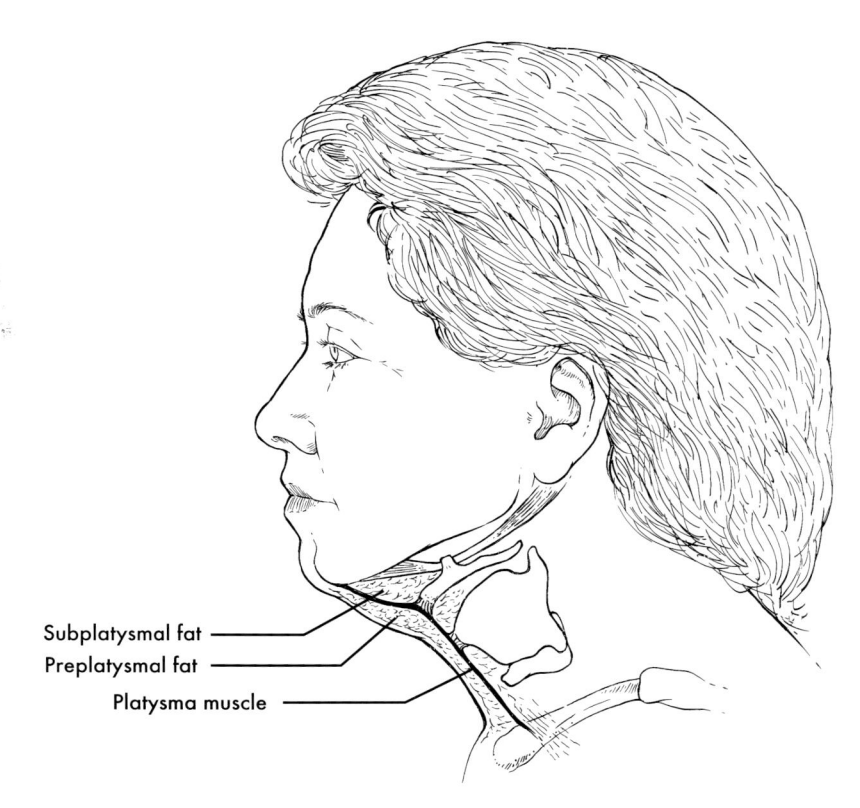

Diagram illustrating the division of neck fat into preplatysmal and subplatysmal compartments. While many patients require some contouring of preplatysmal fat in the submental region (extending from the mentum to the hyoid), it is uncommon, save in the fatty neck, that patients require removal of preplatysmal fat from the hyoid inferiorly toward the base of the neck. Preplatysmal fat in the lower neck should be preserved in most patients. The fat that lies deep to the platysma, within the submental triangle, tends to be more fibrous than preplatysmal fat and is well vascularized. Judicious contouring of subplatysmal fat allows the surgeon to contour the platysma tightly against the underlying deep cervical fascia and floor of the mouth, thereby deepening the cervicomental angle.

Deformities Developing From Attenuation of Deep Layer Support

Many of the deformities seen in the aging face involve more than just degenerative changes within facial skin. The formation of jowls, deep nasolabial folds, and platysma bands have a common theme in that their evolution in the aging face has largely to do with the loss of support from the retaining ligaments of the face and neck (see discussion of anatomy, above). These deformities are best addressed by restoring some type of deep layer support before facial skin redraping.

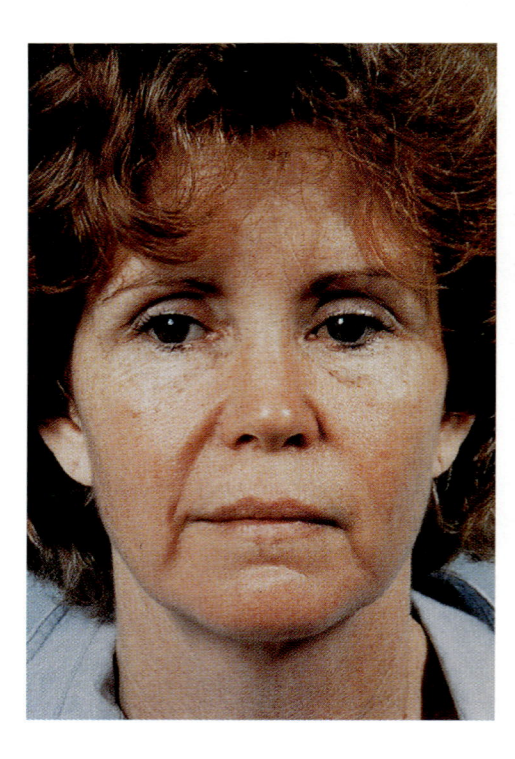

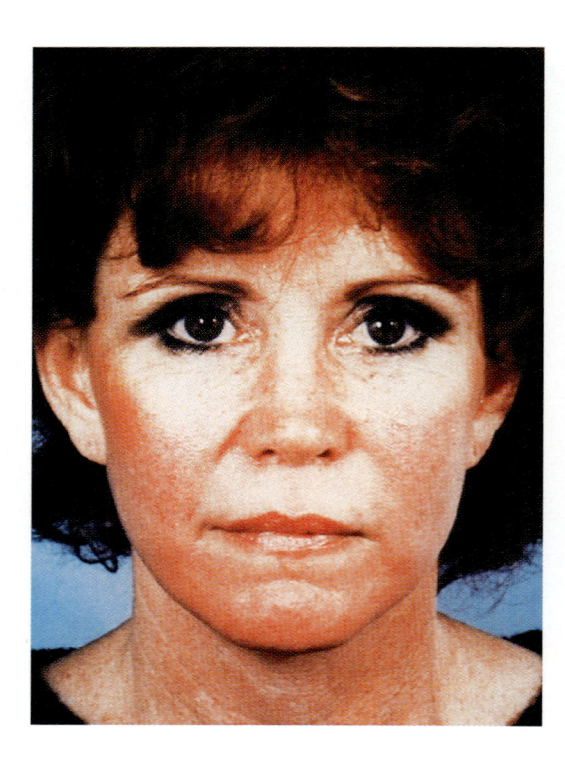

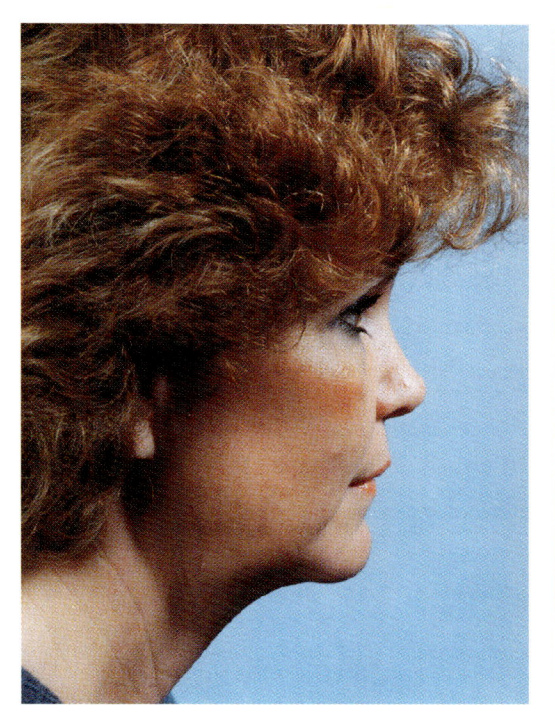

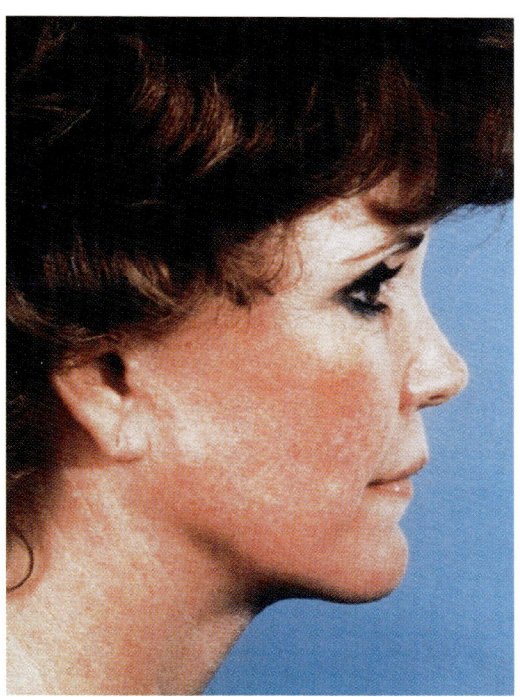

Attenuation of support from the retaining ligaments allows the descent of facial fat and platysma in the aging face, producing what is clinically noted as nasolabial folds, jowling, and cervical obliquity. This tends to blunt the facial contour and imparts a square appearance to the lower face. This patient is seen following extended SMAS dissection, as well as low platysma plication, which has been used to reelevate facial fat cephalad into the face and restore the musculofascial support of the neck. Deep layer support has produced a tapering of facial contour from cheeks to jawline, improving the nasolabial fold, jowl, jawline, and neck. No facial or cervical fat was removed.

■ Jowls

The presence of jowling represents an attenuation of support of the soft tissues of the medial cheek. The cheek soft tissues are largely supported in a superior position by the zygomatic and masseteric cutaneous ligaments. With aging, attenuation of this support can lead to the descent of soft tissues of the cheek (skin, subcutaneous fat, superficial facial fascia, and platysma) below the mandibular body, producing clinically what has been termed the *jowl complex*. An inferior migration of buccal fat can also occur if the deeper fascial support is lost, but, in our opinion, this is uncommon. Buccal fat removal tends to reduce facial fullness, but rarely does it improve a prominent jowl.

Jowling can be of varying degrees. Minor jowls are often improved simply by tightening facial skin. Large, heavy jowls require an aggressive mobilization and tightening of the SMAS, repositioning the ptotic facial soft tissues superiorly within the cheek.

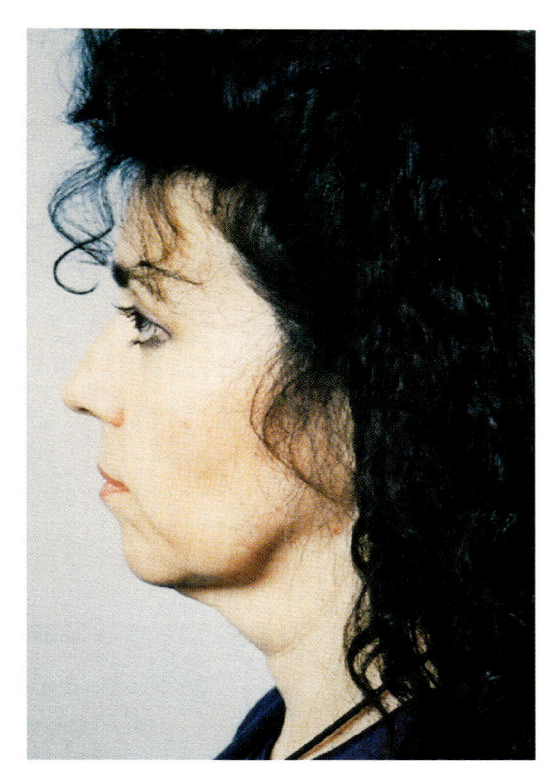

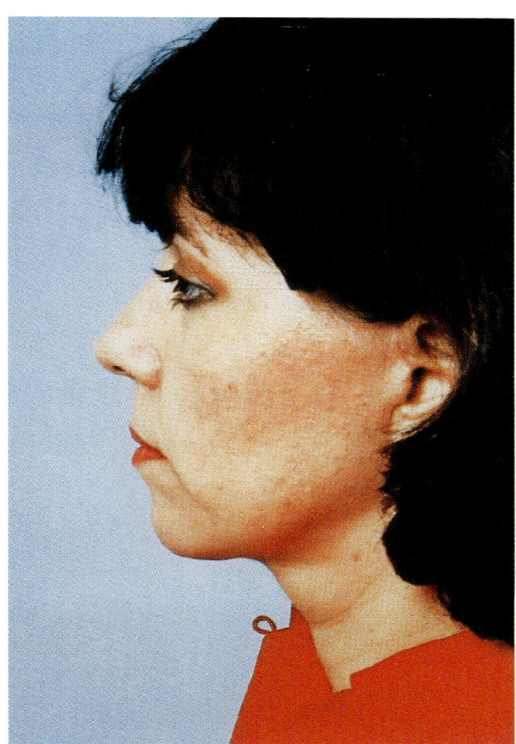

Facial jowling in the aging face is secondary to attenuation of support from the masseteric cutaneous ligament, allowing facial soft tissue to descend inferiorly below the mandibular border. In most patients, jowling can be improved through SMAS rotation. The improvement seen in this patient's postoperative result was obtained solely through resuspension of facial soft tissue. No facial fat was removed, though cervical fat was contoured.

■ Nasolabial Fold

The nasolabial fold is a normal anatomic structure that is essentially present in all persons. As people age, the fold becomes more prominent. This is secondary to many factors, including an inferior migration of both malar and cheek soft tissues lateral to the nasolabial fold. The prominent nasolabial fold should be addressed at the time of rhytidectomy. Although surgeons have attempted to suction the nasolabial fold to reduce its prominence, we have found this technique to produce little lasting improvement. As seen with the development of jowls in the aging face, in most patients the prominent nasolabial fold is not a problem of lipodystrophy, but rather a problem of attenuation of soft tissue support. The prominent nasolabial fold requires restoration of malar support to produce a lasting change in contour. In our experience, extending the cheek SMAS dissection into the malar region to restore malar support has been helpful in improving patients with prominent nasolabial folds.

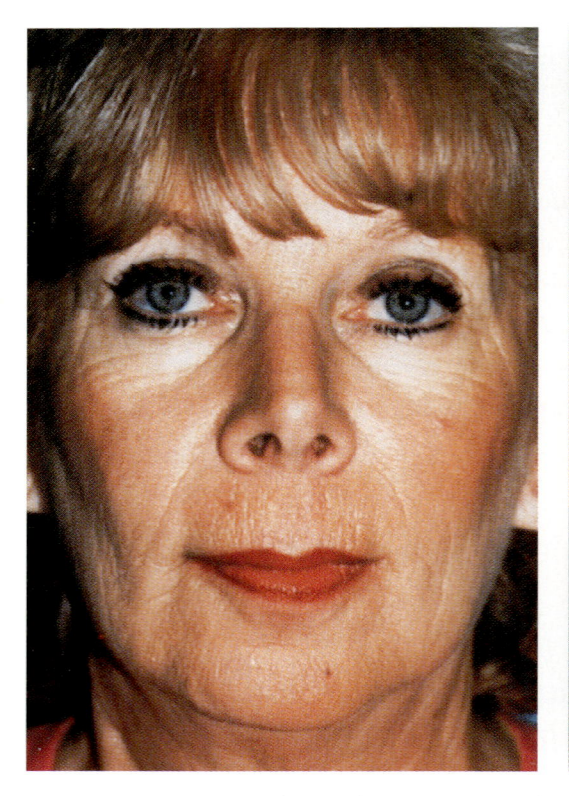

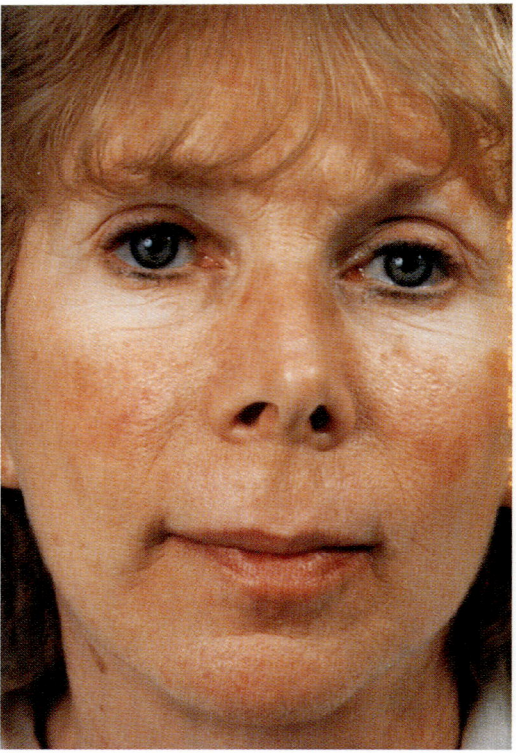

As support from the zygomatic ligaments becomes attenuated, malar fat descends inferiorly into the face, accounting for the prominence of the nasolabial fold and marionette lines. This patient is seen following extended SMAS dissection with reelevation of malar fat back upward over the zygomatic eminence.

Platysma Bands

The presence of platysma bands (bands along the medial edge of the muscle within the anterior neck) and an obtuse cervicomental angle commonly signify an attenuation of support between the platysma and the underlying deep cervical fascia. This is often associated with laxity of submental skin, as well as subcutaneous accumulation of fat within the neck. This loss of cervical support tends to highlight the platysma band, especially with animation. Evaluation of the patient both in repose and with grimacing is an important part of the preoperative evaluation in determining the extent of the problem.

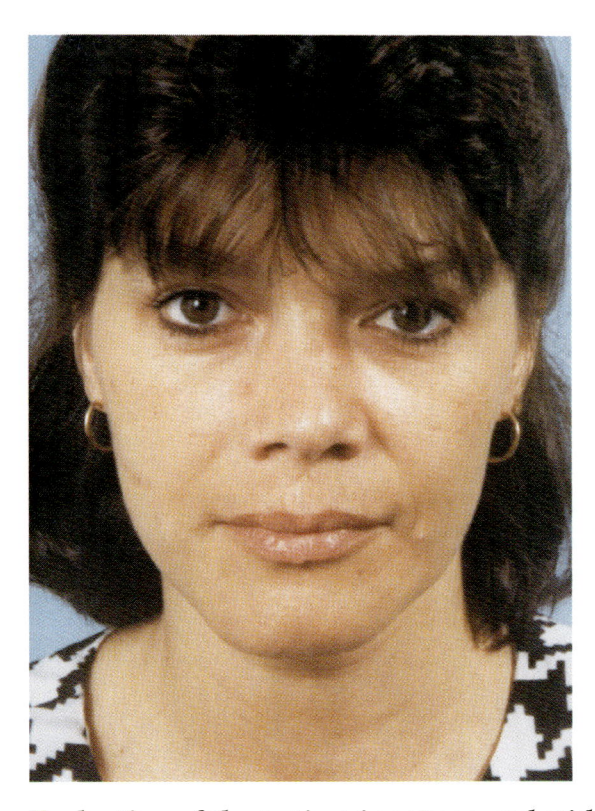

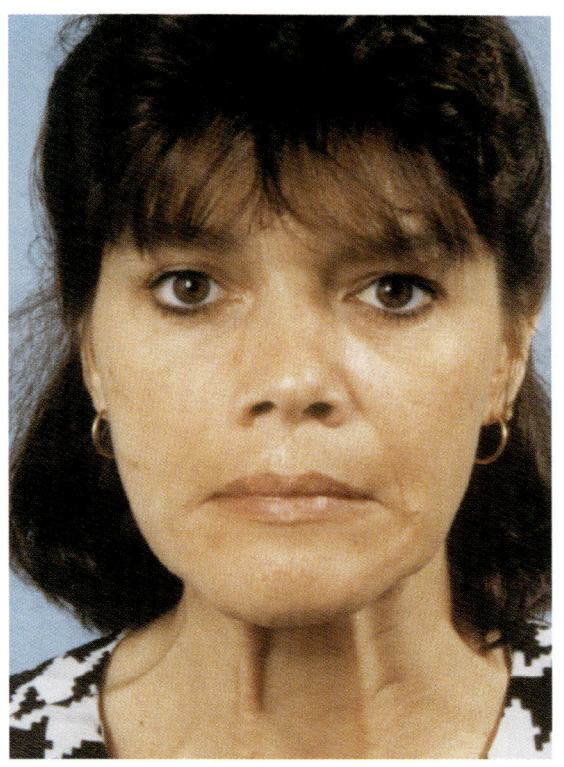

Evaluation of the patient in repose and with animation is important in determining platysma position. As the patient relaxes the platysma, the surgeon is better able to evaluate the location of this muscle at rest, which may be contributing to cervical obliquity. Note the wide separation of the medial borders of the muscle in this patient.

There is a good deal of individual variation in the anatomy of the platysma muscle within the submental region. Vistnes, in cadaver dissections, showed that the medial fibers of the platysma decussate across the midline in 61% of the cases, the decussation extending from the thyroid cartilage to the mandibular symphysis. In the other 39%, decussation was absent and the medial bands of the platysma continued parallel to one another toward their insertion in the mandible.

Cardosa De Castro, in his anatomic studies, observed three different types of platysma muscle configuration within the submental region. Most commonly (75%), a limited platysma decussation was noted extending 1 to 2 cm below the mandibular symphysis. In 15% of the cadavers, decussation of the platysma was noted from thyroid cartilage to mandibular border. In the remaining 10%, decussation of platysma did not occur.

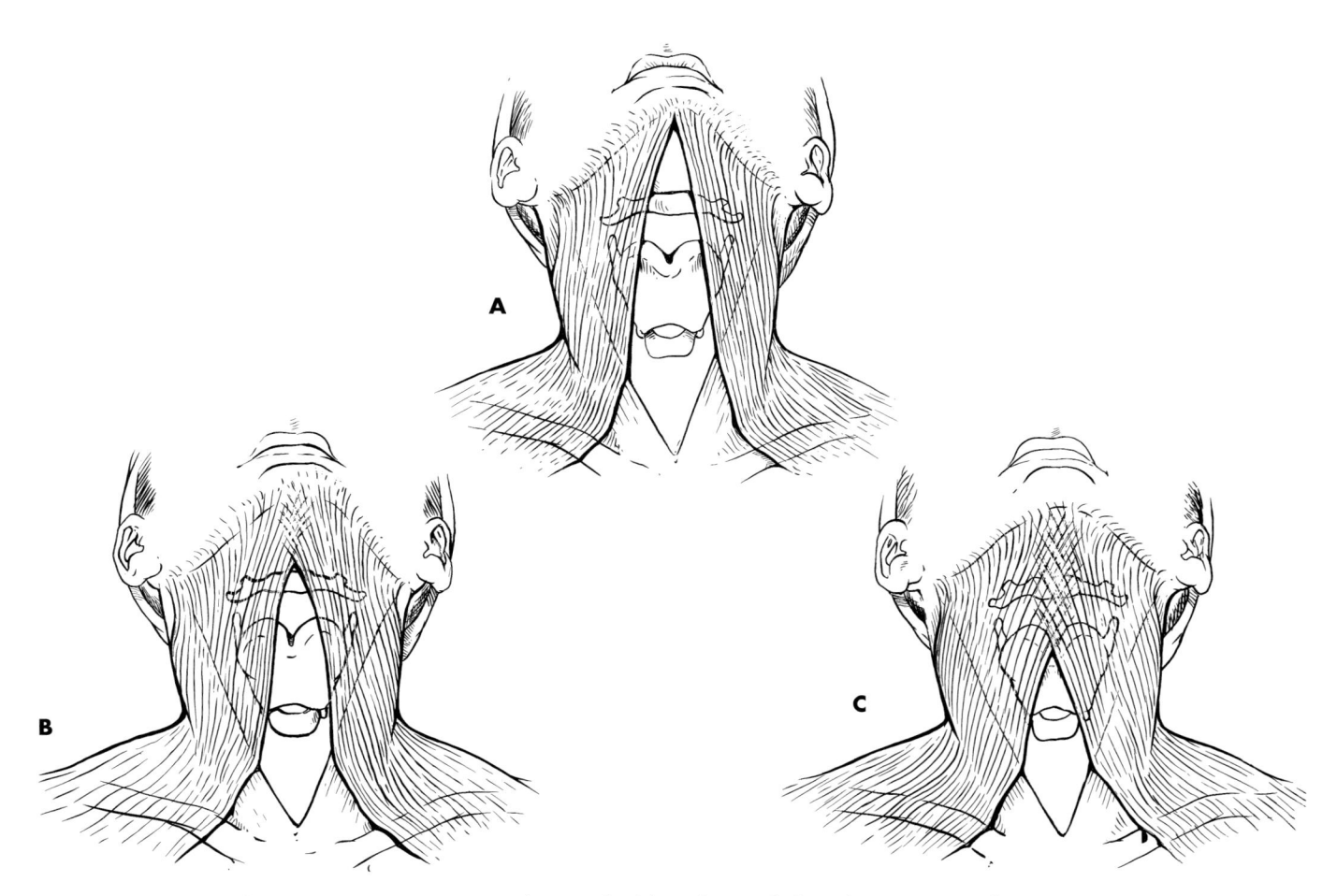

There are variations in the medial borders of the platysma. A shows a complete separation of the medial borders, whereas B and C show different degrees of decussation. Decussation of the platysma in the midline of the neck has little to do with the development of platysma bands as patients age, but rather only the position of the bands in the neck following their development.

It is our opinion, after operating on numerous patients with large platysma bands, that the presence or absence of bands has little to do with the problem of muscular decussation within the midline of the neck. We have noted large platysma bands in patients with complete muscular decussation and, conversely, have seen patients without any muscular decussation who did not exhibit clinical platysma bands. Obvious platysma banding suggests an attenuation of support retaining the platysma to the underlying deep cervical fascia, allowing the medial borders of the platysma to become visible and bowstring across the neck. Muscle hypertrophy and shortening of the muscle with animation also contribute to the presence of the platysma bands and cervical obliquity.

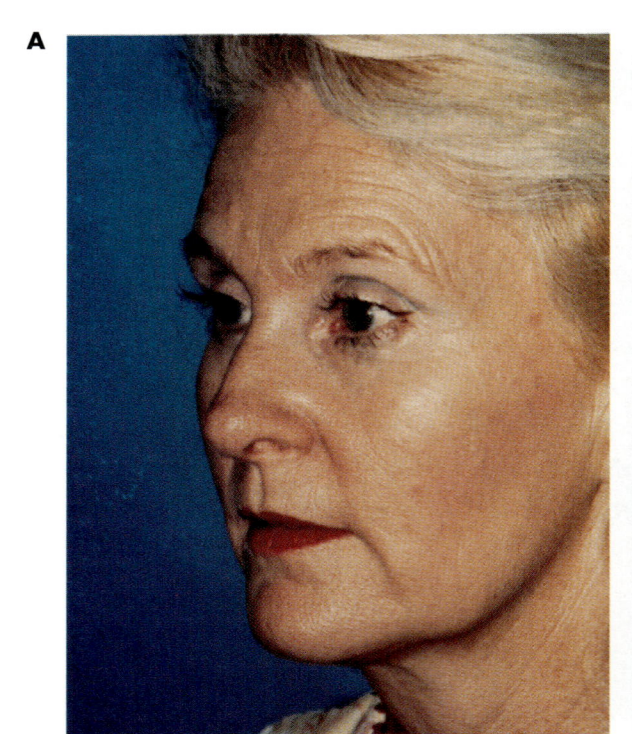

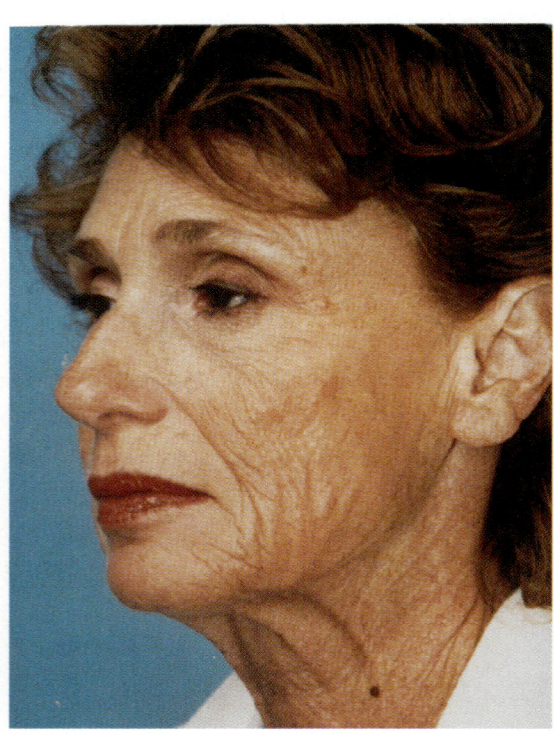

A, This patient is seen in her forties with the early signs of platysma banding. Typically, the earliest signs of platysma descent into the neck are in the region of the superior aspect of the thyroid cartilage and hyoid, accounting for short, flimsy platysma bands. B, This patient, seen in her sixties, has a more complete separation of the platysma muscle from the floor of the mouth and thyroid cartilage, which accounts for the lengthy band.

RHYTIDECTOMY

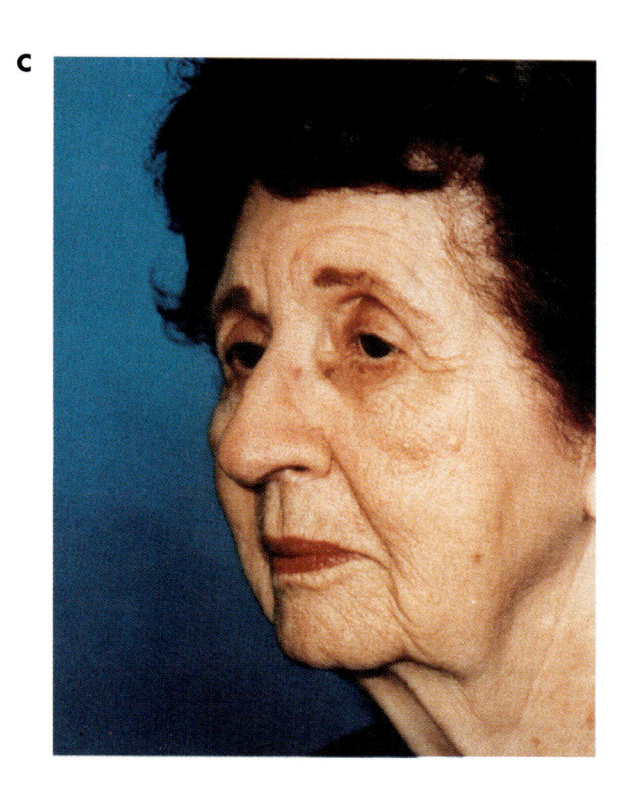

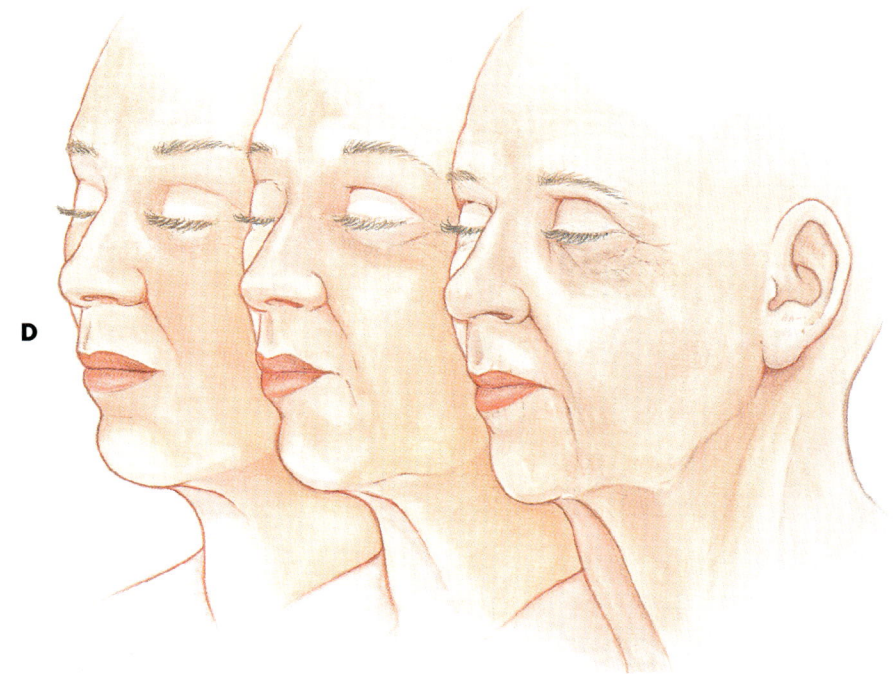

C, This patient is seen in her seventies. At this point, the separation of the platysma from its support along the floor of the mouth and thyroid cartilage is complete, and the platysma muscle is lying essentially vertically in the neck. D, This illustration depicts the descent of the platysma in the aging neck.

SURGICAL REJUVENATION OF THE FACE

There is a great deal of variation among patients in the appearance and quality of the platysma muscle at the time of surgical exploration. In patients who present with essentially a congenital obliquity of the neck, the platysma is short and tethered in the vertical dimension. These patients will usually have some degree of retrogenia, with a short distance between mentum and hyoid. Therefore a small degree of descent of the platysma (often in conjunction with accumulation of subplatysma fat) leads to marked obliquity in cervical contour. As the young platysma becomes vertically positioned in the neck, it shortens to accommodate its bowstringed position. Release of the platysma via a transection myotomy lengthens the muscle and helps to deepen the cervicomental angle.

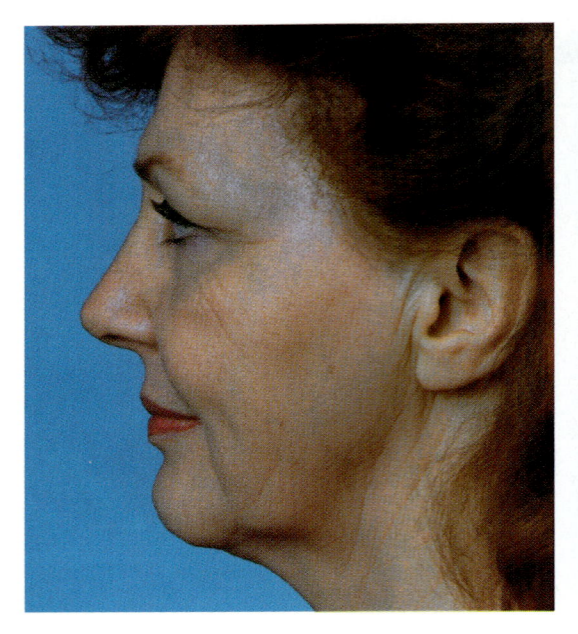

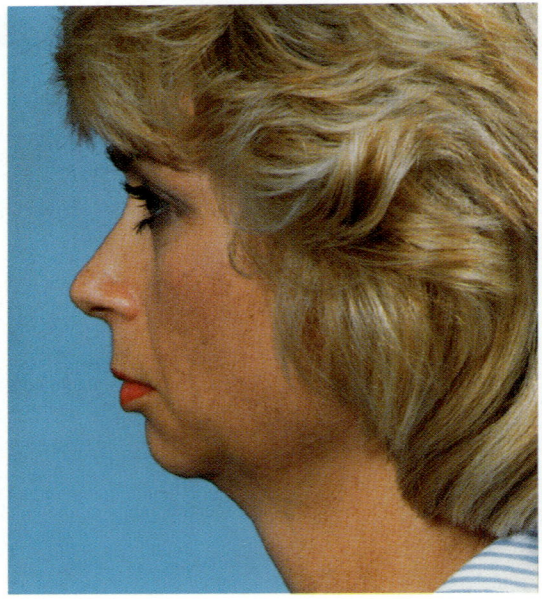

*There is a great deal of variation in length and quality of platysma bands. In the patient seen on the **left**, the platysma band is long, the muscle appears to be somewhat hypertrophic, and there is a normal distance between the hyoid and the mentum. In the patient seen on the **right**, the chin is retrusive and there is a short distance between the mentum and the hyoid. The platysma lies vertically and in this position, it has shortened to what is essentially the shortest distance between two points. The effect of the platysma in terms of cervical contour is thus quite different in these two patients.*

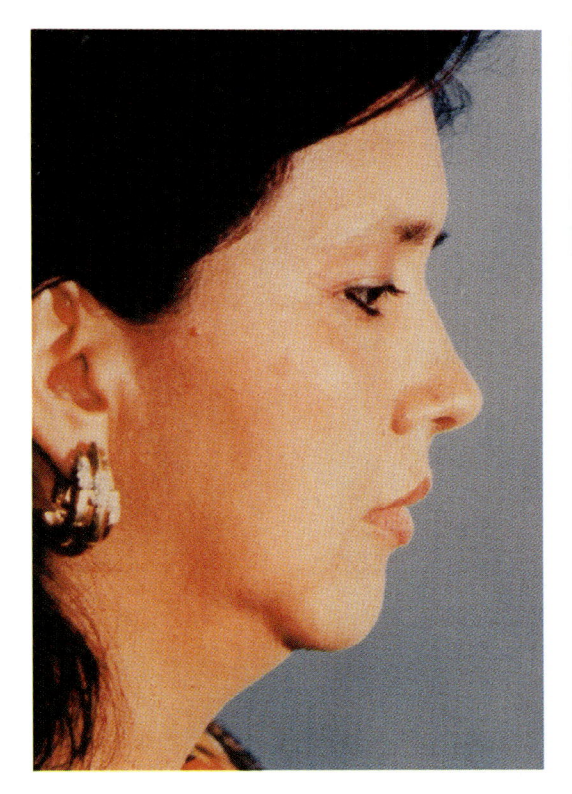

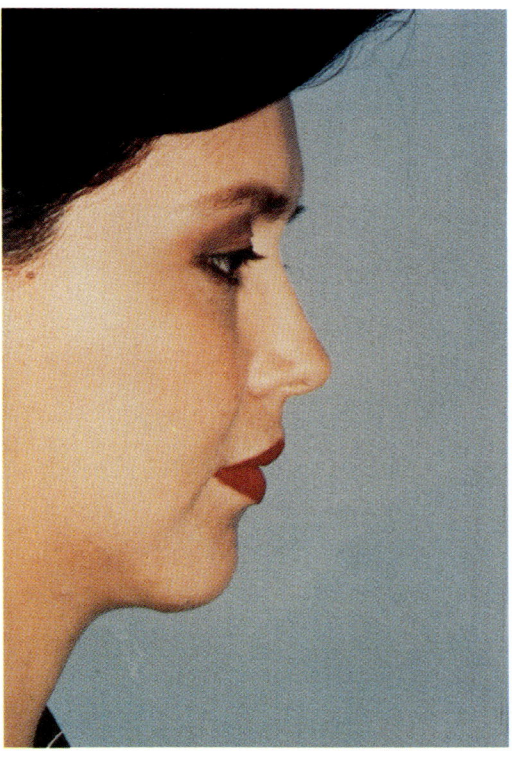

Patients with a retrusive chin and a large degree of cervical obliquity will commonly relate that they had a loss of cervical contour as early as late adolescence or their early twenties. The patient, seen in her early forties, presents with cervical obliquity that is largely secondary to descent of the platysma into the neck. This is commonly associated with accumulation of subplatysmal fat, which forces the platysma to descend into an oblique position. Since there is little distance between the mentum and the hyoid, a slight descent of the platysma muscle is translated into a large degree of obliquity as the platysma becomes vertically positioned. In this position, the young platysma will shorten to accommodate its new bowstringed position. Postoperatively, the patient is seen following long platysma plication, complete muscular transection, and insertion of a chin implant. The improvement seen in the cervicomental angle in the postoperative view is largely secondary to contouring of subplatysmal fat and complete muscular transection (which serves as a lengthening myotomy, allowing the proximal segment of the platysma to shift cephalad, thereby deepening the cervicomental angle).

SURGICAL REJUVENATION OF THE FACE

After years of facial muscular animation, some patients present with hypertrophy of the platysma, which is usually asymmetric. Resection of the thickened medial edge of the larger band to produce an even thickness of muscle throughout the submental region is important in contouring these patients.

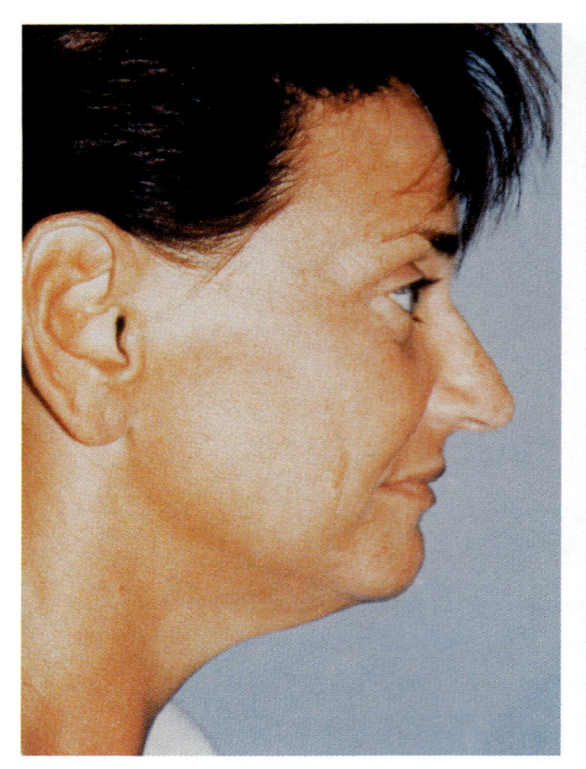

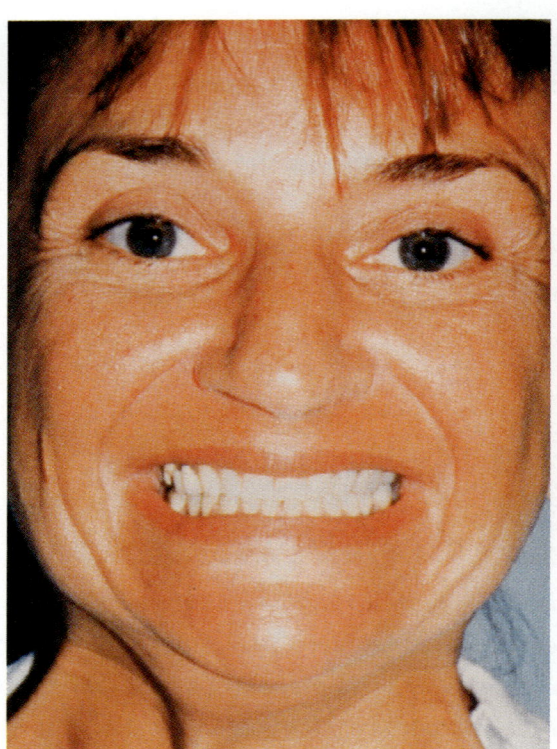

When evaluating a patient with platysmal bands, it is important for the surgeon to understand the position of the platysma within the neck. In this patient the platysma has descended significantly from its support along the floor of the mouth and lies on a straight line from the mentum to the hyoid, accounting for a large degree of cervical obliquity. On animation, the hypertrophy of the platysma is apparent.

In the elderly patient with often prominent banding, the platysma is commonly a thinner muscle than might be appreciated on preoperative examination. In these patients, the thin muscle can provide poor material for suturing. Technical points in handling the patient with an atrophic-appearing platysma include leaving the fascia anteriorly on the platysma intact, preventing undue tension on the anterior plication by minimizing muscle resection, and using numerous sutures placed well away from the muscular edge.

To summarize, patients with obtuse cervicomental angles usually have a combination of problems: lax skin; submental, submandibular, and subplatysmal fat; and attenuation of the fascial support of the neck. Correction of the obtuse neck involves restoration of skin tone, contouring of regional lipodystrophy, and restoration of platysma support.

Certain anatomic factors may exist that make correction of the obtuse cervical deformity difficult. The presence of a low-lying hyoid bone or an anteriorly placed larynx (thyroid cartilage) will interfere with redraping of skin and platysma, and lead to incomplete correction of an obtuse cervicomental angle. Preoperative evaluation of these factors must be noted and explained to the patient to avoid dissatisfaction postoperatively.

Similarly, in patients with retrognathia or microgenia, the distance between hyoid and mentum is short and limits the surgeon's ability to contour the patient's neck. The use of either a chin implant or genioplasty to increase chin projection will often greatly improve the result obtainable in cervical contouring.

SURGICAL REJUVENATION
OF THE FACE

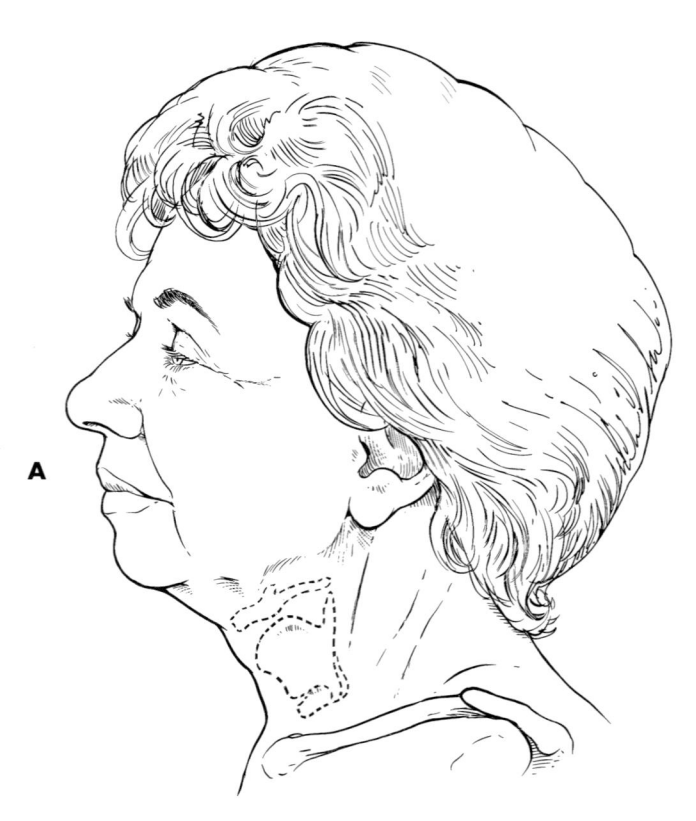

***A**, Patients with a low-lying hyoid bone and anteriorly placed larynx will present with an obtuse cervicomental angle and are a challenge in terms of obtaining proper cervical contouring. Although platysma plication, transection, and subplatysmal fat removal will improve the contour in these patients, it is often difficult to obtain ideal results.*

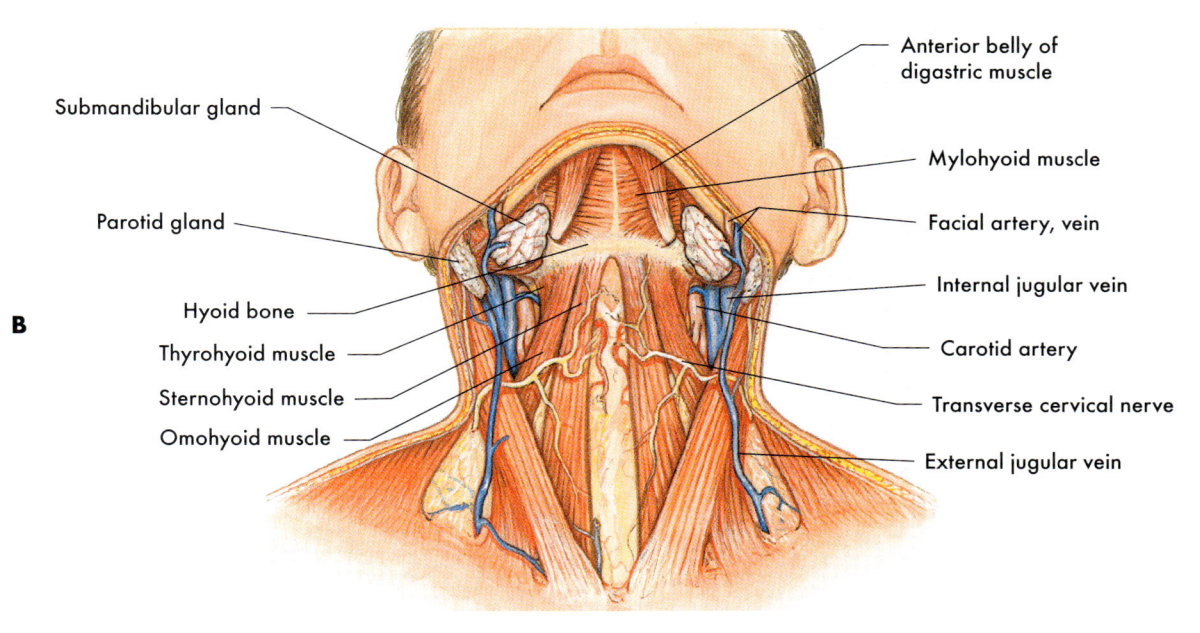

B, Appearance of the anterior neck following platysma removal illustrating the submental triangle that is bordered by the anterior bellies of the digastric muscles just lateral to which is the submaxillary gland. Subplatysmal fat commonly exists within the submental triangle, and in selected patients should be contoured to improve cervical obliquity.

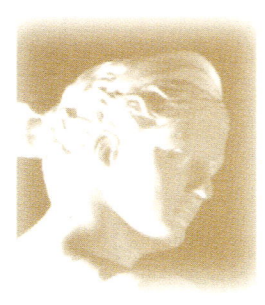

PATIENT EDUCATION

Once the operative plan has been formulated, it should be reviewed in detail with the patient. He or she should be given the details of the surgical plan, expected results, postoperative routine, expected discomfort, and convalescence. Communication frequently breaks down at this point because the patient only hears the positive aspects of the proposed procedure and tends to ignore the negative points. High-quality photographs of the patient are helpful in this situation. As the photographs are reviewed, the patient is often surprised at what the camera reveals. She may say, "I never really looked that bad," or "You have a terrible camera."

Patients are sometimes reluctant to face the reality of their appearance as revealed by the camera. This photographic review not only helps to emphasize the physical findings but also clarifies the objectives of the intended operative procedure.

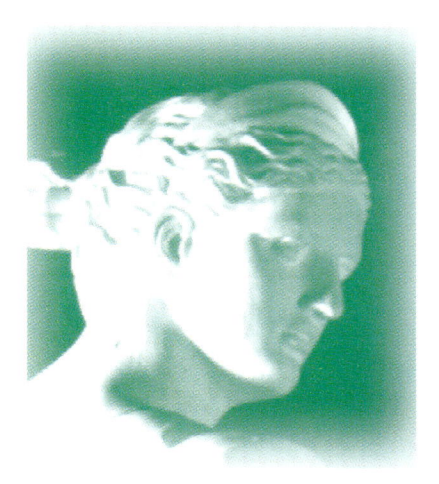

OPERATIVE TECHNIQUE

IMMEDIATE PREOPERATIVE ROUTINE

Immediate preoperative preparation is best completed on a patient that is thoroughly premedicated. The surgeon must first decide if a narrow strip of hair along the anticipated line of incision will be shaved. If the hair is not shaved, it is easier to place the incision parallel to the hair follicles. Many patients prefer their hair to be intact and the operation can be done without shaving however, it is easier for the surgeon when a small strip is shaved. Incisions should be planned to allow the patient to style the hair postoperatively to camouflage the incisions. The patient should have shampooed her hair thoroughly, washed her face, and removed any makeup the night before.

Once the patient has been made comfortable and is properly sedated, povidone-iodine (Betadine) solution is used to prepare the face and neck, including the eyelids and the temporal and posterior cervical hairline.

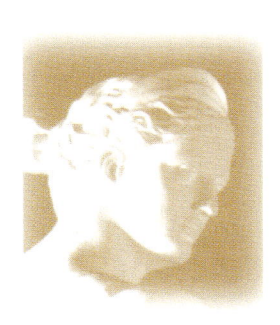

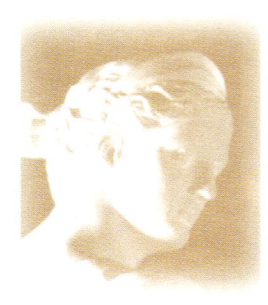

ANESTHESIA

Our policy is to perform all rhytidectomies with the patient under local anesthesia and suitable analgesia and sedation, usually ketamine and midazolam (Versed). (See Chapter 2.) Lidocaine 1% with epinephrine 1:100,000 is infiltrated along the proposed incision lines, and 0.5% lidocaine with 1:400,000 epinephrine is infiltrated into the anticipated plane of dissection. The initial maximum dosage of lidocaine is kept below 500 mg, although it may be safely supplemented later in the procedure if additional anesthetic is required. We routinely block both sides of the face as well as the neck during our initial injection following the administration of ketamine.

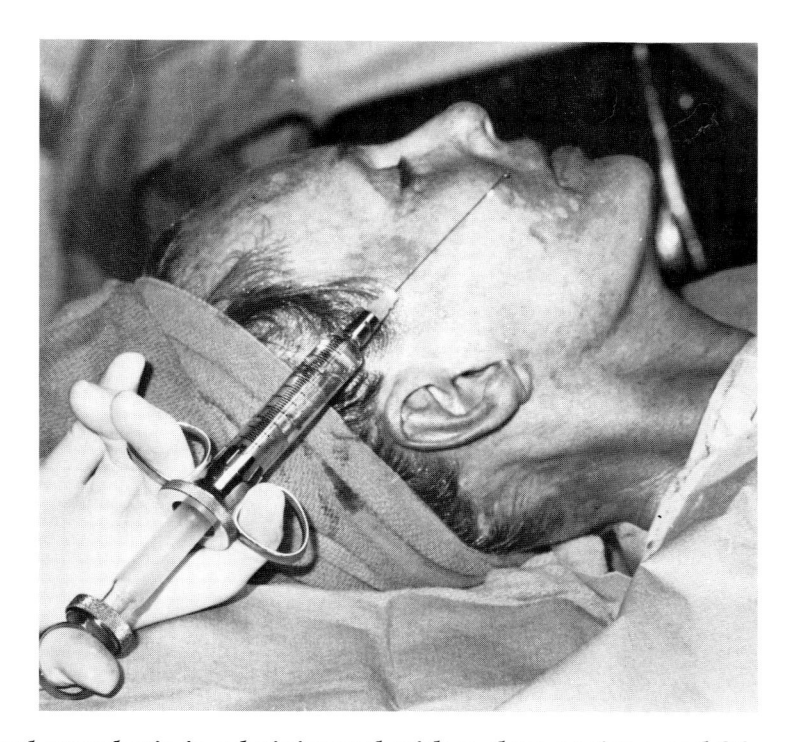

The local anesthetic is administered with a glass syringe and 25-gauge spinal needle. By using the long needle, a sizable area can be infiltrated through a single injection site.

It is important to infiltrate the lidocaine at the proper depth within the subcutaneous layer just beneath the dermis. This provides for maximum hemostasis and serves as an aid to surgery secondary to the hydrodissection that occurs following subcutaneous infiltration in the anticipated plane of dissection.

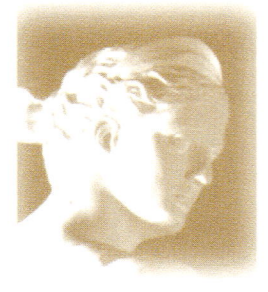

INCISIONS

Most rhytidectomy incisions are similar. The incision is patterned around the ear. The temporal incision is placed within the hairline beginning at a point immediately superior to the junction of the ear with the temporal skin. In women, we prefer to make the preauricular segment of the incision follow the margin of the tragus. Straight-line incisions can be used in front of the ear; however, they are somewhat more visible. Even where a small or almost absent tragus exists, we believe this curved incision to be superior.

RHYTIDECTOMY

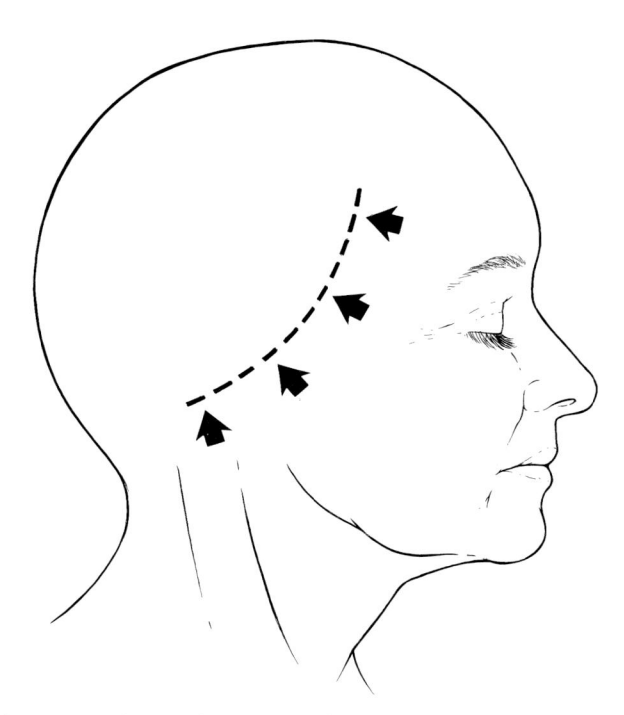

The artist's drawing shows how simple the incision and closure would be if the ear were not present.

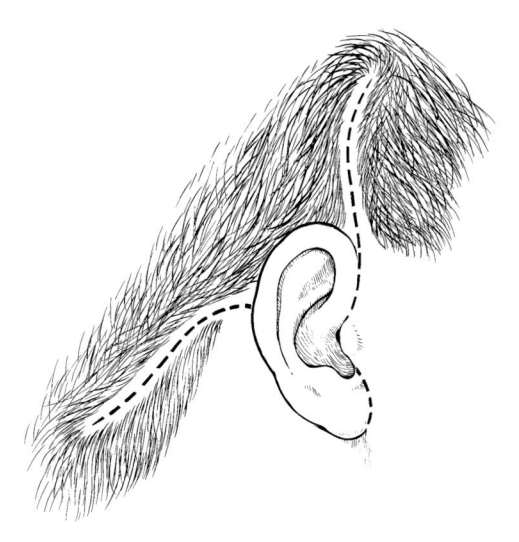

The usual line of incision in the female facelift. The top of the incision is placed paralleling the descending helix. It is important to design the incision directly adjacent to the helix to preserve normal helical width. The incision then conforms to the margins of the tragus and inferiorly contours to the margins of the earlobe.

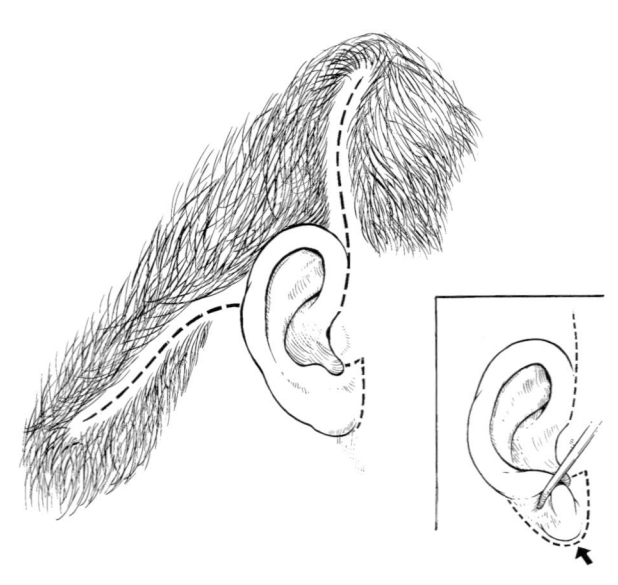

One of the problems with tragal incisions is that they can produce postoperative distortion of the tragus, leading to a more visible postoperative incision. A method of avoiding this distortion is to preserve the incisura of the tragus (i.e., the caudal portion of the tragus at its junction with the cephalad portion of the earlobe). In reality, the tragus is rectangular rather than semilunar and the base of the rectangle is represented by the incisura. Preservation of this structure by extending the incision at a right angle, rather than violating this region of the tragus, will maintain tragal configuration postoperatively and lead to minimal tragal distortion. (Inset) The incision around the earlobe is carried 2 mm distal to the junction of the earlobe with the cheek skin rather than directly at the attachment between the earlobe and the cheek skin. Preservation of this 2-mm cuff along the earlobe allows the surgeon to have enough tissue to tuck the cheek flap beneath the earlobe during flap redraping and prevents the appearance of an attached earlobe postoperatively.

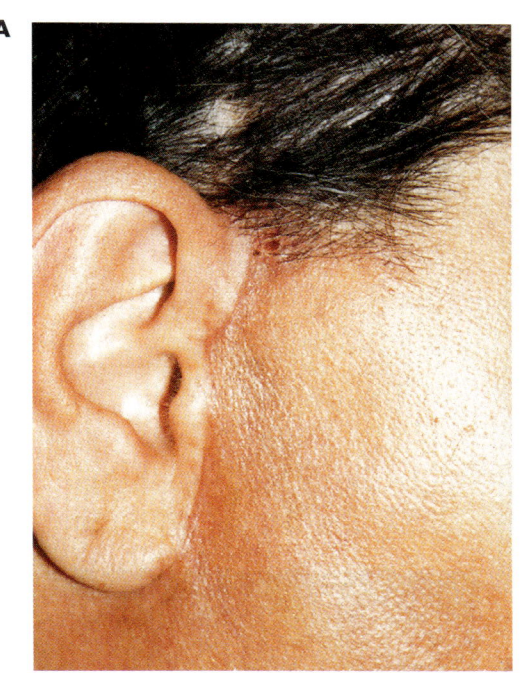

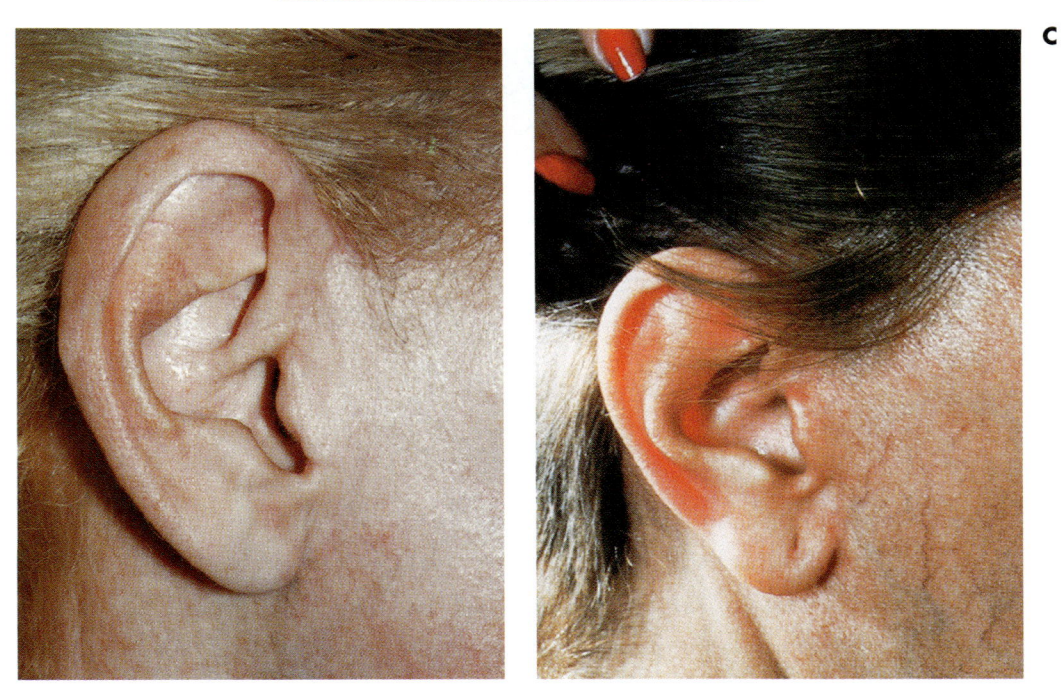

A, Preauricular incision seen 2 months postoperatively. The problem with preauricular incisions is that the difference in color between the skin of the cheek and the skin of the ear is more visible in this anterior incision location. B, Tragal incision seen 5 months postoperatively designed along the methods described in the preceding figure. C, A well-designed and inset tragal incision should produce an imperceptible, normal-appearing tragus which exhibits both a visual beginning and end, and a detached-appearing earlobe. Note that the earlobe has been inset slightly posterior to the longitudinal axis of the pinna.

SURGICAL REJUVENATION OF THE FACE

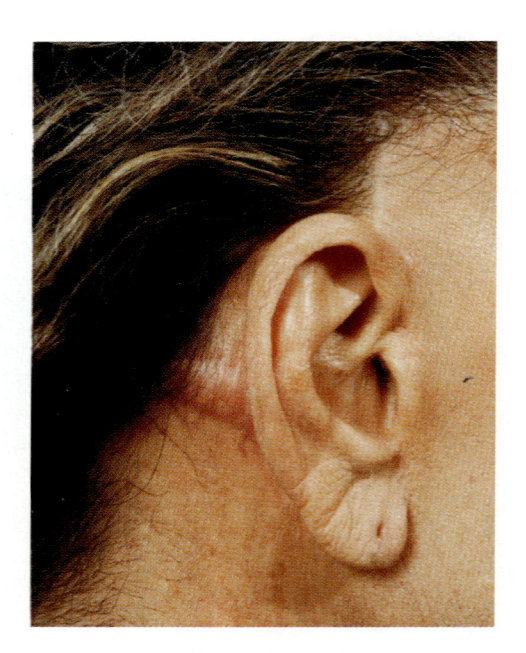

Patient seen following primary facelift performed in another office. She exhibits the characteristics of a poorly designed tragal incision that violated the incisura of the tragus and was redraped with tension at closure. The result is a tragus that is a straight line in appearance, blunted, and pulled anteriorly, opening the external auditory canal.

RHYTIDECTOMY

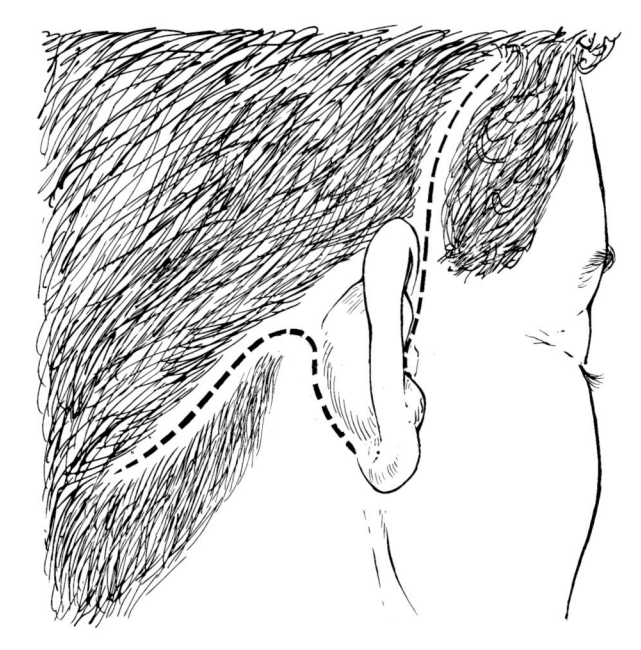

The postauricular incision is placed directly within the conchal groove. The incision should then extend into the hairline where the concha joins the hairline. The angle of the posterior flap should be approximately 90 degrees, if possible. This prevents a sharp angulation and an acute angle at at the tip of the cervical flap, and thus reduces the incidence of skin slough in this area.

SURGICAL REJUVENATION OF THE FACE

There are two basic types of posterior neck incisions. In one technique the incision is directed posteriorly in a transverse manner into the hairline. This technique works well if there is not too much neck skin laxity. However, if the neck skin is extremely lax, and a large amount of redundant cervical skin flap is to be removed, or if the pos-

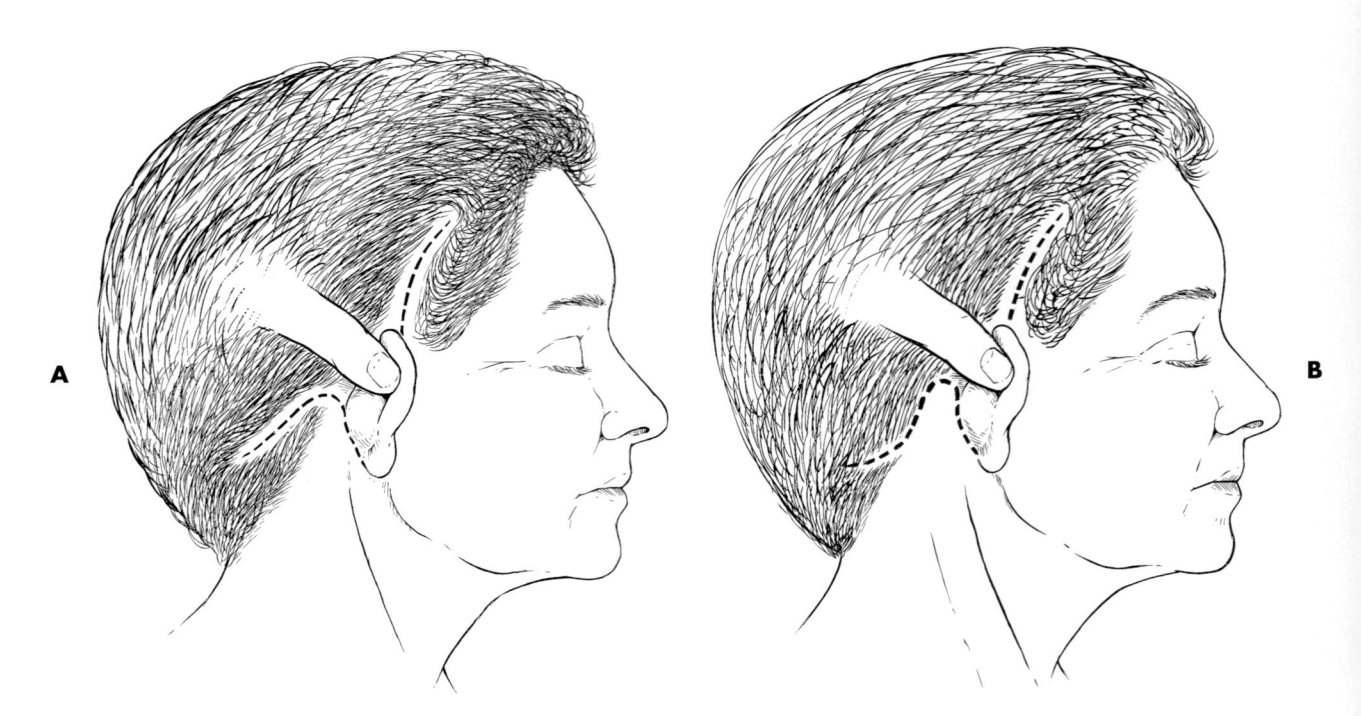

A, The most common incision we use in the posterior hairline is an oblique extension into the occipital hair in the region where the overhang of the pinna meets the posterior hairline. This works quite well in patients who are young, without a large degree of cervical laxity, and in patients with a low postauricular hairline where the hairline lies in close proximity to the postauricular groove. B, In patients in whom a great deal of skin is going to be removed as well as in patients whose postauricular hairline lies quite lateral to the postauricular groove, a partial hairline incision is often used. In these patients stair-stepping of the occipital hair can occur, and it is preferable to use a partial hairline incision superiorly and then, in approximately the midportion of the incision, to extend the incision into the postauricular hair. With closure, the hairline is realigned inferiorly while most of the cervical skin excision occurs within the hairless superior aspect of the incision. This type of incision prevents a compromise in the vector of cervical redraping that can occur in an effort to realign the hairline.

RHYTIDECTOMY

terior hairline lies well lateral to the conchal groove, the posterior cervical hairline may be advanced too far superiorly, creating a bald spot or an obvious "step" in the posterior hairline. In these cases we angle the incision along the posterior hairline, just within the fine occipital hair, for a few centimeters, then curve back into the hairline inferiorly,

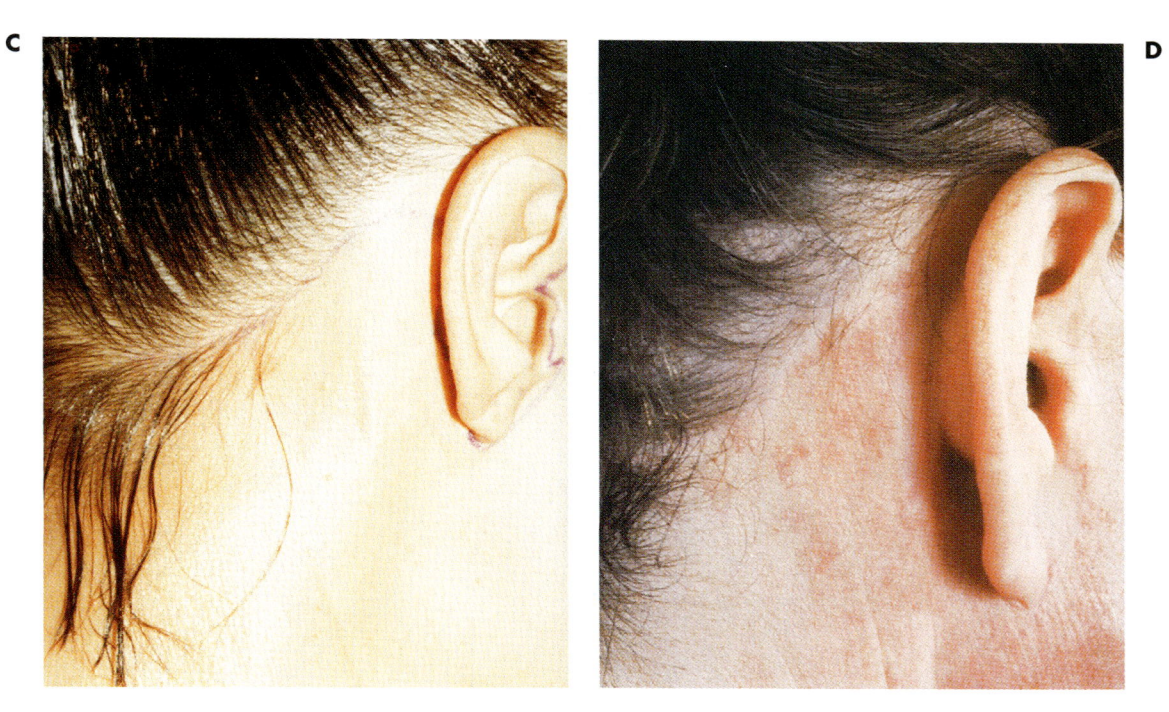

C, Preoperative photograph of partial hairline incision as described in B. D, Postoperative results demonstrating a well-healed postauricular incision. Note that there is no stair-stepping of the postauricular hairline, allowing the patient to wear her hair up off the neck without fear of a noticeable scar.

toward the midportion of the incision. This partial hairline incision prevents a stair-stepping deformity, but must be closed meticulously, without tension, to obtain a fine, inconspicuous scar.

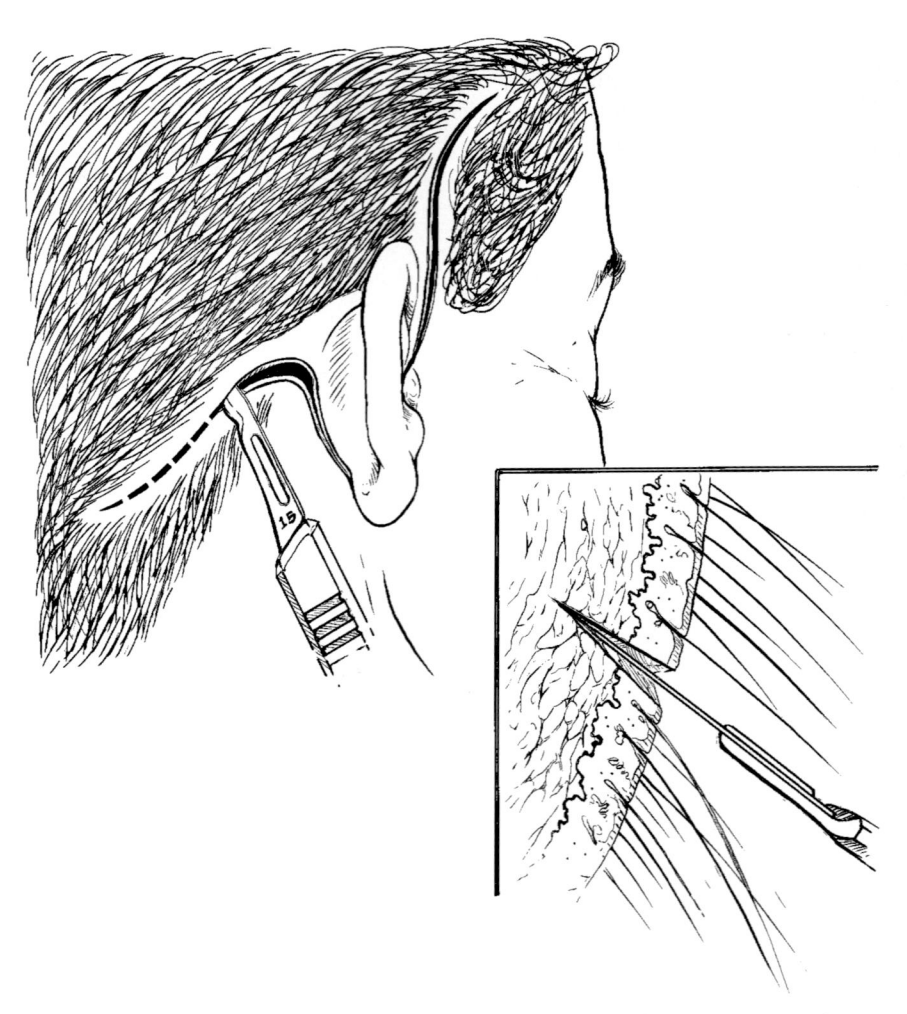

Note that the postauricular incision extends along the postauricular groove and not up onto the conchal surface. The incision then commonly turns into the postauricular hair at the junction where the overlap of the pinna meets the hairline, which usually conforms to the superior aspect of the antihelical cartilage. The incision extends into the hairline for 6 to 9 cm. The scalpel blade is angled inferiorly to parallel the hair follicles, thus destroying fewer of them.

The detachment of the earlobe is an important consideration with reference to how it will be reattached. A small amount of cheek skin, 1 or 2 mm, can be detached along with the lobe, leaving a small cuff or rim of skin immediately inferior to the lobule that can be used for reattachment at the time of closure. It should be noted, though, that this small rim of cheek skin will be different in color and texture from the advanced cheek skin. If this rim is left too wide it will be plainly visible.

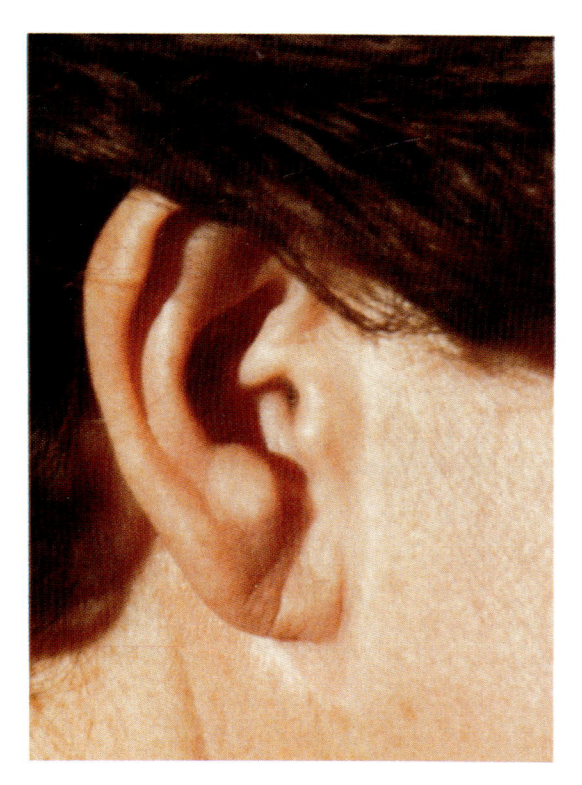

A straight-line scar in a dark-complexioned person is often conspicuous. This patient also had an "island" of skin removed along with the earlobe, which, when replaced, became a telltale sign of a rhytidectomy.

SURGICAL REJUVENATION
OF THE FACE

228

We usually prefer to detach the lobe just caudal (1-2 mm) to its junction with the cheek and to reattach it in a similar manner. As long as there is no downward traction caused by gravitational pull of the cervical flap or excessive skin removed inferior or anterior to the lobe, the earlobe will not be artificially pulled and distorted.

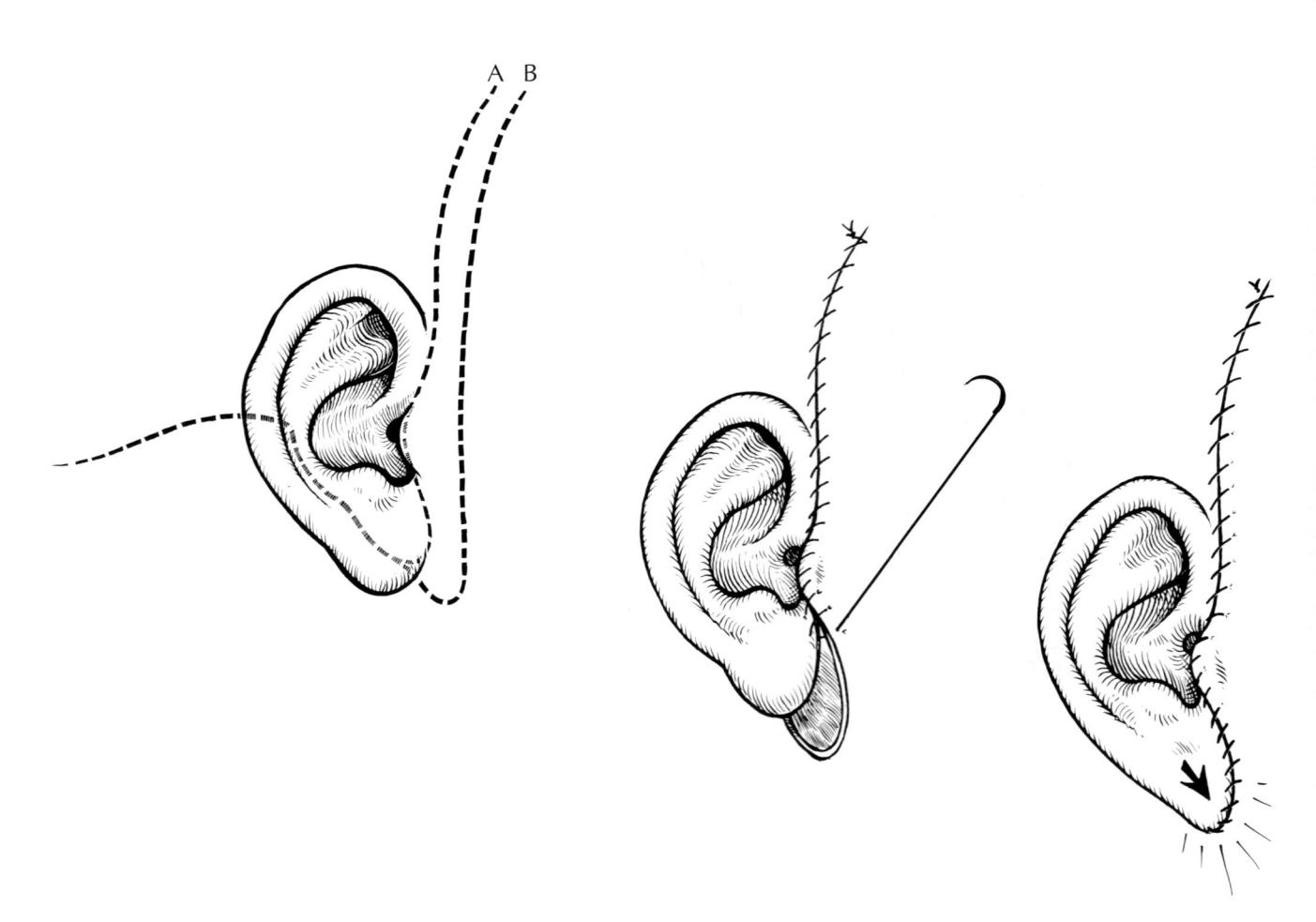

The preferred incision follows the posterior tragal margin. If a straight-line preauricular incision is used, the resulting scar is often more obvious. The straight-line incision is shown extending well beyond the earlobe. If too much skin is removed in this area, the earlobe will be pulled anteriorly and inferiorly at the time of closure, resulting in distortion. Distortion and misplacement of the earlobe result if the preauricular or infraauricular skin excision was too aggressive.

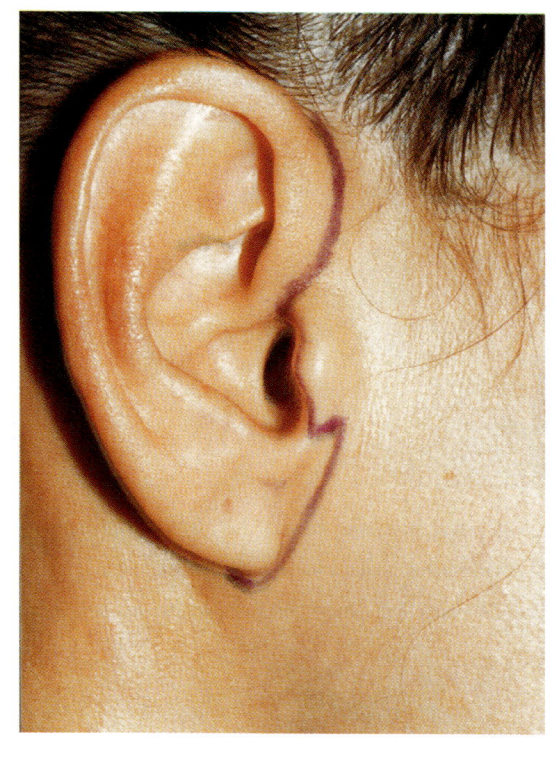

Intraoperative photograph illustrating the standard tragal incision with preservation of the incisura of the tragus. Note that the incision is carried around the earlobe approximately 1 to 2 mm caudal to the junction of the earlobe with the cheek skin.

SURGICAL REJUVENATION
OF THE FACE

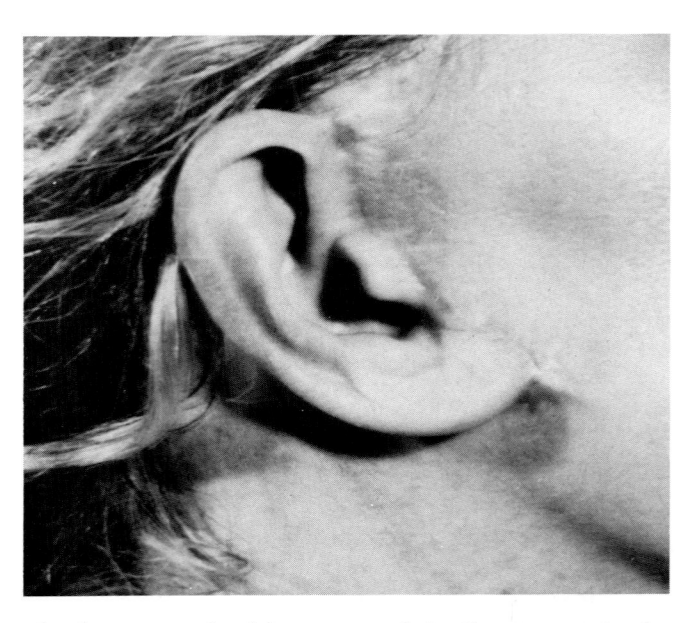

This patient had too much skin removed in the preauricular and infra-auricular area. The earlobe was then advanced into the defect and resulted in distortion. Do not attempt to hang the cheek on the earlobe.

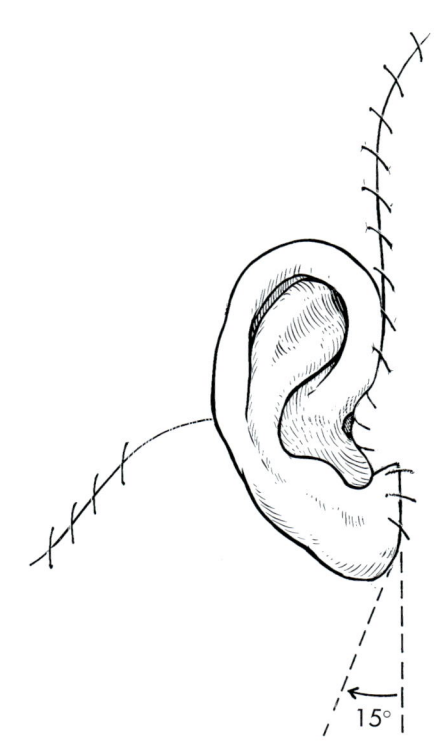

In general, the earlobe should be inset so that it lies approximately 15 degrees posterior to the vertical axis of the pinna. A common error is to attach the earlobe along the vertical axis of the pinna. Secondary to the weight of the cheek flap postoperatively, the earlobe ends up being more forward than the rest of the ear, resulting in a telltale stigma of facelifting.

SURGICAL REJUVENATION OF THE FACE

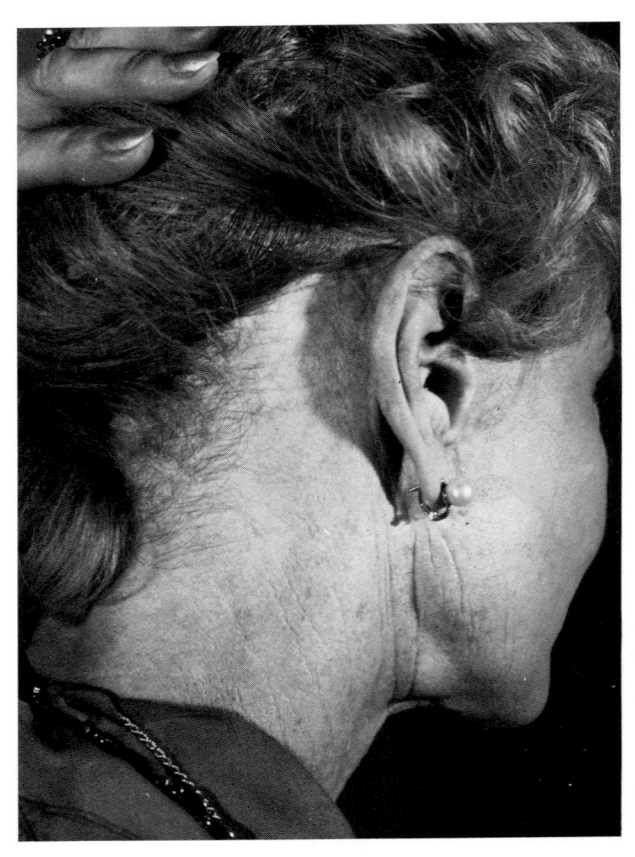

This patient had a posterior cervical incision that was located at the level of the superior pole of the ear. This placement elevated the posterior hairline to an extreme degree and left a large hairless area in the immediate postauricular skin.

DISSECTION

Considerations in Subcutaneous Undermining

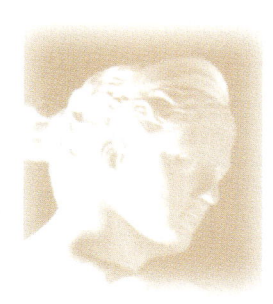

Different problems require differing amounts of subcutaneous undermining. The young patient with minimal submental laxity and shallow nasolabial folds requires essentially only a classic rhytidectomy undermining. The patient with a heavy, obtuse neck, prominent jowls, and a deep nasolabial fold requires a more aggressive approach. In patients with a heavy neck and platysma bands, a through-and-through cervical dissection is usually necessary to allow access to the platysma, proper contouring of cervical fat, and adequate redraping of cervical skin at the time of closure. In patients with a prominent nasolabial fold, we usually undermine the malar region extensively to allow adequate access for malar SMAS elevation. In general, we undermine the skin until it is dissected enough so that it freely redrapes at the time of closure. Dissecting the skin from the restraint of the underlying retaining ligaments is an important technical point in allowing the skin to redrape properly and usually mandates some form of release of the attachments present within McGregor's pad.

Before deciding on the amount of skin undermining that is required, several factors must be weighed. The age of the patient, the degree of degeneration of facial skin, and the smoking history must all be taken into account. In patients with severe actinic damage who are heavy smokers, we favor limiting the amount of subcutaneous undermining to ensure adequate blood supply during postoperative healing.

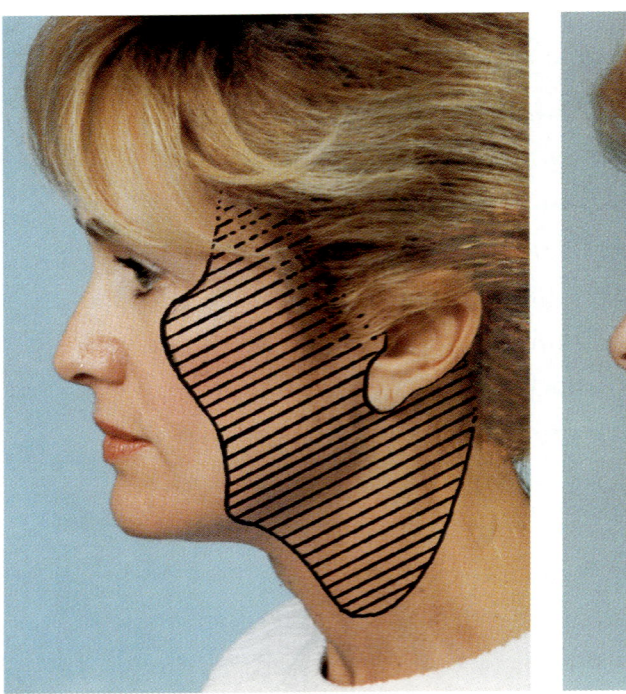

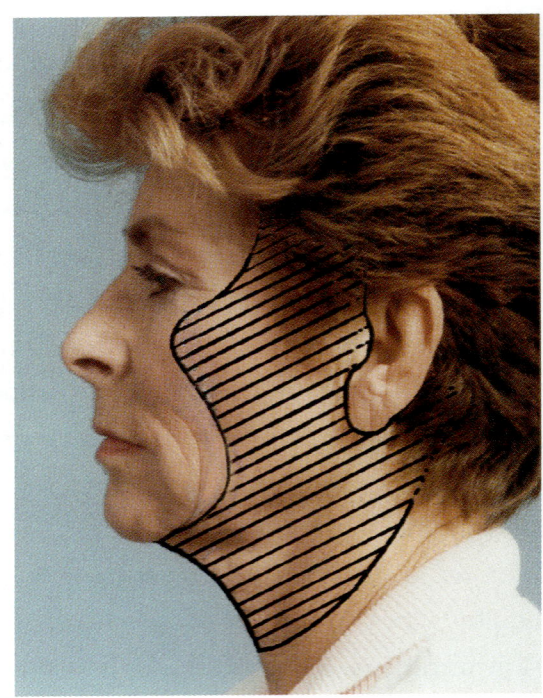

Preoperative photographs illustrate the amount of subcutaneous undermining required in the young patient in her forties versus the amount required in a patient in her sixties with prominent nasolabial folds, jowls, and platysma bands, in whom a greater degree of SMAS mobilization is anticipated.

The undermining required to treat skin laxity must be taken into account. It is interesting that much of the gain in terms of how much skin can be resected at the time of closure occurs quite peripherally in the dissection, usually within the first 6 to 8 cm of skin undermining. From this point forward, in most patients, relatively little extra skin recruitment is gained even if the surgeon undermines well past the nasolabial fold. This most likely has to do with the arrangement between the skin and the retaining ligaments, most of which are divided within the cheek once the dissection has proceeded past the anterior border of the masseter and has extended into the malar region.

If greater skin undermining does not necessarily produce greater skin recruitment, the question remains: Is wide skin undermining a beneficial procedure? It is our opinion that if deep layer support is restored at the time of rhytidectomy, wide skin undermining is contraindicated. This largely has to do with the presence of numerous vertical septa, or so-called skin pulleys, between the SMAS and the overlying facial skin. If some of these skin pulleys are left intact by limiting skin undermining, they provide a vehicle for the resuspension of facial skin as the SMAS-platysma complex is rotated cephalad. If the skin is widely undermined, and all the fibrous septa between SMAS and skin are divided, then SMAS rotation, while tightening the facial foundation, cannot result in a concurrent resuspension of facial skin. In our opinion, the aesthetic results within the midface are greatly improved if the surgeon uses the deep layer support of SMAS rotation to also resupport facial skin, rather than mobilizing and redraping skin and SMAS completely separate from one another. (Figure)

To summarize, undermining of facial skin serves two purposes: (1) it addresses laxity within facial skin itself and (2) allows access to adequate tightening of the SMAS-mimetic muscle layer. Undermining the skin just enough to achieve these purposes produces a more aesthetic contour while ensuring adequate vascularity to the facial flaps.

SURGICAL REJUVENATION OF THE FACE

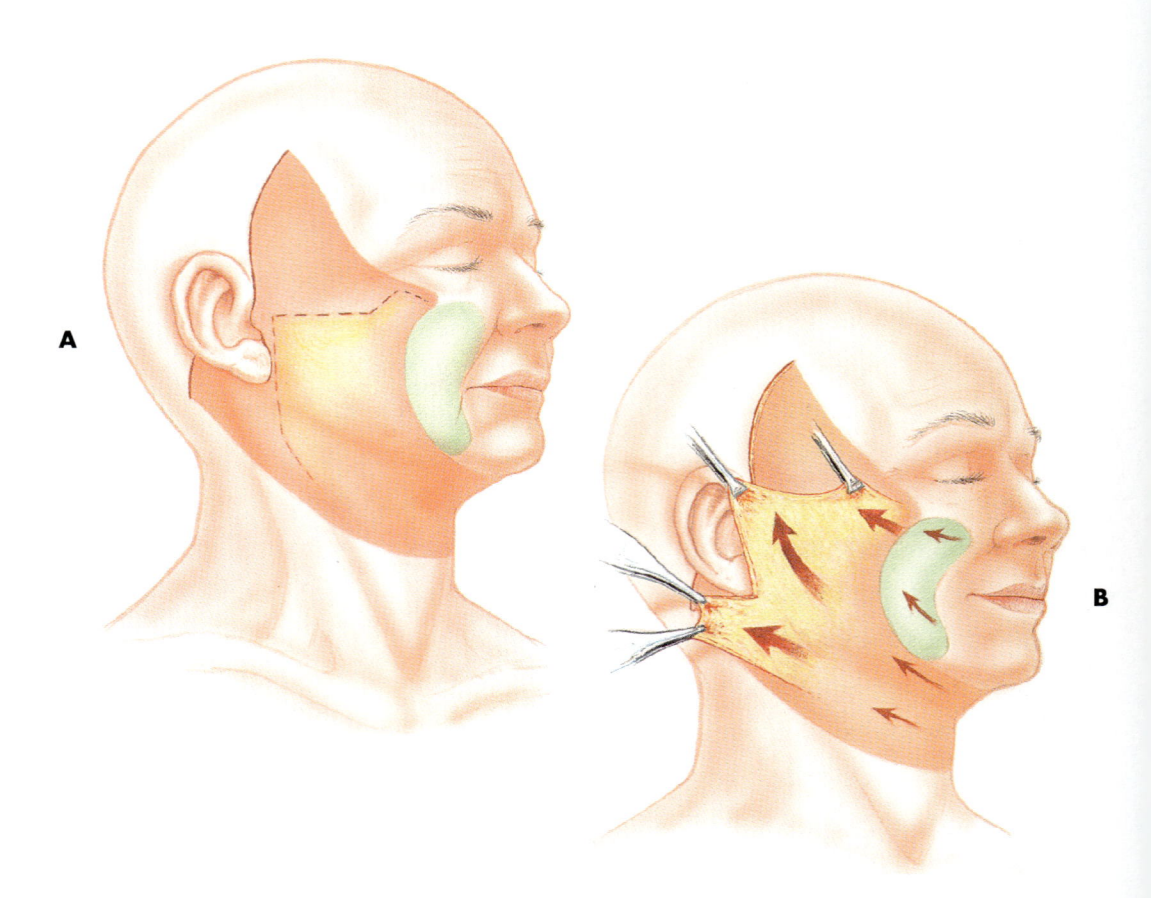

A, If an extended SMAS dissection is to be performed, it is important not to widely undermine the skin all the way to the nasolabial fold, but rather preserve some of the attachments that exist between the skin and the SMAS (the limit of subcutaneous undermining is the shaded area). If these attachments are left intact, this allows the surgeon to simultaneously resuspend undissected anterior facial skin at the time of SMAS rotation and fixation. B, It is important to understand which portion of the SMAS flap will affect facial contouring. In this diagram, the most superomedial aspect of the SMAS dissection affects contour along the nasolabial fold, whereas the more lateral portion of the SMAS dissection is used to reelevate jowl fat back upward into the cheek. A portion of the SMAS flap is rotated into the postauricular region with the vector of rotation of this portion of the SMAS dissection affecting submental and cervical contouring.

Operative Techniques in Subcutaneous Undermining

We begin dissection in the temporal hair-bearing area. After the skin is incised, the dissection is continued through the temporoparietal fascia (SMAS) down to the loose areolar layer (subaponeurotic plane), which overlies the deep temporal fascia. This level of dissection is defined from the attachment of the helix of the ear to the superior extent of the temporal incision. The dissection is then carried medially in the avascular subaponeurotic plane. A combination of sharp and blunt technique, often using gentle finger dissection, leads to rapid development of this area. The medial extent of the dissection is carried as far forward as the region just lateral to the frontal branch of the facial nerve, i.e., (blunt undermining can be carried as far forward as 2 cm above the eyebrow). The inferior extent of the temporal dissection corresponds to a horizontal line parallel to the attachment of the helix, which lies roughly at the level of the superior orbital rim.

The advantage of undermining beneath the temporoparietal fascia is that it produces a thick temporal flap that prevents postoperative alopecia resulting from either ischemia or injury to the hair follicle. Excess tension can still produce alopecia in this hair-bearing area and obviously should be avoided at the time of flap closure. An alternative plane of dissection within the temporal region is subcutaneous, above the temporoparietal fascia and just beneath the base of the hair follicle.

The surgical undermining is continued inferiorly within the cheek, dissecting in the subcutaneous plane superficial to the SMAS. On a horizontal line extending from the orbital rim to the helical attachment, a transition zone exists between the deeper dissection of the temporal region and the more superficial undermining performed subcutaneously within the cheek. This region is termed the *mesotemporalis* and traveling within this transition zone is the frontal branch of the facial nerve. To allow proper redraping with closure, the transition zone be

SURGICAL REJUVENATION OF THE FACE

Labels on illustration:
- Ligated parietal branch of superficial temporal artery
- Frontal branch of superficial temporal artery
- Temporoparietal fascia (SMAS)
- Frontal branch of facial nerve
- Ligated parietal branch of superficial temporal artery

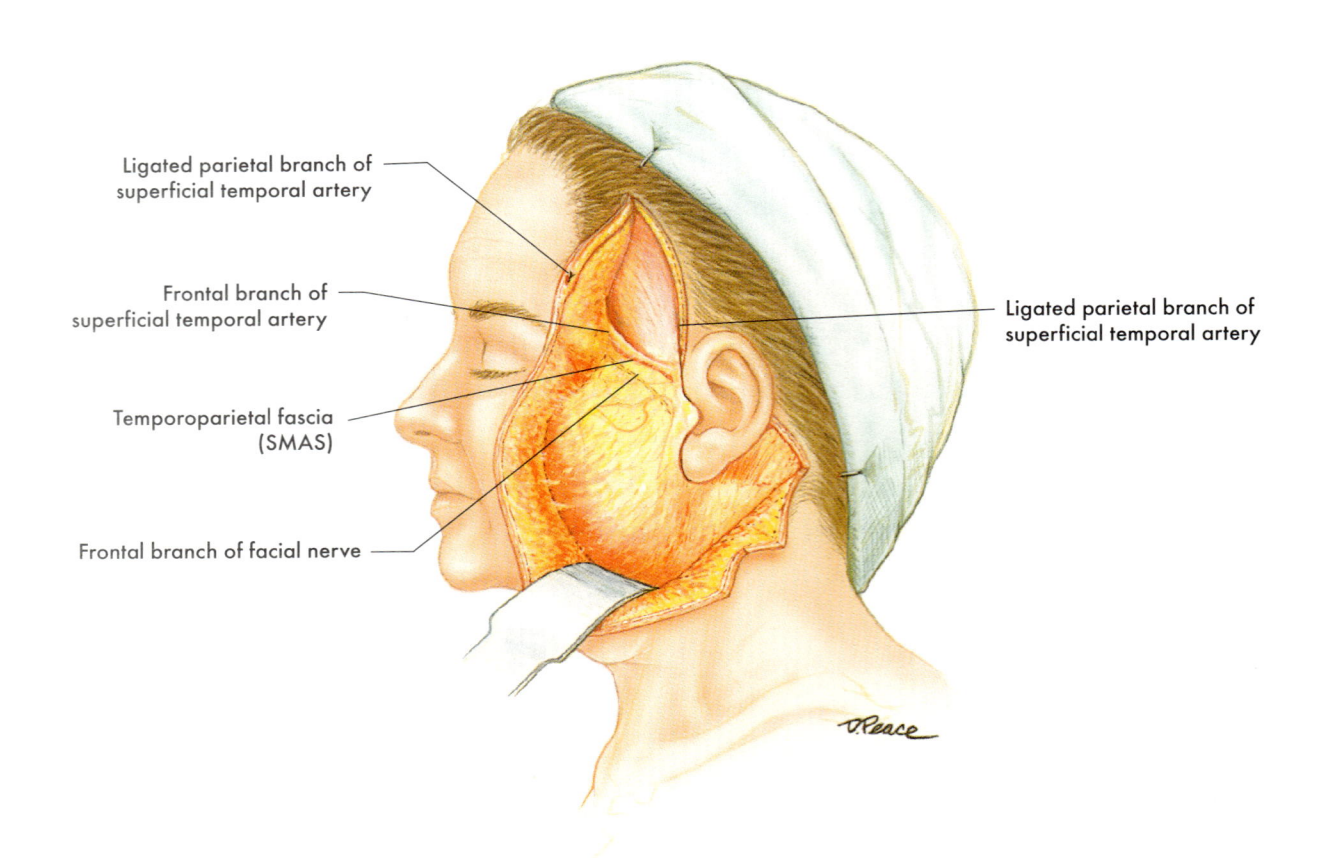

The dissection in the temporal region is carried deep to the temporoparietal fascia, whereas the dissection within the cheek is carried subcutaneously superficial to the SMAS. The transition zone between these two levels of dissection occurs along the helical attachment. Within this mesotemporalis lies the frontal branch of the superficial temporal artery, as well as the frontal branch of the facial nerve. The frontal branch of the superficial temporal artery is a useful landmark because the temporal branches of the facial nerve always lie medial and inferior to this structure. When connecting the areas between the temporal dissection and the cheek dissection, as long as the frontal branch of the superficial temporal artery is preserved, motor branch injury will be prevented.

tween the sub-SMAS, temporal dissection, and the subcutaneous facial dissection must be connected, while preserving the frontal branch. In connecting these two areas of dissection, the parietal branches of the superficial temporal artery and vein, as well as the auriculotemporal nerve, are encountered laterally and should be clamped and ligated. Dissection is then carried medially, usually to the anterior temporal hairline, ensuring that the temporal and facial portions of the dissection are well connected and redraped easily. The frontal branch of the superficial temporal artery is a useful landmark, since it lies immediately superior and lateral to the frontal branch of the facial nerve. Within this transition zone, the medial limit of our dissection connecting the cheek and temporal regions rarely extends medial to the frontal branch of the superficial temporal artery. As long as this vessel is preserved, the frontal branch of the facial nerve will not be injured.

Inferior to the transition zone, the dissection continues within the subcutaneous fat and thus external to the SMAS. The dissection continues medially to allow mobilization of cheek and neck tissues. The dissection is commonly extended into the malar region and toward the nasolabial fold. Because of the attachments between SMAS and skin, which we want to preserve at the time of the SMAS mobilization, we rarely mobilize the skin flap as far peripherally as the nasolabial fold. The fibrous fat present over the most prominent portion of the zygoma is always detached. This area, termed *McGregor's patch,* is freed to allow proper redraping of the skin as well as access for malar SMAS dissection. The blood vessels commonly found within this pad must be carefully controlled. If a malar SMAS dissection is planned, the skin underlying the lateral two thirds of the zygomatic eminence should be undermined.

SURGICAL REJUVENATION OF THE FACE

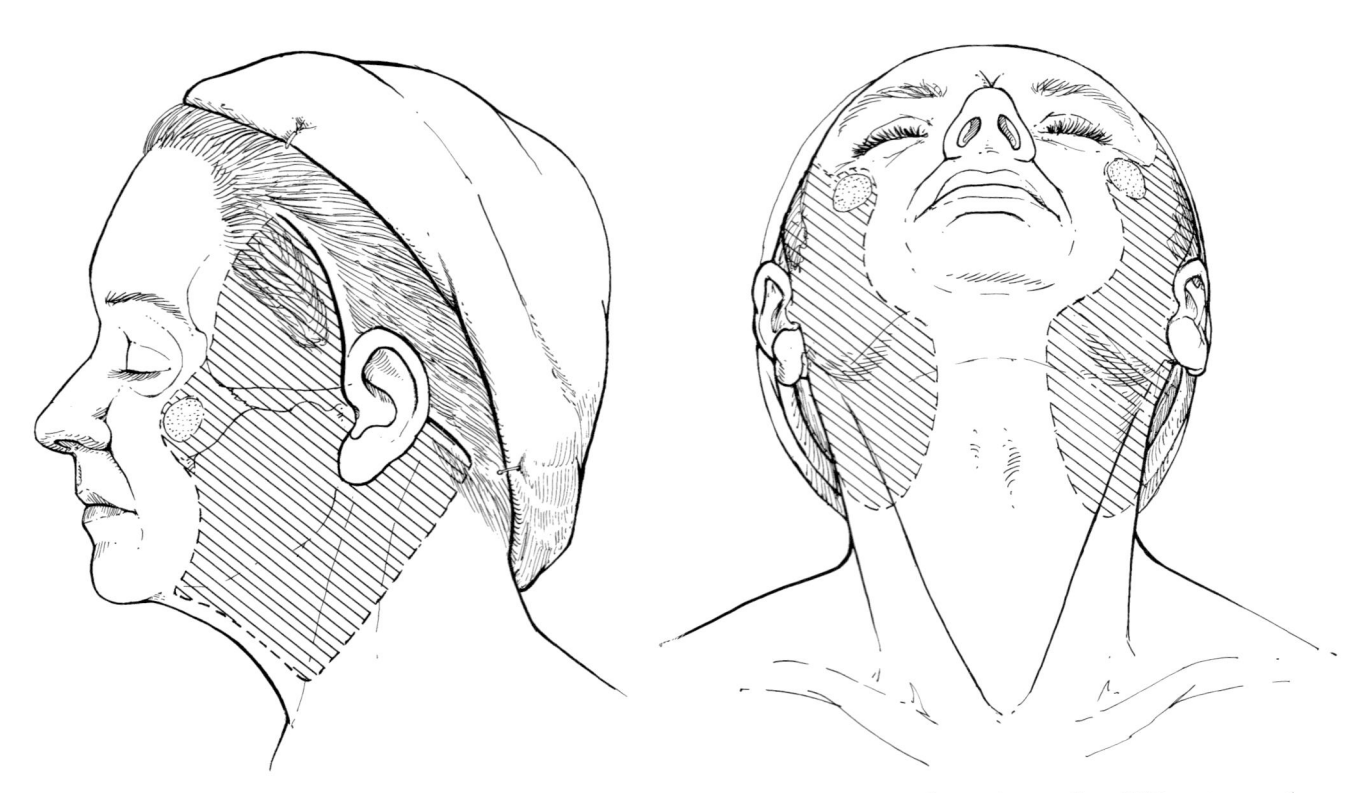

The undermining required in a patient undergoing a facelifting procedure in which the SMAS dissection is planned to extend into the malar region, but in which an anterior approach to the platysma through a submental incision is not required.

The tissue encountered within the cheek in the preparotid region is usually fibrous, but once past the parotid the dissection becomes easier and the subcutaneous fat less dense and fibrous. The subcutaneous fat in the region of the jowls is often bulky, and dissection in this area proceeds easily.

Behind the ear, the plane of undermining is a bit obscure. The dermis is usually firmly attached to the fascia along the sternocleidomastoid muscle. Since the majority of postoperative sloughs occur in the immediate postauricular region, we prefer to keep the postauricular flaps as thick as possible. For this reason, superiorly, the dissection is carried just superficial to the fascia overlying the sternocleidomastoid muscle. This is usually performed with sharp scalpel dissection. Dissection directly on top of the muscle fascia is carried from the postauricular incision inferiorly to the level of the earlobe. Inferior to the level of the earlobe, the dissection becomes more superficial and carries through the subcutaneous fat, to protect the underlying great auricular nerve. The great auricular nerve travels just beneath the superficial fascia overlying the sternocleidomastoid. As long as the dissection over the sternocleidomastoid is subcutaneous and external to the SMAS, the great auricular nerve will not be injured. Superior to the earlobe, the great auricular nerve is not in jeopardy and the dissection can therefore be carried more deeply, producing a thicker and more resilient flap.

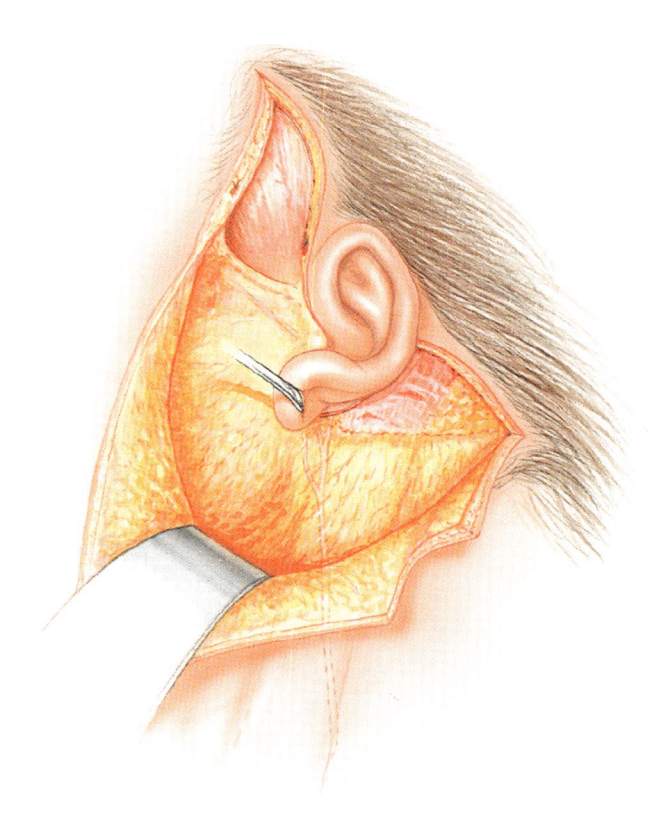

The postauricular dissection superiorly is carried directly overlying the fascia of the sternocleidomastoid muscle. As the dissection proceeds caudad to the level of the earlobe attachment, the surgeon must continue the dissection in the subcutaneous plane to preserve the great auricular nerve, which travels just deep to the superficial cervical fascia overlying the sternocleidomastoid. If the superficial cervical fascia is not violated (the dissection remaining subcutaneous), injury to this sensory nerve will be prevented.

The postauricular and posterior cervical dissection is then made in continuity with the preauricular facial dissection. This is carried forward into the neck as indicated from preoperative surgical planning. This dissection may stop short of the midline if the anterior platysma does not require surgical correction. Usually, mobilization of the cervical skin off the dense attachments along the sternocleidomastoid will allow adequate flap mobility for the redraping of cervical skin, and a through-and-through undermining of the neck is only done if an anterior approach to the platysma is required. In other words, little extra cervical skin recruitment is gained by a through-and-through undermining of cervical skin.

If a submental incision is required for access to the anterior platysma, it should be made just caudal to the natural skin crease in the immediate submental area. The cervical dissection is then made in continuity with the cheek dissection.

Good visibility of the anterior cervical region and platysma borders is obtained by completely undermining the submental area and connecting the midportion of the neck to the lateral dissection. When the dissection is complete, the cervical flaps will redrape without undue tension. The cervical skin flaps should be carefully elevated so that at least 5 to 7 mm of subcutaneous fat remains as a lining of the flaps. When proceeding with dissection of the cervical skin flap, caution should be exercised to avoid injury to the platysma muscle, which can be closely adherent to the cervical skin. An important technical point is to leave the fascia intact along the superficial surface of the muscle; this helps in muscle contouring and in minimizing postoperative contour irregularities.

RHYTIDECTOMY

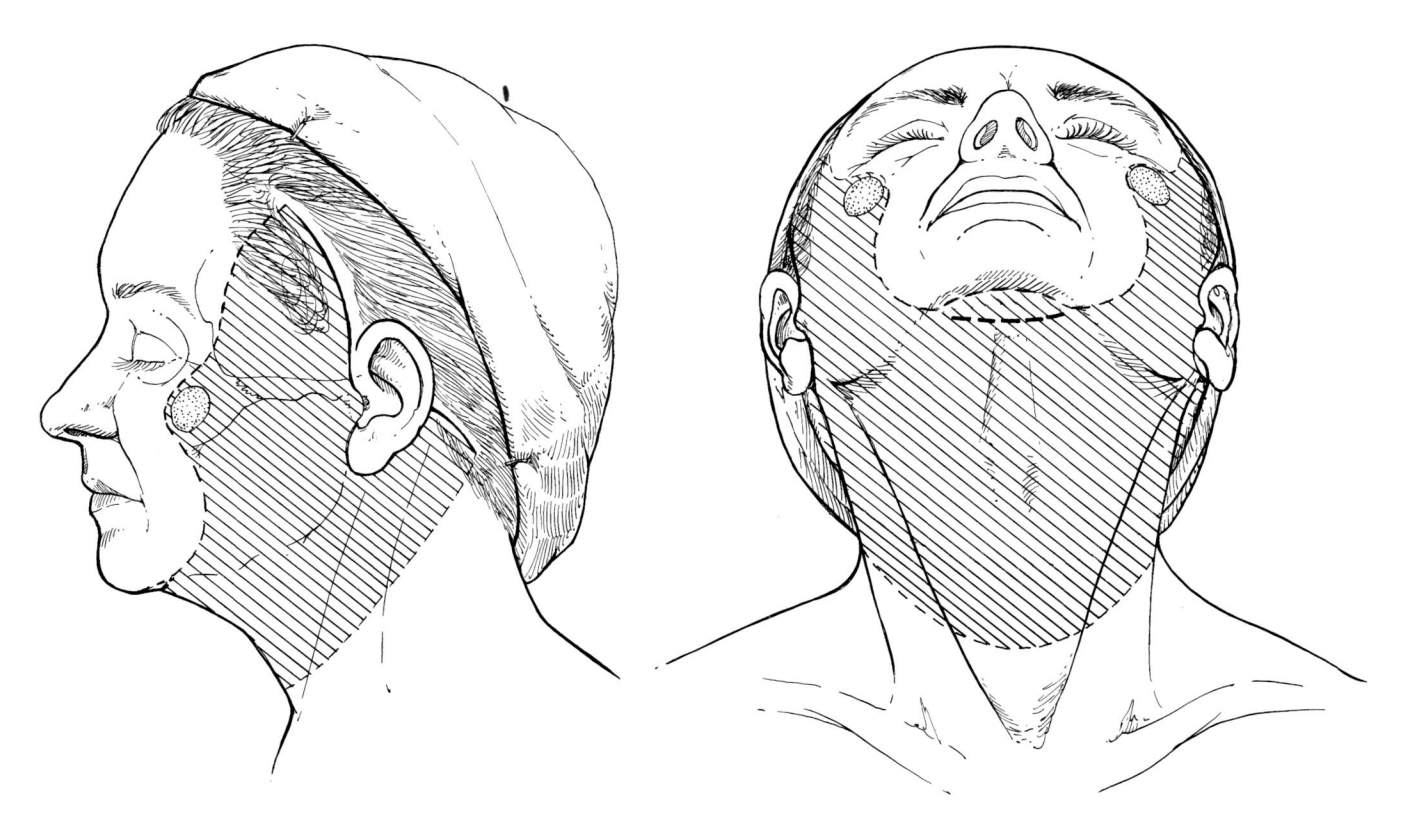

In patients requiring an anterior approach to the platysma, an incision is made in the submental region just caudal to a natural skin crease. Dissection is then continued cephalad to the submental incision toward the mandibular symphysis to free up the attachments of the skin crease to the mandibular border. This is helpful in alleviating a dense submental crease that can be evident on preoperative examination. Following this, dissection is continued caudally in the neck where it communicates with the cervical dissection that has been performed previously through a lateral approach.

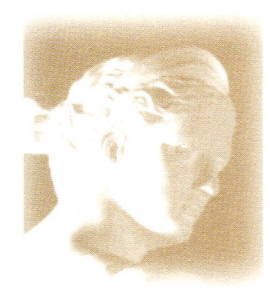

SUPERFICIAL FACIAL FASCIA (SMAS) ELEVATION AND FIXATION

Differential Vectors of Redraping of SMAS Dissection and Skin Flap

Dermal elastosis and the development of skin laxity in the aging face often does not occur in the same direction and at the same rate as aging related to the descent of facial fat. The prime advantage of performing skin undermining separately from SMAS dissection is that it allows these two layers to be redraped along vectors which are independent of one another.

One of the most common aesthetic errors seen in patients presenting for secondary rhytidectomy in which the original surgery has produced a tight, unnatural facial appearance, is that the primary surgeon has used the skin flap as the vehicle to re-suspend facial fat. This requires that the skin flap be redraped along cephalad oriented vectors. Skin that has been over-rotated in a superior direction can produce a distorted facial appearance associated with a tight, masky look, and can also produce distortion of temporal hairlines if incisions are not properly planned.

Using the skin envelope as the vehicle to re-elevate facial fat is not an anatomic approach to the correction of descended facial fat, and thereby can lead to surgical distortion. In preoperative planning, the direction of malar pad and jowl fat elevation (through SMAS flap redraping) should be precisely planned according to the individual patient's needs. In general, we tend to position the malar pad in a direction parallel to the zygomaticus major muscle, as the descent of malar soft tissue most often occurs in this direction. In terms of re-elevation of jowl fat, we commonly re-drape our SMAS dissection in a cephalad direction to produce the optimal re-elevation of descended cheek fat back upward into the face.

We would stress that the direction of the descent of facial fat in aging will vary from patient to patient, and the direction in which this descended fat is re-elevated through the redraping of the SMAS dissection must be individualized for the specific aesthetic needs of the patient. Examining patient photographs taken during youth and analyzing the direction in which the facial fat has descended as the patient has aged is helpful in planning the vectors of SMAS rotation.

The direction of skin flap redraping must also be decided preoperatively, especially when dealing with sundamaged skin. Skin marked by coarse facial rhytides will not tolerate being improperly redraped. This will produce misdirected facial rhytides, which are most commonly seen during animation and as the patient flexes their neck. In general, cheek skin is rotated in a direction a bit more lateral than the cephalad redirection of the SMAS-platysma flap.

The important point to understand is that every patient will age a bit differently in terms of both the direction of facial fat descent and the degree of skin aging. The advantage of doing the SMAS dissection separate from the skin dissection is that it allows the surgeon to precisely redrape these individual layers according to the specific needs of the patient and the aesthetic goals of the surgeon. We would emphasize that while the operative time spent in performing rhytidectomy primarily involves dissection of facial flaps and their subsequent closure, the ultimate result is determined by the vectors of redraping of the superficial fascia and facial skin. Ten to twenty degrees of variability in the direction the surgeon redrapes facial fat and facial skin can make a large difference in terms of postoperative aesthetic appearance.

SURGICAL REJUVENATION OF THE FACE

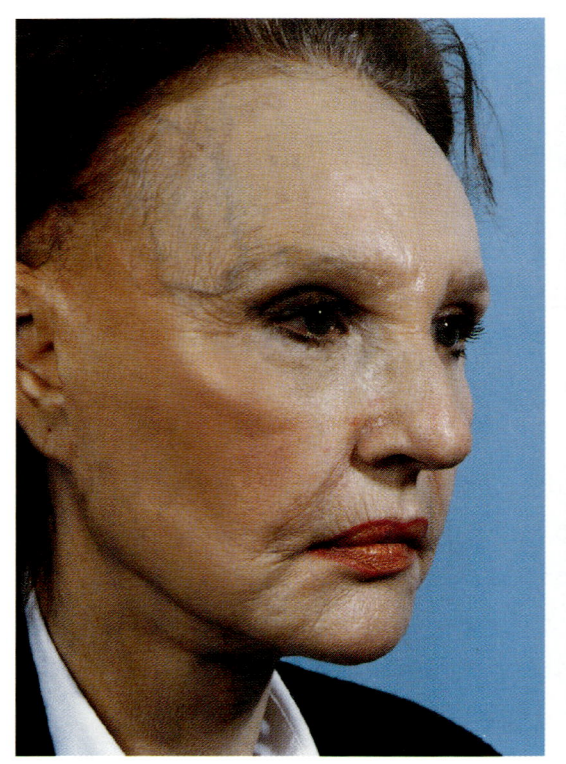

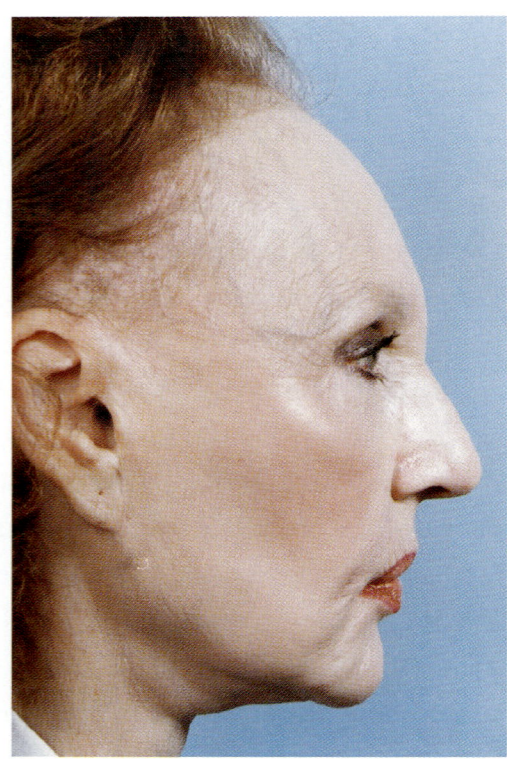

Use of the skin flap as the vehicle to reelevate facial fat commonly may produce postoperative facial distortion by rotating skin in an abnormal (cephalad) direction. This patient, who was operated on in another office, was dissatisfied with her unnatural facial appearance as well as the distortion of her temporal hairline.

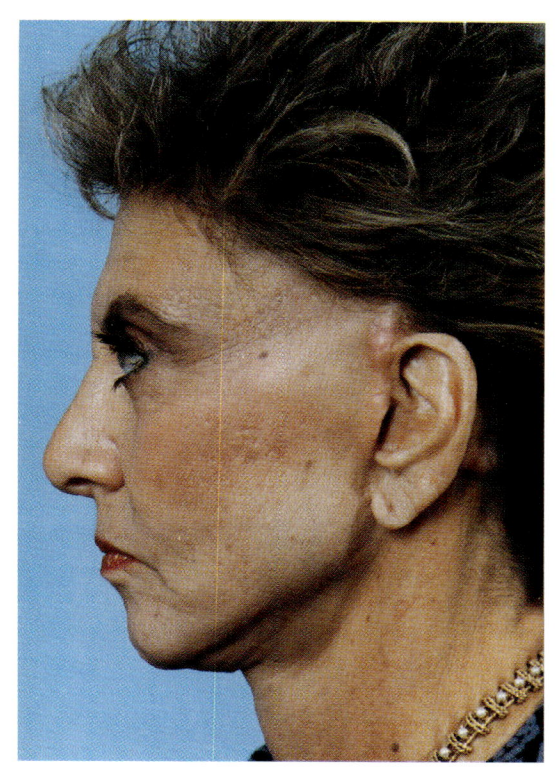

Cephalad rotation of skin in patients with facial rhytides can cause these rhytides to become misdirected, swinging upward into the cheek. This is most notable during neck flexion and with animation. Note also the distortion of the temporal hairline associated with the cephalad redraping of facial skin.

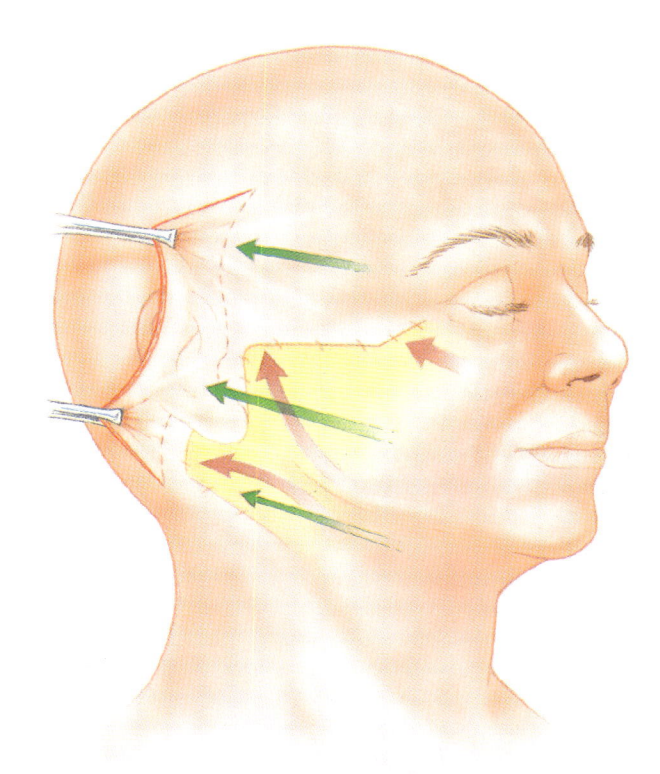

The direction of SMAS redraping in the face tends to be cephalad in its orientation as opposed to skin flap redraping, which is oriented along a more horizontal vector.

Operative Techniques—SMAS

The operative sequence in which SMAS and platysma flaps are dissected and subsequently closed effect the postoperative aesthetic result. The platysma in the neck is in continuity with the platysma and SMAS of the cheek. As this represents a single layer, the sequence in which the surgeon tightens the facial foundation through deep layer support will thereby effect facial and cervical contour. In general, it is our preference to perform cheek SMAS dissection and closure prior to performing cervical contouring of the anterior platysma. If the anterior platysma is contoured at the start of the procedure, then there is a less effective movement of jowl fat back upward into the face with SMAS rotation, as this fat has been tethered into the neck by the prior platysma tightening. For this reason, we prefer to elevate the SMAS of the cheek prior to approaching the platysma, as jowl correction is more complete. Despite significant SMAS mobilization and fixation, the surgeon will find that it is always possible to perform an edge-to-edge approximation of the anterior platysma, although this closure will usually be under more tension than if the platysma has been tightened prior to SMAS elevation

Except perhaps in the young facelift patient, most patients undergoing rhytidectomy will benefit from tightening of the superficial fascia. Aging is more than just skin-deep. Restoration of support to the underlying facial soft tissues has become an integral part of rejuvenation of the aging face. If the SMAS is very thin and tenuous, plication of this layer is a useful alternative to formal SMAS elevation. Nonetheless, in our opinion, better contouring and longer-lasting results are possible following dissection and fixation of the SMAS.

There is little morbidity associated with SMAS dissection as long as the surgeon is knowledgeable in facial soft tissue anatomy. The method we describe here is an attempt to take advantage of the relationship between the SMAS and the underlying parotid gland, parotid-masseteric fascia, and the mimetic muscles. If these relationships are understood, the possibility of facial nerve injury is minimized. *Certainly, if the surgeon becomes uncomfortable as the SMAS is being elevated, or if the*

RHYTIDECTOMY

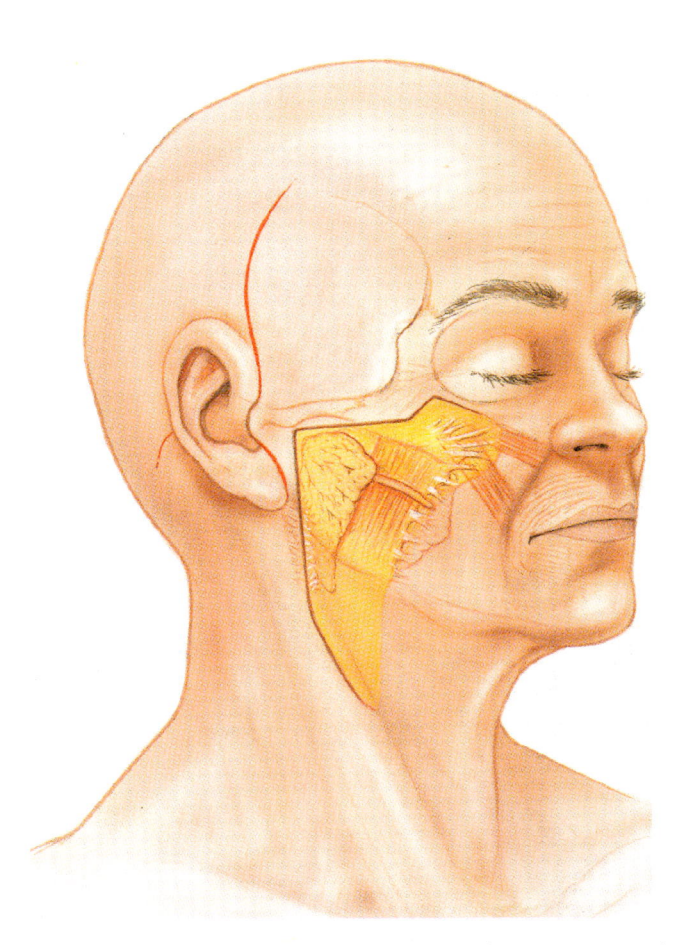

Illustration showing the typical extent of SMAS dissection in the malar region, cheek, and neck. The end point in SMAS dissection is obtaining adequate mobility with redraping. This requires freeing the SMAS in the malar region completely from its zygomatic attachments. To reelevate jowl fat back upward into the cheek usually requires division of both the zygomatic ligaments as well as the upper portion of the masseteric cutaneous ligaments. The SMAS in the cheek below the parotid duct is usually elevated to the anterior border of the masseter, and occasionally division of the lower masseteric cutaneous fibers is required. The SMAS in the neck is elevated off the tail of the gland extending anteriorly within the areolar plane deep to the platysma until adequate mobility is obtained in contouring the submandibular and submental regions of the neck. The key to SMAS elevation is obtaining adequate mobilization to allow reelevation of facial fat without undue tension.

SURGICAL REJUVENATION OF THE FACE

anatomy appears obscured, it is much better to plicate the fascia than risk motor branch injury.

It is helpful when learning SMAS technique to mark the lines where the SMAS is to be incised. The landmarks to note when designing the SMAS flap include the level of the zygomatic arch, the junction of the zygomatic arch with the body of the zygoma, the lateral border of the platysma, and the inferior border of the mandible. Before SMAS elevation, the SMAS is infiltrated with local anesthesia to minimize pain and help with dissection.

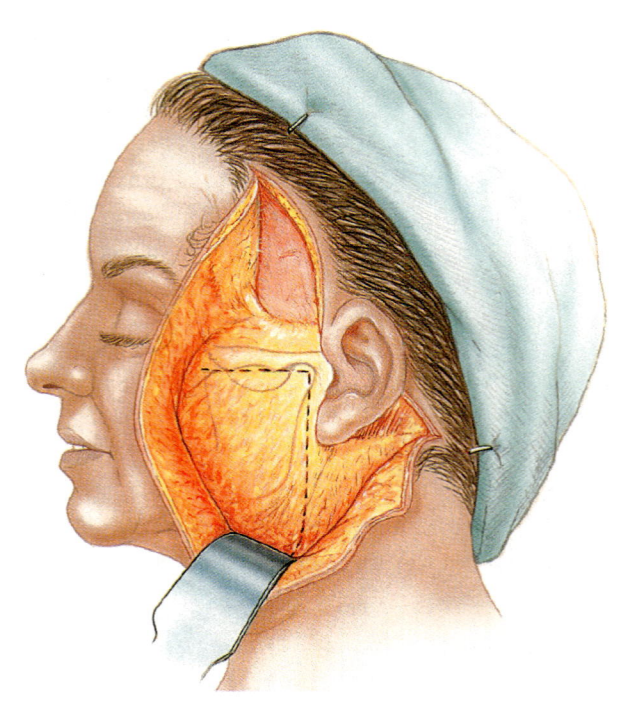

The horizontal incision for SMAS dissection parallels the zygomatic arch and is placed just caudal to it. The mid- to inferior aspect of the tragus serves as a useful landmark for keeping this horizontal portion of the incision below the level of the zygomatic arch (to preserve the frontal branch of the facial nerve). The vertical portion of the dissection extends in the preauricular region inferiorly along the lateral border of the platysma muscle, keeping the incision well posterior to the angle of the mandible (i.e., posterior to the region of the marginal mandibular nerve).

A horizontal incision is made 1 cm inferior to the zygomatic arch (the midportion of the tragus is a usual landmark). This is carried forward toward the malar eminence. A vertical incision is designed along the preauricular region extending along the posterior border of the platysma, to a point 5 to 6 cm below the mandibular border.

SMAS elevation is begun sharply overlying the parotid gland. In some patients, the plane existing between the parotid capsule and the SMAS is easily identified. In other patients, the parotid capsule is elevated with the SMAS flap. This is of no consequence, though it is important to keep the dissection superficial to the parotid parenchyma when elevating the SMAS flap. Entering the parotid gland affords a chance for postoperative parotid fistula, though this is fortunately a rare occurrence.

The dissection is then continued along the posterior border of the platysma. While it is possible to elevate the fascia superficial to the platysma, it is preferable to carry the dissection just along the undersurface of the platysma, which provides a thicker, more useful flap. Identification of the platysma muscle low in the neck, and then continuing the dissection anteriorly and cephalad helps in identifying the proper plane of SMAS elevation.

Dissection proceeds medially toward the anterior edge of the parotid. As the anterior border of the parotid is reached, on careful observation sub-SMAS fat becomes visible as the surgical dissection is carried anterior to the brownish parotid gland, exposing the more medial areolar plane that overlies the masseter muscle. Once this point in flap elevation is reached, dissection can proceed bluntly with gentle finger-gauze dissection or the use of a Kitner dissector. This areolar plane is usually encountered first within the region of the tail of the parotid, since this is the narrowest portion of the gland. The most difficult portion of the SMAS to free up from the parotid is where the parotid duct leaves the gland. The SMAS is commonly adherent at this point, although it can usually be dissected with careful technique.

SURGICAL REJUVENATION OF THE FACE

Once freed from the parotid by dissection, the SMAS flap is rapidly elevated in the areolar plane that exists between the superficial and deep fascia overlying the masseter muscle. Sub-SMAS fat becomes evident and usually obscures underlying facial nerve branches, especially in the region of the marginal mandibular nerve. The dissection can be carried forward with blunt technique to the anterior border of the masseter where the masseteric cutaneous ligaments are encountered. If buccal fat harvesting is planned (a procedure we only occasionally perform in conjunction with rhytidectomy), spreading bluntly through the vertical septa of the masseteric cutaneous ligament will expose the buccal fat lying medial to the masseter.

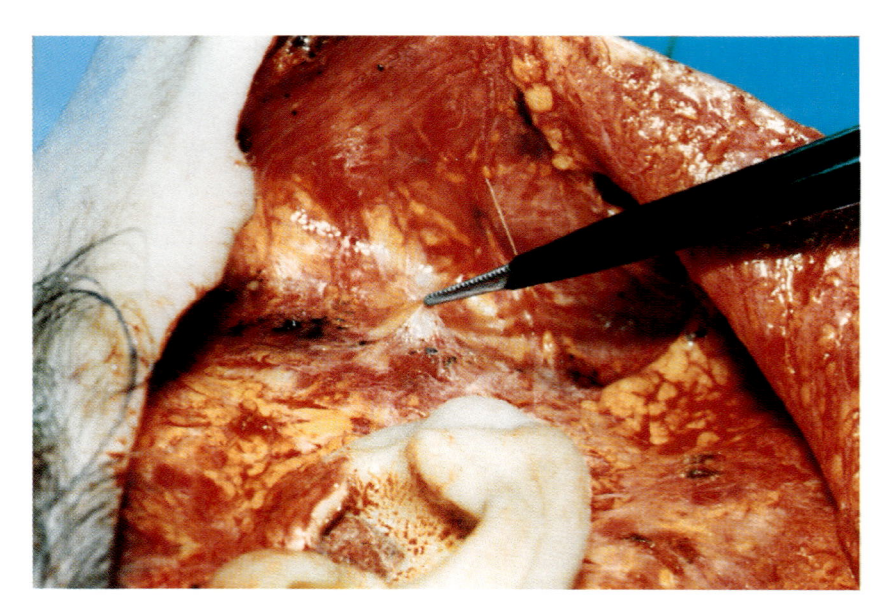

Operative photograph illustrating the SMAS being elevated anterior to the parotid gland, exposing the underlying masseteric fascia (held in forceps). To obtain adequate flap mobility, freeing of the SMAS from the underlying parotid gland is required.

RHYTIDECTOMY

Elevating the SMAS-platysma within the neck proceeds in continuity with the cheek-SMAS dissection. Usually the lateral border of the platysma is undermined for approximately 5 to 6 cm below the mandibular border. A fibrous portion of dissection is encountered in the region of the tail of the parotid (parotid-cutaneous ligament). Anterior to this region the cervical branches of the facial nerve leave the protection of the parotid, traveling to the platysma, and should be preserved. It is important to free the platysma medial to the parotid cutaneous ligament, usually using spreading scissors technique, to ensure flap mobility. Once medial to the ligament, the areolar plane deep to the platysma is encountered and blunt dissection is performed as needed to obtain adequate mobility.

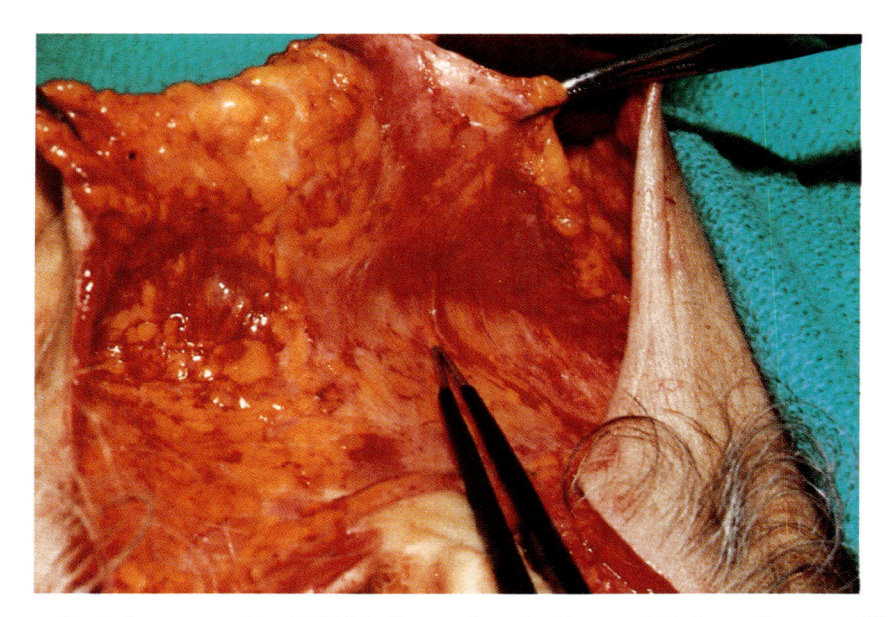

Operative photograph of SMAS dissection in the neck below the mandibular border. It is important to free the SMAS from the underlying parotid cutaneous ligament in this region of the dissection so that adequate flap mobility is obtained. Note that a cervical branch to the platysma is visualized in this portion of the dissection.

In patients with prominent nasolabial folds, we extend the SMAS dissection into the malar region, a procedure we term *extended SMAS dissection.* This malar extension of the SMAS dissection begins in the region of the junction of the zygomatic arch with the body of the zygoma. The incision within the SMAS angles superiorly over the malar prominence toward the lateral canthus for a distance of 3 to 4 cm. On reaching the edge of the subcutaneous skin flap in the region of the lateral orbit, the incision is carried inferiorly at a 90-degree angle toward the nasolabial fold. The SMAS in the malar region is then elevated in continuity with the SMAS of the cheek. On elevating this flap, the fibers of the zygomaticus major and minor are usually evident. It is important to carry the dissection directly external to these muscle fibers where a natural plane exists, remembering that the facial nerve branches lie deep to the muscular bodies. The malar SMAS is elevated until the entire flap is freed from the underlying zygomatic prominence. Freeing of the SMAS completely from its zygomatic attachment is important to obtain the mobility needed to reposition the malar soft tissues superiorly. This usually also requires a division of the upper fibers of the masseteric cutaneous ligament (which will expose the body of the underlying buccal fat pad).

A, In patients with prominent nasolabial folds, we perform what we term an extended SMAS dissection. *By this, we mean we extend the SMAS dissection into the malar region in an attempt to reelevate ptotic malar fat back upward over the zygomatic prominence. The incisions begin at the junction where the zygomatic arch joins the body of the zygoma. From this point, the incision in the SMAS is angled superiorly toward the lateral canthus and along the lateral orbital rim. The incision in the SMAS is then carried medially and inferiorly toward the peripheral extent of skin flap undermining, angling toward the uppermost portion of the nasolabial fold (the amount of subcutaneous undermining is shaded in pink, whereas the amount of SMAS undermining is shaded in yellow.) B, The malar-SMAS dissection is then performed in continuity with the cheek-SMAS dissection. Dissecting in the malar region carries the dissection directly along the superficial surface of the zygomaticus major and usually*

RHYTIDECTOMY

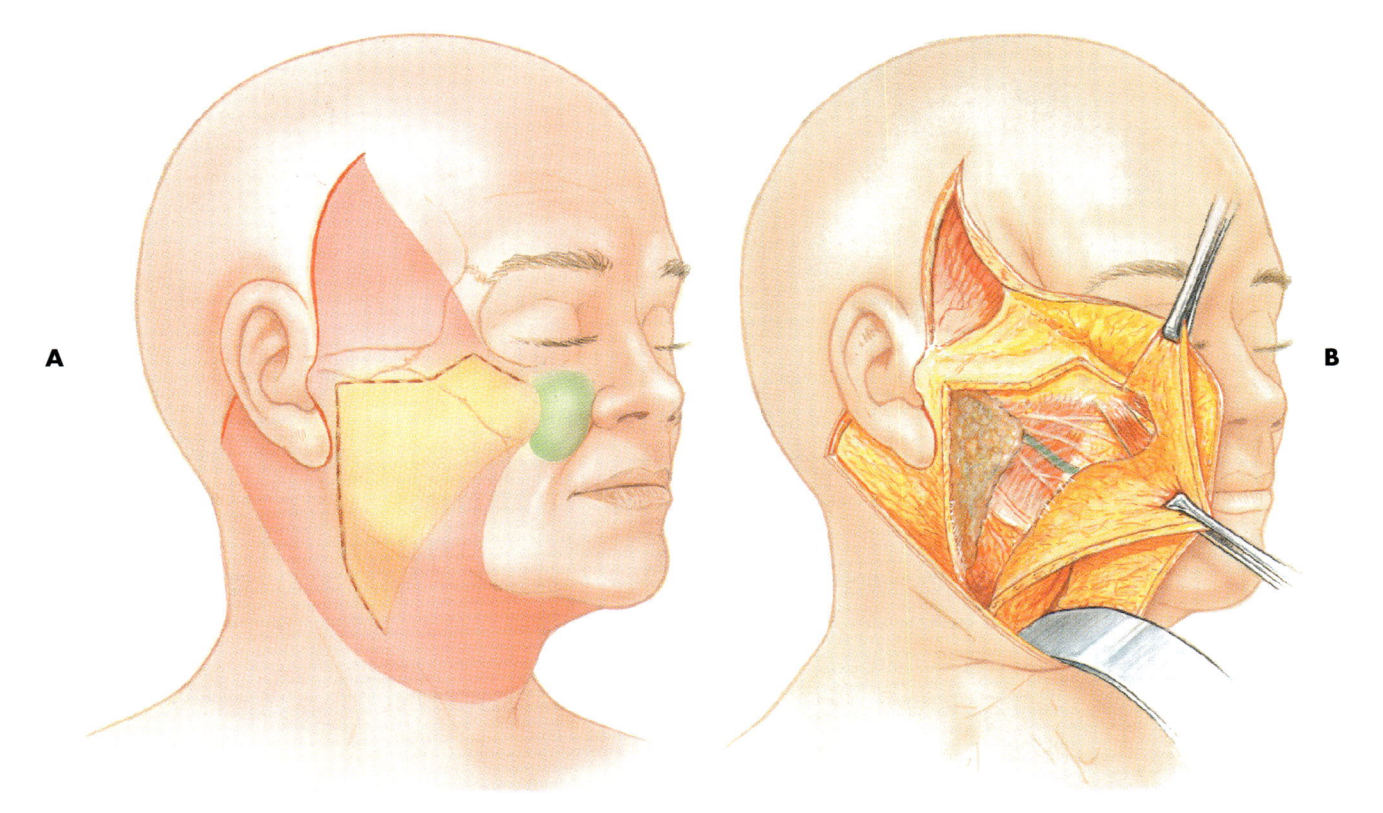

A B

exposes the lateral aspects of the zygomaticus minor as well. To obtain adequate mobility in terms of SMAS dissection, it is necessary to elevate the malar portion of the dissection completely from the zygomatic eminence and free it from the zygomatic ligaments. To obtain mobility in terms of SMAS movement affecting jowl contour, the uppermost portions of the masseteric cutaneous ligament commonly are divided, especially where they merge with the zygomatic ligaments of the malar area. If these fibers are not divided, they will restrict the upward redraping of jowl fat. Upon division of the upper portion of the masseteric cutaneous ligaments, the buccal fat pad becomes evident, and commonly the zygomatic nerve branches traversing toward the undersurface of the zygomaticus major muscle are visualized. This diagram illustrates the typical degree of mobilization performed in our extended SMAS dissection.

Continued.

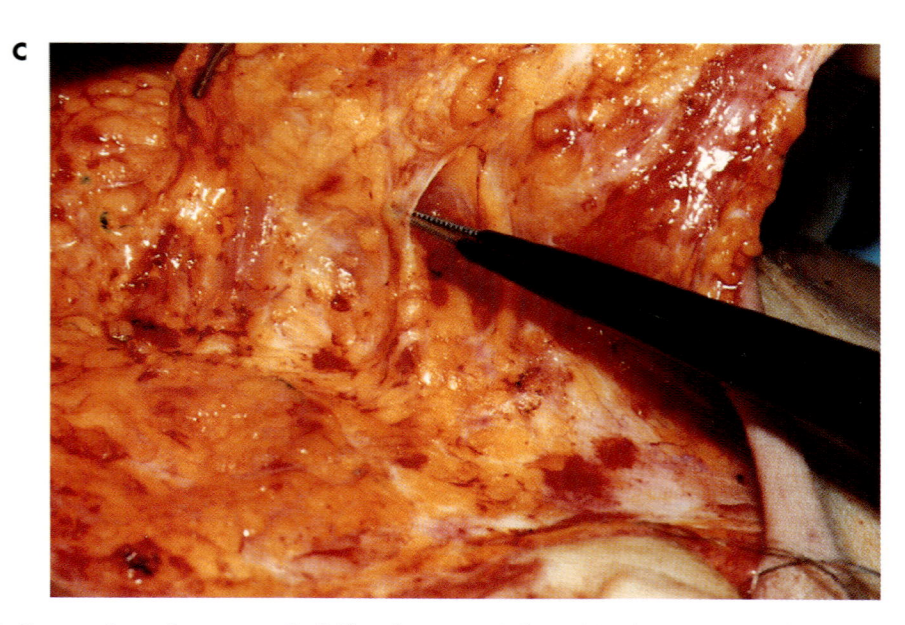

C, Operative photograph following partial SMAS elevation in the malar region. Note the origins of the zygomaticus major and minor muscles visualized in the region below the hemostat along the medial portion of the dissection. Dissection in the region overlying the junction of the malar eminence with the origin of the masseteric muscle exposes the stout fibers of the masseteric cutaneous ligament (overlying the forceps) that must be divided to obtain adequate flap mobility. In some patients it can be difficult to differentiate ligamentous fibers from small nerve bundles, and this portion of the dissection must be performed with great care.

In most patients, following extended SMAS dissection of the cheek and malar region, mobility of the soft tissues lying lateral to the nasolabial fold will remain restricted unless the dissection is carried more medially. This restriction in movement results from undivided retaining ligaments, which originate medial to the zygomaticus minor. To improve mobility, we commonly continue the sub-SMAS elevation toward the medial portion of the cheek, in an area where we have not subcutaneously undermined the skin. This dissection is carried directly in the plane between the SMAS and the elevators of the upper lip. It is usually easy to delineate this level of dissection after the malar SMAS elevation is complete and the plane of the elevators of the upper lip is visualized. The scissors are then inserted directly superficial to the elevators of the upper lip, and blunt dissection is quickly performed by pushing the scissors in a series of passes past the nasolabial fold. We find that when we insert the scissors in the proper plane, the dissection glides quickly through the malar soft tissues and we usually feel a "snap" as we dissect through the remaining retaining ligaments. Once these structures are divided, one notes greater mobility when traction is applied to the malar portion of the SMAS flap.

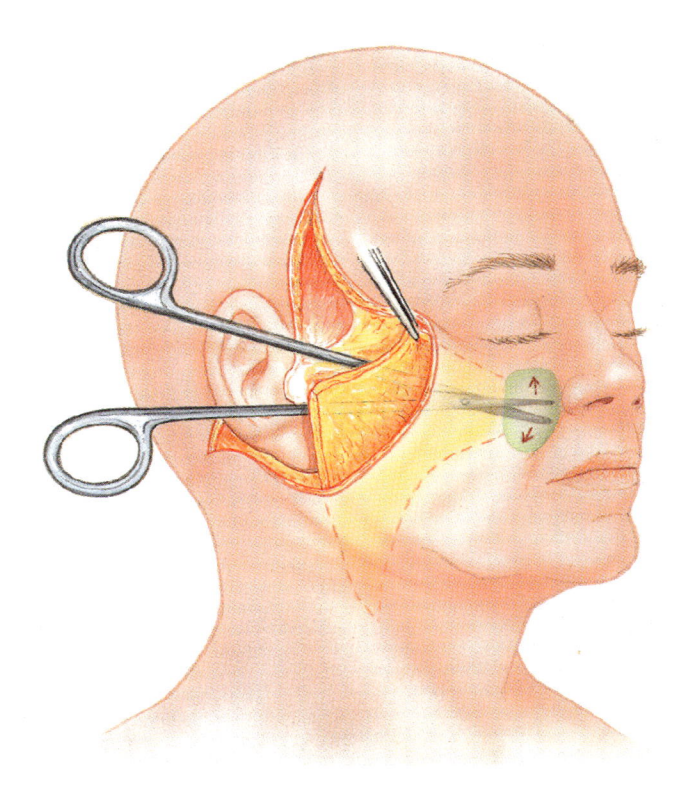

It is commonly necessary to extend the malar SMAS dissection more peripherally than the subcutaneous dissection to obtain adequate flap mobility of the soft tissues lateral to the nasolabial fold. This portion of the dissection is easily performed by simply inserting the scissors in the plane between the superficial surface of the elevators of the upper lip and the overlying subcutaneous fat. Once the scissors are inserted in the proper plane, the surgeon bluntly dissects in a series of passes past the nasolabial fold (area marked in green). As long as the scissors remain superficial to the elevators of the upper lip, motor nerve injury will be prevented. Usually two or three passes are required to obtain adequate flap mobility.

Repositioning and closure of the SMAS is then performed. The malar SMAS flap is advanced superolaterally over the zygomatic prominence in a direction perpendicular to the nasolabial fold. After superior and lateral advancement, the excess tissue can be excised and the flap securely fixated to the zygomatic periosteum with interrupted sutures.

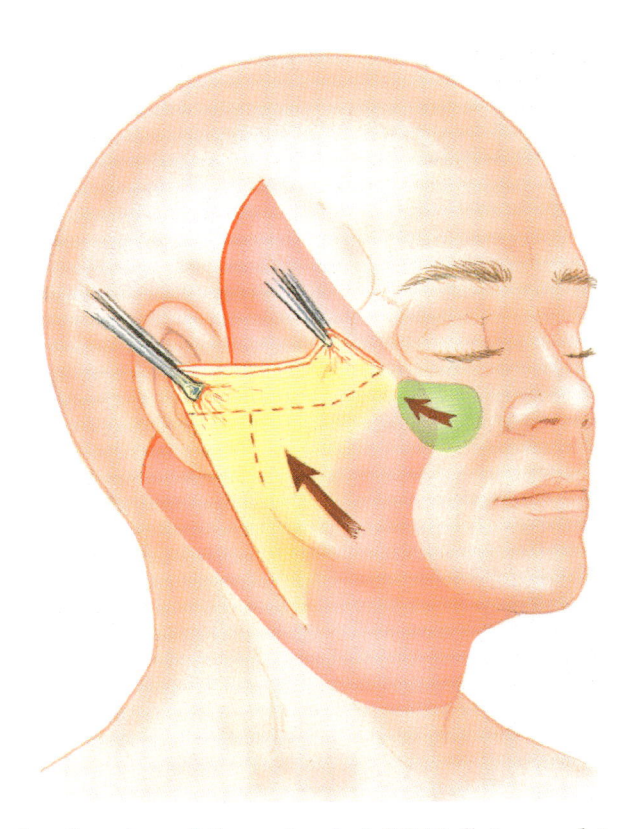

The vectors of redraping of the extended SMAS flap are determined according to the preoperative evaluation of the patient and are generally more cephalad than skin flap redraping.

SURGICAL REJUVENATION OF THE FACE

Once the malar flap is secure, the cheek-SMAS flap is rotated superiorly, perpendicular to the mandibular border. This portion of the SMAS flap is used to contour jawline and jowl. The SMAS flap overlying the preauricular region and ear is then treated as a transposition flap and carried posteriorly behind the ear, helping to restore tone to the submental region and neck. Following trimming, the SMAS flap is

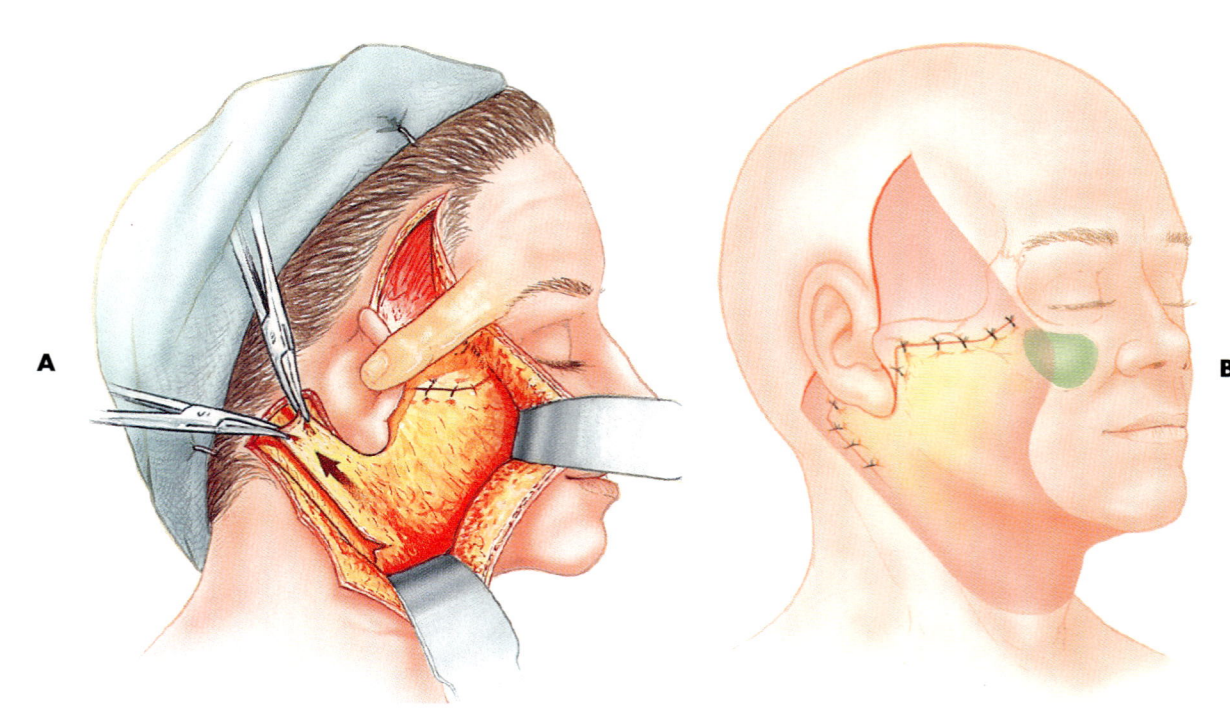

A, Following SMAS redraping in the cheek, the excess SMAS is transposed posterior to the ear to effect contour in the submental and submandibular region by tightening the platysma through lateral tension. It is important to secure this flap to the immobile mastoid fascia, rather than to the mobile fascia overlying the sternocleidomastoid. B, The final closure of the extended SMAS dissection.

carefully secured with multiple interrupted sutures. Occasionally, skin dimpling is noted after securing the SMAS flap. This results from the forces of SMAS rotation on resuspended facial skin. Skin dimpling is treated by simply performing a bit more subcutaneous undermining before skin flap redraping.

That the SMAS has been adequately mobilized can be determined by observing the effect of facial contouring when traction on the SMAS is applied. In general, freeing the SMAS past the restraint of the retaining ligaments provides the mobility necessary to obtain consistent facial contouring through SMAS redraping.

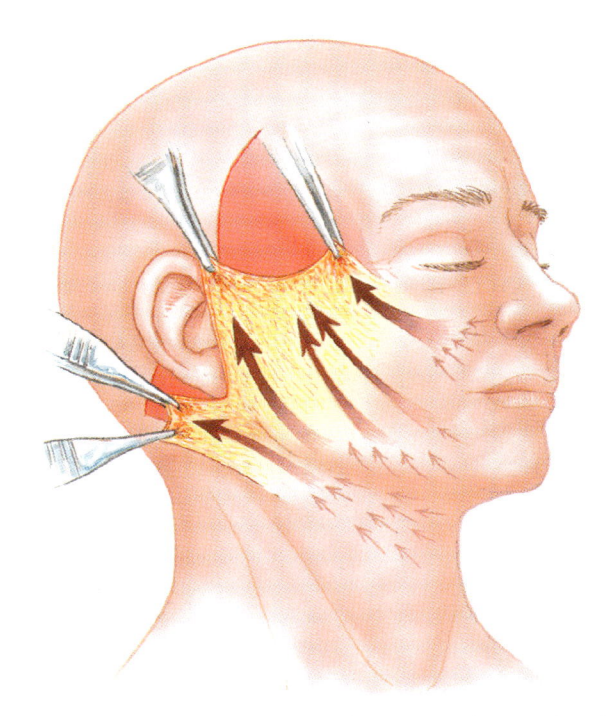

Illustration of the various portions of the SMAS dissection in terms of affecting facial contour. The vectors of redraping can be adjusted according to the needs of the individual patient.

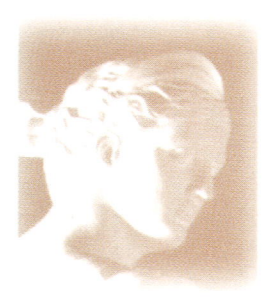

PREVENTING RELAPSE AND SMAS FIXATION

Over time it has become apparent that one of the difficulties in obtaining lasting results using deep layer, or SMAS, techniques is not only inadequate mobilization of this layer but also in the difficulty in obtaining long-lasting fixation. Numerous forces are working to bring the facial fat back down into the face. Forces exerted by smiling, mastication, and animation act as tension factors that can result in a loosening of the suture fixation of the SMAS, resulting in an early relapse and loss of contour. Individual patients show a good deal of variation in terms of the thickness of the SMAS layer, and this is especially true in the secondary or tertiary facelift patient. For this reason, over the last several years, we have concentrated on improving our methods of SMAS fixation. The method that we have found to be most useful is a technique suggested by Dr. Val Lambros. In this method, instead of discarding the excess SMAS following mobilization, the excess soft tissue is doubled onto itself to create a thicker layer for suturing, and a better tissue substrate for suture fixation. The SMAS is redraped along the proper vectors of rotation and marked as if excision is to be performed. The excess tissue is then rolled under itself along the marking and a roll of the doubled-over SMAS is created. This thickened roll of tissue is then fixated under moderate tension using permanent nonabsorbable 4-0 sutures (Mersilene). Fixation is usually begun in the malar region, securing the SMAS roll to the periosteum of the zygomatic buttress. The closure is then continued more laterally in the face, beneath the zygomatic arch, with care taken not to suture the periosteum of the arch out of concern for the underlying frontal nerve branch. The transposition flap is then formed as described above and secured in the postauricular region to the underlying mastoid fascia. We have noted that as we have improved our methods of SMAS fixation, postoperative relapse, with descent of facial fat, has become less common and the results of SMAS contouring have improved. An added benefit of preserving the excess SMAS, rather than excising it, is that as the thickened SMAS layer is secured to the zygomatic eminence, it leads to highlighting of the malar region, serving as an autologous malar augmentation.

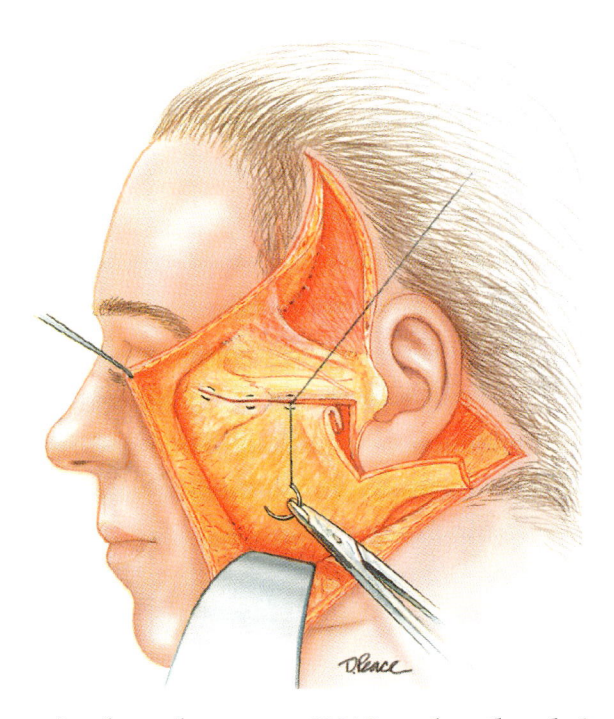

Diagram illustrating how the excess SMAS, rather than being excised, is rolled onto itself (forming a double layer of SMAS thickness). Once the roll has been formed, it is fixated to the periosteum of the zygomatic buttress using permanent sutures. It is important to obtain a secure intraoperative fixation, and we emphasize that fixation is as important as adequate SMAS mobilization.

Morbidity and Complications

We have noted little morbidity associated with extensive SMAS dissection, although to be performed safely requires a working knowledge of the subtleties of facial soft tissue anatomy. Our technique of SMAS undermining represents an attempt to take advantage of the relationship which exists between the SMAS and the underlying protection offered by the parotid gland and deep facial fascia. If these relationships are understood, the possibility of facial nerve injury is minimized. We would emphasize that if the surgeon becomes uncomfortable as the SMAS is being elevated or the anatomy appears obscured, it is better to plicate the fascia than risk motor branch injury.

The most difficult portion of the SMAS to raise in performing extended SMAS dissection is in the transition zone between cheek SMAS and malar SMAS directly inferior to the zygomatic eminence. This area represents the transition zone between the zygomatic ligaments and the masseteric cutaneous ligaments, and anatomic variances are common in this area. Specifically, in approximately 10 percent of patients, the zygomatic nerve branches will penetrate the deep fascia a few cm lateral to the zygomaticus major and lie in the sub-SMAS plane in this region, rather than continuing deep to the deep fascia on their path to the elevators of the upper lip. Because these nerves penetrate the deep fascia early in some patients, and because of the presence of both zygomatic and masseteric ligaments in this region of the face, it can be difficult in some patients to differentiate between the zygomatic nerve branches and the facial ligaments. Great care is required in this area so that the zygomatic branches are protected and only the ligaments divided.

The other problem that occurs in this region of the fascial soft tissue area is that the transition zone between cheek SMAS and malar SMAS often represents the thinnest portion of the flap dissection and the easiest area to tear the flap. Experience is required to safely elevate the superficial fascia in the region directly inferior to the zygomatic eminence, and we could urge conservatism in the dissection until the surgeon becomes completely familiar with the anatomic nuances which occur in this area of facial soft tissue anatomy. *No amount of improvement in facial contouring is worth an injury to the facial nerve.*

In terms of postoperative morbidity, we would note that patients who have had an extended SMAS dissection usually are a bit more swollen than patients who have had a simple plication of the superficial fascia. Most of our patients are socially acceptable within a ten day period and are able to return to work within two weeks, although the use of covering cosmetics is occasionally required. Full recovery requires approximately three months in most patients.

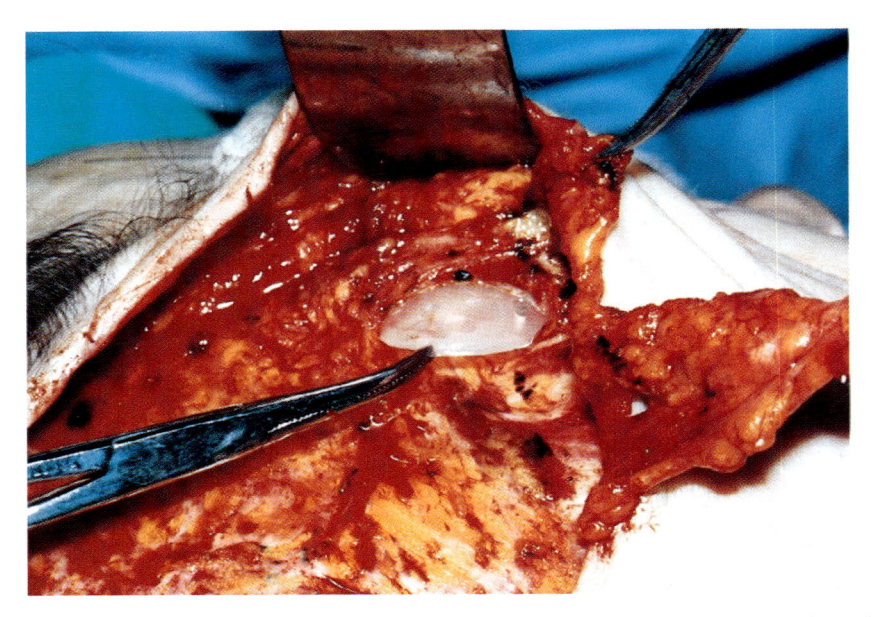

Extended SMAS dissection in a patient who had previously placed malar implants and wanted them removed during the secondary rhytidectomy. Note the zygomaticus major overlying the implant. The malar deficiency following implant removal was reconstructed by using the excess malar soft tissue doubled on itself as described in the preceding figure.

Continued.

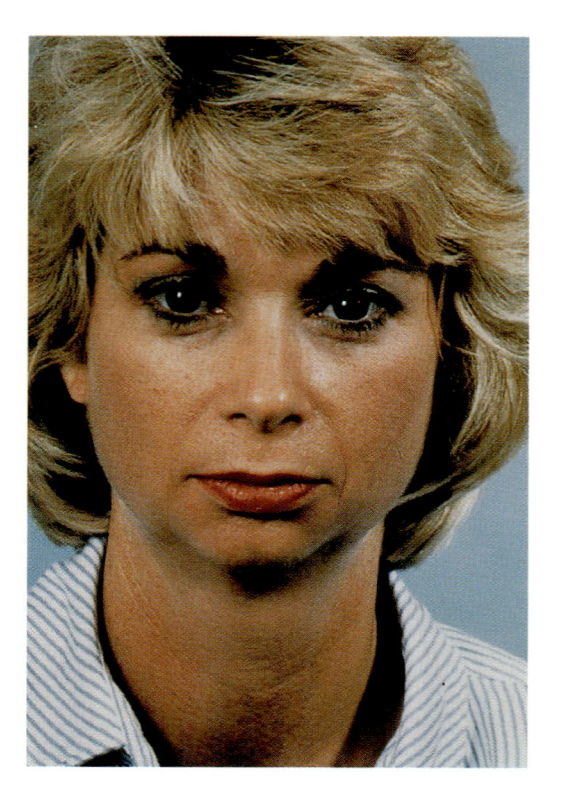

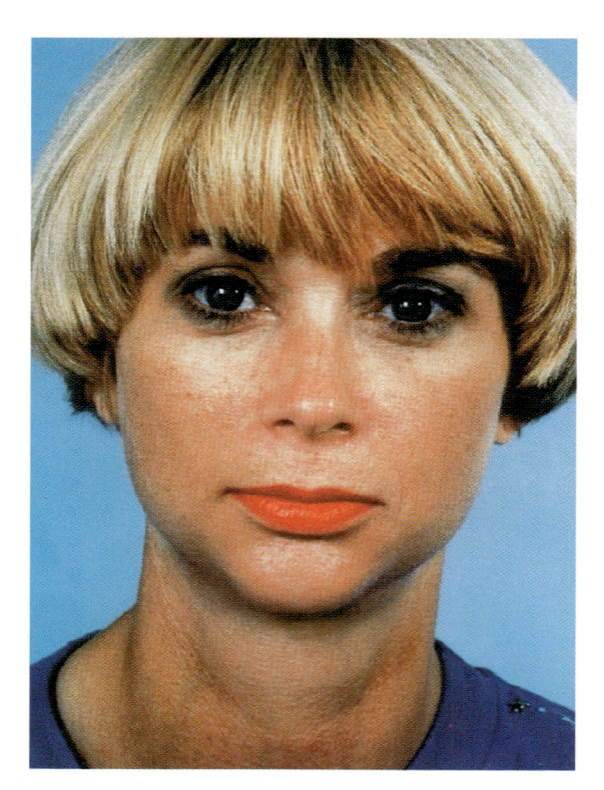

A, Preoperative appearance. *B,* Postoperative result following extended SMAS dissection in which the recruited excess malar soft tissue was used to highlight the malar eminence by the technique described in the text.

RHYTIDECTOMY

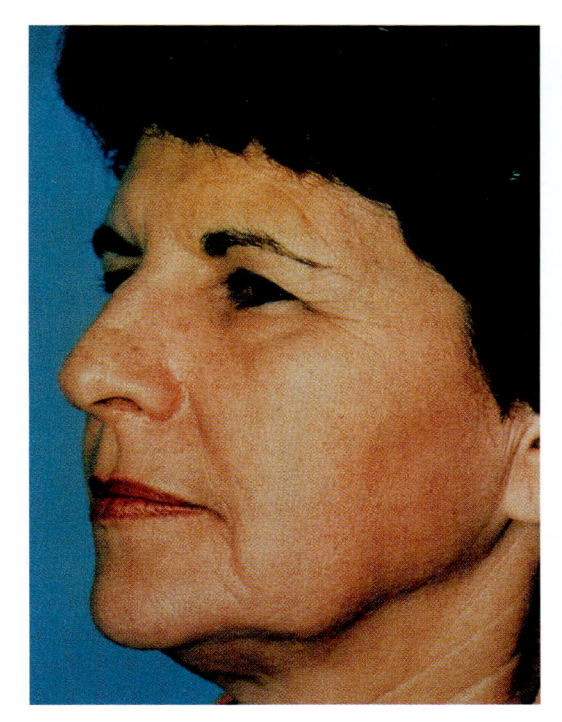

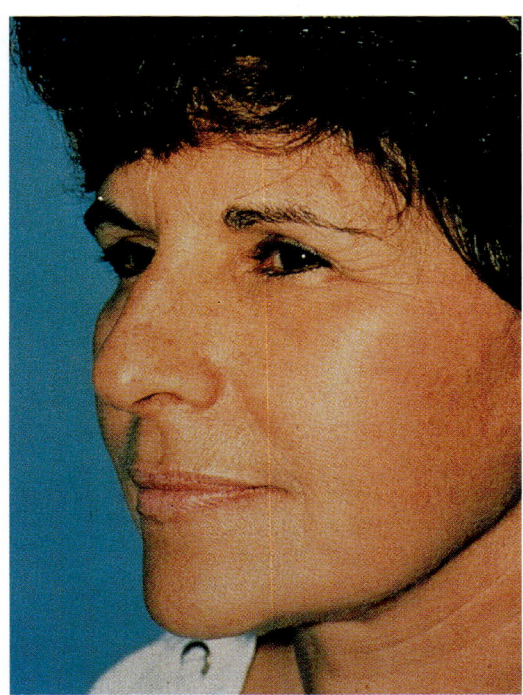

One of the prime advantages of an SMAS technique is that it allows elevation of facial fat in a direction independent of skin flap redraping. In this patient, the improvement of the jowl and jawline is largely secondary to resuspension of facial fat back upward in the face by SMAS techniques. No facial fat was removed.

SURGICAL REJUVENATION OF THE FACE

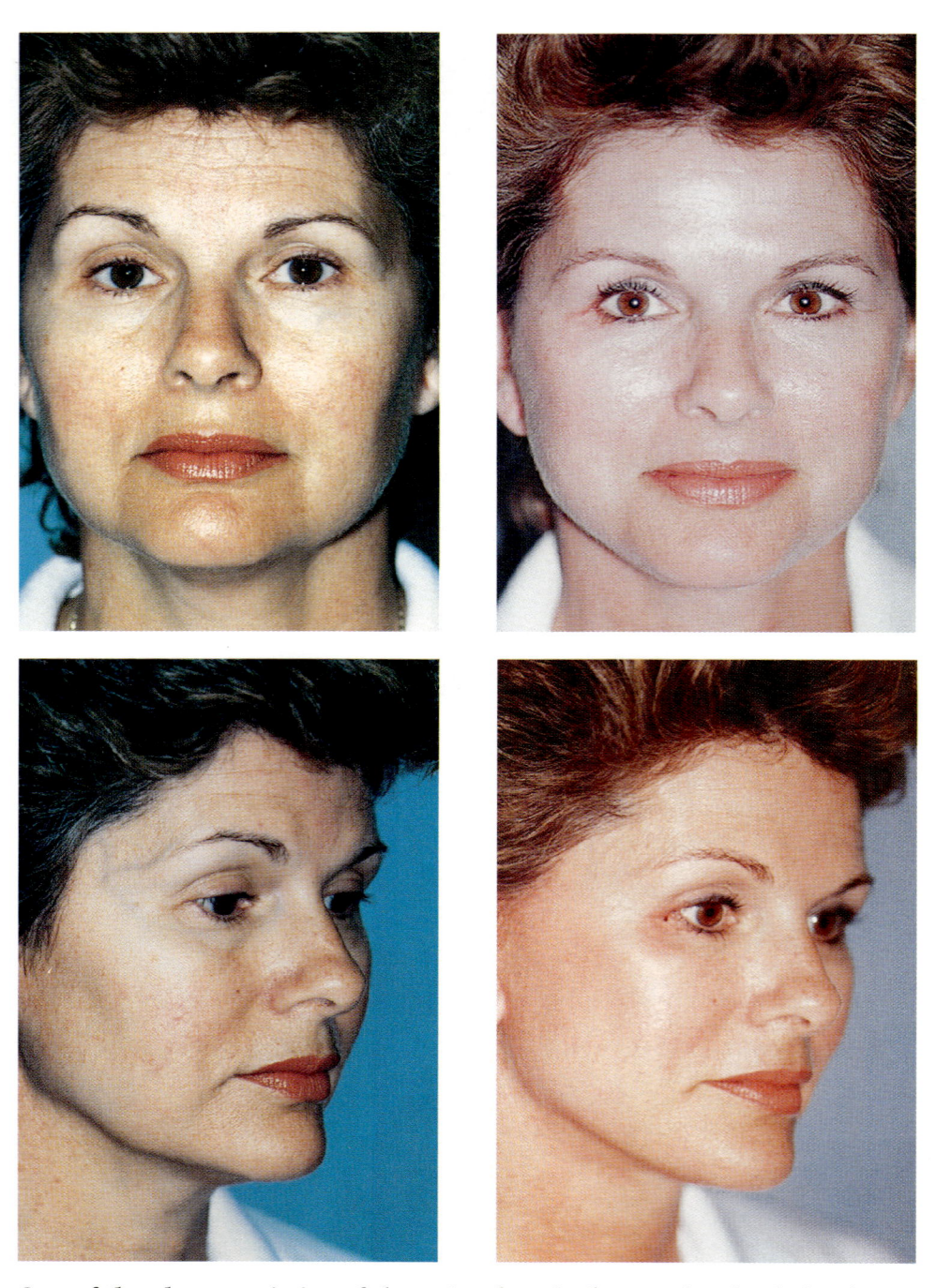

One of the characteristics of the aging face is that as the cheek fat descends to form jowls, the facial contour changes from an oval shape to one more square. Through elevation of facial fat using SMAS techniques, it becomes apparent on the postoperative view that a tapering in facial contour has been obtained without the removal of facial fat.

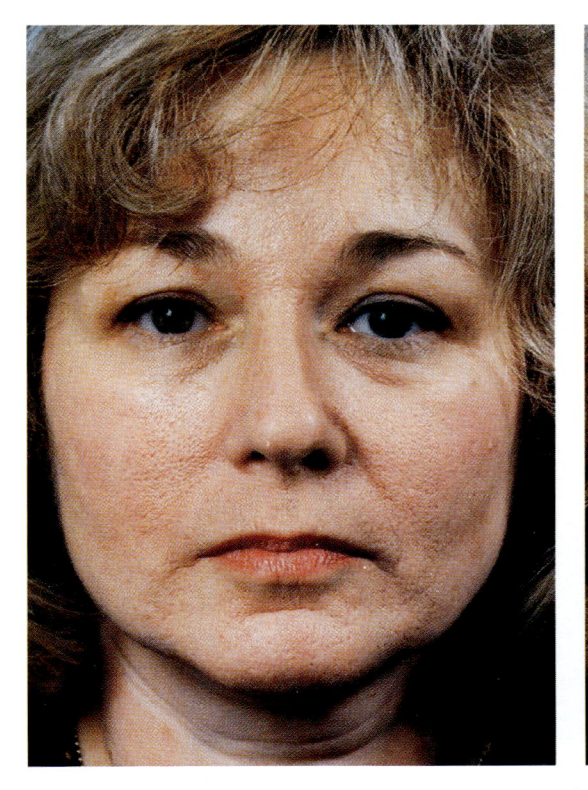

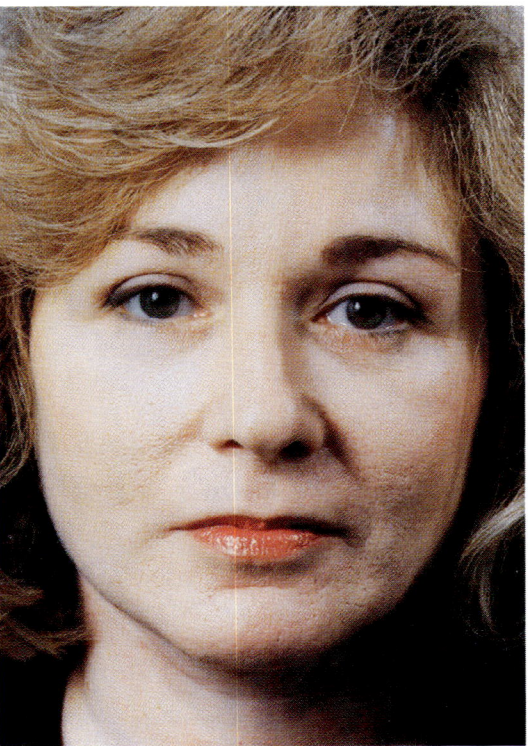

As people get older they tend to gain weight, and this can result in a change of facial contour. In this patient with a round, fatty face, removal of jowl fat in conjunction with restoration of muscular support through a standard SMAS dissection has produced a tapering in facial contour. The decision to remove facial fat should be made preoperatively, and we emphasize that in general it is better to reelevate facial fat to its normal anatomic location rather than remove it from an abnormal location.

SURGICAL REJUVENATION OF THE FACE

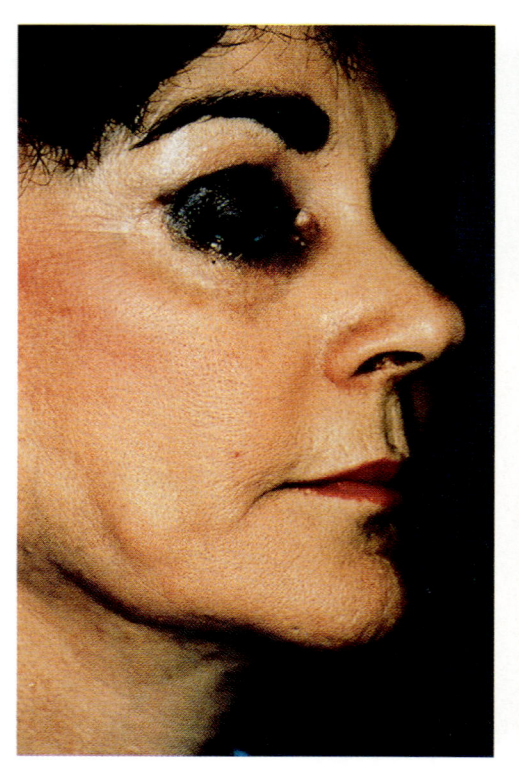

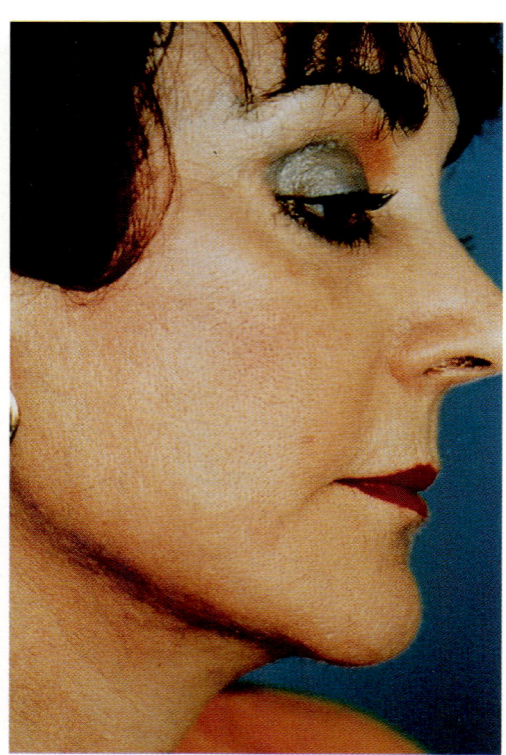

The decision to remove jowl fat must be made judiciously. The patient seen here had two facelifts done in another office. The surgeon attempted to improve the jowls by removal of facial fat using an open-type suction technique. This resulted in attenuation of support of both the superficial and deep facial fascia overlying the buccal fat pad, allowing the buccal fat to prolapse into an unsightly postoperative bulge. The patient is shown postoperatively following reexploration with removal of buccal fat and imbrication of the weakened SMAS layer overlying the buccal fat pad.

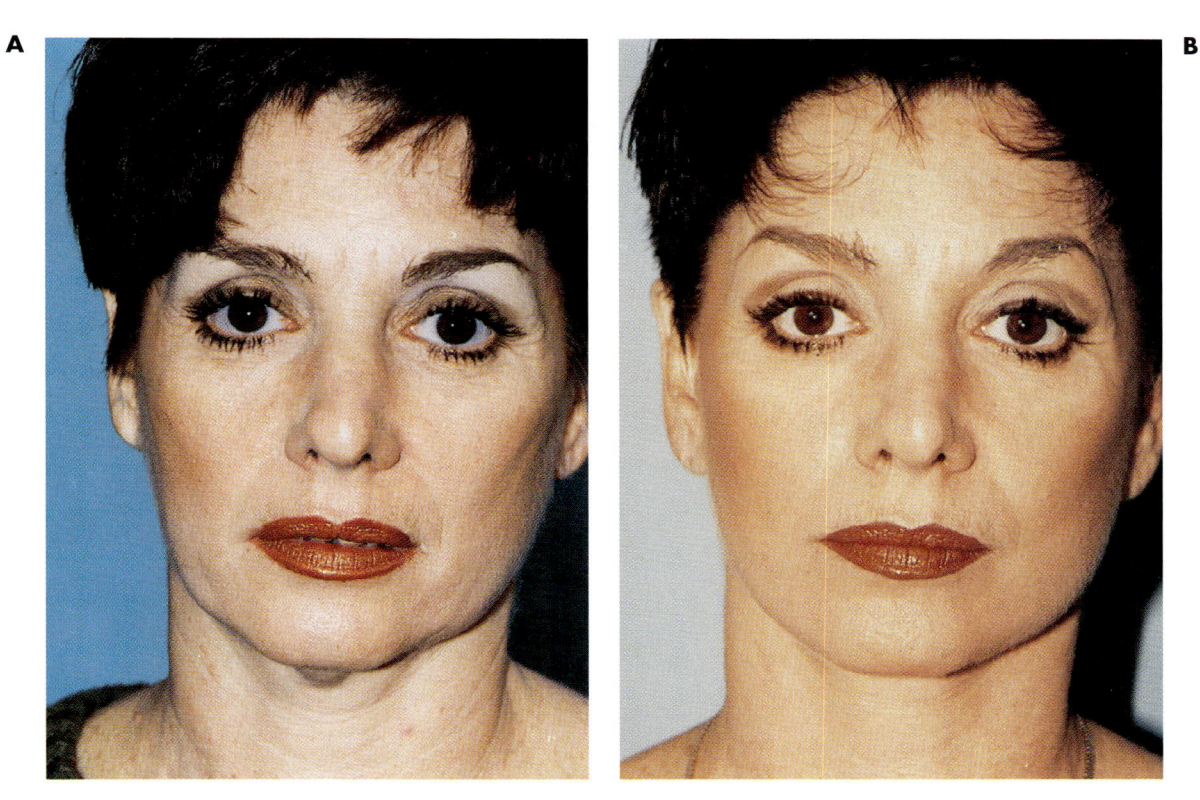

A, This 49-year-old woman shows early signs of facial aging. B, Result following rhytidectomy with extended SMAS dissection.

SURGICAL REJUVENATION OF THE FACE

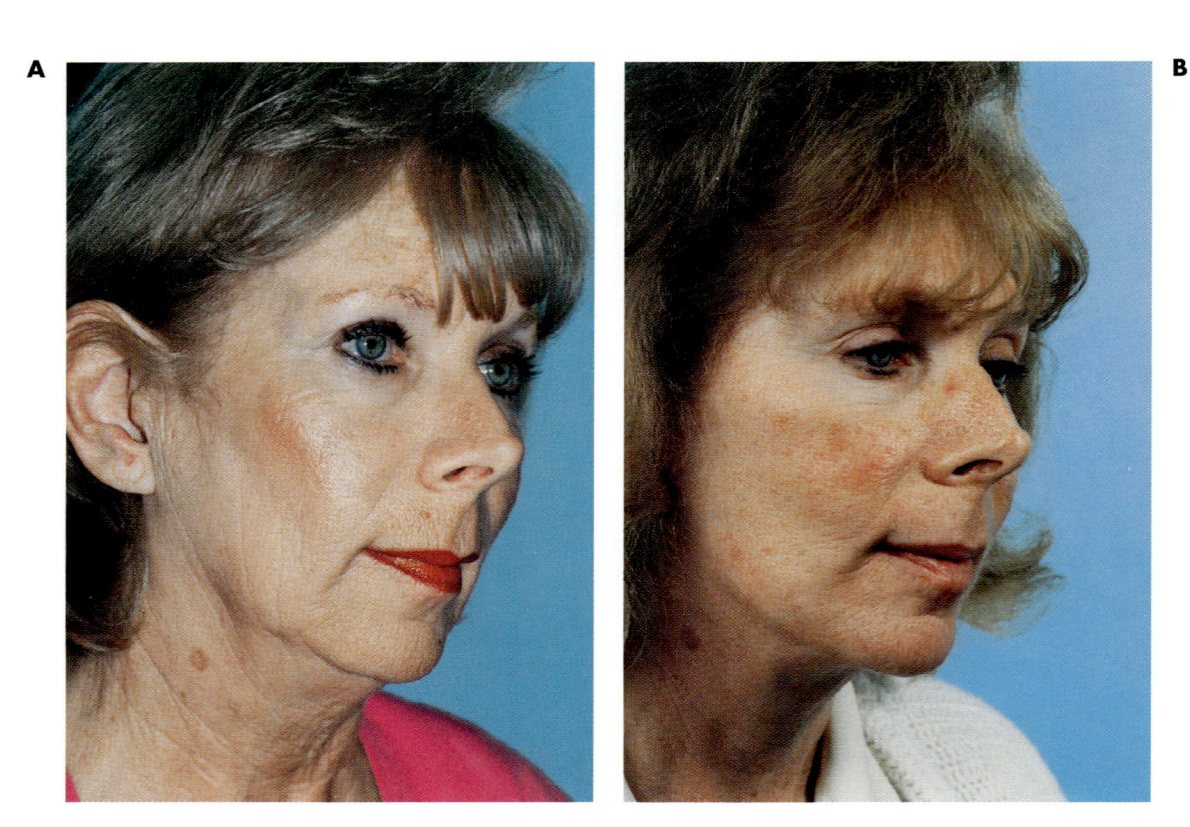

A, Preoperative appearance. *B*, Postoperative appearance following extended SMAS dissection.

A, Preoperative appearance. B, Postoperative result following extended SMAS dissection.

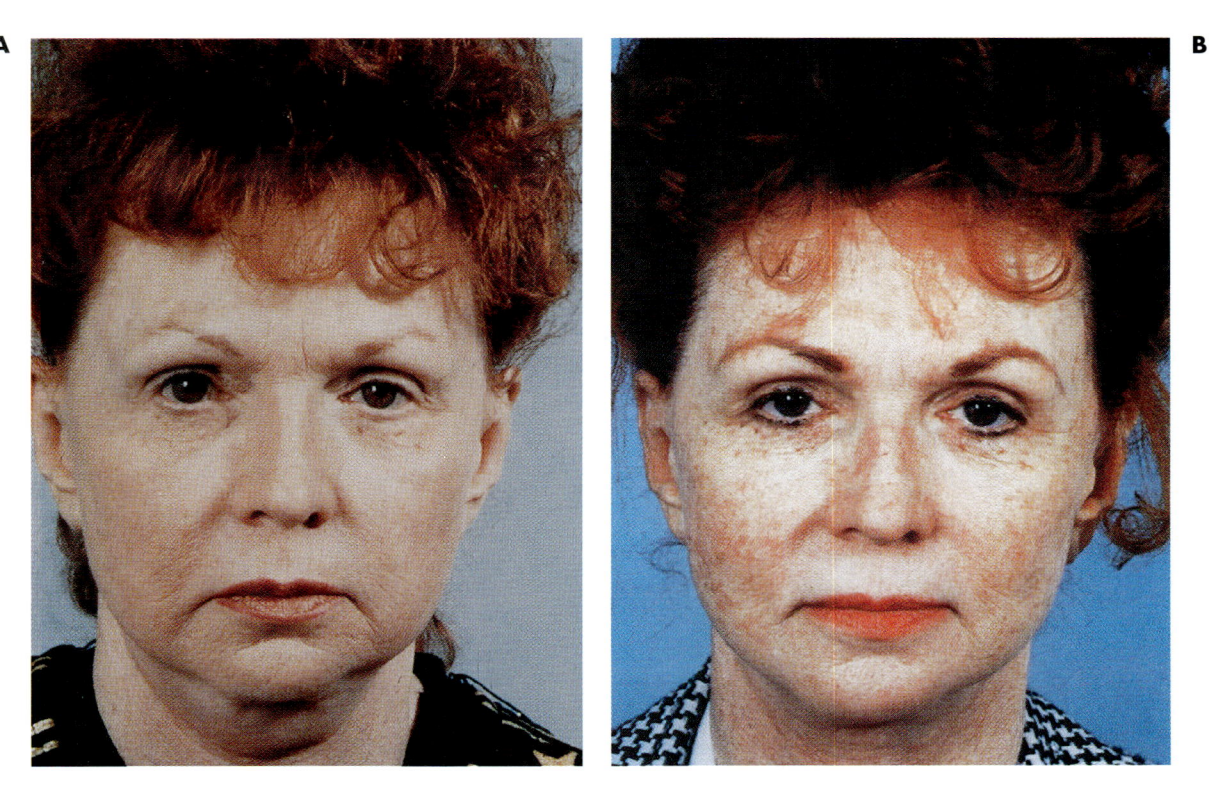

A, Preoperative appearance of a patient with a prominent nasolabial fold, B, Result following rhytidectomy with extended SMAS dissection. No facial fat was removed.

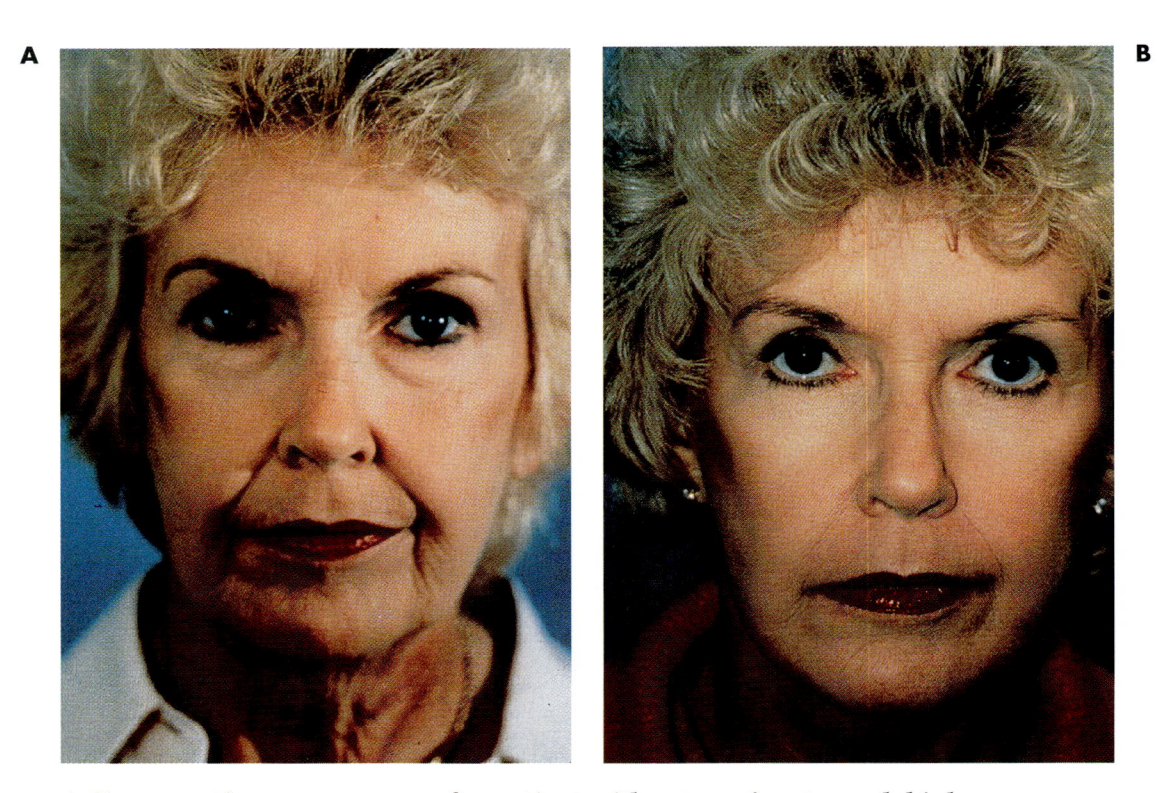

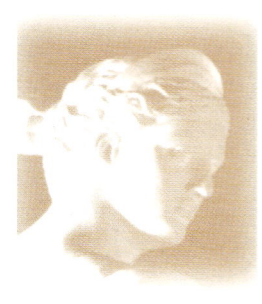

CERVICAL CONTOURING—LIPECTOMY

Contouring of cervical fat has become a common adjunct to rhytidectomy due to the large number of patients exhibiting varying degrees of cervical lipodystrophy. Before every lipectomy areas within the neck requiring contouring should be marked, and a decision on the amount of fat to be removed should be made. In the last several years, suction-assisted lipoplasty has become a less common method of removing cervical fat. We have returned to shape scissor removal of fat, which is more precise and less traumatic than blunt aspiration.

If cervical defatting is contemplated in patients who do not require surgical contouring of the anterior platysma or complete cervical skin flap elevation, we routinely treat these patients via closed suction technique. This is usually performed through a small submental incision, followed by introduction of a small cannula. The suction cannula can alternatively be introduced for a lateral approach by cannulas inserted from the most anterior portion of the facelift dissection, sparing the need for a separate submental incision.

In patients requiring complete cervical dissection, flap undermining is performed before lipectomy, so that a proper amount of fat is left intact along the base of the skin flap. Following undermining, the remaining cervical fat from the superficial surface of the platysma can be removed via scissor dissection.

Suction lipoplasty of the submandibular region can be performed through the lateral facelift dissection. Submandibular fat contouring should always be performed following SMAS flap elevation. The reason for this is that if lipoplasty is performed before developing the SMAS flap, the defatted platysma may be elevated above the mandibular border, producing an unsightly contour line above the jawline. Lateral defatting should be performed just inferior to the mandibular border so that the delineation between face and neckline is accentuated.

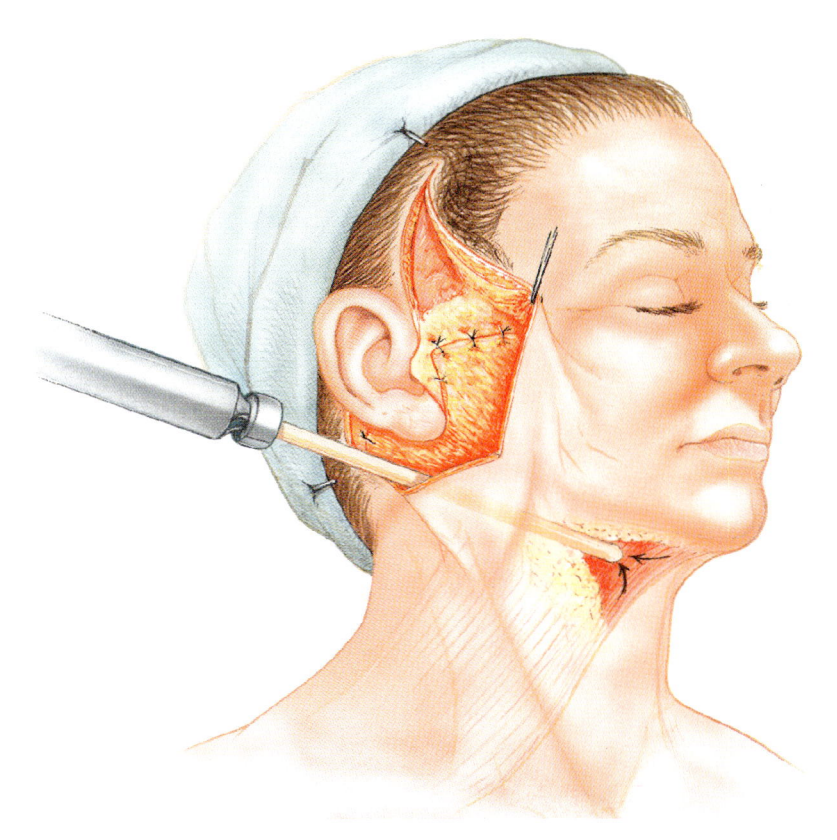

The technique of submandibular defatting at the end of the procedure following SMAS redraping. Lateral defatting should be performed just inferior to the mandibular border so that the delineation between face and neckline is accentuated, and should always be performed following SMAS redraping.

After a decade of using suction lipoplasty to contour cervical fat, we find ourselves relying less on this technique and more on sharp scissor dissection. Sharp dissection of fat offers several advantages over suctioning:

1. Sharp removal is more precise and allows for greater control in removal of fat from specific regions of the neck.
2. Sharp dissection is less traumatic than blunt aspiration of fat and patients seem to have a more rapid recovery in terms of edema and induration when fat is removed via scissor dissection.
3. Suctioning fat glazes the appearance of the superficial surface of the remaining fat and can make the distinction between fat and platysma more difficult in the final tailoring of cervical contour.

Suction-assisted lipoplasty offers the advantage of being rapid and fairly hemostatic. Because of the ease and widespread use of this technique, we are now seeing a new generation of secondary facelift patients who present with an overly defatted neck. This is an uncorrectable problem and makes it difficult in the reoperative situation when the neck must be dissected to correct platysma bands in the face of virtually no tissue (fat) interposition between platysma and skin.

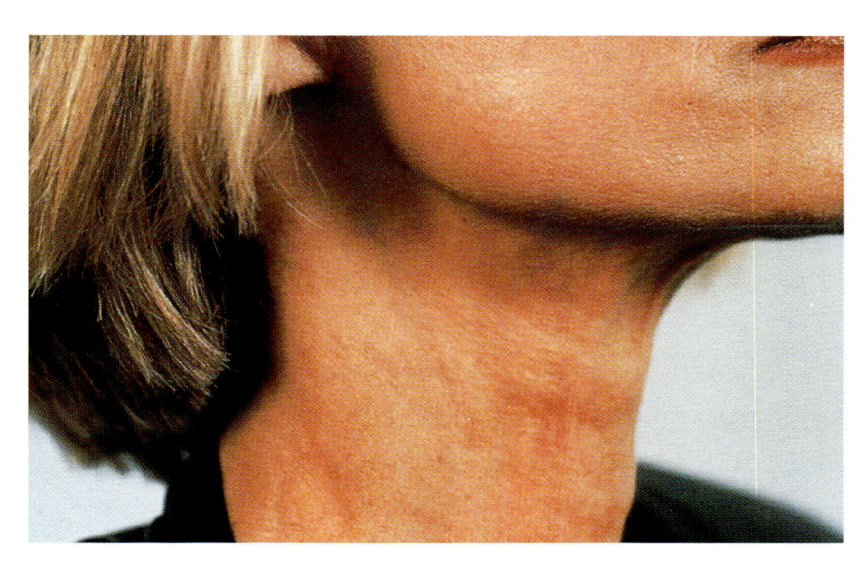

This patient is seen following previous facelifting where preplatysmal fat was aggressively removed, leaving the patient with an overthinned skeletonized-appearing neck with apparent irregularities. This makes secondary surgery much more difficult, especially if work on the anterior platysma is required, since there remains little tissue interposition between the skin and the platysma to disguise any postoperative irregularities on the muscle.

Most patients do not require cervical defatting caudal to the level of the hyoid, and submental lipectomy is commonly limited to the submental and submandibular regions. It is apparent that the youthful-appearing patient with a good cervical contour has a significant amount of fat between the skin and the platysma. Cervical fat is a precious resource and must be precisely contoured. In our opinion, a common error in facelifting is to substitute preplatysmal fat removal for restoration of muscular (platysma) support. *Preoperative evaluation should focus not only on the amount of preplatysmal fat that must be removed but also on the amount of preplatysmal fat that should be preserved.*

In an effort to preserve preplatysmal fat, we commonly do much of the cervical dissection from a lateral approach. The lateral approach allows the surgeon greater exposure when dissecting into the neck compared with the exposure obtained via a submental incision. As the subcutaneous dissection proceeds into the neck anterior to the sternocleidomastoid muscle, it is simple to identify the interface between the platysma and the overlying cervical fat. Using a combination of sharp and blunt dissection, we then proceed directly along the superficial surface of the platysma muscle, keeping all the cervical fat attached to the base of the flap. The dissection is continued as far anteriorly as possible, and usually with the use of a fiberoptic retractor, the surgeon is able to dissect within 2 cm of the cervical midline. A similar procedure is performed on the contralateral side. Following this, the submental incision is made and a complete dissection is

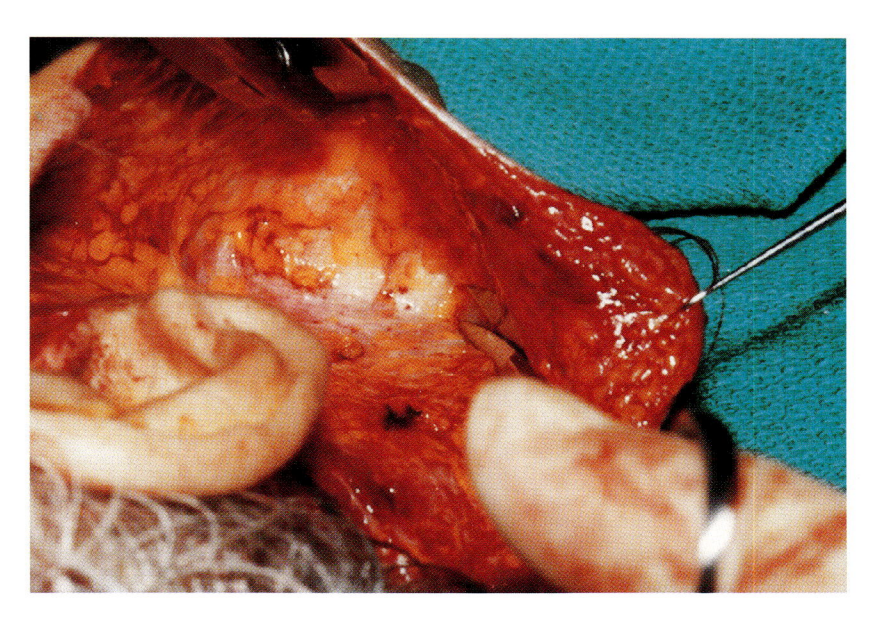

Intraoperative photograph demonstrating that most of the cervical undermining can be performed through the lateral facelift approach. The interface between the platysma and the overlying cervical fat is easily identified low in the neck once the dissection has proceeded anterior to the sternocleidomastoid muscle. Following this identification, the dissection can proceed rapidly using a combination of vertical spreading technique and sharp dissection so that all of the fat is dissected from the superficial surface of the platysma muscle and left intact to the base of the cervical skin.

achieved. Any remaining fat on the platysma can then be removed using suction-assisted lipoplasty, sharp dissection, or both. After platysma muscle modification is performed, if the cervical flaps are judged to be too thick, it is quite simple to thin these flaps using sharp scissor dissection.

We emphasize that in most patients the cervical contour obtained in a facelift results from muscular work on the platysma, as well as the modification of subplatysmal fat. It is interesting that as we become more adept at platysma muscle manipulation, how little preplatysmal fat removal is required to obtain consistent cervical contouring.

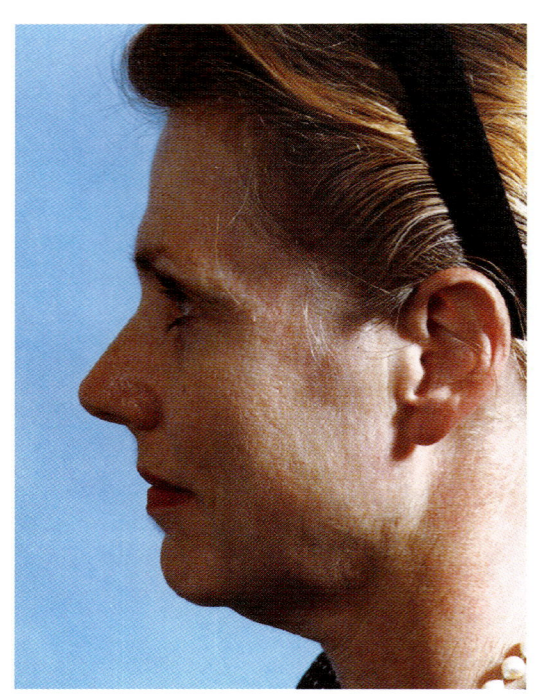

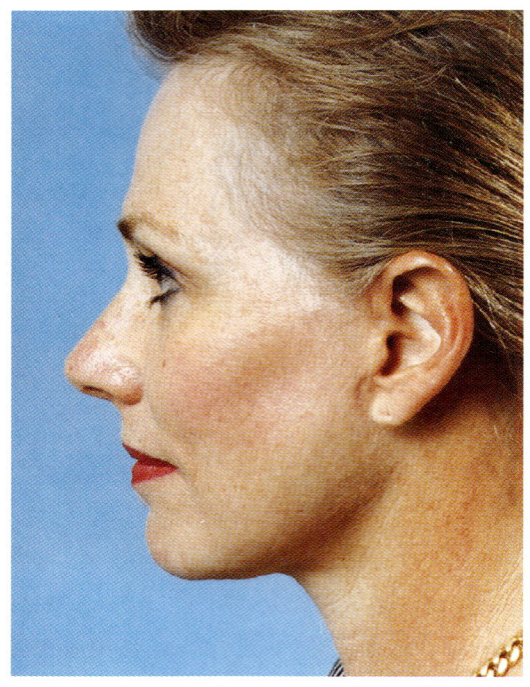

Preoperatively, this patient is seen to have a significant degree of cervical obliquity that is largely secondary to attenuation of support of the retaining ligaments, allowing the platysma to descend inferiorly in the neck. Postoperatively, the patient is seen following long platysma plication performed with a partial muscle transection. No cervical fat was removed.

Some patients require contouring of subplatysmal fat. If fat accumulation below the platysma produces a problem with cervical contour, then this problem should be corrected. An aggressive resection of subplatysmal fat should be avoided, since this can produce an over-hollowed appearance of the midline of the neck. If removal of subplatysmal fat is required, the decussating fibers of the platysma are bluntly separated in the midline, exposing the underlying fat. Numerous small veins are usually present within this fat pad and attention to hemostasis is important. It can be difficult to decide how much subplatysmal fat to remove when the patient is recumbent. We have found that during surgery, on flexing the neck, if the subplatysmal fat slightly bows anteriorly, then adequate contouring of the area is usually evident postoperatively. In general, we rarely contour the fat below the

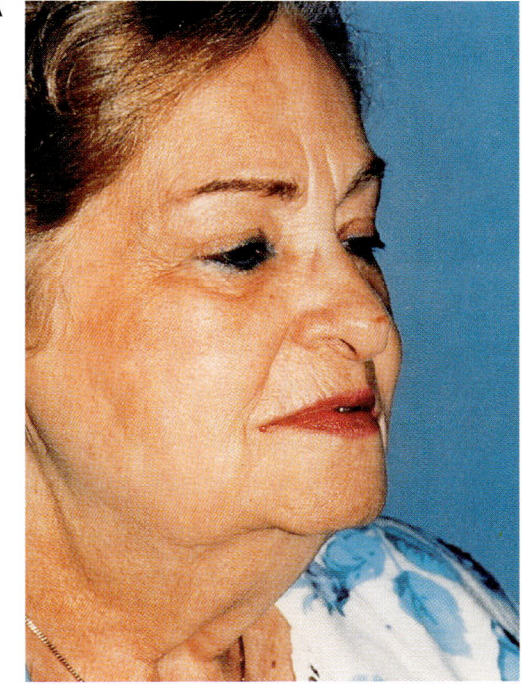

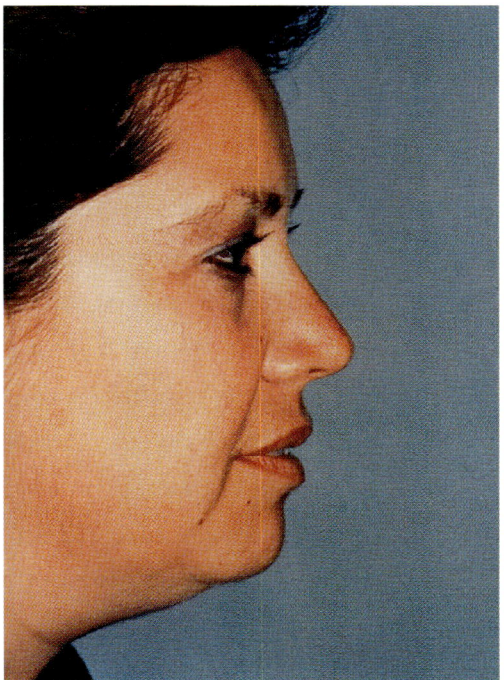

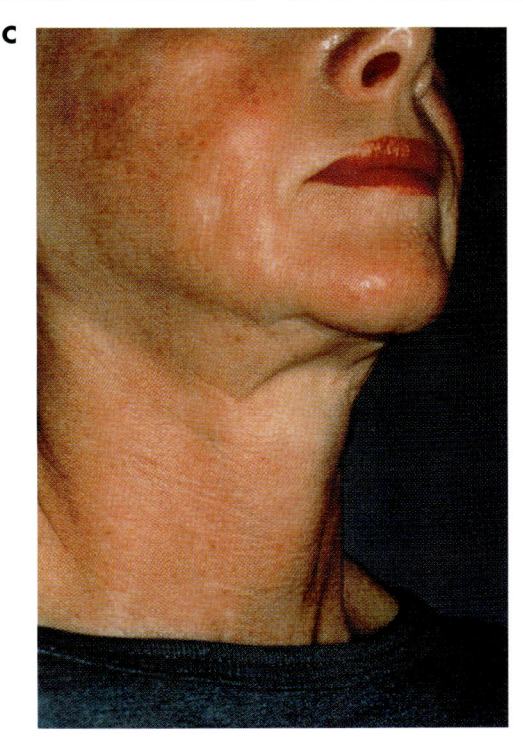

A and B, Two types of patients in whom subplatysmal fat removal should be considered as an adjunct to improving cervical contour. C, Patient following an agressive removal of both preplatysmal and subplatysmal fat. Note the severe degree of submental hollowing which has occurred, leading to a submental depression. The outlines of the depression are formed by the caudal borders of the anterior belly of the digastric muscle, which have become outlined postoperatively because the platysma is now adherent to the underlying floor of the mouth and mylohyoid.

level of the caudal margin of the anterior belly of the digastric muscle, and almost never remove subplatysmal fat to the extent that the mylohyoid muscle is completely exposed. We urge precision in resection of subplatysmal fat. A hollowed-out submental appearance following overresection is essentially impossible to correct. We would note here that it is perhaps more forgiving to resect a greater amount of subplatysmal fat in the region of the hyoid (where it will help to deepen the cervicomental angle) than it is to resect fat more cephalad in the submental triangle. Following removal of subplatysmal fat, the medial borders of the platysma should be reapproximated with interrupted sutures.

RHYTIDECTOMY

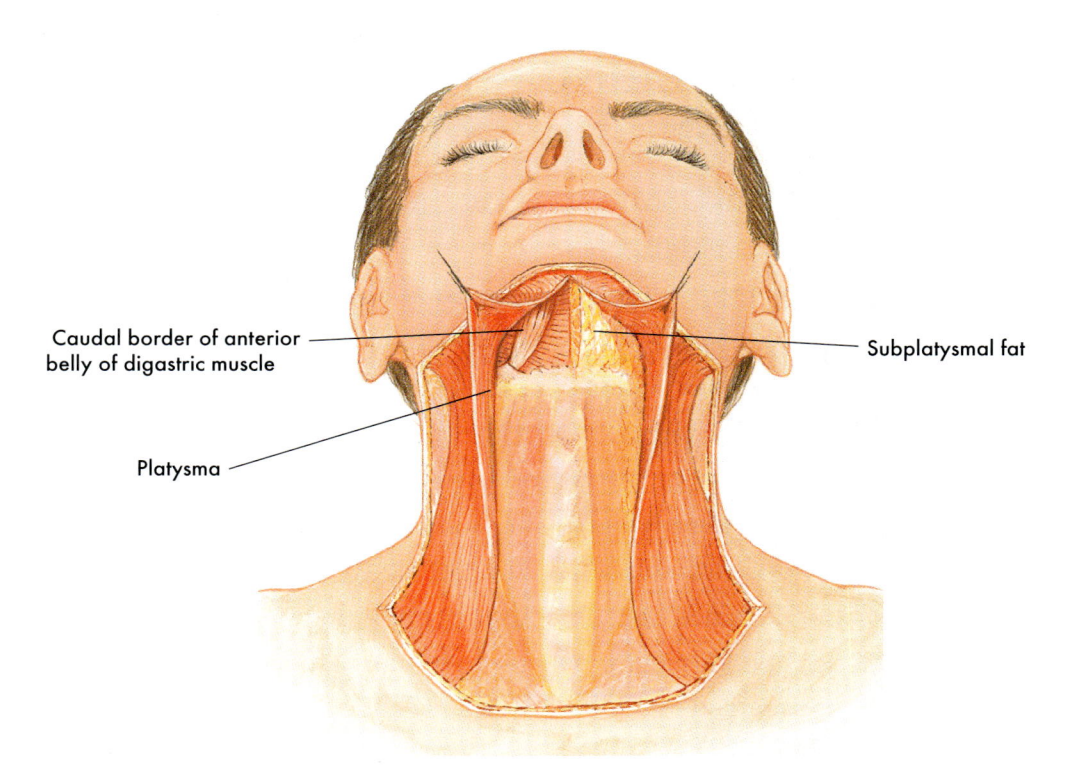

Caudal border of anterior belly of digastric muscle

Platysma

Subplatysmal fat

Mobilization of decussating platysma fibers in the midline through a submental incision will expose subplatysmal fat. In general, we rarely contour subplatysmal fat deep to the level of the caudal margin of the anterior belly of the digastric muscles and rarely remove all the subplatysmal fat so that the mylohyoid is completely exposed. Proper contouring of subplatysmal fat remains a powerful force and will effectively allow the surgeon to deepen the cervicomental angle following long platysma muscle plication.

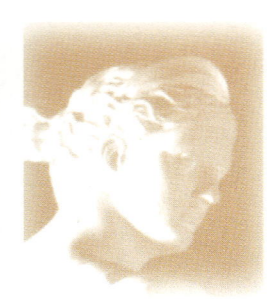

CERVICAL CONTOURING—TREATMENT OF PLATYSMA BANDS

Laxity within the platysma usually presents as two problems: platysma bands or an obtuse cervicomental angle. Both problems can be addressed by approaching the platysma anteriorly through a submental incision.

If platysma bands are slight or present only with exaggerated grimacing, then surgical correction of this problem through an anterior approach is probably not warranted. Improvement in these patients is usually achieved by simply tightening submental skin and restoring lateral tension to the platysma at the time of SMAS undermining and closure. If platysma bands are obvious on preoperative examination at rest, however, then surgical correction should be undertaken.

In some patients, the decision whether to address platysmal laxity anteriorly is difficult. Some patients present with what appears to be no evidence of banding at rest, but as the patient is observed animating during the preoperative interview, obvious banding becomes apparent. In this type of patient, if platysmal laxity is not addressed at the time of rhytidectomy, it can be anticipated that within a few years more obvious platysma bands will become apparent. We favor anterior platysma surgery in this type of patient.

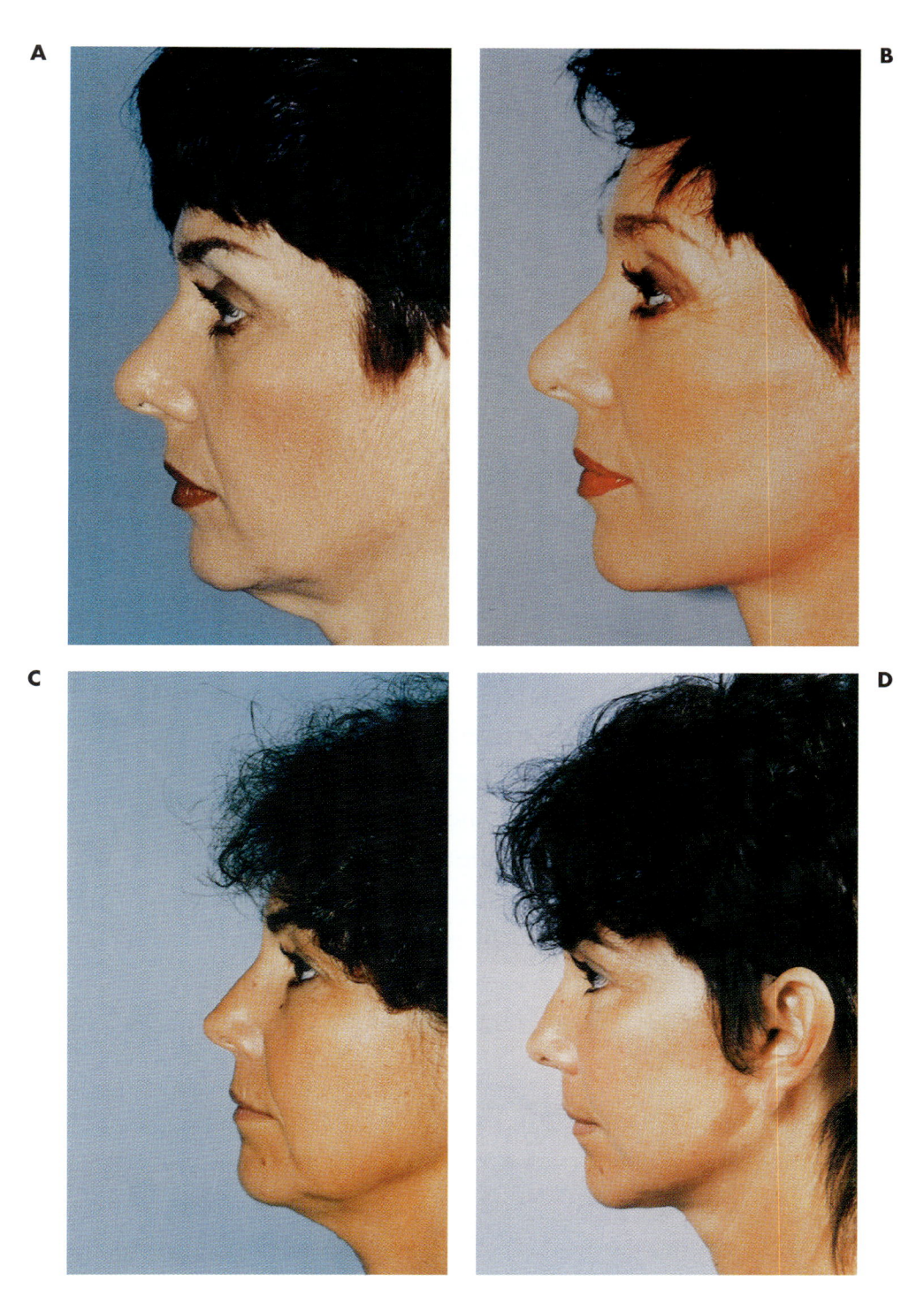

Pre- and postoperative photographs of a patient with short platysma bands that were treated by lateral tension on the platysma through the SMAS transposition flap. No anterior approach was performed.
A, Preoperative appearance in young patient showing moderate descent of the platysma from its attachments to the deep cervical fascia. B, The postoperative result following long platysma plication. Of note, no cervical fat was removed in this patient.

It can be difficult to evaluate the presence of platysma bands in elderly patients with heavy necks and obtuse cervicomental angles. Although not clinically evident, it is our belief that an attenuation of support for the platysma and concomitant descent of the platysma caudad into the neck commonly occurs in patients with significant cervical obliquity. We have noted that addressing the anterior platysma at the time of rhytidectomy is often very helpful in improving cervical contour in the elderly, heavy-necked patient. Because of the low morbidity associated with the treatment of platysma bands, we tend toward the side of correcting platysma bands in our surgical treatment.

The important point in deciding whether to approach the platysma anteriorly via a submental incision is not just the presence of platysma bands, but rather the degree of cervical obliquity.

■ Correction of Platysma Bands

The best approach to the anterior platysma is via a submental incision, placed just caudal to the submental skin crease. If this crease is very deep, we commonly elevate the skin cephalad toward the base of the chin pad and along the caudal mandibular border to free any retaining mandibular ligaments, which tend to accentuate the crease. Following this, the cervical skin is carefully elevated. The cervical skin is usually undermined at least to the level of the cricoid.

RHYTIDECTOMY

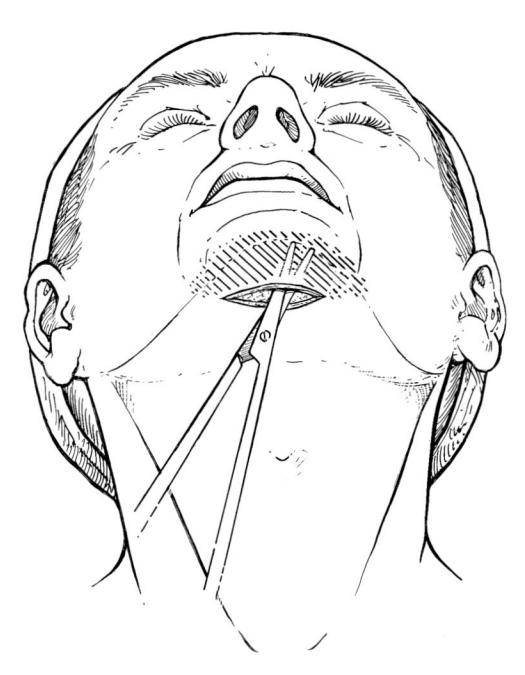

Illustration of the release of a deep submental crease that is performed by dissecting cephalad from the crease toward the base of the mandibular symphysis. This frees up the retaining ligaments that go from the bone to the cervical skin and allows for release of a crease postoperatively. Care should be taken to perform this dissection in the subcutaneous plane. We emphasize that the submental incision is placed just caudal to the naturally occurring skin crease.

Upon exposing the platysma muscle anteriorly, most patients exhibit a decussation of platysma fibers across the midline, at least for a few centimeters below the mentum. When platysma band surgery is contemplated, these decussating fibers must be sharply divided with scissor dissection directly in the midline. Following this, the medial edge of the platysma is mobilized from the mentum inferiorly at least to the hyoid and commonly as caudal as the cricoid cartilage. Mobilization, usually performed using a combination of sharp and blunt dissection, separates the platysma from the underlying subplatysmal fat, the anterior belly of the digastric muscle, and the strap muscles overlying the thyroid cartilage. At times numerous small venules are encountered within the subplatysmal fat and careful hemostasis must be obtained. Following mobilization of the medial

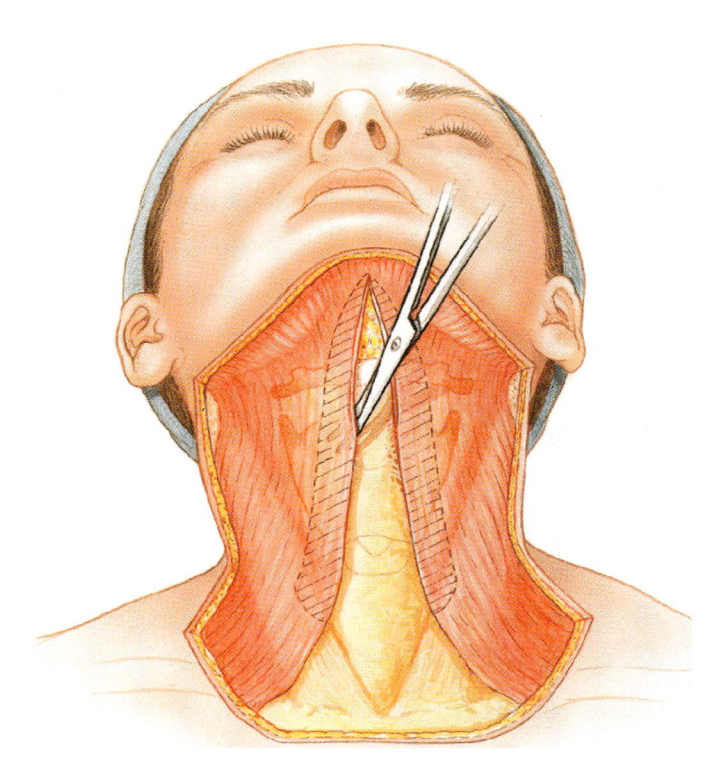

After cleaning the platysma of all preplatysmal fat, mobilization of the medial 2 cm of the muscle is performed, using sharp scissor dissection. It is important to mobilize the band from the mentum as far inferiorly in the neck as possible, usually carrying the dissection at least to the level of the cricoid cartilage.

edges of the platysma, the subplatysmal fat is contoured according to preoperative planning.

Following mobilization, the medial edge of the platysma muscle is grasped on either side and overlapped in the midline in order to estimate the amount of excess muscle present. This will vary from

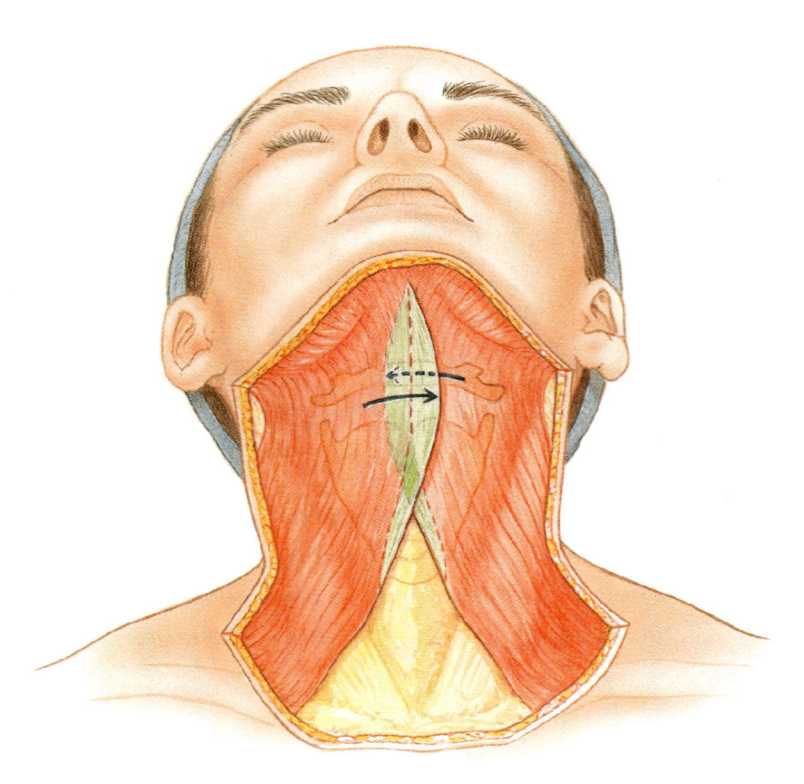

After the platysma has been mobilized, the muscle edges are overlapped and the excess amount of muscle is excised. It is important to be conservative in this resection so that the edge-to-edge approximation of the platysma will be performed under not too great tension.

patient to patient. A portion of the medial edge is then excised to remove redundancy within the platysma and this resection is carried along the entire edge of the mobilized muscle. A conservative resection is performed so that undue tension is not present at the time of suture plication.

We then begin our muscular plication beginning at the mentum and extend this edge-to-edge approximation using multiple interrupted sutures at least to the level of the hyoid. Suture placement back from the leading edge of the muscle, in areas of intact muscular fascia, is an important technical point in preventing suture pull-through postoperatively.

In most patients we continue the edge-to-edge suturing below the hyoid inferiorly toward the base of the thyroid cartilage. This lower muscle plication is especially useful in long-necked patients with long platysma bands. It is also useful in patients with hypertrophied and redundant platysma muscle, to help in taking up the excess slack that exists within the platysma. The goal of muscular plication is to produce an even, smooth contouring of the platysma that is tightly adherent to the underlying floor of the mouth and thyroid cartilage providing a proper framework for redraping of cervical skin. A low plication

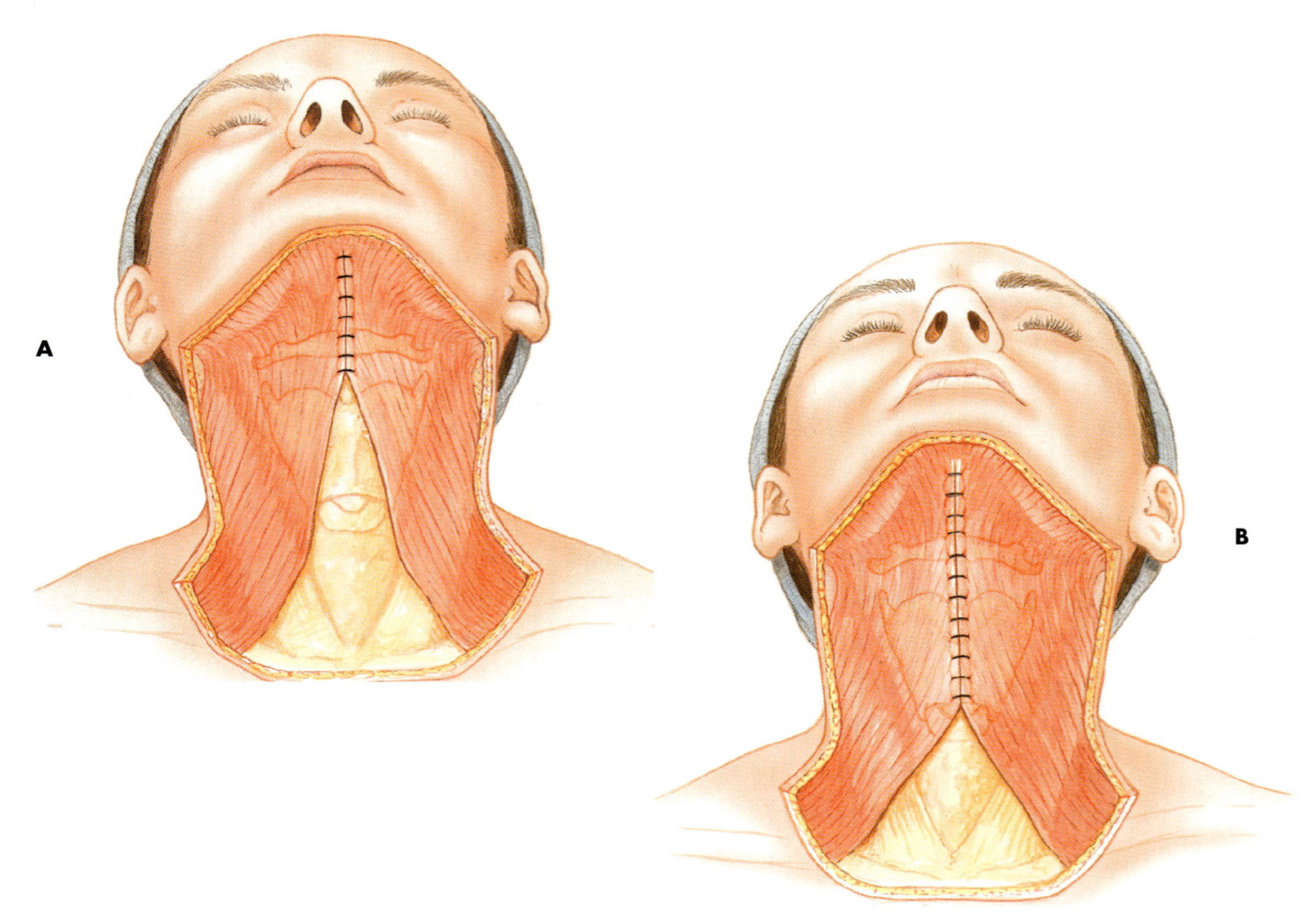

SURGICAL REJUVENATION OF THE FACE

A, An edge-to-edge approximation is then performed of the platysma muscle. In the past, this most commonly extended from the mentum to the superior aspect of the thyroid cartilage. We rarely use a short plication at this time and rather perform a longer plication that extends from the mentum to the base of the thyroid cartilage. *B,* This longer plication greatly enhances the surgeon's ability to tighten and contour the platysma so that it is adherent to the floor of the mouth and the thyroid cartilage. This produces a better foundation for redraping of cervical skin.

joining a widely separated platysma over a prominent thyroid cartilage also tends to blunt a prominent larynx and produce a rounder, more feminine appearance to the neck.

Following edge-to-edge approximation of the platysma, we usually perform some form of muscular release. This muscular release commonly involves a partial transection of the platysma muscle with the myotomy performed inferiorly within the neck.

Platysma transection is a powerful tool in the treatment of platysma bands and obtaining the desired cervical contour. The procedure must be performed meticulously because the early experience with transection was fraught with complications. Specifically, if the transection is performed at a high level, it can be associated with unveiling of the submaxillary glands and denervation of the platysma associated with lower lip dysfunction. Also, obvious contour depressions associated with divided muscular edges can be noted in the overly thin neck.

The key to platysma transection is that the horizontal portion of the transection be performed as low as possible, at least as inferior as the level of the cricoid cartilage. We usually begin this portion of the transection from the submental incision where it is easy to identify the level of the cricoid cartilage and ensure that this portion of the transection is kept low. The rest of the platysma transection is then performed from the lateral aspects of the facelift incision. In most patients, only partial division is required. The myotomy is performed from the midline laterally to approximately the anterior border of the sternocleidomastoid muscle.

SURGICAL REJUVENATION OF THE FACE

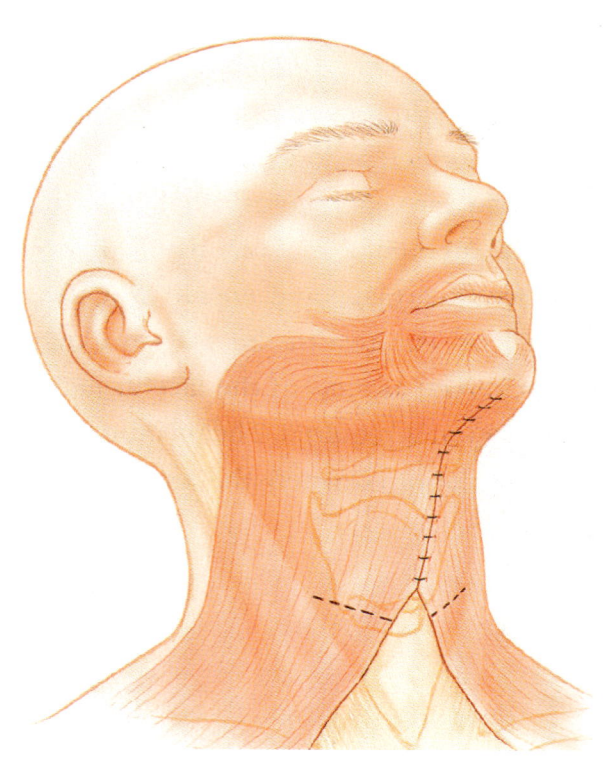

Following edge-to-edge approximation of the platysma from the mentum to the cricoid cartilage, some form of muscular release is performed. This usually consists of a horizontal cut extending from the midline to the anterior border of the sternocleidomastoid muscle. The key to platysma transection is to perform it as low in the neck as possible.

The muscular release seen following platysma transection serves many purposes:

1. It alleviates tension along the medial portion of the platysma transection following plication.
2. It allows the platysma to shift superiorly, producing a deeper cervicomental angle.
3. It prevents the conversion of two platysmal bands to a single band following edge-to-edge approximation, which can be visible when the neck is extended.

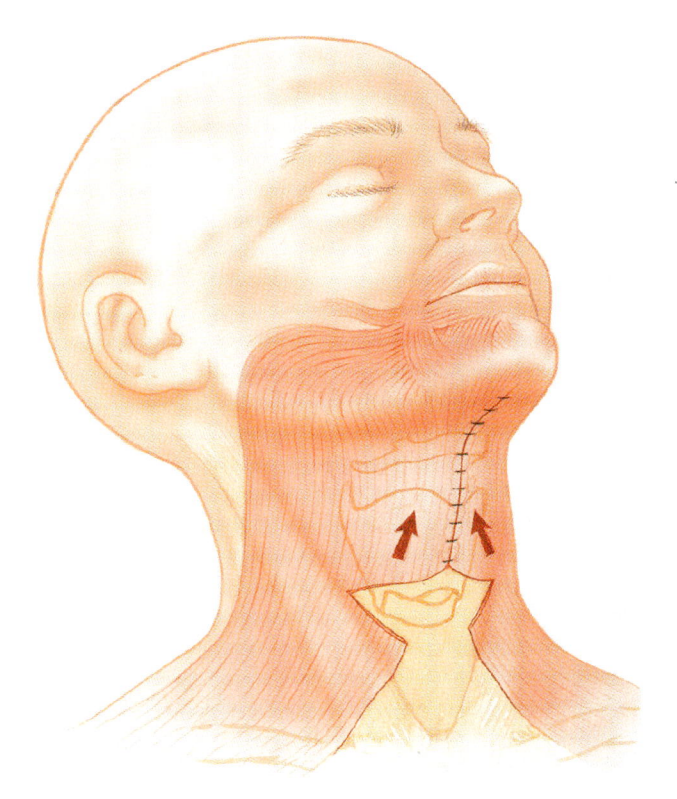

The effects of partial platysma transection include: (a) alleviating tension along the closure, (b) allowing the platysma to shift superiorly to deepen the cervicomental angle, and (c) the prevention of a single band following edge-to-edge approximation that can be visible when the neck is extended.

SURGICAL REJUVENATION OF THE FACE

Complete platysma transection is required in some patients. An important concept regarding platysma transection is that most of the transection is vertically oriented rather than horizontally, as traditionally conceived. When we perform platysma transection, we usually continue it as a downward extension of our SMAS dissection. The traditional SMAS dissection descends vertically from the preauricular region along the lateral border of the platysma muscle. Approximately 5 to 6 cm below the mandibular border, well away from the marginal mandibular nerve, we then continue our incision within the platysma in an oblique fashion paralleling the anterior border of the sternocleidomastoid muscle. This oblique and vertically oriented cut within the platysma continues inferiorly to the level of the cricoid cartilage. The

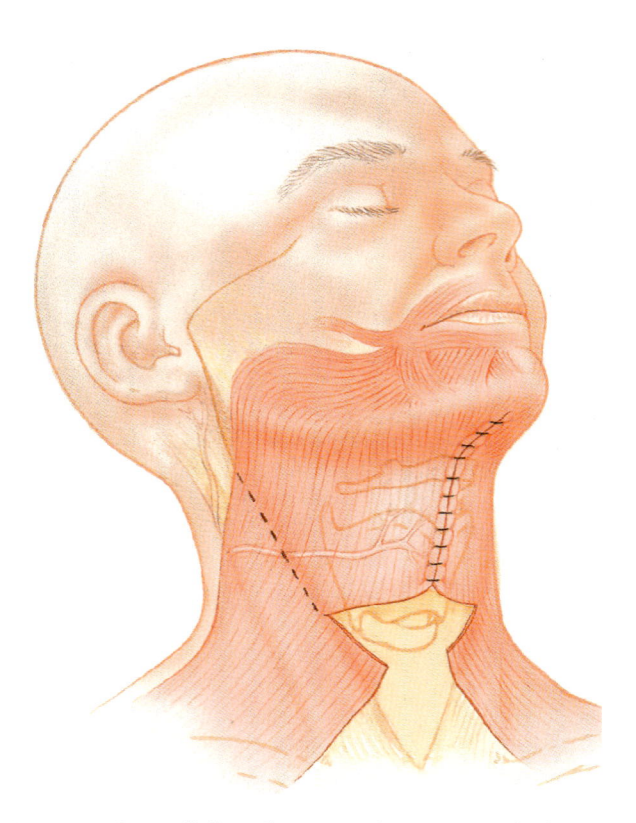

If a complete transection of the platysma is required, the greater portion of the cut in the platysma is oriented obliquely along the anterior border of the sternocleidomastoid muscle. The only horizontal portion of the incision extends from the midline of the platysma at the level of the cricoid to the anterior border of the sternocleidomastoid muscle.

horizontal cut within the platysma is then made at the level of the cricoid cartilage, extending from the anterior border of the sternocleidomastoid to the midline. Following complete platysma transection, the muscle will usually be found to gap several centimeters. This is especially marked along the lateral aspect of the transection. This gap in the muscle serves essentially as a lengthening myotomy and as the platysma shifts superiorly this is accompanied by a deepening of the cervicomental angle. Full-width platysma transection is also effective in treating patients with heavy, multiple platysma bands, since all of these bands are divided during transection. It is also useful in the patient with a short, contracted platysma.

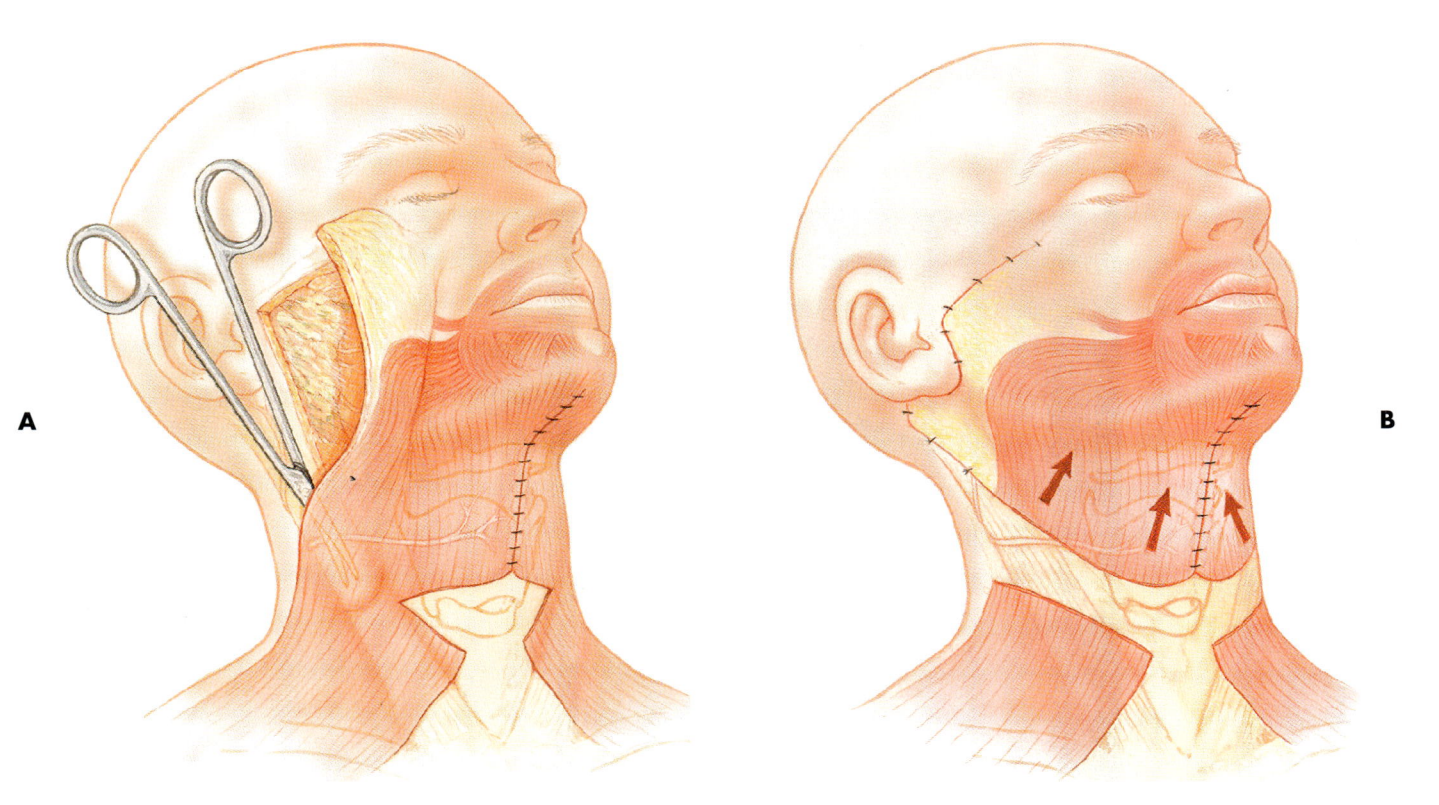

A, Before transecting the platysma muscle, it is important to bluntly elevate the platysma from the underlying deep cervical fascia. This ensures that only the platysma is divided during the transection and will prevent injury to the underlying transverse cervical nerve. B, Following complete transection of the platysma, the muscle is seen to gap several centimeters. This superior shifting of the platysma will tend to deepen the cervicomental angle as well as highlight the submandibular region and the angle of the mandible.

SURGICAL REJUVENATION OF THE FACE

We cannot overemphasize the importance of performing the platysma transection in essentially an oblique fashion. The division of the muscle along the anterior border of the sternocleidomastoid will not only release the platysma muscle but will serve to accentuate the anterior borders of the sternocleidomastoid, a feature associated with a youthful-appearing neck. Similarly, by performing the transection predominantly vertically, well away from the area of the submaxillary gland, this will prevent the platysma from retracting above the level of the submaxillary gland, producing unveiling of these structures.

Several technical points are important in performing platysma transection. First, we bluntly elevate the platysma from the underlying deep cervical fascia before muscle division. As long as the underlying deep cervical fascia is left intact, then the transverse cervical sensory branches, as well as the anterior and external jugular veins, will not be injured, since these structures lie just deep to the deep cervical fascial

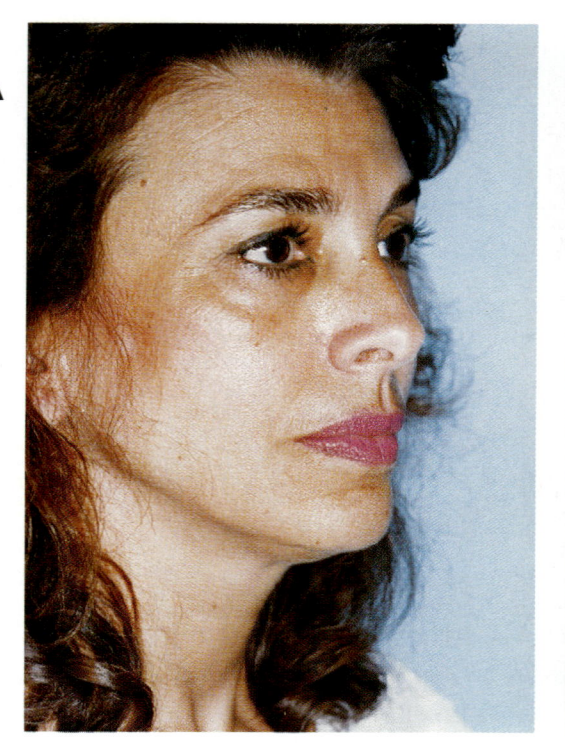

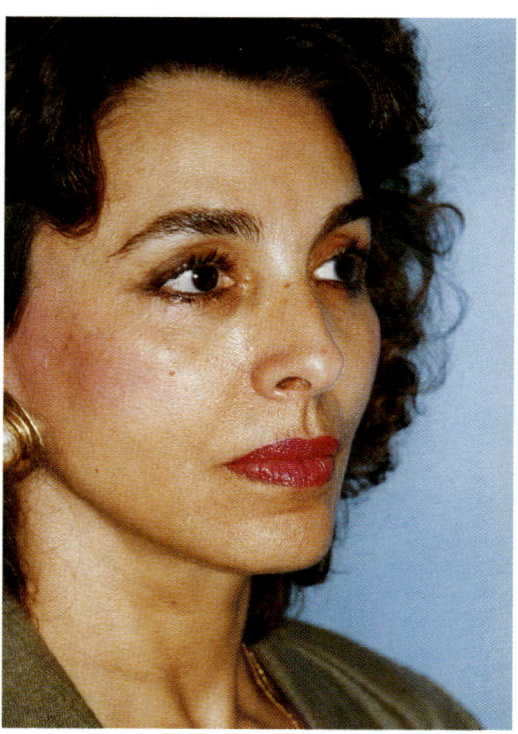

(A) Pre- and (B) postoperative appearance following closed suction of the neck and tightening of the platysma via a lateral approach through the use of the transposition flap during SMAS dissection.

layer. The transverse cervical nerves are usually encountered in the lateral portion of the transection and must be carefully preserved.

Following transection, the edges where the muscle has been transected must be carefully feathered so that a smooth cervical contour is produced. This will prevent unsightly contour depressions and obvious muscular edges in the postoperative result. Careful hemostasis along the cut muscle edge should be ensured before closure. We emphasize that complete muscular transection is reserved for specific patients (and most patients do not require full-width transection to obtain proper cervical contour). These patients include:

1. The patient with the fat, heavy neck where an attempt is made to make the neck thinner than the face.
2. The patient with a short, tethering platysma.
3. The patient with multiple prominent platysma bands.
4. The patient in whom partial platysma transection intraoperatively has not produced the desired cervical contour.

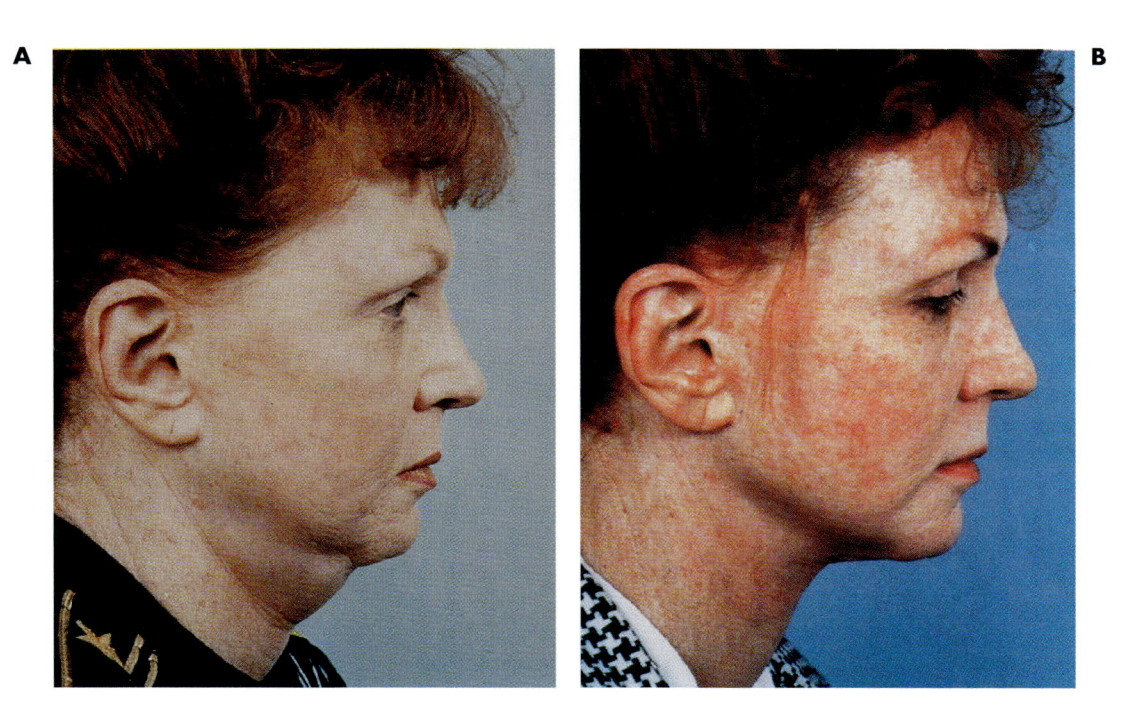

A, Preoperative appearance. B, Postoperative appearance following submental contouring with contouring of both preplatysmal and subplatysmal fat in conjunction with long platysmal plication from mentum to cricoid, associated with partial platysma transection.

SURGICAL REJUVENATION OF THE FACE

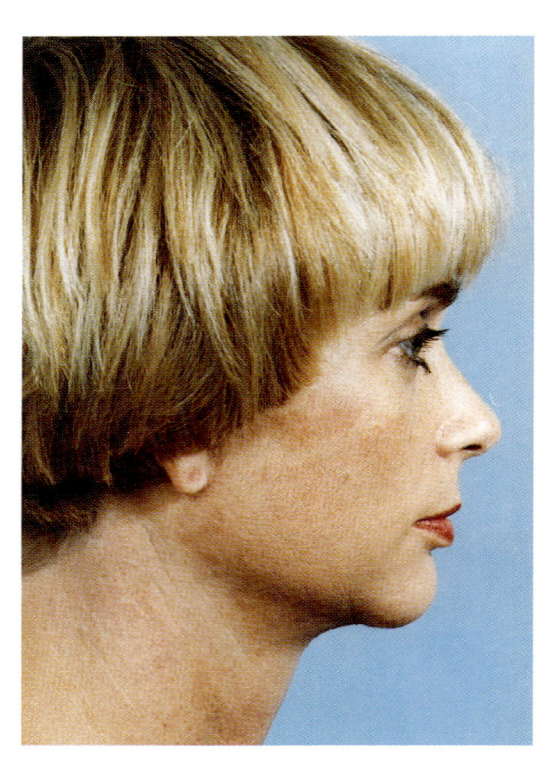

A, This patient with a retrusive chin and short platysma related a history of having had poor cervical definition since adolescence. B, Postoperative result following long platysma plication, complete muscular transection, and insertion of a chin implant. The deepening of the cervicomental angle and the apparent lengthening of the neck are a result of the lengthening myotomy associated with complete platysma transection.

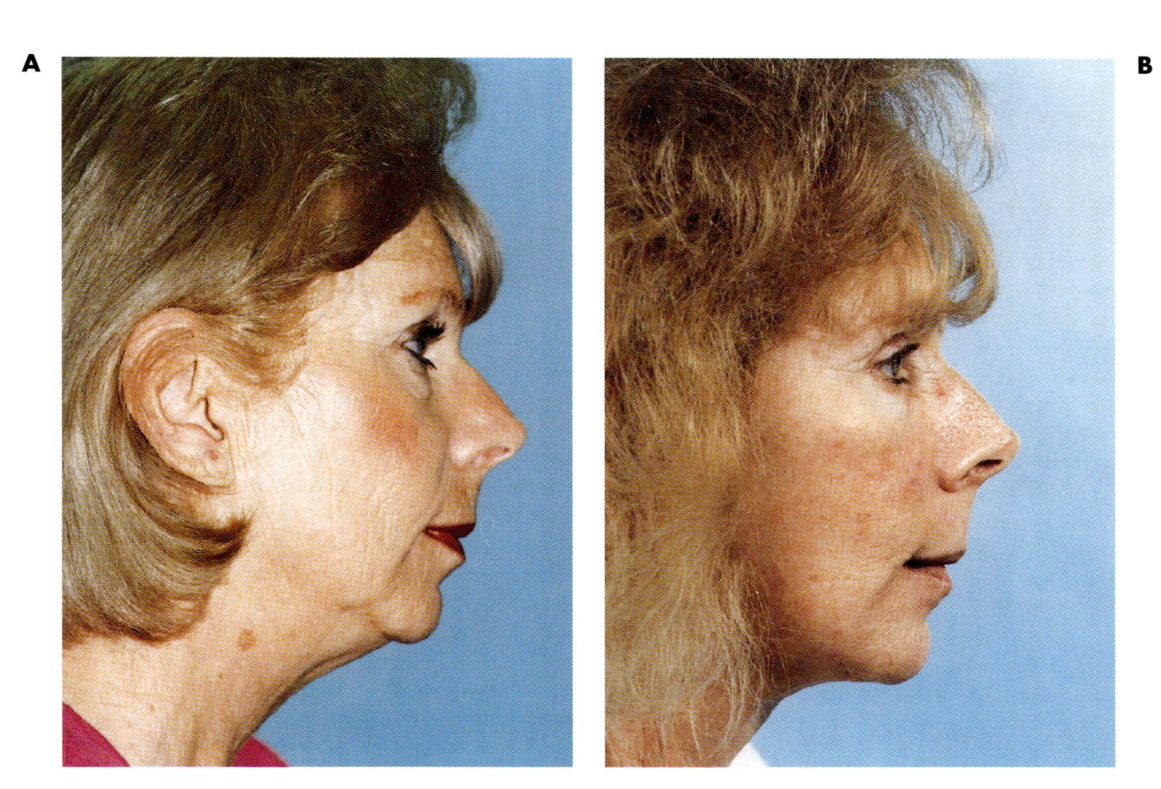

A, Cervical obliquity associated with a retrusive chin and short tethering platysma. B, Postoperative result following long platysma plication, preservation of preplatysmal fat, and complete muscular transection. No chin implant was placed in this patient.

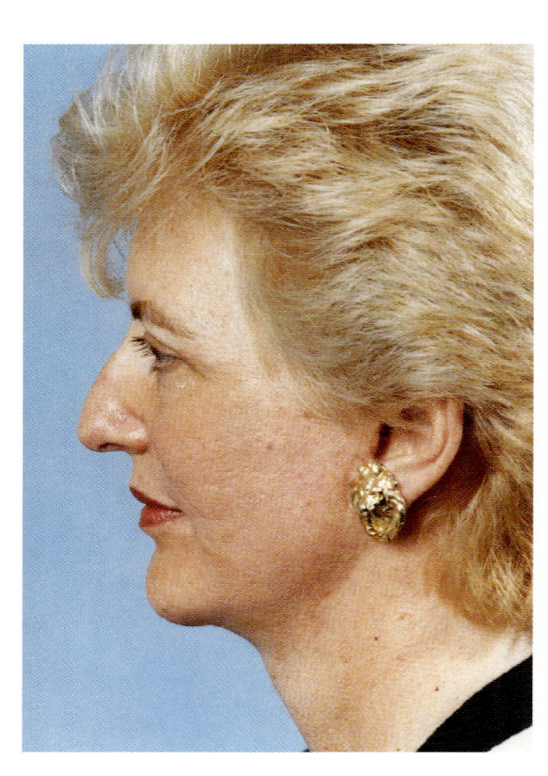

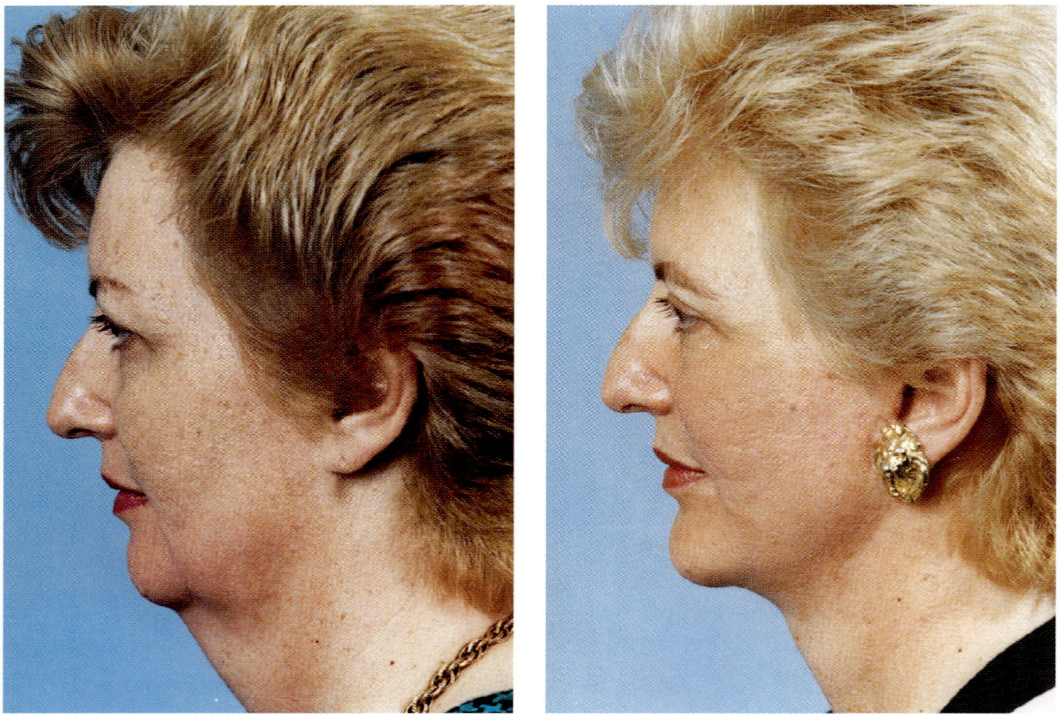

A, This patient has a large degree of cervical obliquity associated with preplatysmal fat, subplatysmal fat, and loss of muscular support of the platysma. The platysma is short and lies vertical in the neck. B, Postoperative result following long platysma plication, contouring of preplatysmal and subplatysmal fat, and complete muscular transection. A chin implant was also placed.

CLOSURE—SKIN FLAP REDRAPING

The direction of skin flap redraping is extremely important. Many of the unsightly changes seen in facial appearance, as well as hairline distortion following rhytidectomy, are associated with redraping of the skin flap in an improper direction, usually too cephalad. In our opinion, this represents an abnormal direction of pull on the skin flaps in an attempt to compensate for inadequate deep layer support. In general, the direction of skin flap redraping in the aging face is slightly cephalad and predominantly lateral. In a primary facelift, redraping in this direction rarely results in the hairline being elevated above the helical attachment. A key suture is placed between the flap and the base of the helical attachment in the preauricular region.

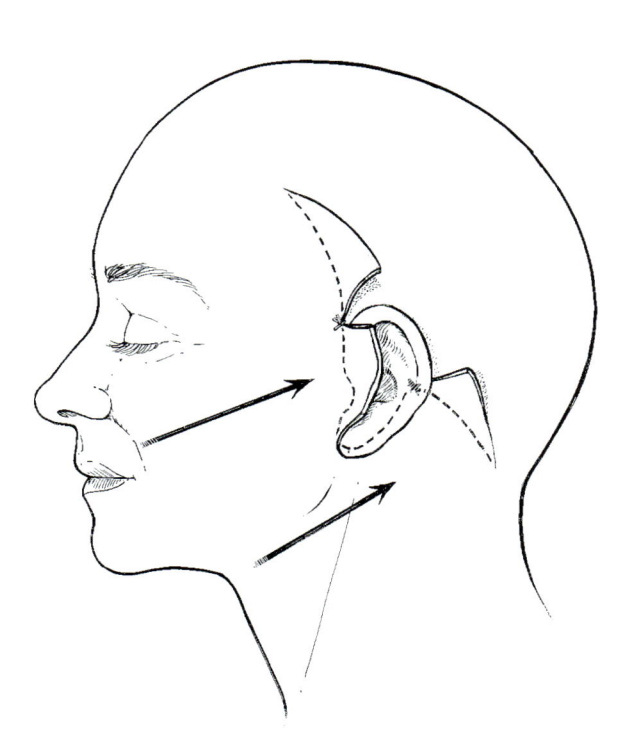

The direction of skin flap redraping is illustrated. In general, the vector of rotation of skin flap redraping is slightly cephalad but predominantly lateral. In the neck, the direction of redraping should be parallel to the cervical creases. Key sutures are placed along the helical attachment and at the superior aspect of the postauricular incision.

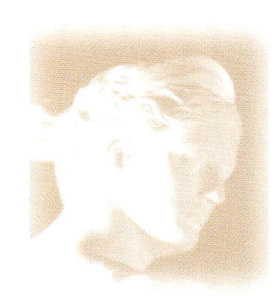

The cervical portion of the dissection is usually redraped in predominantly a posterior direction, paralleling the cervical creases. A key suture is then placed at the apex of the postauricular flap.

Although some tension is present along both key sutures, excess tension should be avoided. In general, the skin flaps are inset with a minimum degree of tension placed along the key sutures and then the skin flaps are trimmed with a degree of redundancy between the key sutures to minimize tension along the incision sites. We favor restoring contour in our face lifts through our deep layer support, placing the tension on the SMAS and platysma closure, and minimizing the tension on skin flap closure to obtain consistency in terms of scar perceptibility. Stated in other terms, we prefer to obtain the bulk of facial contouring through deep layer support rather than through tension in skin flap redraping.

RHYTIDECTOMY

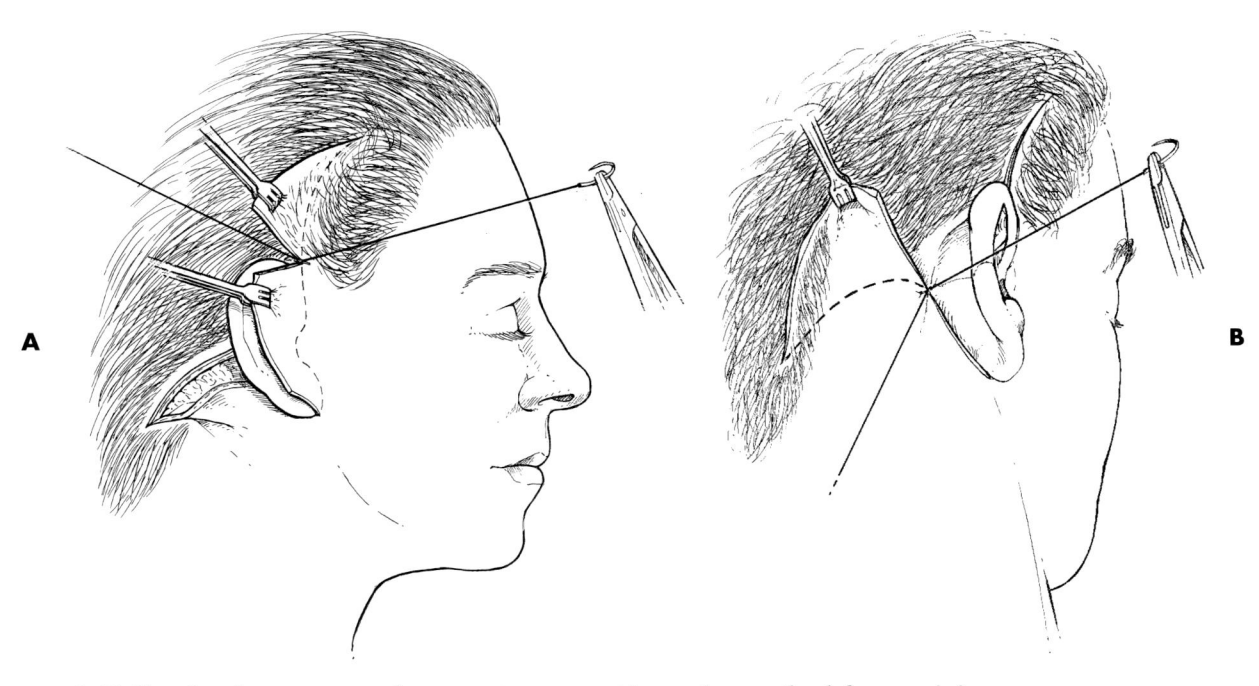

A, Following key suture placement, excess tissue is marked for excision. It is important that in the preauricular region the design for excision conform exactly to the underlying contour of the helix, tragus, and earlobe. There should be little tension or gapping following skin excision. Tension in this region will only lead to wide scars and tragal distortion. B, The postauricular skin is redraped and marked for excision.

Following placement of the key sutures, the excess facial and cervical skin is marked for excision. It is important that the skin resection in the preauricular region conform exactly to the tragal incision and contour of the earlobe.

Following excision of excess skin, we commonly resect the subcutaneous fat and SMAS directly in front of the tragus to form a pretragal hollow. If a tragal incision has been used in a male patient, the hair follicles should be removed to prevent a problem in shaving.

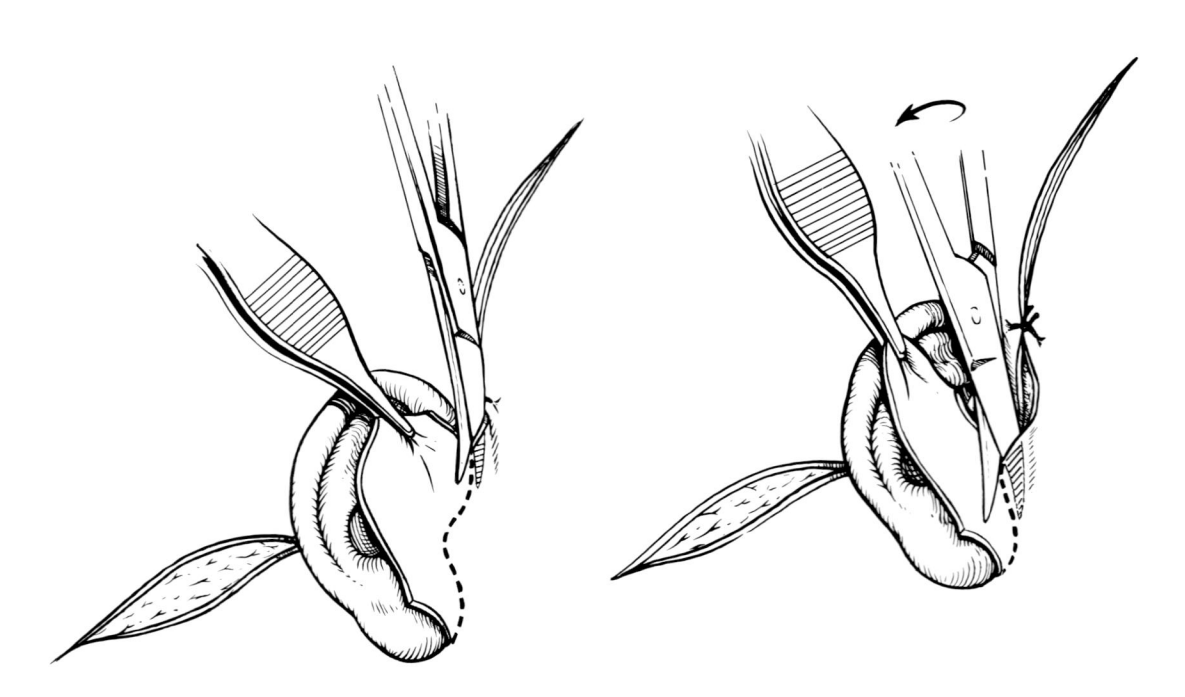

Trim the preauricular skin to create a thin flap and cover the tragus. Bevel with the scissors to remove the subcutaneous fat.

RHYTIDECTOMY

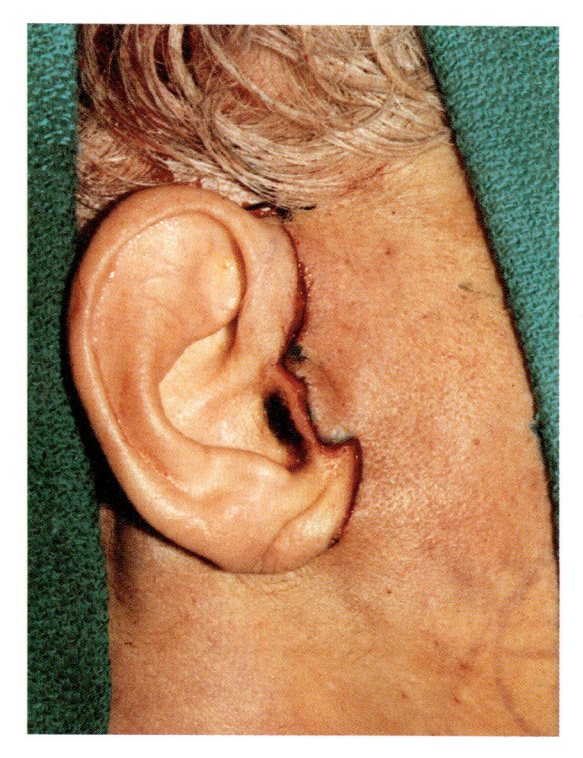

Intraoperative photograph following redraping of preauricular skin. To avoid postoperative distortion, no tension should exist on the preauricular closure. Note the creation of a pretragal hollow. Also note that following limited detachment of the earlobe, this structure tends to lie parallel to the axis of the ear. An effort should be made to reattach the earlobe posterior to the axis of the pinna to prevent the common postoperative appearance of an anteriorly situated lobule.

SURGICAL REJUVENATION OF THE FACE

Closure of a posterior neck incision is begun at the most inferior portion, to avoid leaving a "dog ear" in this area that would be subsequently "chased down onto the neck."

The posterior hairline is realigned with a single suture. We close the posterior portion of this incision within the hairline using an interrupted 4-0 nylon monofilament suture. Since the area is camouflaged

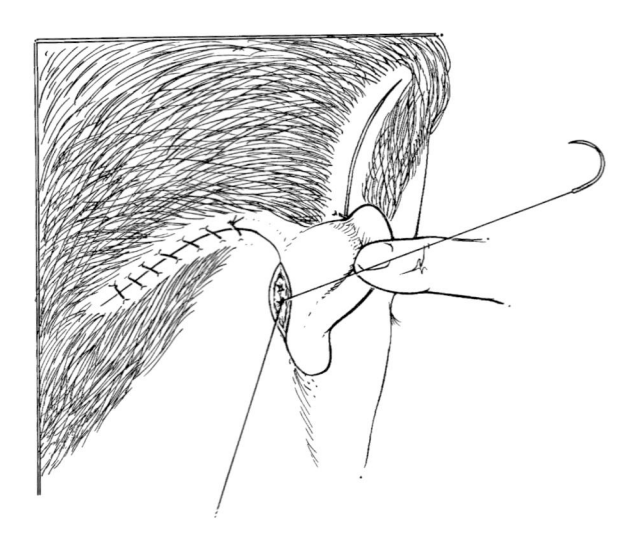

Postauricular closure is begun by realigning the hairline. Following this, the first suture is placed posteriorly and then interrupted sutures are placed all the way to the end of the hairline. Further suturing in the bare area behind the ear is then performed either with buried interrupted polyglactin 910 (Vicryl) sutures or half-buried nylon mattress sutures. If a small amount of excess tissue remains in this region because of different lengths of the flap, we prefer to excise the dog ear in the region behind the ear.

by subsequent regrowth of hair, some cheating can be done by placing the skin sutures closer together on the scalp portion of the incision and a bit further apart on the cervical flap. This maneuver helps to make up the difference between the length of the surgical flap and the length of the incision along the scalp. Once the posterior hairline incision is closed, the suture technique is changed. No sutures should cross the line of incision on the non–hair-bearing portion of the postauricular region, since this would result in crosshatching, an undesirable sequela. The immediate postauricular incision in the non–hair-bearing portions of the scalp is closed with a single layer of 4-0 polyglycolic acid sutures with the knot on the downside, or alternatively, half-buried mattress sutures of 4-0 nylon with the knot tied on the cephalad aspect of the incision.

As the closure proceeds superiorly toward the concha, any additional skin can be trimmed from the cervical aspect of the flap and the necessary adjustments made. This is preferable to a dog ear at the inferior portion of the incision.

Crosshatching is not a problem in the preauricular area, since these sutures are under little or no tension and are removed by the fifth postoperative day. In dark-complexioned patients in whom suture marks might be visible, pull-out or buried sutures are used to avoid crosshatching in the line of preauricular closure. Our preference for closure within the temporal hairline is a running suture of 4-0 monofilament nylon. Closure of the temporal flap is done with minimal tension on the suture line to avoid necrosis and subsequent alopecia.

Staples may be used for closure in the hair-bearing areas of the temporal and postauricular incisions; however, we have seen no particular advantage to this and prefer sutures. Staples are more uncomfortable for the patient, are more expensive, and save little time.

Elevation of the short temporal flap does not appreciably alter the position of the eyebrow. If the intention is to elevate the lateral portion of the eyebrow, a coronal approach is usually required. In our experience, the application of tension in the temporal closure will not substantially elevate the outer canthus, or eliminate crow's-feet.

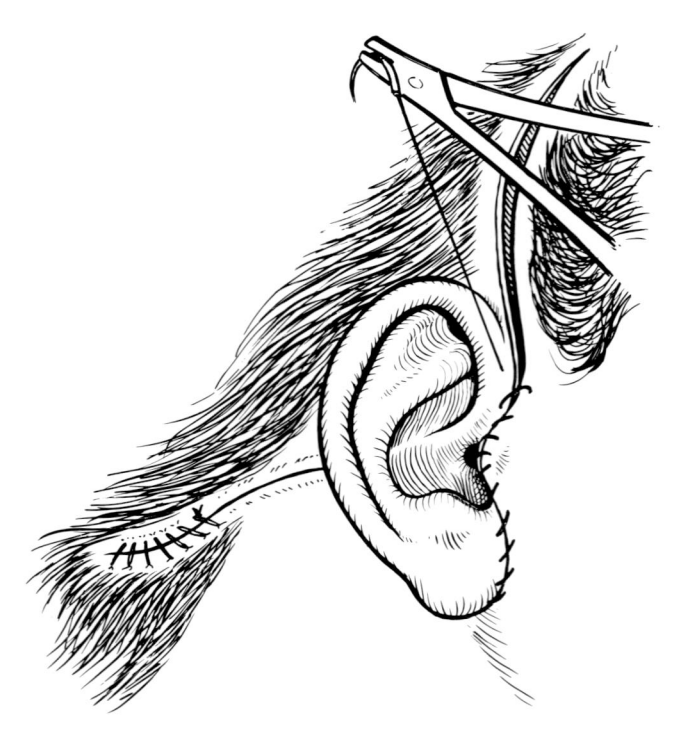

The preauricular incision is closed with nylon suture. Since there is very little tension on this portion of the flap, crosshatching does not occur. These sutures should be removed in 5 days.

RHYTIDECTOMY

DRAINS

The decision to use drains—Penrose, ribbed, or suction—is a matter of personal preference for the surgeon. Unless the patient's wounds are oozing considerably at the end of the procedure, we prefer not to use drains. Ironically, a few of the most severe hematomas we have seen were associated with the use of drains. Drains *will not* prevent formation of an expanding hematoma. They will, however, help to eliminate some serum, as well as small collections of blood. When the surgery involves a significant degree of neck work associated with platysma plication and transection, we use closed suction drains on these patients for 24 to 48 hours.

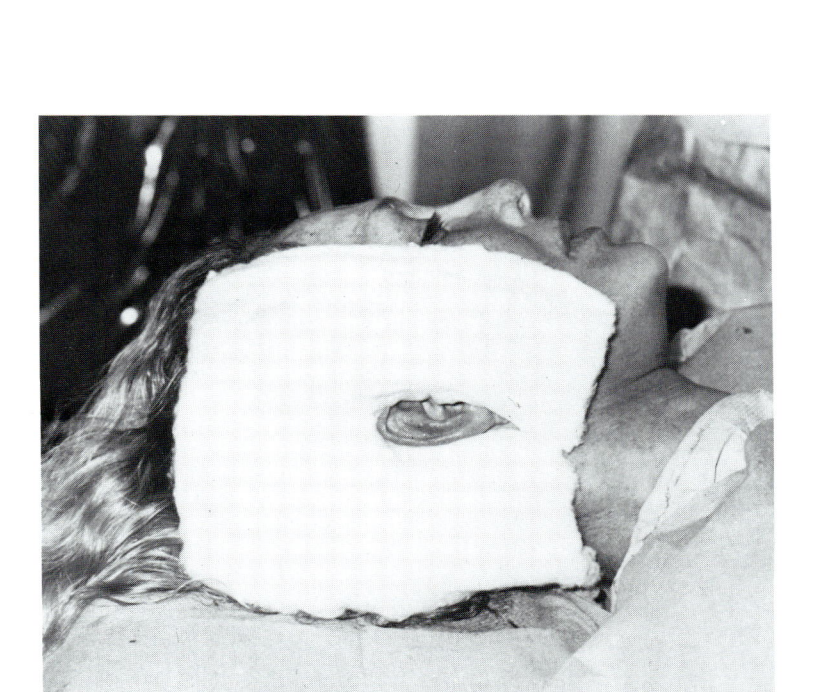

Cotton squares soaked in mineral oil are used to dress the wound. Open an area for the ear to protrude and splint the posterior aspect of the concha with the oil-soaked cotton.

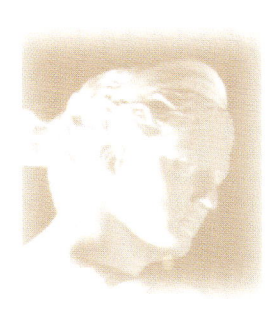

SURGICAL REJUVENATION OF THE FACE

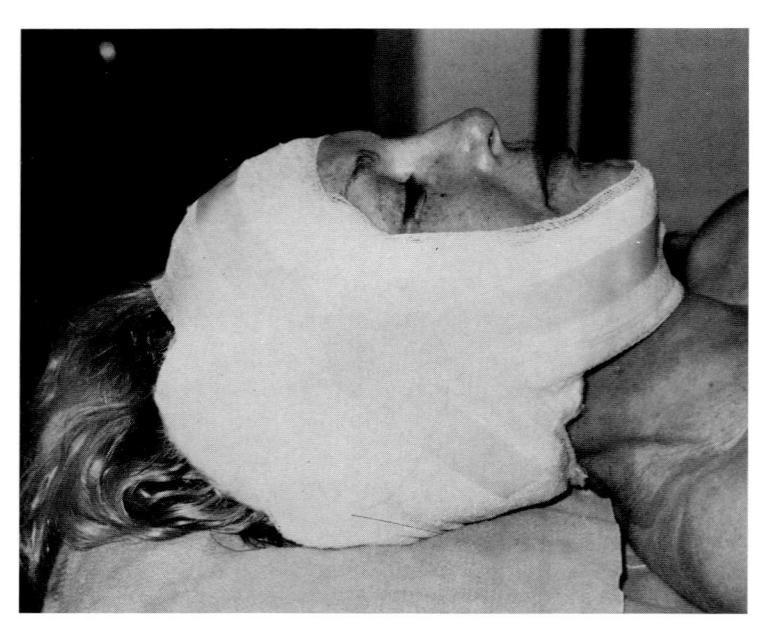

Soft gauze (Kling) is used to hold the cotton squares in place. No pressure is necessary; in fact we believe it is contraindicated. Pressure on flaps is rarely indicated and the face is no exception. The soft dressing is also more comfortable for the patient. Remove this dressing in 24 hours and inspect the operative site.

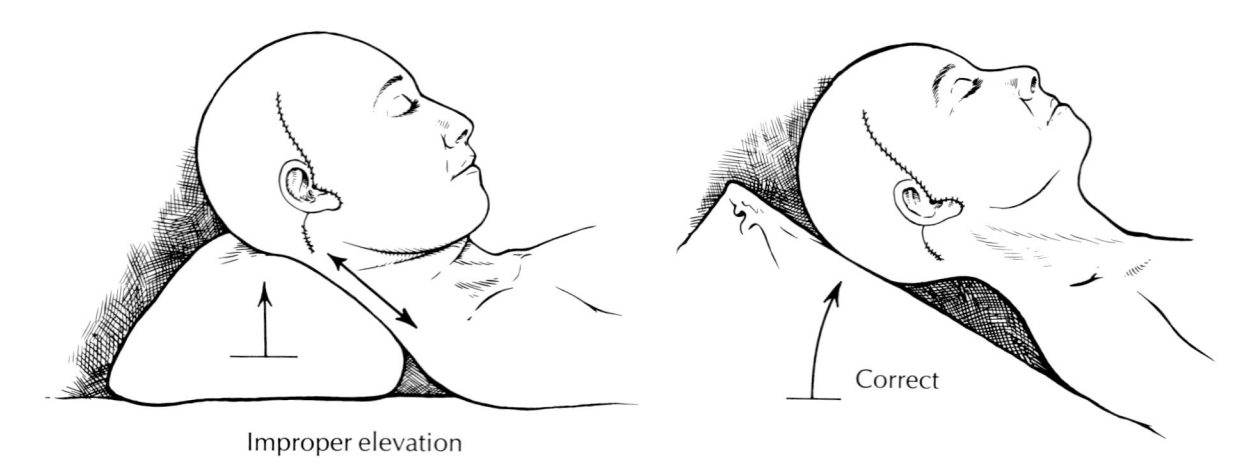

Improper elevation

Correct

The head should be elevated without neck flexion postoperatively, since extreme flexion could result in skin necrosis in the undermined area because of pressure or ischemia.

IMMEDIATE POSTOPERATIVE ROUTINE

The patient will want specific instructions about her postoperative care. Some surgeons provide the patient with a printed list, whereas others prefer to give the instructions orally. The following postoperative recommendations have proved to be helpful:

1. Pressure dressings are not used.
2. The head of the bed is elevated at all times, but avoid flexing the patient's neck since this may compromise circulation to the cervical flap.
3. Appropriate pain and sleep medications are given; narcotics are rarely required.
4. The patient may go to the bathroom with assistance on the first postoperative day and as desired thereafter.
5. The first dressing is changed after 24 hours. At this time the wounds are inspected and a light dressing is reapplied for an additional 24 hours.
6. All dressings are removed after 48 hours, and the patient's hair is shampooed daily during the first postoperative week.
7. Preauricular sutures are removed on the fifth or sixth postoperative day.
8. All sutures are removed by the seventh or eighth postoperative day.
9. Antibiotics are routinely used. Cephalexin (Keflex), 1 g/day, is given 24 hours preoperatively and 4 days postoperatively.
10. If crusty or oozing, wounds are cleaned with hydrogen peroxide and coated with a topical antibiotic ointment.

If the patient is healing well at the end of a week or 10 days, she is advised to return in 2 to 3 weeks for a routine postoperative visit and again in 3 months. She is instructed to return or call at any time if she has any questions regarding the postoperative course.

During the first week the patient is allowed to walk and is encouraged to be up and about as much as is reasonably possible. Strenuous physical activities such as tennis, water-skiing, and golf are not permitted for 5 or 6 weeks. A good basic rule is: "If it hurts, don't do it."

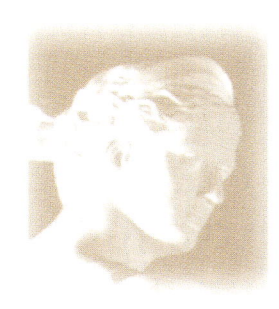

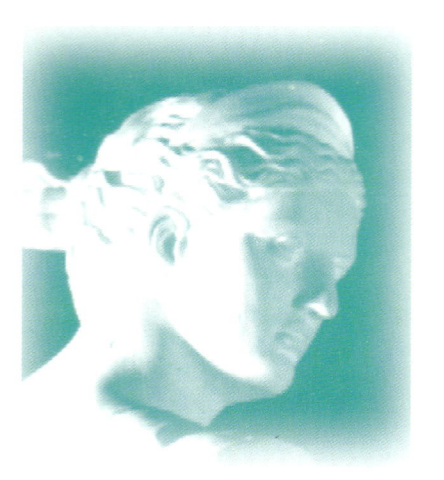

D

REOPERATIVE RHYTIDECTOMY—STAYING WITH IT

After one has been in a plastic surgical practice for a number of years, there develops a considerable backlog of previously operated rhytidectomy and blepharoplasty patients who present for a secondary operation. These persons have undergone successful procedures, were initially pleased with their results, and often request the secondary surgical procedure because they want to maintain their best possible physical appearance. Approximately 35% of the patients in our practice who request rhytidectomy have undergone this procedure at least once previously. Some patients have undergone two or three previous facelifts.

Although most of the considerations for primary rhytidectomy apply to patients seeking reoperative surgery, there are specific problems associated with treating a patient who has undergone a previous surgery—especially if it was done by another surgeon and there is a question of exactly what was done during the initial procedure. Usually, though, additional intervention is beneficial in terms of facial contour and appearance.

One of the most frequent questions asked by patients in the upper age brackets is, "Am I too old to undergo a facelift?" The suitable answer is, "Not if you are in good physical (and mental) health, and if it is determined after examination that surgery would be of significant benefit." Chronological age is not a deterrent to aesthetic surgery.

How often have we heard this type of patient say, "This is my last shot at youth," and then see the same patient return for additional surgery several years later. The oldest patient seeking treatment in our surgical experience was 91 years of age. She had been a patient for other procedures over a number of years and when asked, "Why do you want more treatment at this point in your life?," she replied, "I want to look good when I go." Since her health status was satisfactory and there were no medical contraindications, a limited chemical peel was done, which seemed to satisfy her.

Advances in medical knowledge have increased life expectancy and since prospective patients are living longer, we as plastic surgeons will get more and more requests to assist them in the challenge of physical self-improvement through reoperative surgery.

PATIENT EVALUATION

■ General Considerations

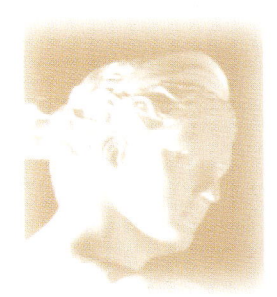

Most of the patients seeking secondary or tertiary rhytidectomy are elderly and often have the concomitant ailments seen in their age-group. A careful medical history should be obtained to rule out such common problems as hypertension, angina, previous myocardial infarction, or cerebral ischemic events. It is important to ascertain the general level of activity of the patient to see if there is any limitation of normal activity or exercise secondary to underlying health problems. We ask most of our elderly patients to see their personal physician before surgery for a complete physical examination and obtain a letter of medical clearance. A consultation with the patient's internist, as well as the anesthesiologist preoperatively, is helpful in obtaining information that allows for a smooth intraoperative and perioperative course.

Incision Placement

The scars in secondary rhytidectomy may pose a challenge. Usually the surgeon is forced to follow the incision line that was made during the first intervention. If a preauricular scar was used in the first procedure, we discuss with the patient whether she prefers that incision as opposed to an incision placed within the tragal margin. In our experience most patients prefer tragal margin incisions and if there is enough laxity present within the skin envelope, the preauricular incision is converted to a tragal incision during the secondary procedure. The greatest problem with incisions seen in secondary rhytidectomy involves hairline shifts. In our experience most patients presenting for secondary rhytidectomy have had significant stair-stepping of the posterior hairline, leaving them with a large hairless area behind the ear. This is essentially impossible to correct at the time of secondary rhytidectomy and usually forces the surgeon to accept it and simply use the old postauricular scar.

RHYTIDECTOMY

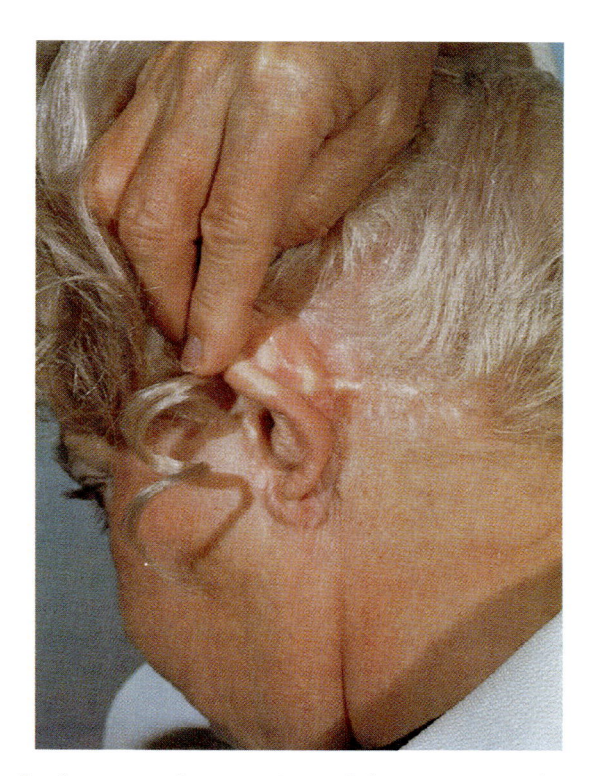

This photograph shows stair-stepping of the posterior hairline, associated with hypertrophic scars. The surgeon performing a secondary facelift often must accept this hairline distortion and simply use the patient's original incision, though a finer scar is usually obtainable.

SURGICAL REJUVENATION OF THE FACE

Another common problem with hairline shift is seen in the temporal region if the cervicofacial flap has been advanced in an exaggerated cephalad direction at the time of the initial procedure. The redraping of facial skin in a superior direction elevates the sideburn above the helical attachment, leaving what appears as a bald spot above the level of the ear. It is occasionally possible at the time of reopera-

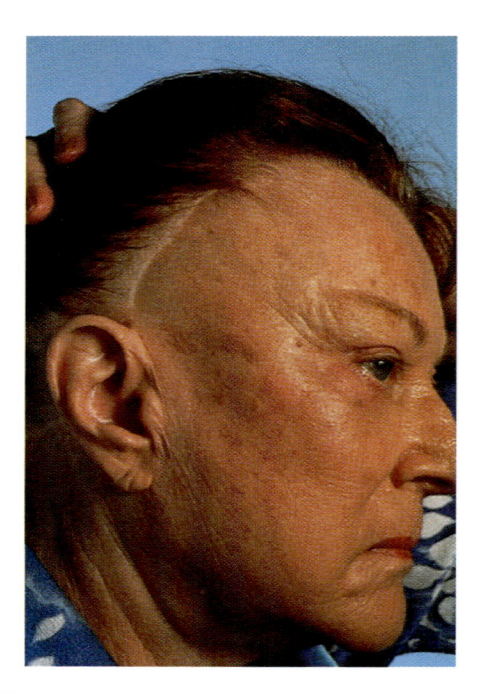

This photograph shows temporal balding following a primary facelift and coronal browlift resulting from cephalad rotation of the facial skin. Note the misdirection of facial rhytides associated with this vector of skin flap redraping.

tion to rotate the temporal hair inferiorly and partially lower the sideburn. Another alternative to this in patients with a high temporal hairline is to shift the secondary incision along the temporal hairline. Since the secondary incision is placed in front of the temporal hair, there is no shift of the hairline at the time of cervicofacial flap advancement.

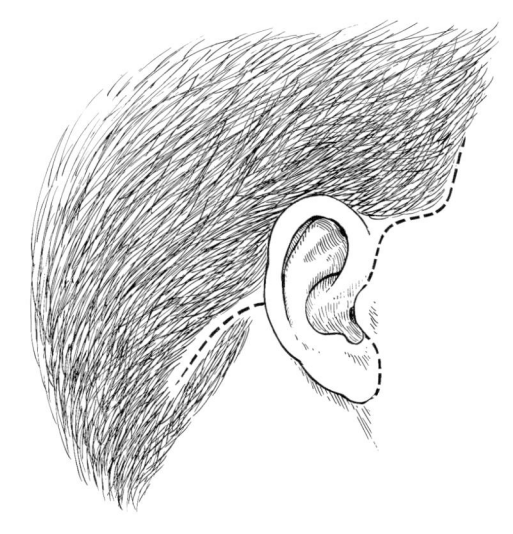

As an alternative to distorting the temporal hairline, the temporal incision can be placed directly anterior to the temporal hair.

Another common problem secondary to poor incision placement is the formation of the pixie ear. This results from excess skin being removed caudal to the earlobe during closure in the primary procedure. This forces the surgeon to use the earlobe to close the resulting defect, producing a distorted and malpositioned earlobe. The correction of this problem usually involves reincising the earlobe to a more rounded appearance and then removing any tension around the lobe following advancement of the cervicofacial flap. It cannot be stressed enough that tension around the earlobe must be avoided at the time of closure and that the surgeon should never attempt to hang the cheek on the earlobe to minimize this potential problem.

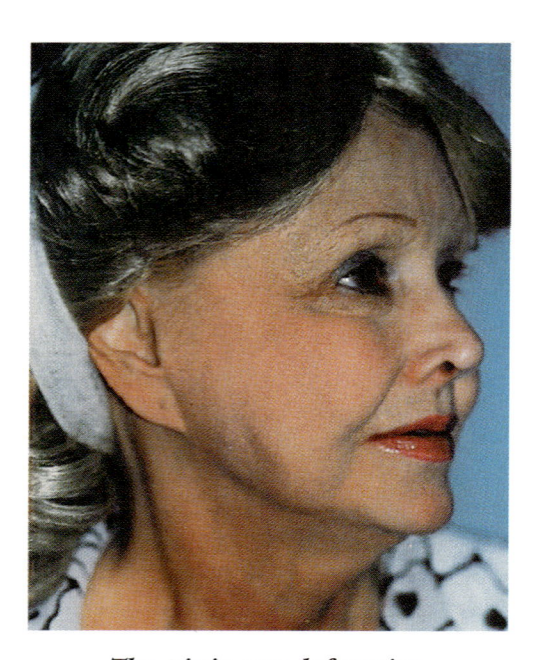

The pixie ear deformity.

Skin Laxity and Associated Rhytides

Commonly, in the secondary or tertiary rhytidectomy patient, there exists little laxity within the skin envelope. The reason for this is that most of the excess skin present was removed at the previous procedure. How much skin laxity is present will, of course, vary from patient to patient, but in general much of the contour deformity seen in the secondary patient has to do with attenuation of the deeper facial soft tissue support rather than within the skin envelope itself. Because the skin has been tightened during the primary procedure, skin resection in a secondary facelift results in less skin excision compared with the initial operation.

Many patients undergoing a secondary procedure show further evidence of degenerative changes from continued actinic exposure, smoking, gain and loss of weight, and intrinsic aging. The ongoing process of dermal elastosis, with the formation of inelastic and poor-quality skin, has a definite effect on the long-term results seen in patients undergoing a secondary procedure.

Facial rhytides are not removed by a facelift and are usually evident postoperatively. In some patients presenting for a secondary procedure, facial rhytides will have been rotated in an abnormal direction during the initial procedure, producing an unnatural appearance. It is important to examine this situation closely and, in patients with obvious rhytides, to decide in what direction the facial flaps will need to be rotated at the time of closure. Rotation of cervicofacial flaps too cephalad will commonly place these rhytides running in an upward direction. It is better to redrape the cervicofacial flaps in a more horizontal direction than to displace facial rhytides to an even more abnormal position.

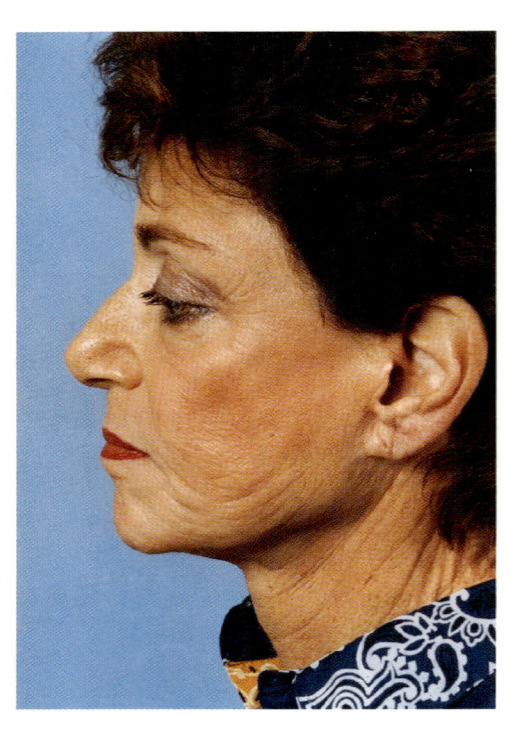

Photograph of a patient with sun-damaged skin and facial wrinkling. The wrinkles run in cephalad following a previous facelift. This problem usually becomes more evident with animation and as the patient flexes her neck.

■ Fat Accumulation

With the advent of liposuction, plastic surgeons have become aggressive in removing cervical and facial fat. One of the most common problems we see now in patients seeking reoperative surgery is that their necks have been excessively defatted, leaving little soft tissue present between the skin and the underlying platysma. This becomes a difficult problem in that many patients seeking secondary rhytidectomy often require platysma surgery, and there is little cover to disguise any postoperative irregularities that may occur following platysma manipulation. Similarly, when elevating the cervical flaps in these patients, since there is little subcutaneous tissue to work in, it is easy to violate the fascia overlying the platysma, or the platysma muscle itself, and increase the possibility for cervical irregularities in the postoperative period. While some patients presenting for secondary rhytidectomy require further defatting, especially if they have gained weight in the ensuing period, cervical problems in reoperative rhytidectomy commonly do not include excess preplatysmal fat. The more common problem in cervical contouring centers around laxity within both platysma and skin. Sorting out these factors is an important part of the preoperative evaluation.

As patients age, they commonly lose facial fat. This is often seen in the cheek contour of the elderly, where atrophy of buccal fat leads to a gaunt facial appearance. It will help in these types of patients if one is able to relocate the jowl fat back over the buccal recess at the time of SMAS advancement. Again, in terms of contouring facial fat, the same caveat applies to secondary patients as was discussed in primary rhytidectomy. It is better to relocate facial fat to a normal location than to obtain contour by removing fat that is present in an abnormal position. Nonetheless, some secondary or tertiary patients will require very judicious removal of jowl fat at the time of reoperative rhytidectomy. This should be decided upon based on the preoperative evaluation and performed following SMAS advancement and closure.

Attenuation of Deep Layer Support

The most common scenario in patients presenting for secondary rhytidectomy is that while their skin envelope has been tightened from the previous surgery, they remain with the stigmata of an attenuation of deep layer support (i.e., with prominent nasolabial folds, jowls, and platysma banding). Although very little skin is often removed at the time of reoperation, most of these patients will have a significant amount of laxity present within the SMAS and platysma, and will benefit from a tightening of the deeper facial soft tissues.

SURGICAL REJUVENATION OF THE FACE

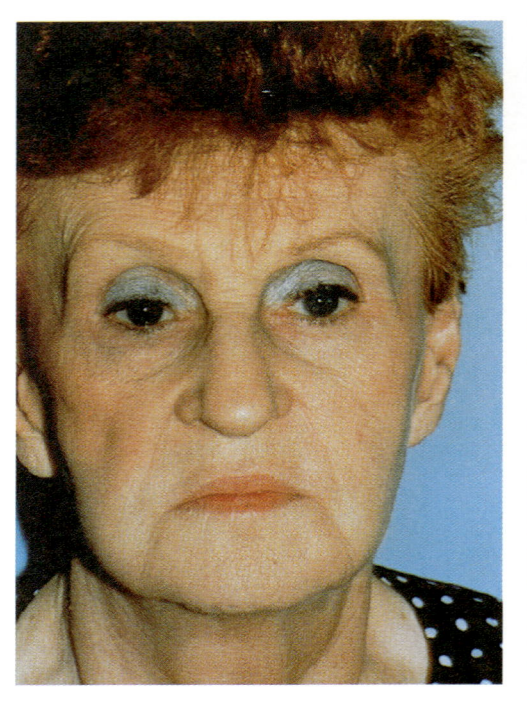

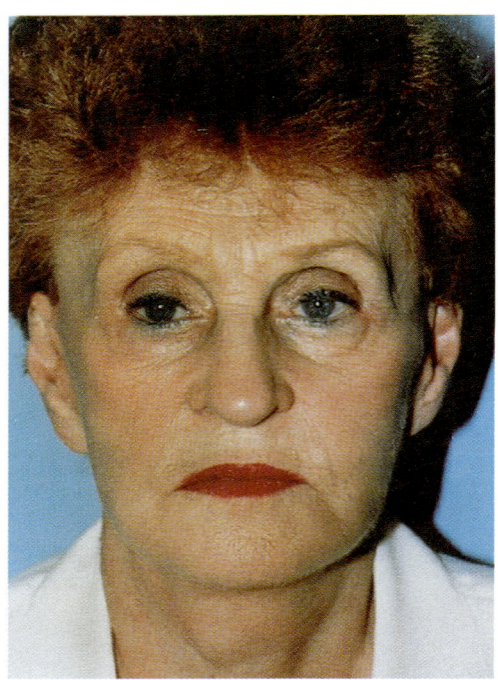

Pre- and postoperative photographs of secondary rhytidectomy and extended SMAS dissection. Note the improvement in the nasolabial folds following malar pad resuspension, after a procedure in which essentially no skin resection was performed.

In some of these patients, at the time of reexploration the SMAS is found to have been previously undermined. Reelevation of the SMAS can be attempted at the time of secondary rhytidectomy as long as the planes are not obscured by scarring. Most commonly, the cicatricial distortion is encountered overlying the parotid gland, where there is fortunately good protection for the underlying facial nerve. Usually, SMAS elevation was limited during the primary procedure and once the SMAS is freed up past the parotid, the areolar plane overlying the masseter muscle is encountered and can be rapidly bluntly dissected. Similarly, usually little SMAS elevation has been performed in the malar region and by extending the SMAS dissection into this area, significant mobilization can be performed in a region free of surgical scarring. Although secondary SMAS elevation is most commonly performed without problems, it should be emphasized that if the anatomy is obscure or the surgeon becomes uncomfortable with the anatomic relationship between the superficial and the deep facial fascia during the dissection, we favor simply plicating the SMAS in these patients.

In some patients undergoing secondary or tertiary rhytidectomy, the SMAS is extremely thin and attenuated from the previous operation. The thin SMAS layer is difficult to raise and commonly tears as it is elevated. In this situation, one may find the SMAS unsuitable for elevation and advancement, and again we favor plication in these patients.

Platysma Bands and Cervical Obliquity

As previously noted, a common approach to cervical contouring during primary rhytidectomy involves removing preplatysmal fat along with tightening the cervical skin. Commonly, little attention was given to the platysma during the primary procedure and, with aging, platysma bands have become more obvious. This problem should be addressed at the secondary procedure. The treatment of cervical bands in the reoperative patient is similar to what was discussed previously under primary rhytidectomy. We emphasize that every effort must be used to keep as much fat as possible along the base of the cervical flaps during undermining. This can often be difficult when operating on a thin-necked patient through a submental incision. For this reason, in the secondary patient, we commonly perform the cervical undermining from the lateral approach, because dissection is better controlled through this broader-based incision. Great care is taken to keep as much fat as possible attached to the cervical skin flap. After dissecting well into the neck in a bilateral fashion, the submental incision is opened and through-and-through dissection of the neck is completed. Following this, mobilization of the platysma bands, anterior edge-to-edge approximation, and inferior transection can be easily completed as described previously.

SURGICAL REJUVENATION OF THE FACE

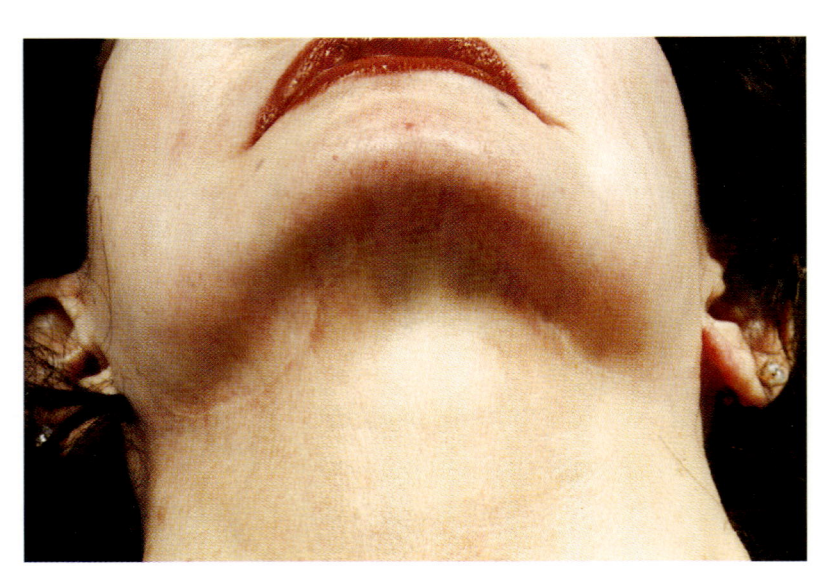

In this patient the primary surgeon performed a direct excision of cervical skin paralleling the mandibular border. We prefer to retighten cervical skin through a classic incision rather than produce the permanent deformity associated with these highly visible scars.

We disapprove of direct cervical skin excision as a technique of tightening neck skin. This commonly produces an unsightly scar that can prove difficult to revise and causes, in our opinion, greater morbidity than performing a secondary tightening via standard incisions.

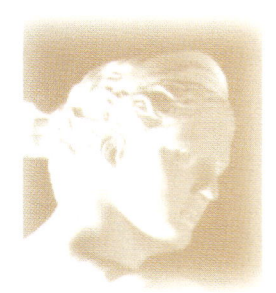

TECHNIQUE

Technically, it is often easier to dissect a secondary rhytidectomy flap, since the plane has been defined from the previous surgery. Undermining a secondary facelift flap tends to be less bloody, since most of the small crossing vessels between the SMAS and skin have been divided during the primary procedure and the flaps have been subsequently delayed. In the patient with a moderate amount of subcutaneous fat, it is usually quite easy to reenter the previous operative plane and quickly dissect the flaps peripherally. The amount of dissection required in the secondary rhytidectomy is similar to that in primary rhytidectomy patients.

A word of caution is advised in regard to thin patients undergoing a reoperative procedure. In these patients, there is commonly a paucity of subcutaneous fat, since normal cheek fat has been replaced by a fibrous layer of fat and scar, and there is little tissue interposed between the skin and the underlying SMAS. In these patients it is easy to penetrate the superficial fascia and elevate the SMAS with the cervicofacial flap. If the SMAS is violated significantly during cervicofacial flap undermining, not only is the possibility of facial nerve injury present but the possibility of using a SMAS flap to contour the deeper facial soft tissues has been eliminated.

One great advantage in secondary rhytidectomy patients is that as the flaps have been delayed, they are quite hardy in terms of vascularity. It is rare to see a skin slough or even superficial necrosis in a secondary rhytidectomy patient. This allows for a greater margin of safety when determining the amount of skin undermining required or in working with patients who have a smoking history.

We perform the SMAS dissection in secondary patients in a fashion similar to that in primary rhytidectomy patients. As noted, much of the contouring obtained in secondary rhytidectomy patients has to do with restoring deep layer support. Although the SMAS is usually thinner in the reoperative situation, it is usually possible to elevate this layer if the dissection is performed carefully and meticulously.

During closure several factors must be noted. We prefer to rotate our cervicofacial flaps in a direction perpendicular to the nasolabial fold, but we also consider other factors. If rotation of the skin in this direction causes facial rhytides to run in an abnormal pattern, skin flap redraping should be adjusted to minimize this problem. Also, if cephalad rotation of the flaps produces a hairless area above the ear, an attempt to correct this can be made by performing a transverse incision

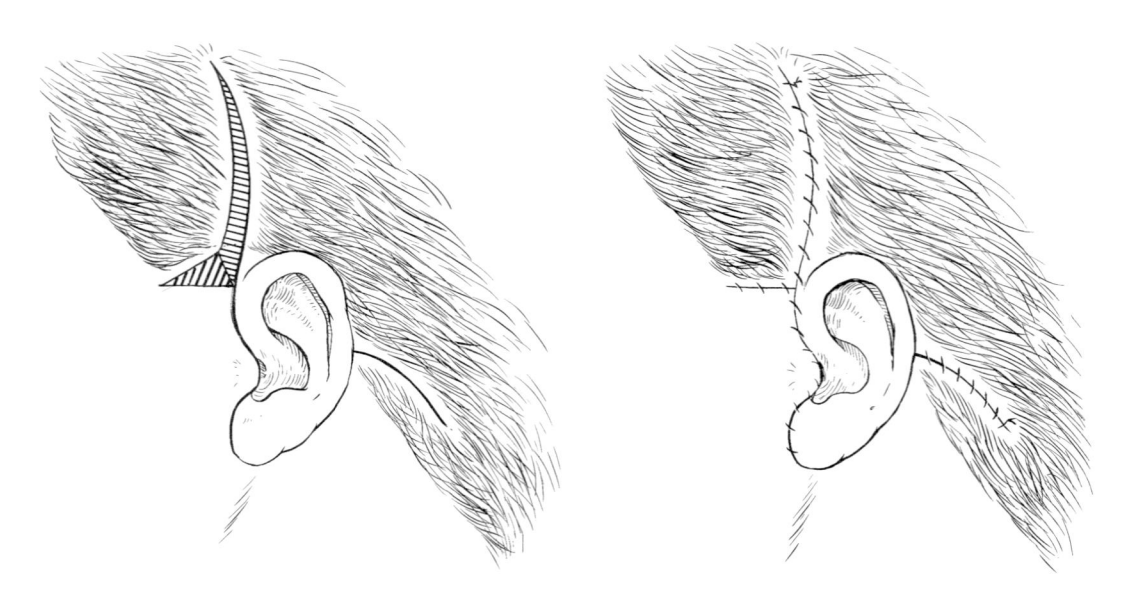

To prevent temporal balding, a transverse incision can be made along the base of the sideburn; a local flap of temporal hair is then rotated inferiorly at the time of flap redraping.

along the base of the sideburn and then rotating the temporal hair inferiorly to the same level as the base of the helical attachment. Alternatively, a temporal hairline incision can be used to prevent an unwanted hairline shift in secondary facelift patients.

In general, we prefer to restore contour with deep layer support, via the SMAS and platysma, than to rotate skin flaps in an exaggerated cephalad direction, which produces an unnatural, tightened look. Contouring the skin flap around the tragus, earlobe, concha, and postauricular region is given the similar considerations noted in primary rhytidectomy. If the posterior hairline can be aligned at the time of closure, we recommend that it be done. Unfortunately, most patients presenting for secondary rhytidectomy have a large stairstep in their postauricular hairline, and it is difficult to improve this at the time of secondary closure.

POSTOPERATIVE CARE

Postoperative care of the secondary rhytidectomy patient is exactly the same as that in the primary patient. The healing time, bruising, and appearance of the scars in secondary rhytidectomies are comparable or even somewhat less than those seen in primary procedures. Certainly the hematoma rate is less in secondary patients than in primary patients, and flap necrosis is almost nonexistent in secondary rhytidectomies. The less edema and bruising seen in the secondary rhytidectomy patient is countered by the older age of the patients in this group. Overall we have noted little difference in terms of convalescence between groups of patients undergoing either primary or reoperative rhytidectomy.

SURGICAL REJUVENATION OF THE FACE

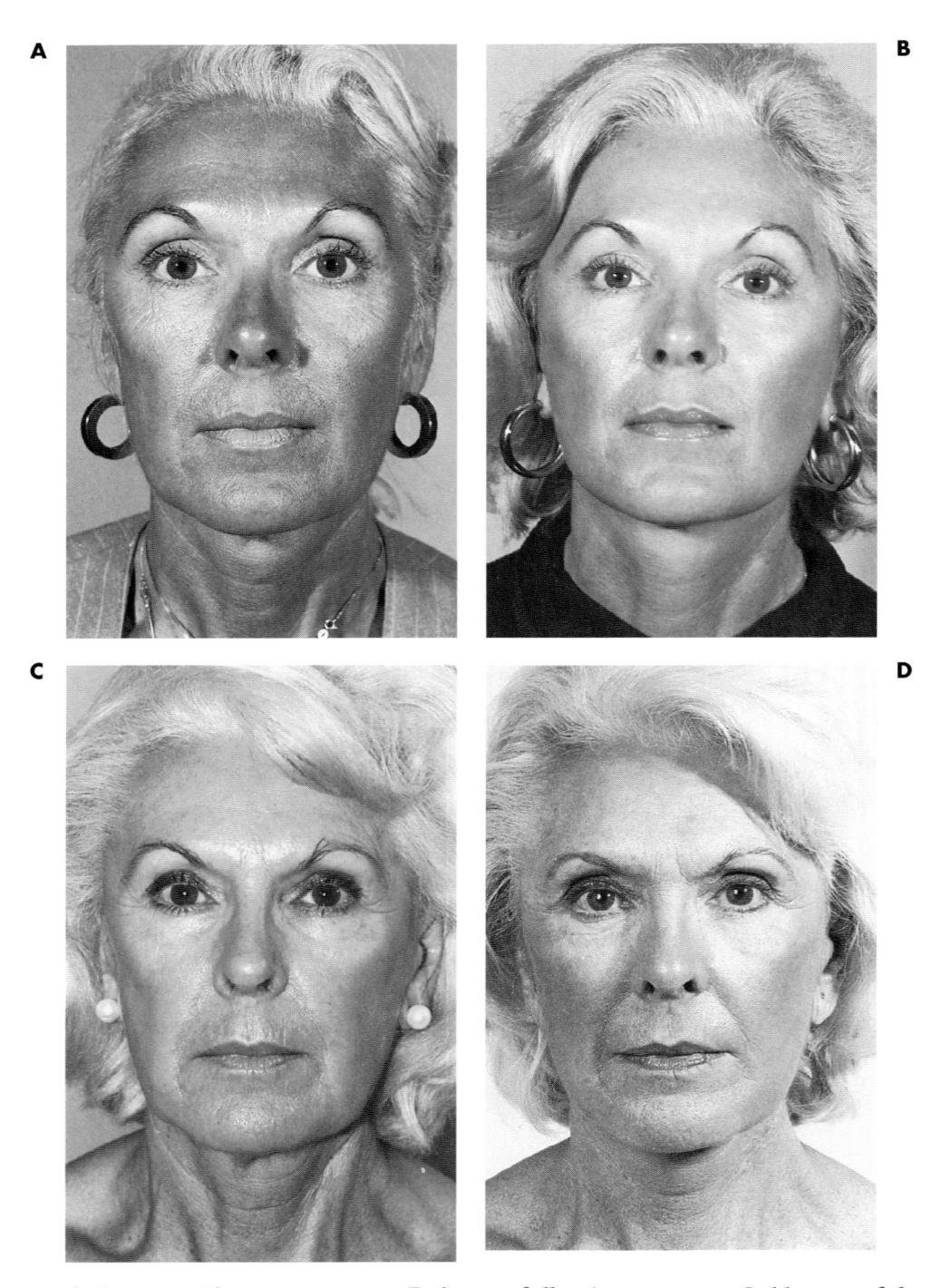

A, Preoperative appearance. B, 1 year following surgery. C, 11 years following the primary procedure. D, 6 months following secondary rhytidectomy. A desire to look youthful is a common request of patients wanting a secondary facelift.

RHYTIDECTOMY

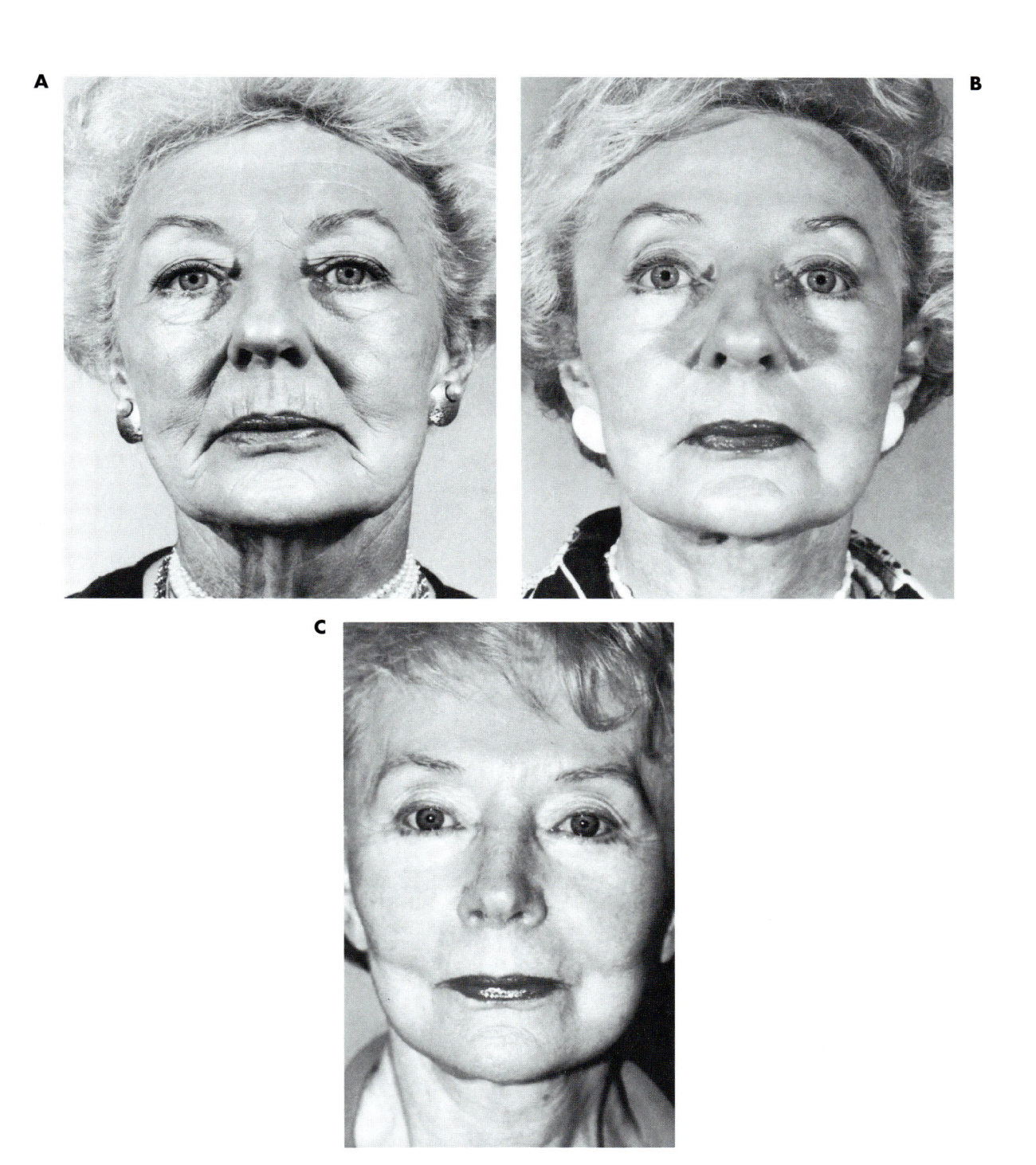

A, Preoperative appearance. B, 1 year following the primary procedure. C, 6 months following secondary rhytidectomy. The patient is now seen 11 years after the primary procedure.

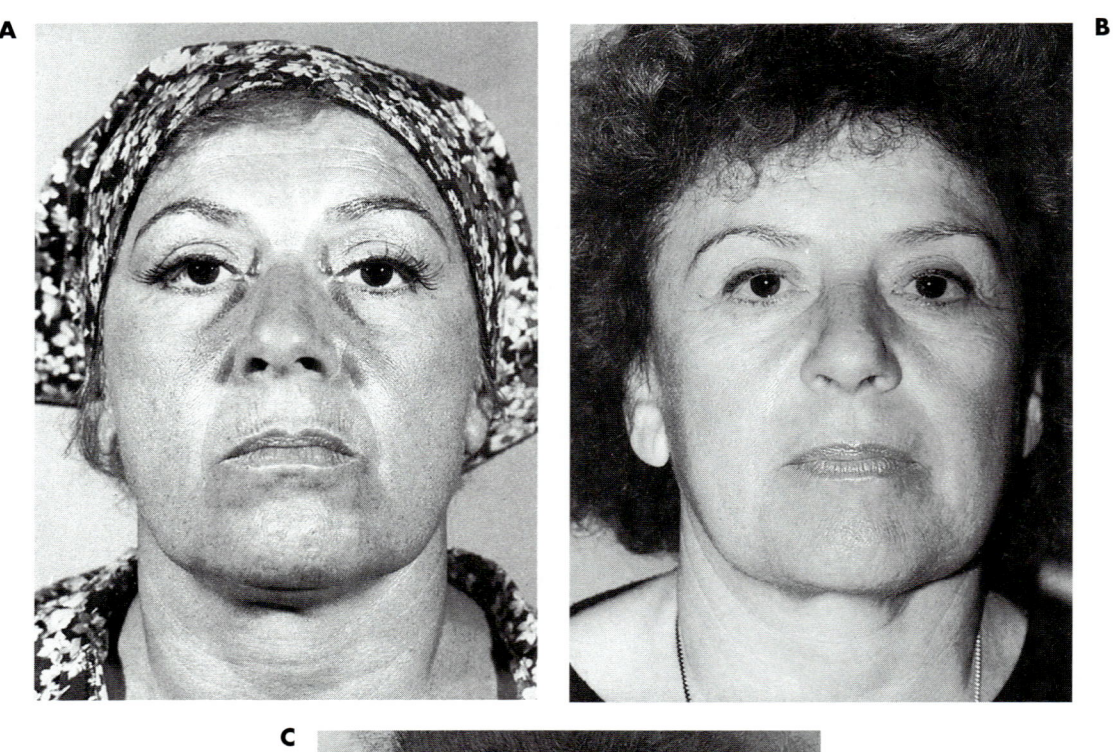

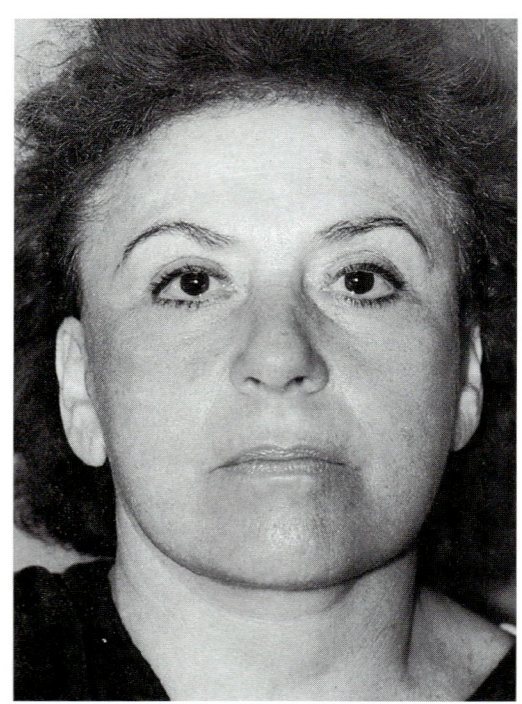

A, Preoperative appearance. B, 14 years postoperatively. C, 1 year following the secondary rhytidectomy.

E

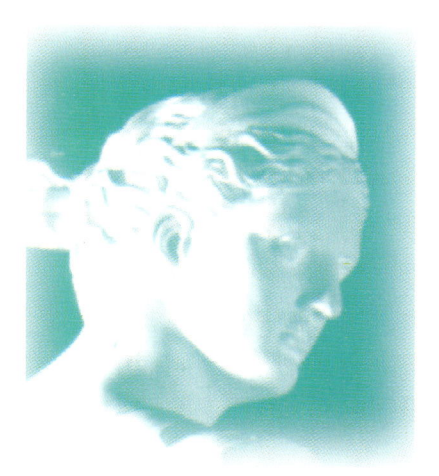

THE MALE FACELIFT

Some plastic surgeons are reluctant to perform rhytidectomy in male patients, but any well-trained plastic surgeon who has the ability to do a facelift in the female patient can do the same operation in a male patient. There is no mystique about the technique of male rhytidectomy. There are a few simple differences between the procedures in the two sexes, and these principally involve accommodating the change in the beard pattern and the slight modification of the basic incisions. Requests for male facelifts have increased during the past few years and, in our practice, men now constitute approximately 10% of all patients seeking the operation.

In an earlier report, we reviewed 100 consecutive male facelifts in our practice, of which 80 procedures were primary facelifts, and 20 were secondary. An additional 50 consecutive male facelifts were reviewed subsequently. The average age of the men undergoing rhytidectomy remained the same at 60 years. The ages ranged from 37 to 83 years. The incidence of hematomas requiring evacuation was approximately 6% in this group. The major difference in the most recent series reviewed was that 70% of patients had a direct repair of the platysma bands by suturing in the midline as contrasted to only eight patients (8%) in the first series that was surveyed. In addition, more attention is being given to support of the cheek and neck by SMAS advancement, as has been described earlier.

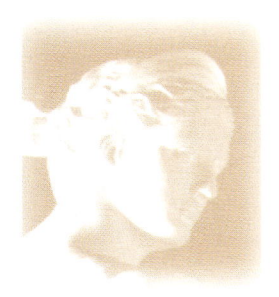

BASIC DIFFERENCES IN TECHNIQUE

Most of the technical details of rhytidectomy are almost identical in the male and female facelift, but some of the differences are:

1. The beard pattern.
2. Thicker male skin.
3. Male tendency toward more bleeding intraoperatively and postoperatively.
4. A higher incidence of hematomas in males.
5. Slightly more pronounced edema in the initial postoperative period in the male.
6. A need to modify the incision slightly in the male.

PREOPERATIVE EVALUATION

The evaluation of the male patient is similar to the evaluation of females. Predictable results can be achieved through careful preoperative planning. A frontal view photograph should be obtained and discussed with the prospective patient, and if any asymmetry is present this should be pointed out preoperatively. Many patients are not aware that their faces are asymmetric, and this can lead to some patient disappointment in the postoperative phase. The use of a reversing mirror is helpful in illustrating these irregularities. The incisions should be drawn on the face and demonstrated to the patient so he knows exactly where the scars will be. It should be emphasized that the beard pattern will be changed and that it is likely that the sideburns will be thinner. Some hair-bearing skin will be rotated into the postauricular area and, therefore, it may be necessary to shave behind the ear. It should also be emphasized that the facelift is not a permanent operation and that the aging process will continue after surgery. The patient will either age with the face as it is now or with the one that is present postoperatively. As with the female patient, the preoperative visit must be cordial, relaxed, and thorough. It is helpful to paint a complete scenario beginning from day 1 until the patient can return to social and business activity. This initial consultation must have adequate time for a complete give-and-take between the physician and patient. Men often are very concerned about when they can return to physical activity, such as jogging, workouts in the gymnasium, or sports such as tennis and golf, and definite guidelines should be drawn. Before returning to strenuous physical activity, it is probably best to wait 5 to 6 weeks.

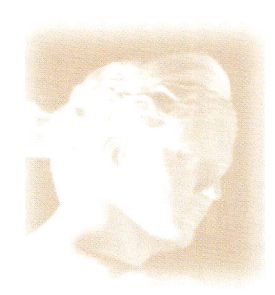

As in the female, the surgeon should assess whether or not the patient's request is realistic. The surgeon must decide whether the patient's desires are reasonable and discuss their feasibility with the patient. It is often helpful to find out what motivated the individual to seek this consultation at this particular time in his life. If there are psychological problems, divorce proceedings, employment difficulties, or other stressful situations, it is probably best to postpone surgery until these conditions are rectified or until the surgeon believes the patient is coping with them in a stable manner. The conversation between the patient and the physician must lead to the point where they feel like they are on the same wavelength. Communication is all-important.

Our goal is not to make the patient happy (he may well not have been happy when he sought the consultation), but to carry out a surgical procedure that will try to meet the objectives of both patient and surgeon and, by doing so, enhance the quality of the patient's life. It is a good idea to rediscuss the alterations of the male beard pattern and the significance of the altered position of the hair growth in the postoperative phase. The patient should not be surprised postoperatively if he discovers that he has to shave behind the ears. The surgical consent form should be gone over thoroughly and the common complications explained. Hematoma is not a true complication, but it is a calculated risk, and it is seen with approximately two to three times the frequency in males.

As in females, the medical history is important. Listing any drugs that the patient is taking on the front of the chart is a good policy. If there are any medical problems, a medical consult must be obtained. Our office policy requires a medical clearance for all patients 65 years of age or older.

In examining the patient, any previous scars from facial surgery need to be assessed, and the revision of these scars or the creation of new scars should be documented in the medical records, photographed, and discussed with the patient.

Other procedures that may be done at the time of the facelift include the following:

1. Chin implant or sliding osteotomy.
2. Direct excision of nasolabial folds.
3. Blepharoplasty.
4. Rhinoplasty.
5. Otoplasty.
6. Browlift.
7. Hair transplantation.

Although the surgeon should not pressure patients into undergoing additional surgical procedures, if it is apparent that some of these ancillary procedures would significantly improve the end result, it is best to discuss them preoperatively and either plan to do them at the time of the initial surgery or plan a subsequent procedure or procedures at predetermined intervals.

With reference to patients who request a direct excision of cervical laxity, such as a Z-plasty, T-plasty, or M-plasty, it is best to avoid them, if possible, except under very unusual circumstances. These procedures leave visible scars and significantly alter the beard pattern, making the resultant deformities almost impossible to correct. By using a submental incision and aggressive undermining from the lateral incisions in the cervical area, platysmal laxity and contouring of the neck can usually be adequately done without direct excision of skin in the midline.

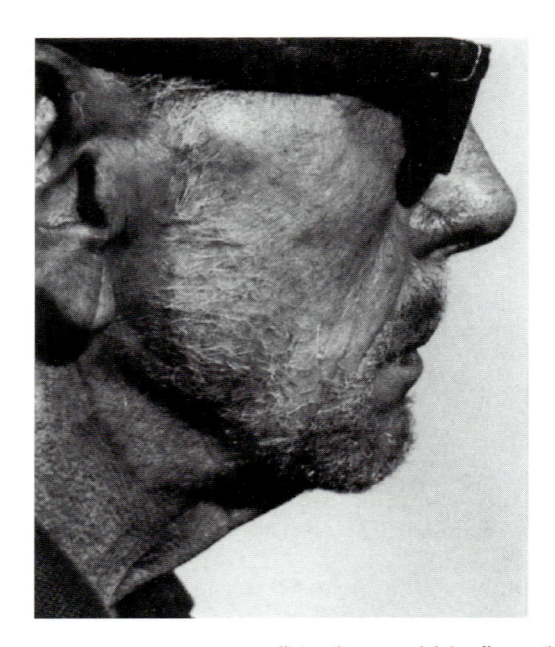

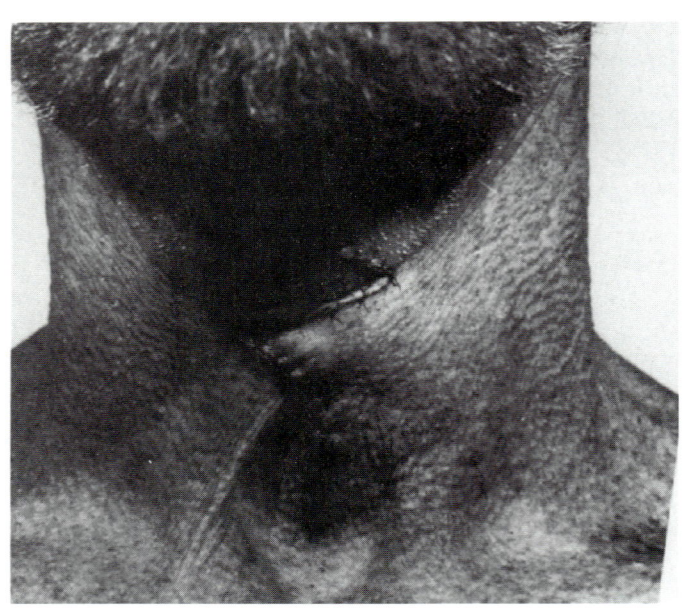

"Turkey gobbler" neck web in a man who wears a beard at all times. He accepted the probability of neck scarring if a Z-plasty were done and stated that his beard would hide the scars. In the photograph on the right, the patient is shown with sutures in place after a cervical Z-plasty.

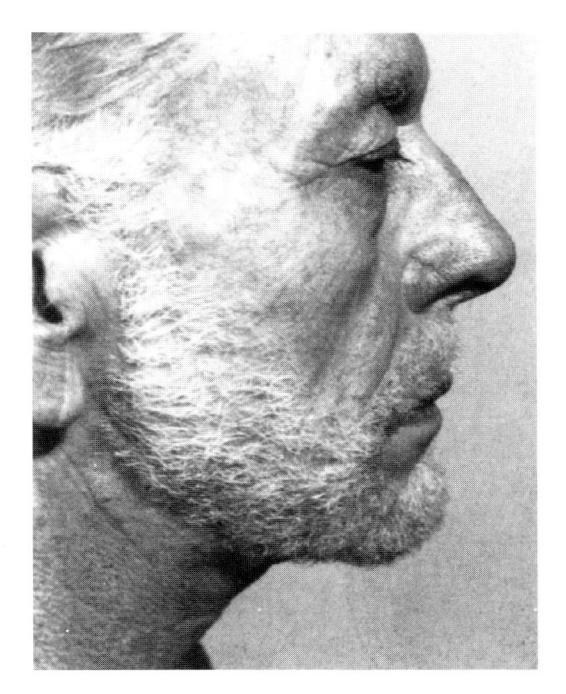

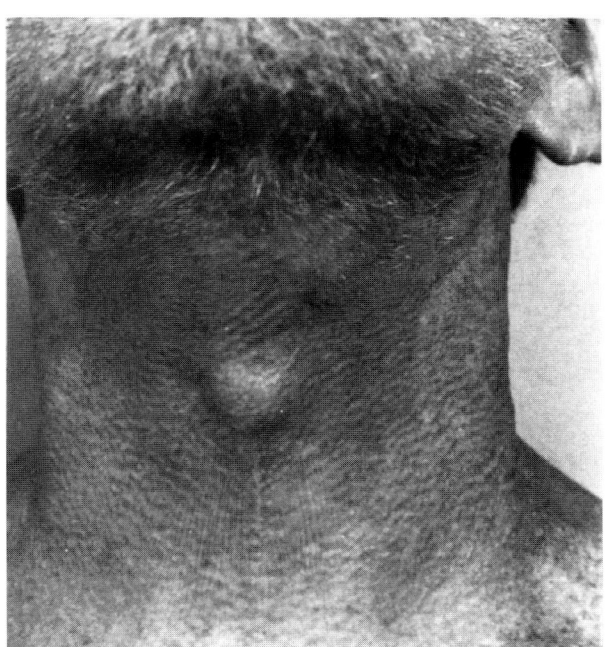

Only minimal scarring occurred after the cervical Z-plasty. This result is the exception rather than the rule. In our opinion, external incisions in the neck should be avoided because when unsightly scars develop they are almost impossible to correct. A classic cervical rhytidectomy would have worked in this case, and the scars would have been better camouflaged.

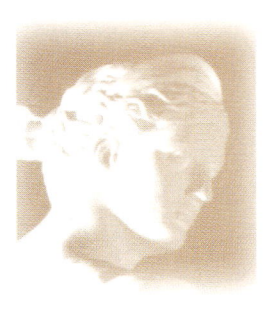

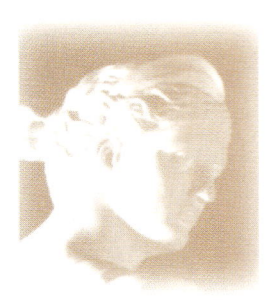

PREOPERATIVE PREPARATION

All of our male patients receive local anesthesia with adequate analgesia. Our local anesthesia of preference is 1% lidocaine with 1:100,000 epinephrine along the lines of incision and 0.5% lidocaine and 1:400,000 epinephrine in the anticipated plane of dissection.

INCISIONS

In contrast to the usual incision used in women (our personal preference is to follow the tragal margin), a male facelift incision is most often placed in the non–hair-bearing preauricular skin. The incisions can follow the tragal margin, but this advances the beard pattern over

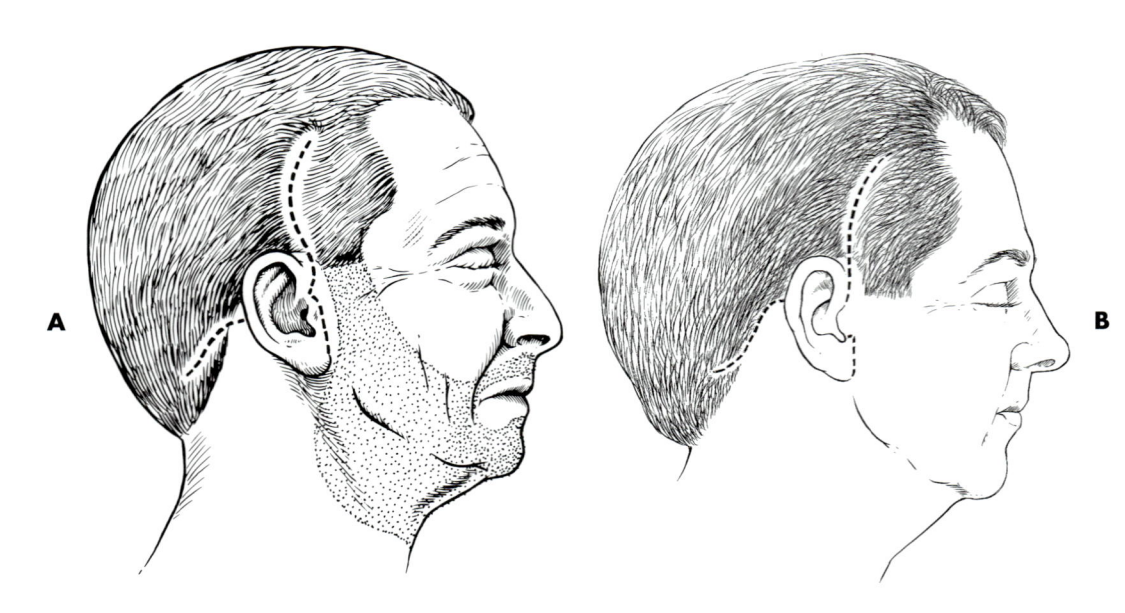

Two types of incisions in the male are illustrated. A, The classic preauricular incision avoids bringing bearded skin within the tragal contour. B, The tragal margin incision requires the surgeon to excise the base of the hair follicle prior to closure.

the tragus at the time of closure and the hair follicles must be dissected from the tragal flap. If the hair follicles are carefully removed, particularly in patients with a sparse beard pattern, the tragal incision works quite well. The postauricular incision does not usually extend into the hairline as in females, since men do not generally wear their hair up. Thus it is easy to camouflage the posterior cervical scar by placing it superiorly along the posterior hairline, just barely within the hairline,

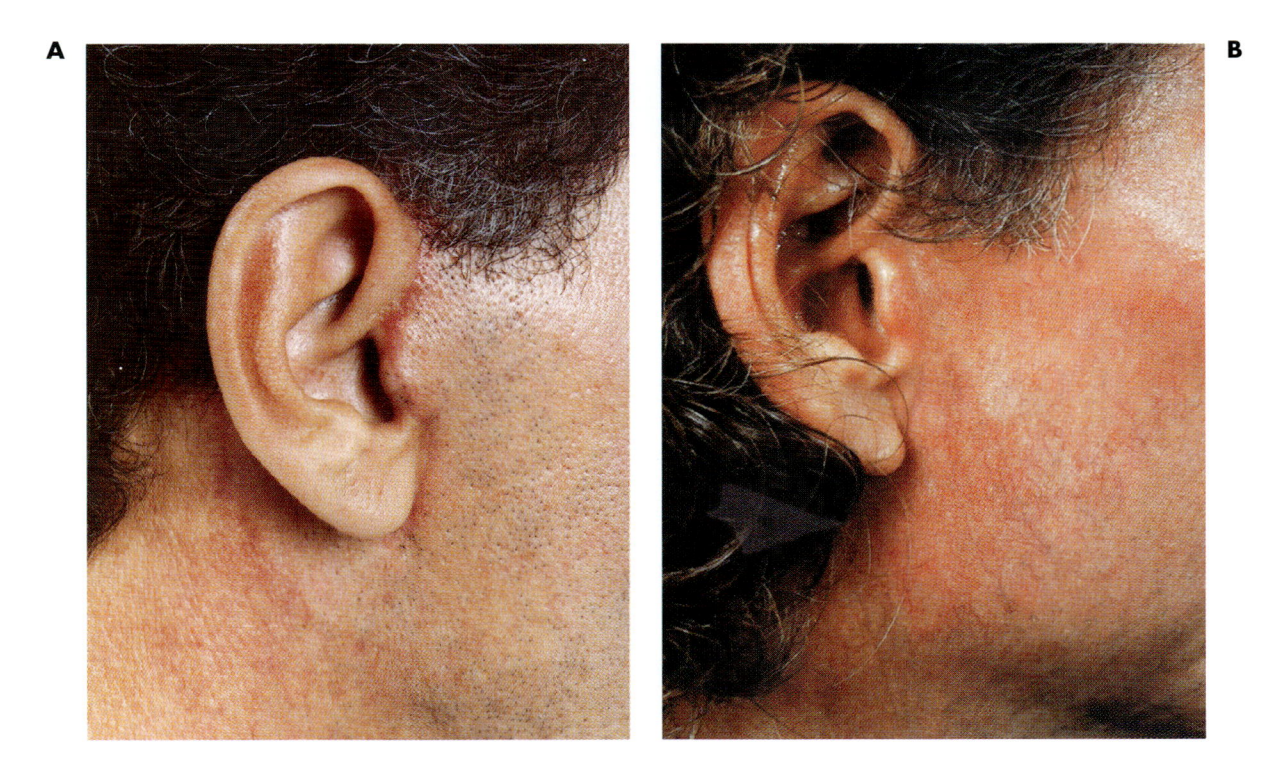

A

B

Early postoperative appearance of the tragal incision with removal of hair follicles along the base of the tragus. B, Late postoperative appearance of a tragal incision another patient. A well-designed and well-inset tragal incision will usually produce an imperceptible scar that is visualized as a color differential between the blush skin of the cheek and the more pale skin of the ear.

SURGICAL REJUVENATION OF THE FACE

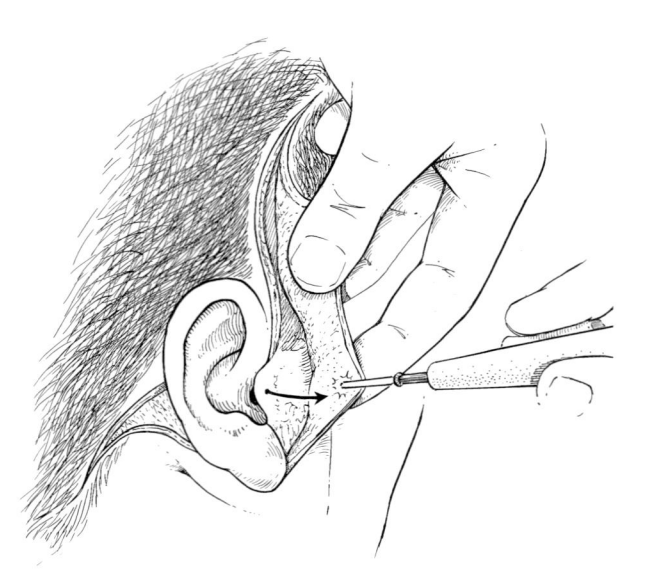

The roots of the hair follicles are removed with the electrocautery when a tragal margin incision is used.

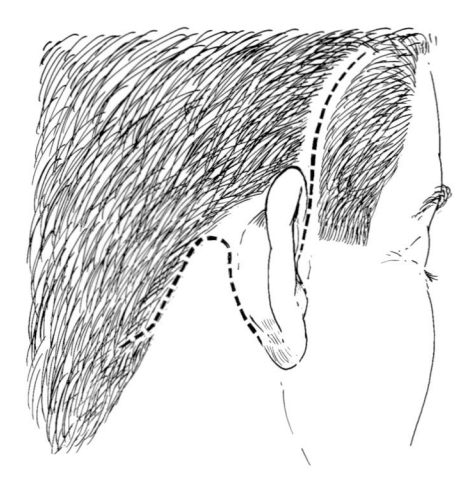

The postauricular incision in the male extends superiorly along the hairline and then sweeps back inferiorly into the postauricular area.

and then lower on the neck swept back into the posterior hairline. If the patient has an extremely low hairline, it may be possible to place the incision completely within the postauricular hair, but this is rarely the case. Since men do not employ an upswept hairdo, the incision at the hairline along the back of the neck is easily concealed because of the downward growth of the hair follicles. The length of the postauricular incision averages 8 to 10 cm in length. If a submental incision is necessary, it is usually placed just caudal to a natural crease.

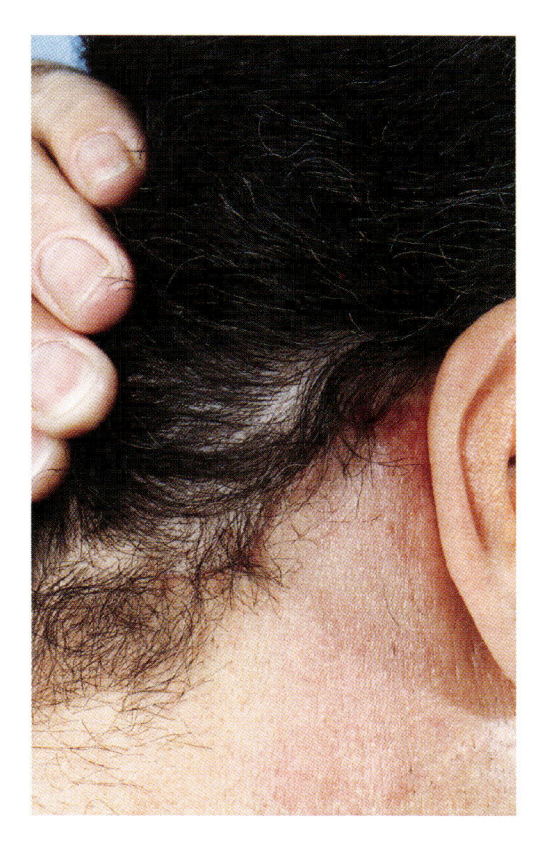

Early postoperative appearance of postauricular incision carried along the hairline as illustrated in the preceding figure. Note that when hair is worn down, this incision is well camouflaged.

Bleeding is controlled throughout by electrocautery. Meticulous hemostasis is essential. The amount of undermining in the male patient is similar to that in the female patient, and in most patients a through-and-through cervical dissection is performed. Contouring of preplatysmal fat is done if indicated, and subplatysmal fat is contoured as required. If platysma bands are present clinically, they must be dealt with. We prefer to suture the bands together in the midline and trim them appropriately before suturing. The plication is carried at least to the base of the thyroid cartilage. The anterior platysma is then partially transected at the level of the cricoid, usually as far laterally as the anterior border of the sternocleidomastoid muscle.

The management of the SMAS depends on the preoperative findings. A SMAS dissection is done in most male patients and is similar to what has been previously discussed. One of the important aspects of the SMAS flap is the transposition flap that is created to aid in deepening the cervicomental angle and "cleaning up" the jawline. In some men, the nasolabial folds are quite prominent and fatty, and in these patients, after performing the extended SMAS dissection and fixation, we occasionally follow this with defatting of the nasolabial fold, using a small suction cannula.

After adequate hemostasis is secured, the two large cervicofacial flaps are rotated laterally and slightly superiorly. In the neck, the rotation follows the cervical creases posteriorly.

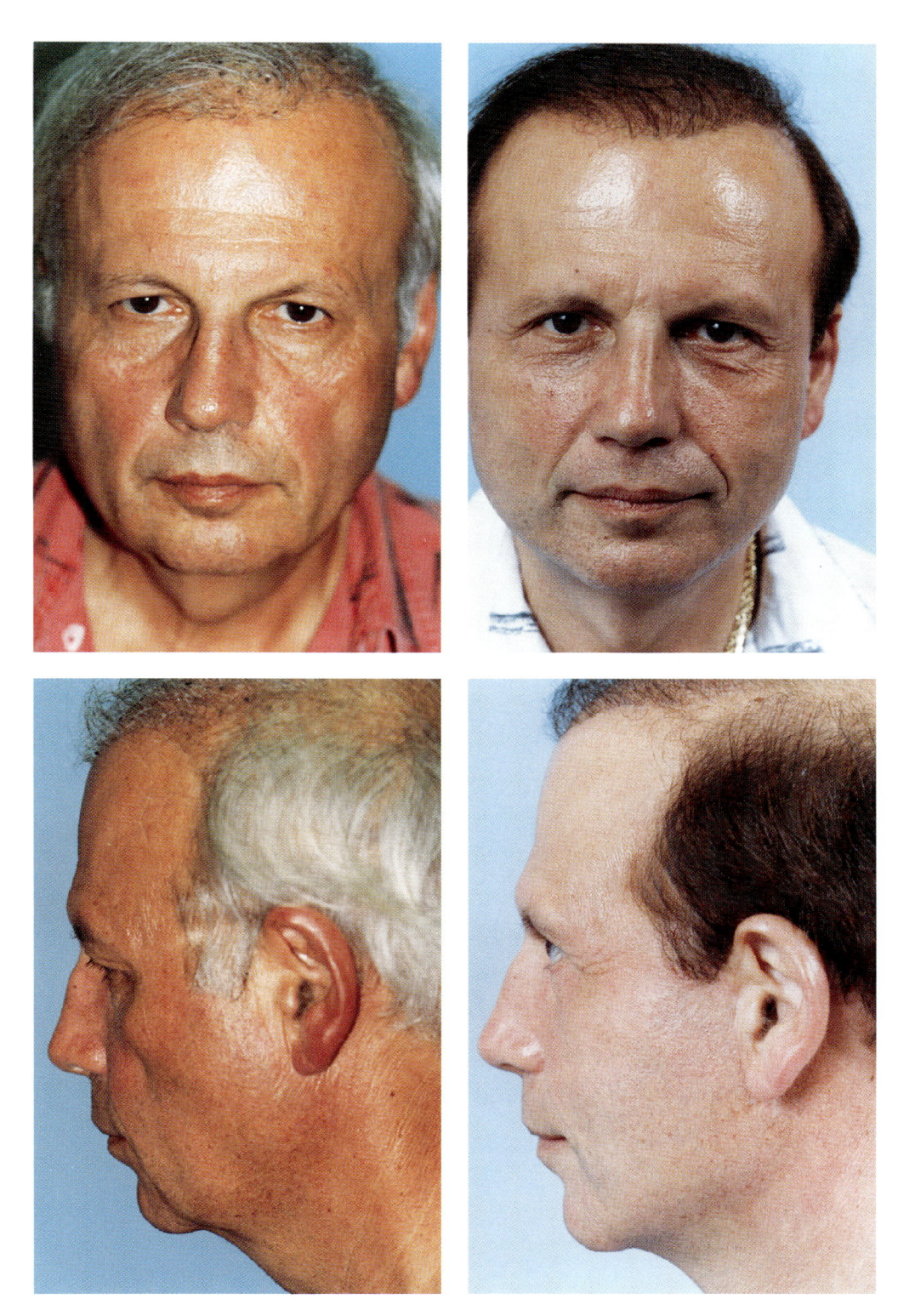

Patient seen before and after primary rhytidectomy with SMAS dissection and low platysma plication.

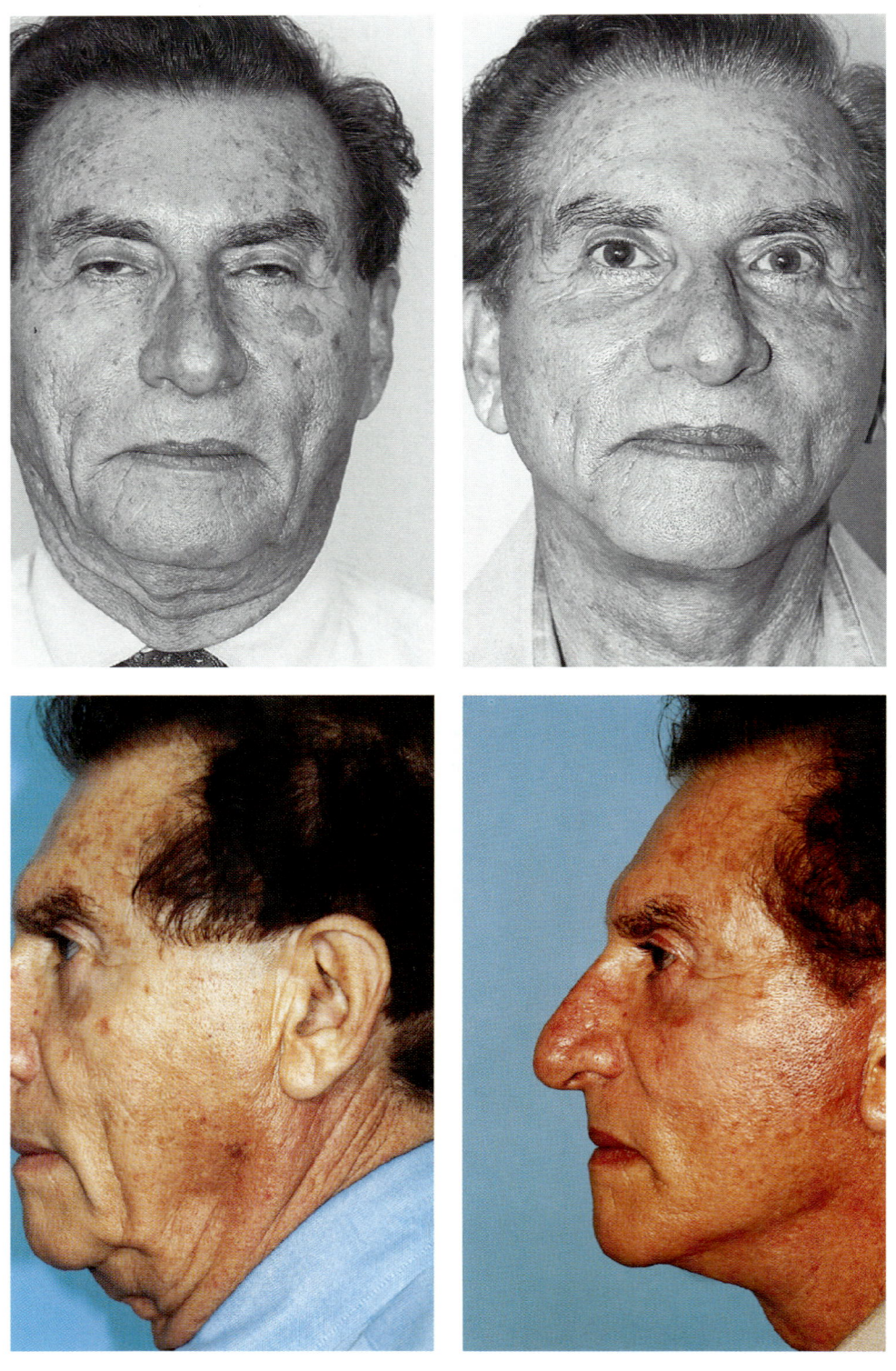

SURGICAL REJUVENATION OF THE FACE

Pre- and postoperative appearance following primary rhytidectomy with SMAS dissection and platysma plication.

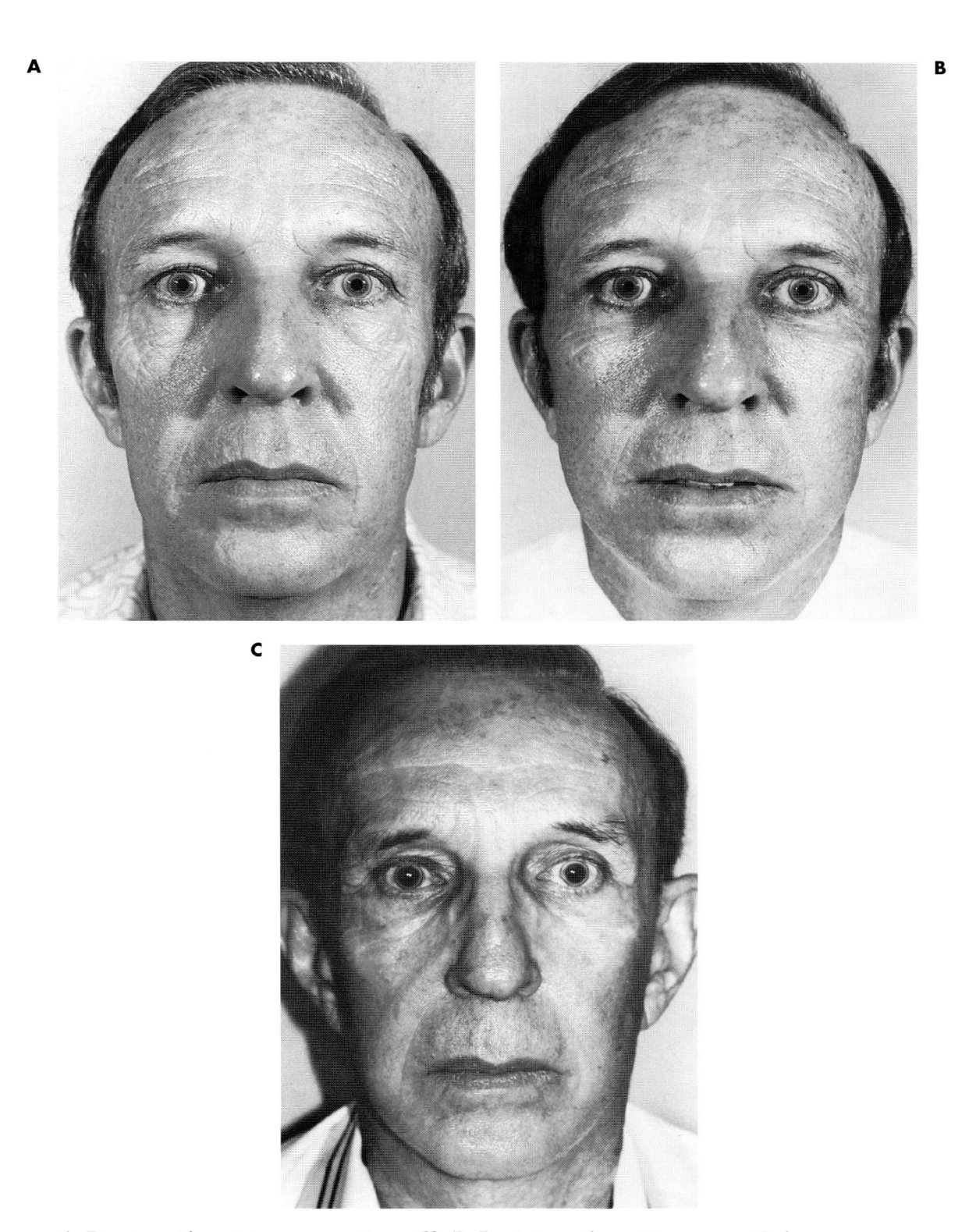

A, Preoperative appearance at age 52. B, Postoperative appearance. C, 1 year following secondary facelift. This patient is now 69 years old.

Closure in the male patient is identical to that in the female. Dressings and postoperative management are also similar. It should be emphasized that it is essential to keep the patient free of pain. In anticipation of rebound pain, it is our policy to give pain medication before the patient requests it. The blood pressure must be carefully monitored so that it does not exceed 150/90 mm Hg. For control of hypertension, chlorpromazine (Thorazine) is administered IV in increments of 1 to 2 mg at 10-minute intervals. With this drug, patients can be adequately titrated to maintain their blood pressure within normal levels. By keeping the patient free of pain, relaxed, and calm, and by keeping the blood pressure within normal limits, the incidence of hematoma should be extremely low.

After the patient has been stable for 3 to 4 hours in the recovery area, he is discharged to a recovery facility or to the care of a family member with explicit postoperative instructions. As with their female counterparts, male patients are given a prescription for pain relief. All patients are also given oral antibiotics, usually cephalexin unless contraindicated.

Male patients, like females, are seen the day after surgery for dressing changes and wound inspection. If drains are used they are removed at this point, and after the wounds are adequately cleaned with peroxide, the bandages are replaced for an additional 24 hours, after which time they are removed and the patient instructed to wash his hair in the shower on a daily basis. The preauricular sutures are removed on the fifth postoperative day, and all remaining sutures are removed on the seventh or eighth postoperative day. During the postoperative phase the patient is reminded about limiting his physical activities. It is especially the case with men to emphasize this, since most men want to get back to a strenuous routine rather quickly.

LATE POSTOPERATIVE CARE

During the next 3 to 4 weeks, moderate physical activity is allowed and the patient may engage in some social activities, depending on his personal appearance. The first follow-up examination following suture removal is usually done at approximately 2 to 3 months, after which the patient is seen at intervals as deemed necessary.

CONTRAST AND SATISFACTION

There are a few more challenges that present in the male patient such as the tendency toward a bit more intra- and postoperative bleeding. In addition, the change in the beard pattern remains a challenge, but by careful planning and preoperative education of the patient, this can be adequately handled. Men tend to complain less in the postoperative period. Most men accept the improvement gained and rarely require revision.

Even though there is more oozing in the male patient, they commonly have less bruising than female patients. While most men will not use makeup to cover bruises or scars, it is our observation that their recovery is a bit quicker than the average female patient and most men are able to return to work within 2 weeks.

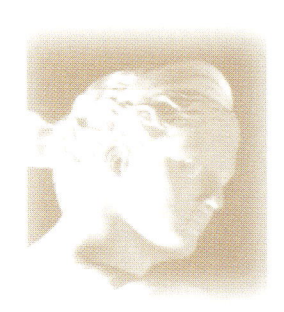

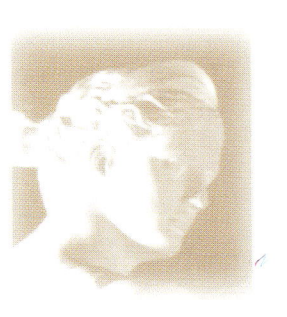

F

COMPLICATIONS

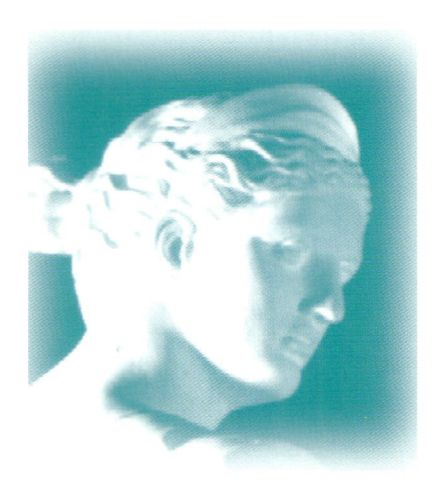

No surgical procedure exists without complications. The surgeon must be able to recognize and deal with these problems. The most common complications following rhytidectomy include the following:

1. Hematoma (70% of all rhytidectomy complications).
2. Postoperative edema.
3. Ecchymosis.
4. Nerve injury.
5. Unacceptable scarring (hypertrophic).
6. Skin slough.
7. Seromas.
8. Contour irregularities.
9. Infection.
10. Patient dissatisfaction (see Chapter 1).

RHYTIDECTOMY

HEMATOMA

Hematomas are the most common complication of rhytidectomy. Some may think it unjust to classify them as complications. It has been said that the only way to prevent a hematoma after a facelift is not to do the operation. Our incidence of expanding hematomas is around 1%, the minimum incidence that we have been able to attain. It is not a catastrophe for a patient to have an expanding postoperative hematoma; the catastrophe occurs when it is not recognized and properly managed.

The rhytidectomy patient should be observed and monitored closely, especially during the first 6 to 8 hours following the procedure. Almost all expanding hematomas occur during this initial period, and the surgeon should be aware of any patient exhibiting symptoms

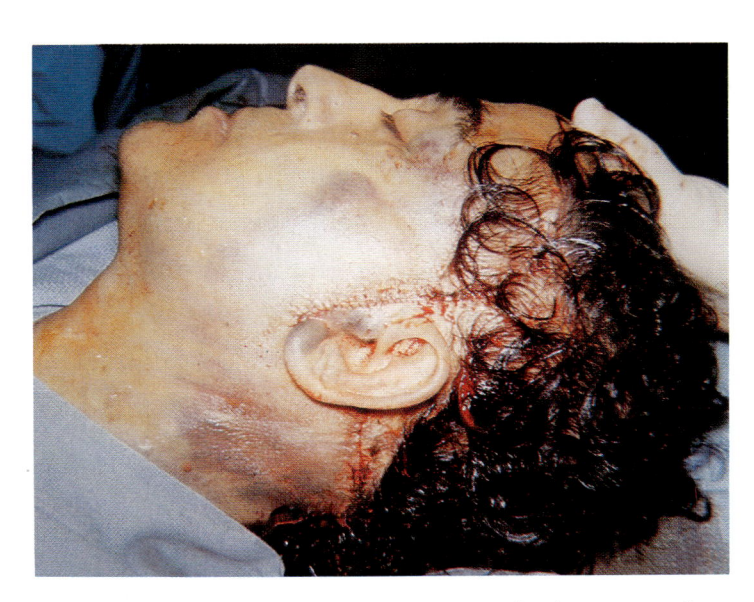

This man has an early expanding hematoma which occurred approximately 2 hours after surgery. It is at this stage that early recognition is important. By removing the sutures, evacuating the clots under direct vision, coagulating the bleeding points, and resuturing, there should be no significant sequelae.

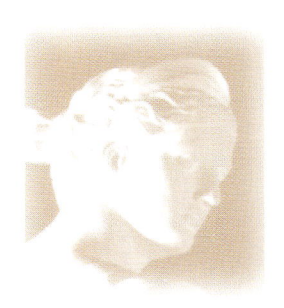

of pain, restlessness, nausea, or elevation of blood pressure, all typical findings in a patient prone to the development of a hematoma. A patient with any of these symptoms must be carefully observed and have appropriate treatment initiated to reverse these findings. Other physical findings include eversion of the lips, hardness of the neck and cheek, and bluish discoloration of the buccal mucosa on the affected side.

Prevention

To lower and control the incidence of hematoma, it is mandatory for the surgeon to have the patient's blood pressure and other vital signs carefully monitored. If the patient develops hypertension during surgery, medication is administered IV to maintain the pressure at the desired level. It is unnecessary to reduce the blood pressure immediately after the administration of the lidocaine-epinephrine local anesthetic or with the elevation produced by the ketamine response. These responses are temporary, and a normal or near-normal blood pressure reestablishes itself spontaneously within minutes.

Our preference for the maintenance of blood pressure during rhytidectomy is the preoperative administration of Clonidine, between .1 mg and .3 mg by mouth one hour prior to surgery. Clonidine represents a selective alpha-2 adrenergic agonist that exhibits both peripheral as well as central effects in lowering blood pressure. The effects of Clonidine are usually apparent within one hour after administration, and because of the long duration of this drug, a systolic blood pressure in the range of 90 mm to 110 mm mercury is apparent for up to 12 hours following administration. In our opinion, this represents the ideal blood pressure range in patients undergoing a long and potentially bloody procedure such as rhytidectomy and offers blood pressure control in the early postoperative period, when hematoma development is most common. Of note, since we have begun the routine administration of Clonidine in our practice, we have not had to return a patient to the operating room for an expanding hematoma over a period of approximately three years.

Intraoperatively, if hypertension becomes a problem, there are several drugs available to the surgeon for maintenance of blood pressure. Chlorpromazine is an extremely reliable and safe drug in our experience, usually administered in 2-3 mg intravenous dosage, given at ten minute intervals, until the blood pressure has been lowered to normal. Alternatively, standard hypertensive medication including Labetalol, Vasotec and hydralazine hydrochloride (Apresoline) can be administered in incremental doses.

The second factor in reducing the incident of hematoma is to keep the patient free of pain. Almost all patients will have some discomfort during the first few hours after surgery as the effect of the anesthetic wears off. The surgeon should anticipate the pain and administer analgesics prior to the patient requesting medication. If the medication is delayed until the patient requests it, she may begin to thrash around unnecessarily and precipitate an expanding hematoma. Prochlorperazine (Compazine) has proved to be of benefit in reducing postoperative nausea. We prefer to administer 5 mg of prochlorperazine IV at the end of the operative procedure. This reduces nausea and vomiting to a minimum and so increases the patient's comfort, thereby reducing any postoperative bleeding because of this drug's antiemetic property. An antiemetic is recommended for use on all patients unless contraindicated.

Narcotics seem to induce nausea. Therefore, if narcotics are used preoperatively and intraoperatively, although this is commonly unnecessary, then the use of prochlorperazine as a precaution against nausea and vomiting seems worthwhile.

Treatment

When an expanding hematoma is recognized, it is time to take action. Early hematoma recognition is the key to preventing disaster postoperatively. This close observation is easier to carry out in an office surgery setup, since the surgeon can have his own well-trained personnel attend the patient during the immediate postoperative phase. This early intervention will prevent subsequent necrosis of the flaps caused by ischemia. There may be times when the operating surgeon is not immediately available; in these cases, emergency treatment by

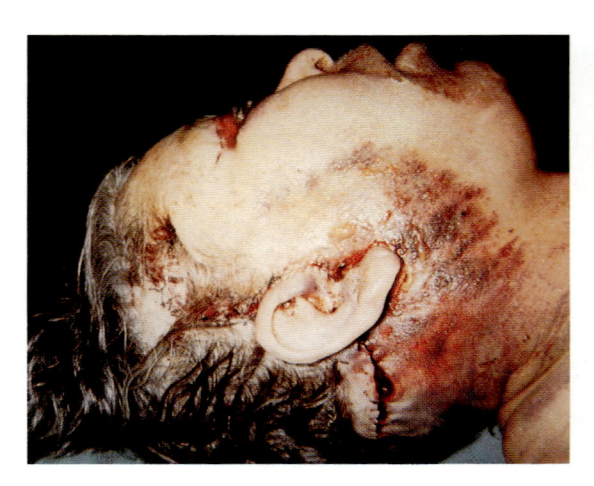

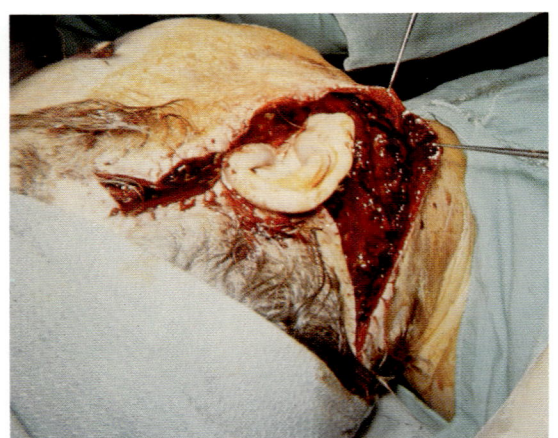

This patient has an expanding hematoma that went unrecognized for approximately 20 hours. The patient was on an obstetric floor where the nurses were unfamiliar with facelifts. When the patient complained of pain and swelling, she was given narcotics to ease her discomfort. Inadvertently, the resident did not see her on evening rounds and the stage was set for tissue necrosis. When the tension was released from the flap, the tenacious clots were gently removed from the operative site. However, some tissue necrosis had already occurred, as evidenced by the superficial blistering seen on the skin surface.

the operating room personnel allows adequate time for the surgeon to return to the operating suite for definitive therapy. The patient is returned to surgery as soon as it is practical, monitoring equipment is applied, and an IV route is established. The sutures are completely removed on the involved side, and the flaps are retracted to permit adequate inspection of the area beneath the flaps. The clots that have formed are tenacious and can be removed with sponge forceps. The wound is packed with sterile gauze sponges moistened with a solution that is 50% saline and 50% hydrogen peroxide. This mixture facilitates the breakup of clots and exposes the bleeding points for easy identification. Patient comfort is ensured during the evacuation by reinjecting the individual bleeding points before electrocoagulation.

Patients who undergo evacuation of expanding hematomas will usually have a significant drug hangover from the initial surgery and, with the administration of a small amount of IV diazepam, may not even remember the second trip to the operating room. After hemostasis has been secured, the skin incisions are reapproximated as described earlier.

Incidence

A review of our experience with more than 4,000 facelifts demonstrates a downward trend in the incidence of expanding hematoma that now seems to have plateaued. In 1975 we reported an analysis of 1,500 consecutive cases of rhytidectomy. The incidence expanding hematomas requiring evacuation was 4.2%. From 1975 to 1980 the incidence dropped to 2.5%, and in the 1980 to 1982 group the incidence was 2%. In our practice, between 1988 and 1992 the incidence of hematoma was approximately 1% of all cases.

There are several reasons for the reduction in the incidence of hematomas. Eliminating the intake of aspirin and ibuprofen preoperatively has been a definite factor. Narcotics have also been eliminated as preoperative medications. A more concentrated effort in monitoring patients in the immediate postoperative period, giving special attention to the prevention of nausea, pain, and hypertension, has also been helpful. Attention to detail by experienced personnel is the best "antihematoma" insurance. A patient who is normotensive, pain-free, and nausea-free is not apt to develop a hematoma.

If an expanding hematoma is properly managed, there should be no serious sequelae other than the possibility of a slight increase in the amount of postoperative ecchymosis and edema. All plastic surgeons performing rhytidectomies will have patients who develop hematoma. This is no reflection on the surgical ability of the individual physician. It is the recognition and proper management of hematoma that proves the surgeon's expertise. If a hematoma has been adequately evacuated, there does not appear to be any significant difference in the rate of healing when comparing one with the other.

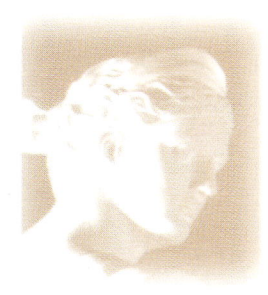

POSTOPERATIVE EDEMA

When postoperative edema occurs, attempts should be made to reduce it, primarily by elevating the head of the bed. Pressure dressings are of doubtful significance in reducing the incidence of edema and are more uncomfortable than loosely applied bandages. Therefore we do not use pressure dressings on facelifts. Since pressure dressings are not used on flaps in other parts of the body, it seems illogical to use them on the large cervicofacial flaps and they may in fact be harmful.

We have tried postoperative enzymes for edema, and because their effectiveness remains questionable, we no longer use them. We administer 8 mg of dexamethasone (Decadron) IV during and immediately following the operative procedure. In our clinical experience we have found that this helps to reduce postoperative edema. Patients often experience feelings of euphoria for 1 or 2 days after this drug is given.

The application of cold compresses in the first 24 to 48 hours may offer the patient some pain relief. It is also psychologically beneficial to the patient because she is doing something to help speed her recovery.

Time and elevation of the head are the two most important factors in reducing edema. The patient may get impatient when the swelling does not disappear rapidly.

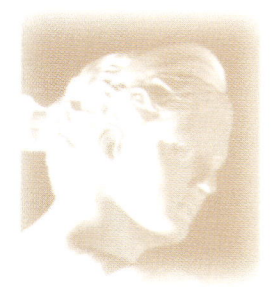

ECCHYMOSIS

Extensive ecchymosis either with or without hematoma is annoying for the patient. The patient's clinical history is of importance in treating these patients, because if she has indicated that she bruises easily, she should be informed preoperatively that discoloration may remain for several weeks after surgery.

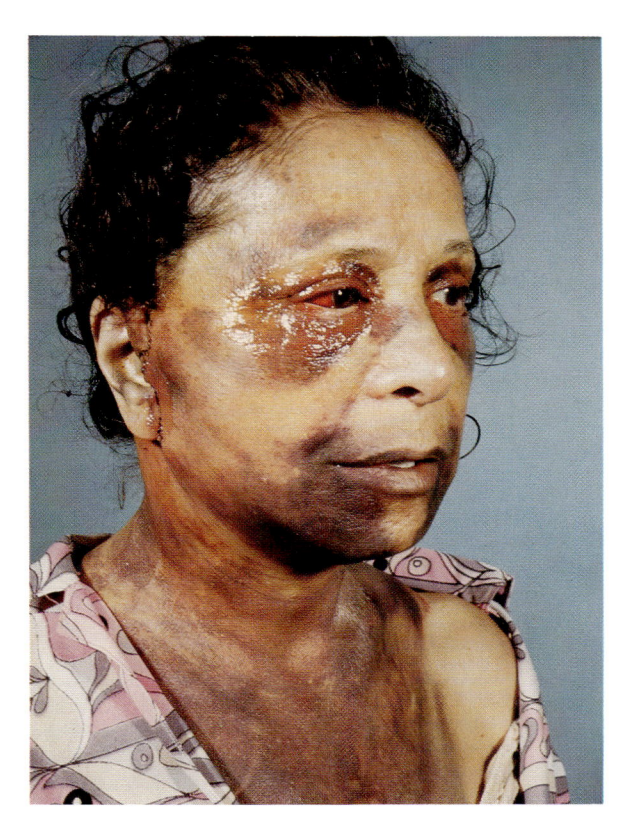

This patient gave a history of "bruising easily." Routine blood studies were within the normal range. She required several weeks for the discoloration to disappear. In rare instances, the patient may be aware of medical problems that can contribute to the severe bruising, and so a detailed medical history is very important. Known conditions such as thrombocytopenia, blood dyscrasia, or a clotting disorder should be thoroughly investigated. If there is a question about such matters, secure a consultation with a hematologist. Even after all avenues have been explored, a small number of patients will exhibit extensive ecchymosis and the cause will never be found. Fortunately, the appearance is of more concern than the sequelae.

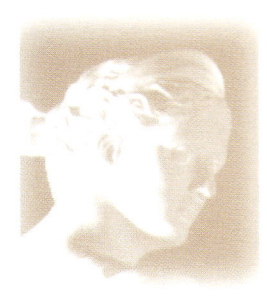

NERVE INJURY

Sensory Nerve

The major nerve most commonly injured in rhytidectomy is the great auricular nerve. Special care must be taken to elevate the cervical flap from the underlying sternomastoid muscle to avoid this injury. In slender persons the great auricular nerve is often closely adherent to the skin flap and can be easily injured. The great auricular nerve can be identified as it crosses the midbelly of the sternocleidomastoid muscle between 6 and 7 cm below the external auditory canal.[55] If the nerve is inadvertently cut during the dissection, it is repaired primarily using magnification and fine sutures. The return of function is to be expected.

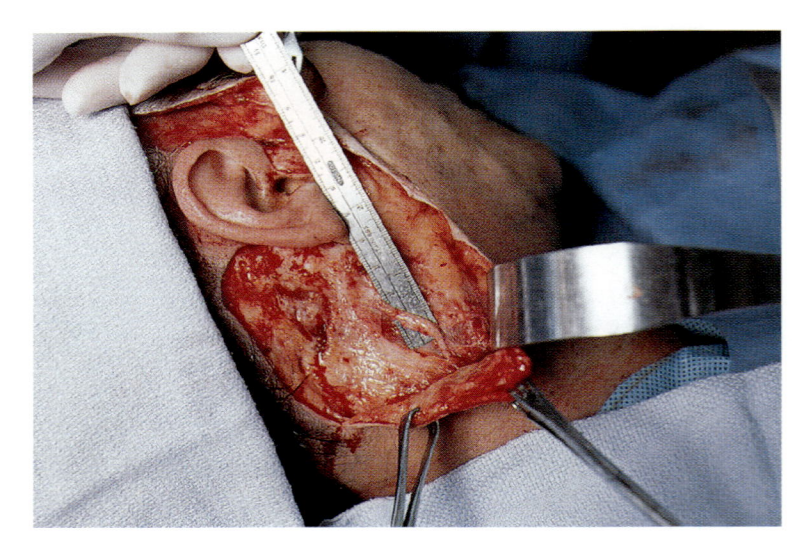

The great auricular nerve crosses the midbelly of the sternocleidomastoid muscle 6.5 cm inferior to the external auditory canal. This landmark should be kept in mind as the cervical skin flap is elevated. Injuries to this nerve can cause two troublesome consequences—permanent anesthesia in the ear and preauricular region, or development of a painful neuroma. This intraoperative photograph was taken in a patient who developed painful dysesthesia following a facelift. A neuroma of the great auricular nerve was identified and buried within the sternocleidomastoid muscle.

The superficial sensory nerves supplying the cheek and temporal skin are divided during elevation of the cervicofacial flaps, and no attempt is made to identify these small branches. All patients have a temporary loss or alteration in sensation in the areas of dissection, as well as the earlobes and ear margins. Sensation returns spontaneously within a relatively short period of time and is usually complete in 3 to 4 months. Patients should be informed of this preoperatively. Only in rare instances will the sensation fail to return to normal.

If the great auricular nerve has been injured, it is possible that a painful neuroma may form, but this sequela is fortunately rare. We have observed only two cases, and in only one patient was it so disabling that the nerve was subsequently sacrificed to relieve the pain.

Motor Nerve

The most commonly injured motor nerve is the buccal branch of the facial nerve. Though return of function can be expected within a 3- to 4-month period, injury to the frontal branches tends to produce longer-lasting facial weakness. The reported incidence varies, but it is probably less than 1% and in our practice is 0.1%. The obvious neurologic signs of injury are present, such as inability to elevate the eyebrow and forehead on the involved side, ptosis of the eyebrow, and loss of forehead wrinkles. The injury can be caused by trauma from the cautery, a suture inadvertently encircling the nerve, or most likely, neuropraxis because of stretching. Almost all temporal nerve weaknesses will improve with time. This recovery period varies from 2 to 6 months. If a nerve weakness is noted postoperatively, it is discussed with the patient and she is informed of what has happened and what to anticipate.

These patients are reexamined at 3- to 4-week intervals until full function has returned. In only one case in our series did nerve function fail to return completely. After a period of 1 year, a decision was made to sever and partially resect the temporal branch of the facial nerve on the normally functioning side. This was discussed with the patient and her husband and was carried out. The wife preferred the appearance of the paralyzed side to the nonparalyzed side before the secondary procedure, stating that the absence of wrinkling on the paralytic side was more acceptable.

Injury to the marginal mandibular nerve can occur either in subcutaneous or SMAS dissection in the region along the angle of the mandible and mandibular border. Fortunately, this nerve lies deep beneath

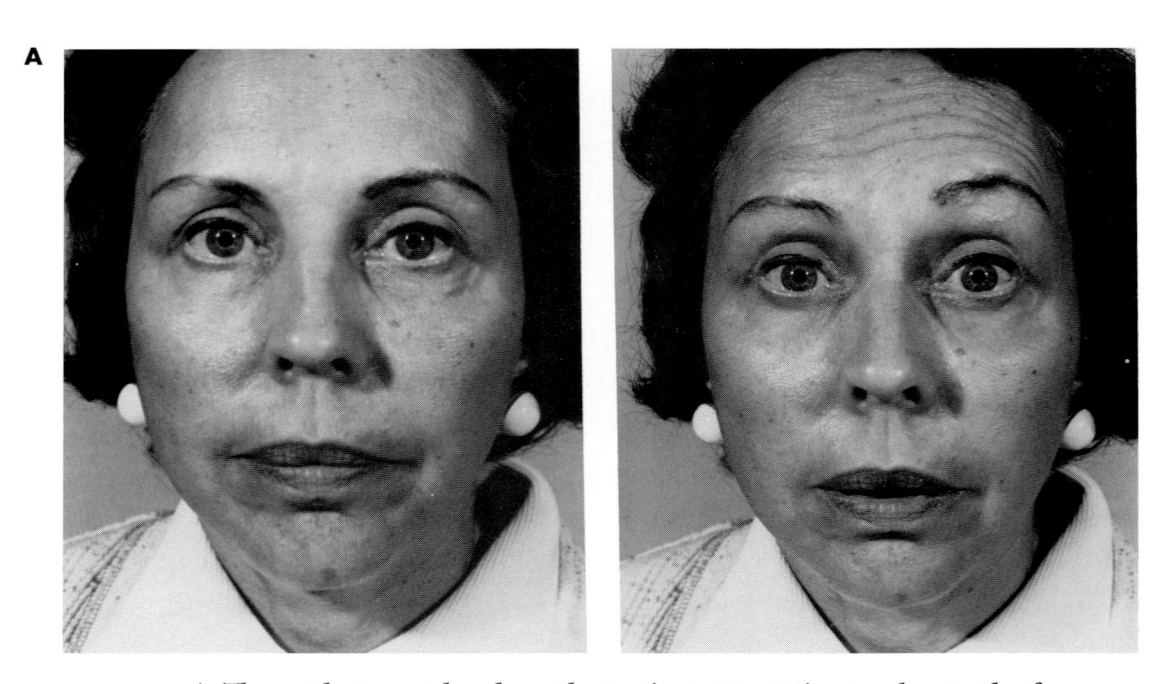

A, These photographs show the patient attempting to elevate the forehead, with little or no muscular activity on the right side. This temporary paralysis most likely resulted from stretching the temporal branch of the facial nerve or from injury by the electrocautery.

the deep facial fascia and as long as this layer is not violated, motor branch injury will be prevented. Injury to the marginal mandibular nerve produces weakness of the lower lip depressors as well as the mentalis muscle. Although this injury can be permanent, as with other facial nerve injury, spontaneous recovery within 6 months is the expected outcome in most (80%) patients.

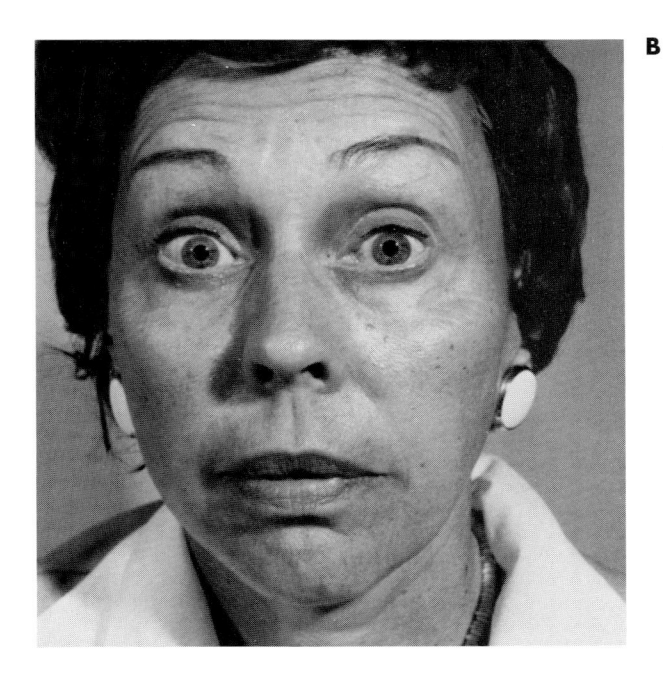

B, The patient now exhibits a total return of function of the temporal branch of the facial nerve. This branch of the facial nerve will almost always spontaneously return to normal function. In this instance the time interval was approximately 6 months.

Fortunately, motor nerve injuries are rare following facelifts. Nevertheless, it is imperative that this potential complication be mentioned during the preoperative consultation and included in the surgical consent form.

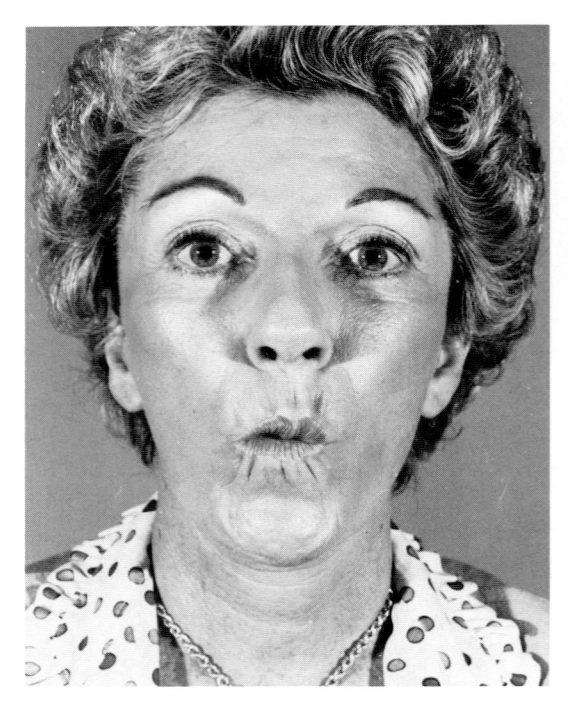

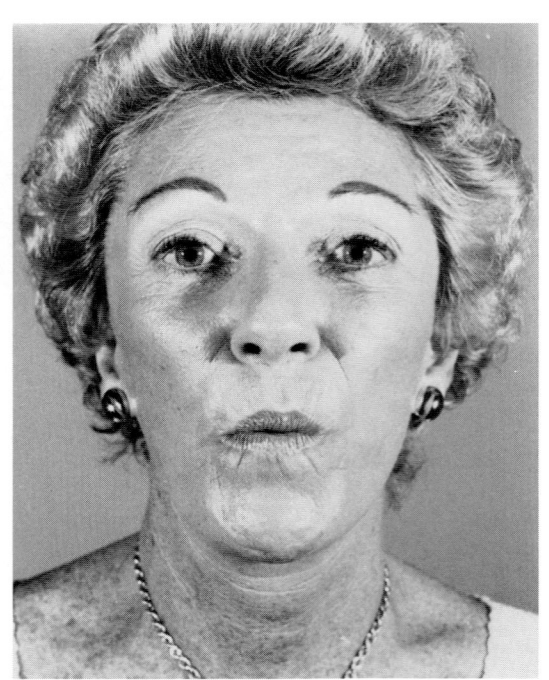

A, This patient is shown 2 months postoperatively. She exhibits weakness of the right upper lip because of buccal nerve injury. B, The patient is shown 4 months after surgery. The function of the buccal branch has almost completely recovered, as it eventually did.

We have observed two cases where the spinal accessory nerve was permanently injured resulting in muscle atrophy. It would seem that extensive posterior dissection would be necessary to injure this nerve. Since the nerve passes beneath the sternocleidomastoid muscle and exits along the deep surface of the posterior border, the incision would need to be quite far posterior in the neck for this to happen.

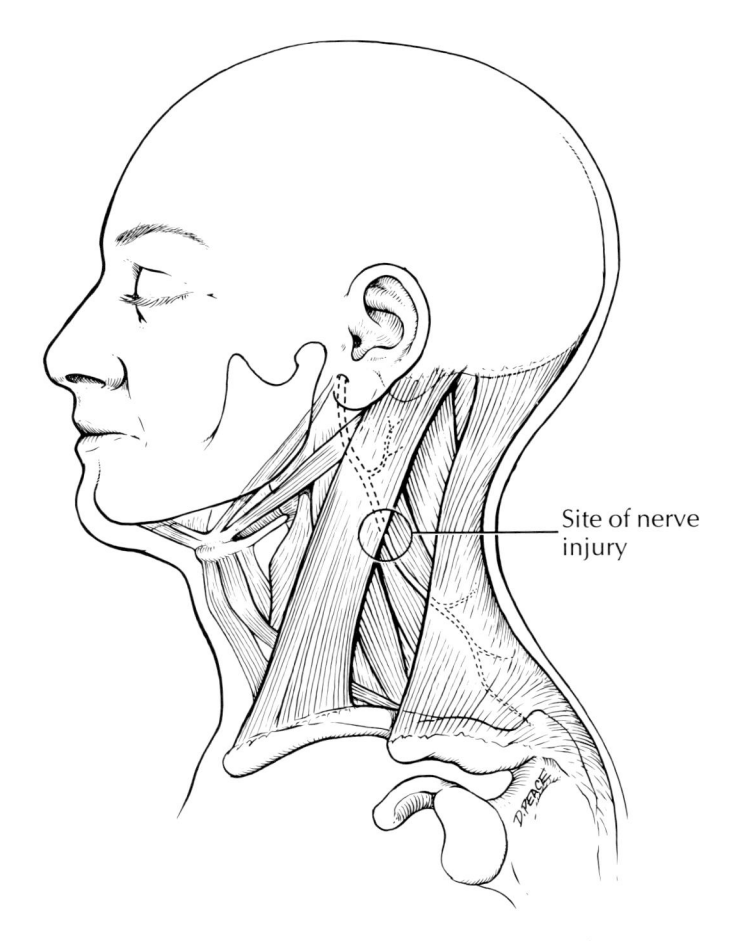

Although rarely injured, the spinal accessory nerve can be encountered along the posterior border of the sternocleidomastoid muscle on its way to innervate the trapezius muscle.

SURGICAL REJUVENATION OF THE FACE

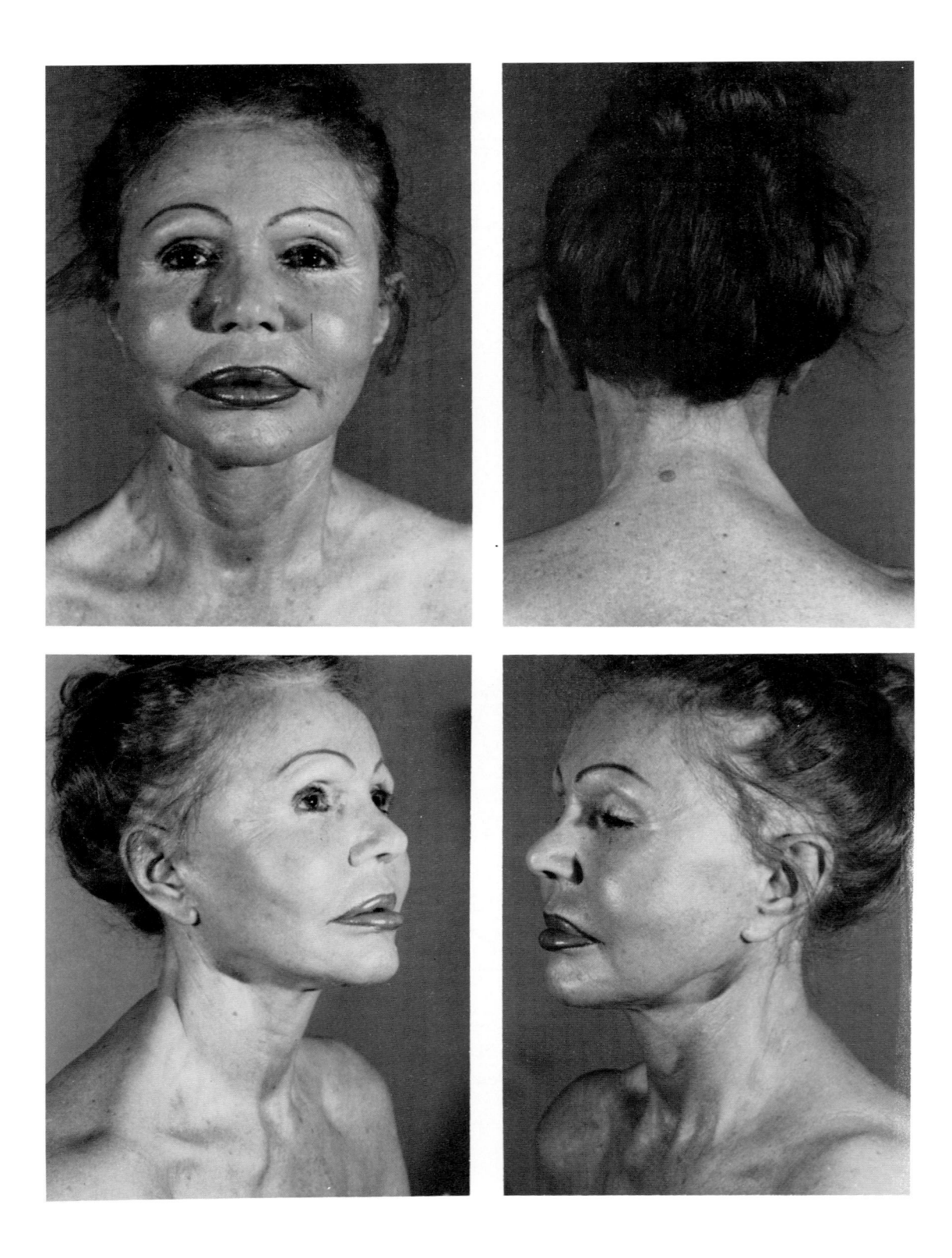

364

RHYTIDECTOMY

This patient came for consultation 2 years after a rhytidectomy. Her complaint was asymmetry of the neck muscles and a posterior neck deformity. Examination revealed atrophy of the left trapezius muscle. The spinal accessory nerve has been injured. This error required that the dissection extend deep in the posterior neck and posterior to the sternocleidomastoid muscle.

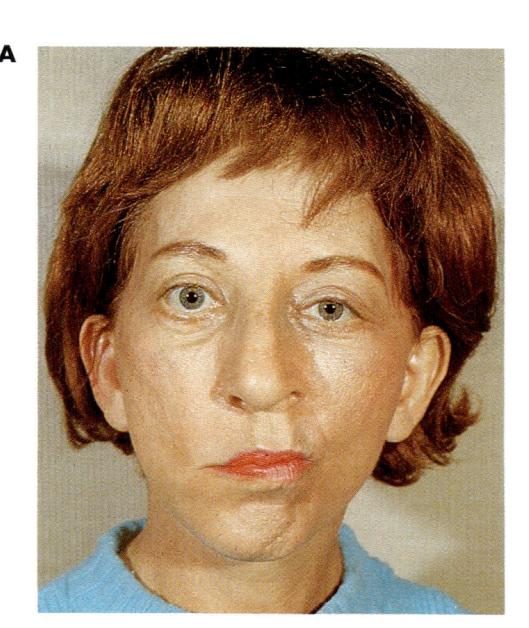

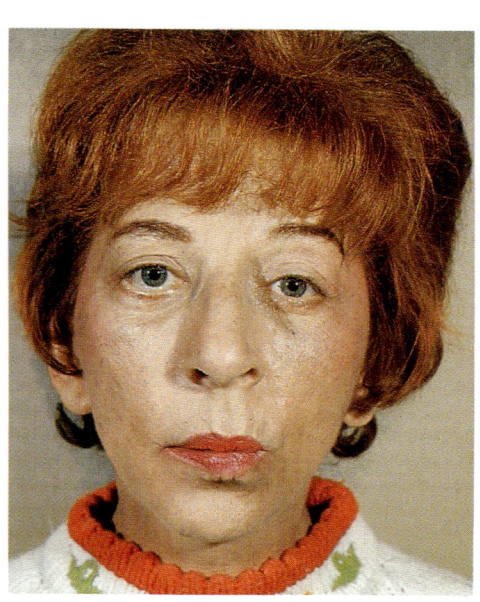

A **B**

A, This patient had a rhytidectomy 7 days previously. There was no evidence of motor nerve damage in the first few days after surgery. On the fourth postoperative day a facial nerve weakness was noted. Neurologic consultation verified the diagnosis of Bell's palsy that was coincidental with the facelift. B, 6 weeks after the diagnosis, the facial muscles are gaining activity. Muscular function returned completely within 3 months.

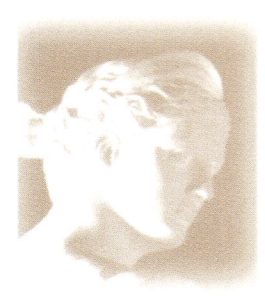

HYPERTROPHIC AND UNDESIRABLE SCARS

Despite meticulous technique and attentive postoperative management, a small percentage of patients develop some undesirable scarring. The scars may become wider over a period of several weeks or months or possibly exhibit true hypertrophy.

Persons most apt to exhibit this phenomenon are dark-complexioned patients and those with ruddy, freckled skin. True keloids have not been observed, even in black patients.

When hypertrophic scars are encountered, we prefer to inject intralesional steroids directly into the scar tissue under pressure utilizing a Luer-Lok syringe. We currently use triamcinolone (Aristocort) acetonide, 40 mg/mL. We previously used triamcinolone acetonide suspension (Kenalog), but occasionally a patient exhibited yellow crystals that were later visualized in the area of the atrophic scar. Intralesional injections of steroids result in atrophy of the hypertrophied scar tissue, and occasionally no subsequent scar revision is necessary. Steroid injections also reduce redness, itching, and discomfort within a few days. Some of these patients with hypertrophied scars will need subsequent scar revision, and, if so, the scar is excised and the wound is closed primarily. It does seem, however, that in some patients a suitable solution cannot be found for the correction of wide or thickened scars. Recurrence is common, especially in the posterior cervical scar where the tension is greatest.

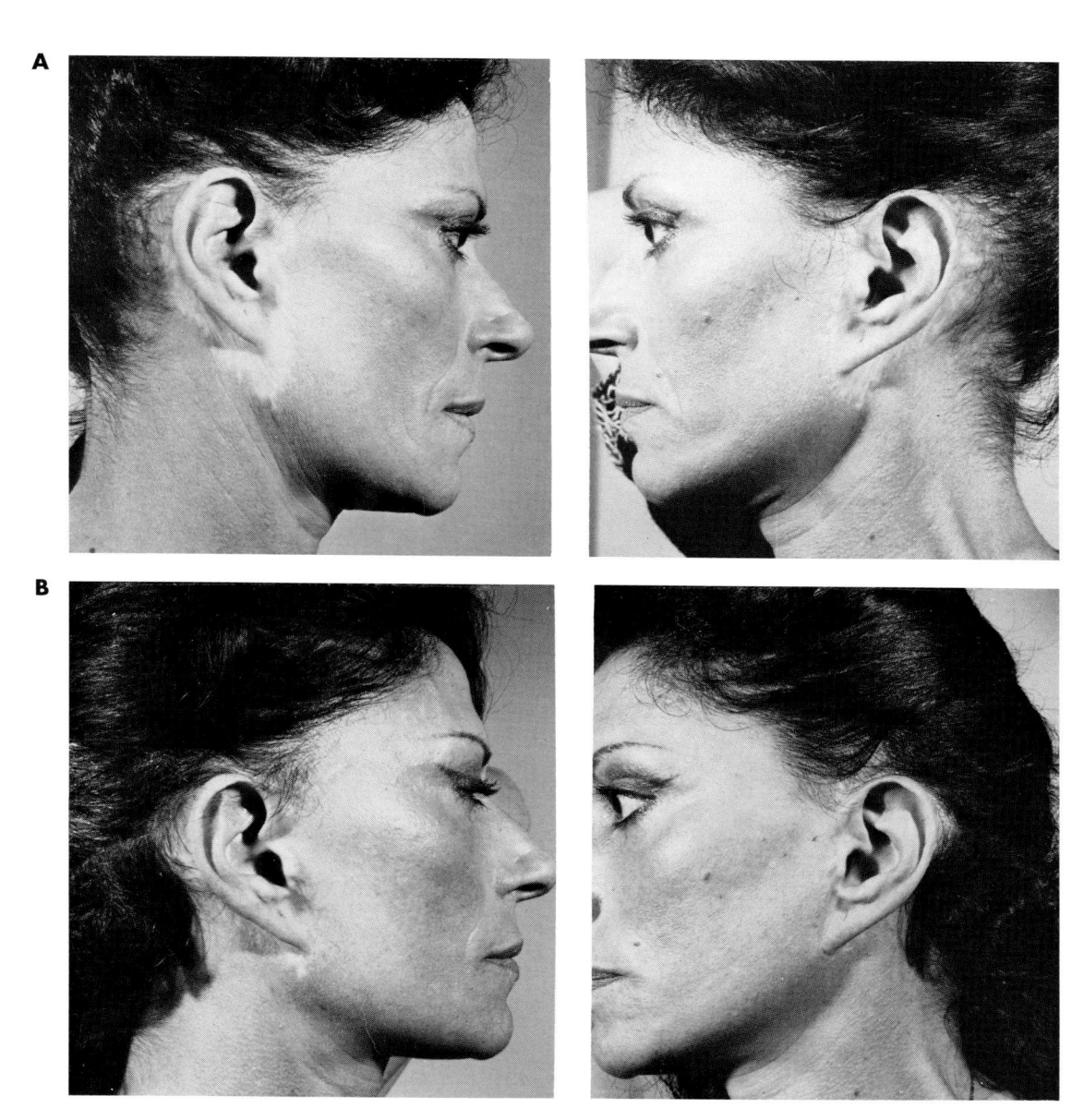

A, This dark-complexioned patient had a rhytidectomy and came for consultation requesting removal of her unsightly scars. She gave a history of "poor healing" and stated that the crusts remained for several weeks in the area of the incisions. She also said that the sutures were not removed for approximately 11 or 12 days. **B**, The depigmented areas were excised insofar as possible, and the neck and facial areas were undermined and advanced. Additional improvement could probably be achieved by a secondary advancement of the cervicofacial flaps and reconstruction of the earlobes.

SURGICAL REJUVENATION OF THE FACE

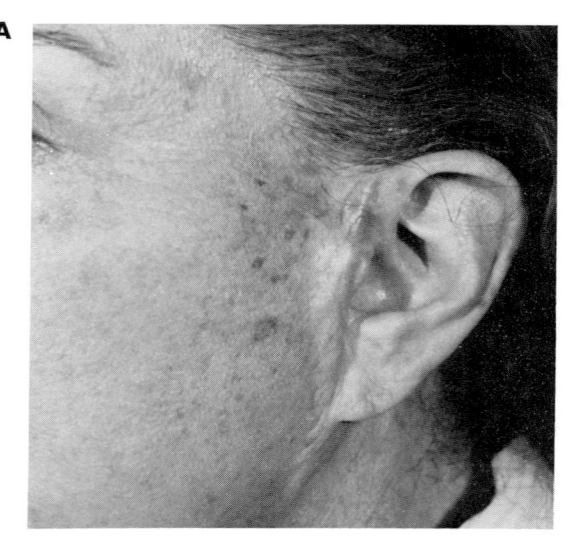

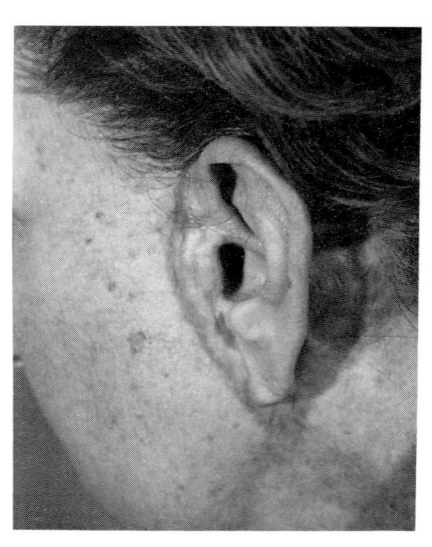

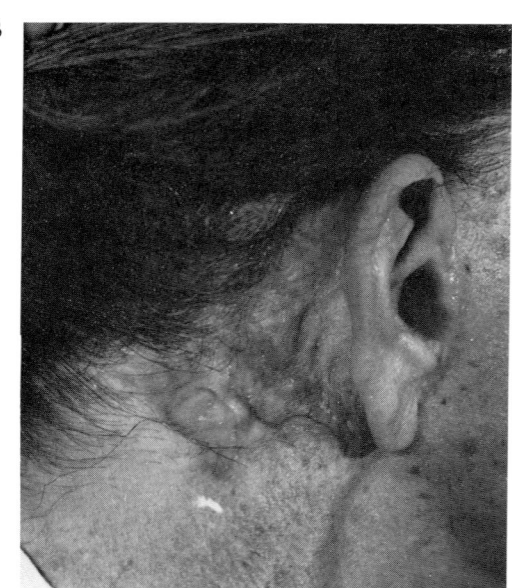

A, This patient exhibits idiopathic scarring after a rhytidectomy. B, This patient experienced "delayed healing" from an unexplained cause. The hypertrophic scarring needed revision. While the undesirable result is rare, it does occur. Most patients understand when it is explained and discussed with them. Intralesional steroids shrink the scars, but the scar remains and is best treated by excision-revision.

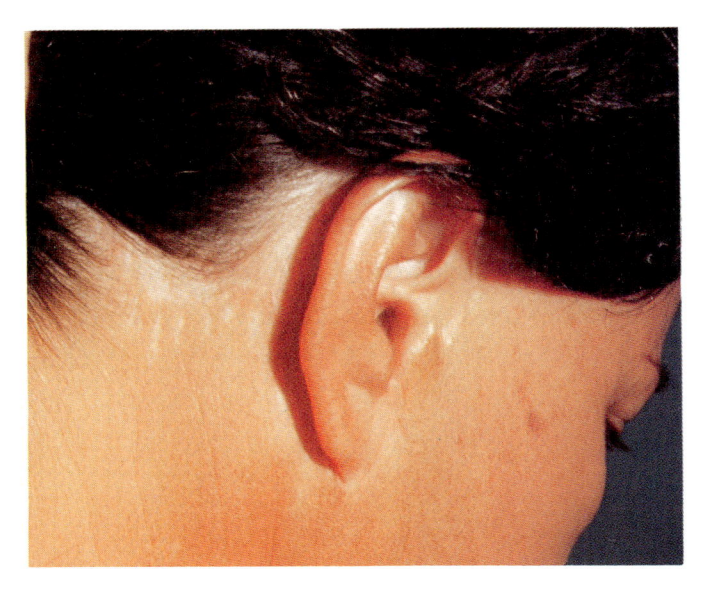

Unacceptable scarring in the posterior cervical incision resulting from sutures cutting into the wound margins. This crosshatching is preventable by not allowing the sutures to cross the line of incision when closing the wound.

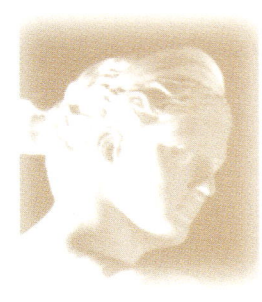

SKIN SLOUGH

The primary cause of skin necrosis following rhytidectomy is tension. This may be the result of hematoma, a superficial infection, or most likely, the effect of closing the wound under too much tension at the time of the initial reapproximation. Heavy cigarette smoking has also been implicated, and it probably is a factor in the reduction of the circulation to the distal margins of the skin flaps. We advise patients to stop smoking before surgery, but this admonition is difficult to enforce. Pressure dressings may be a factor in the constriction of blood flow to the distal margins of the flaps. Patients with excessive edema may also develop enough tension along the suture line to cause some local tissue necrosis with subsequent superficial skin loss. If a skin slough does occur, the wound is allowed to granulate and reepithelialize spontaneously. Skin grafting and debridement of necrotic areas should be done only after nature has had an opportunity to correct the problem.

RHYTIDECTOMY

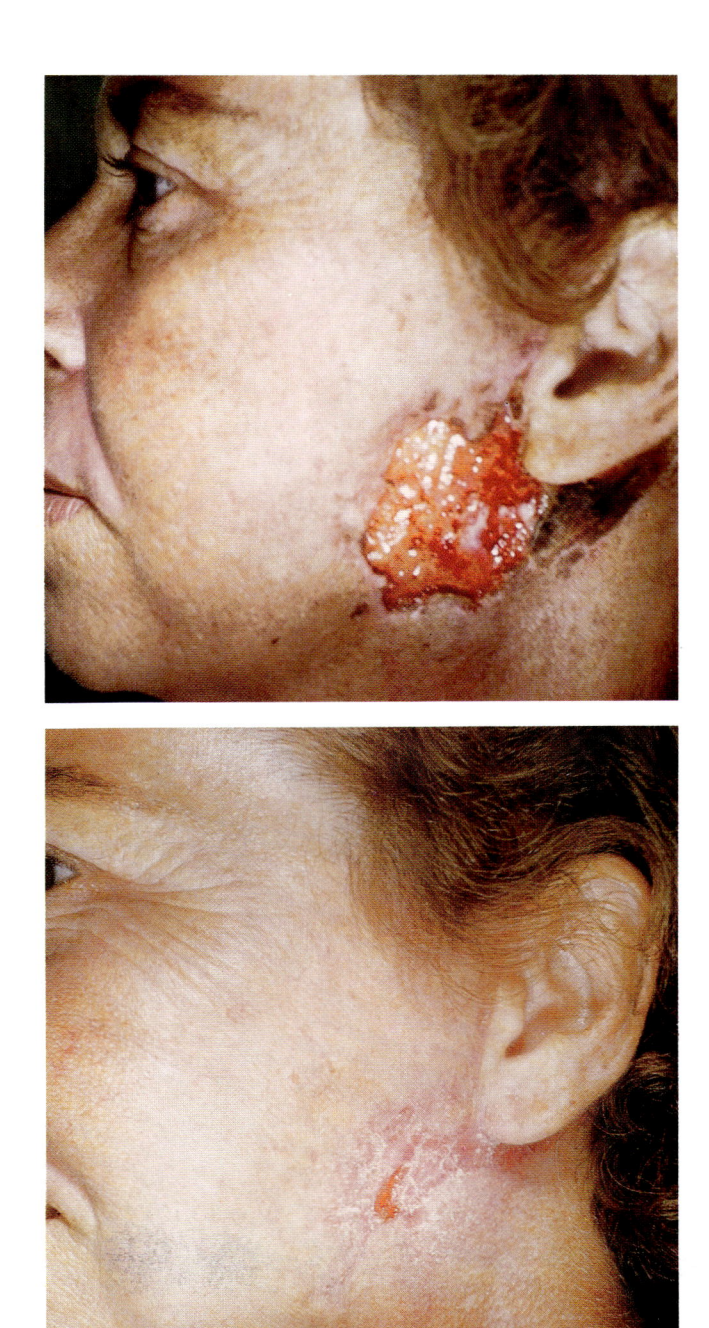

This patient developed a staphylococcal infection shortly after her discharge from the hospital and a portion of the left cheek sloughed. The wound was cleaned daily and allowed to reepithelialize spontaneously. The photograph below shows the appearance of the wound 6 weeks later. It eventually improved sufficiently so that no scar revision was necessary.

SURGICAL REJUVENATION OF THE FACE

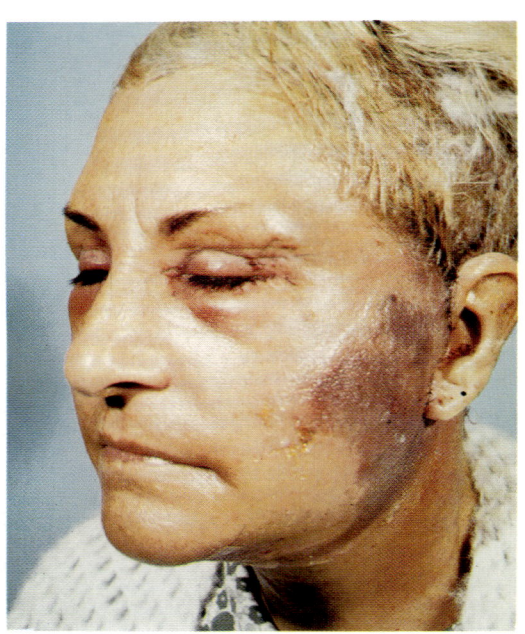

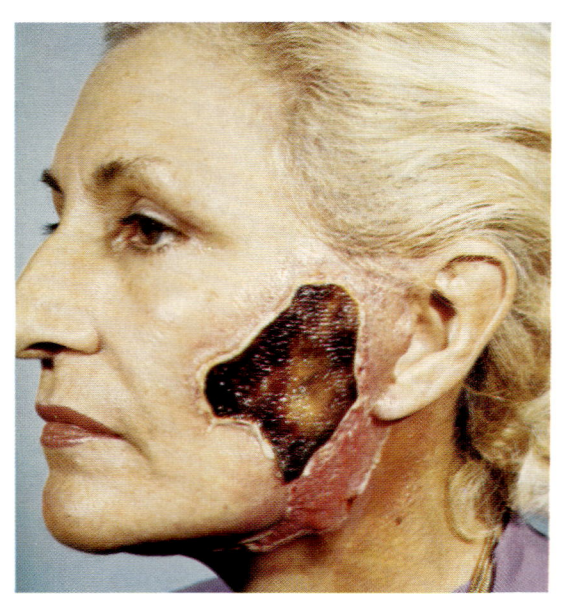

A, Frontal view of a patient who had a facelift, upper and lower eyelid blepharoplasty, and submental lipectomy 24 hours previously. B, Oblique view 24 hours postoperatively. There appears to be a line of demarcation and early tissue necrosis. There is no indication of infection, and no hematoma is present. C, The patient is shown 3 weeks after surgery. The eschar is ready for debridement. We elected to merely keep the wound clean and allow reepithelialization to occur.

RHYTIDECTOMY

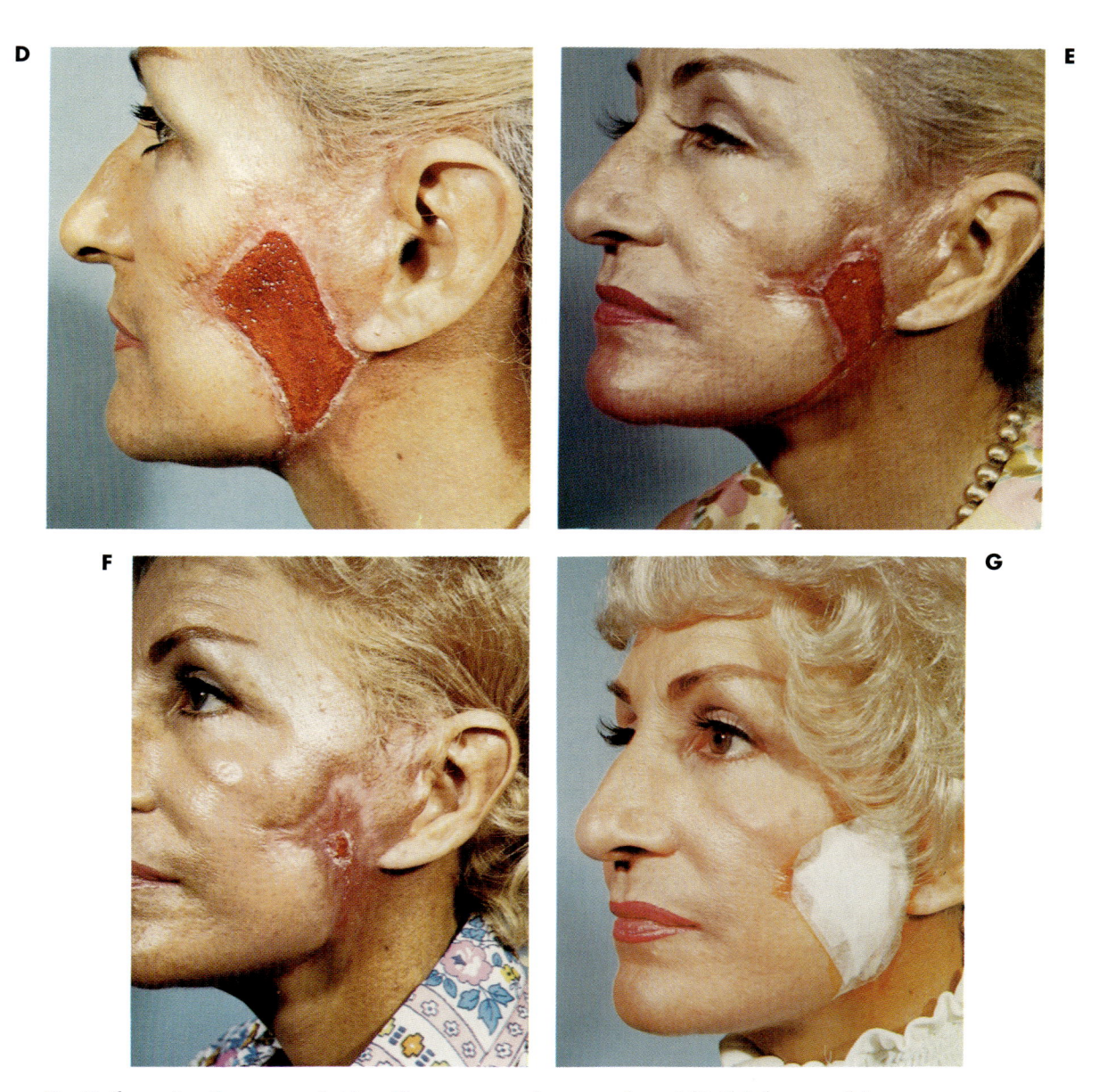

D, At 6 weeks the granulation tissue was clean and a split-thickness skin graft was considered. E, At 9 weeks the size of the granulating area was being reduced by contracture and ingrowth of new epithelium from the periphery of the wound. F, At 12 weeks the area is almost completely covered by new epithelium and there is further evidence of scar contracture. G, The patient wore a small bandage to cover the healing wound and returned to work.

SURGICAL REJUVENATION OF THE FACE

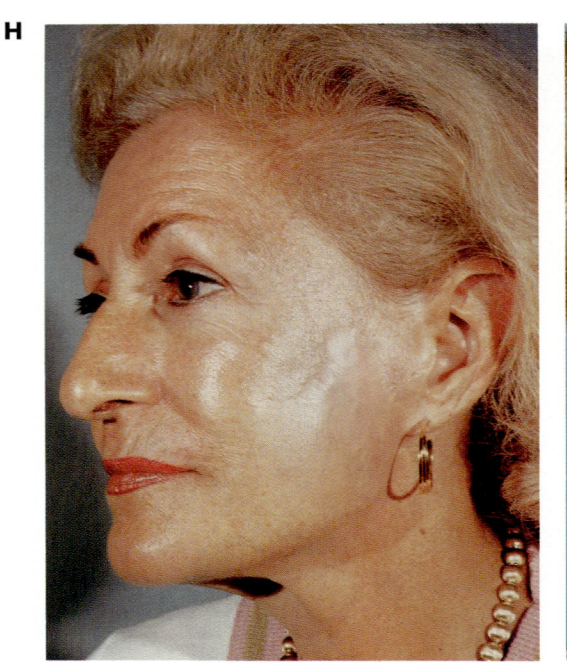

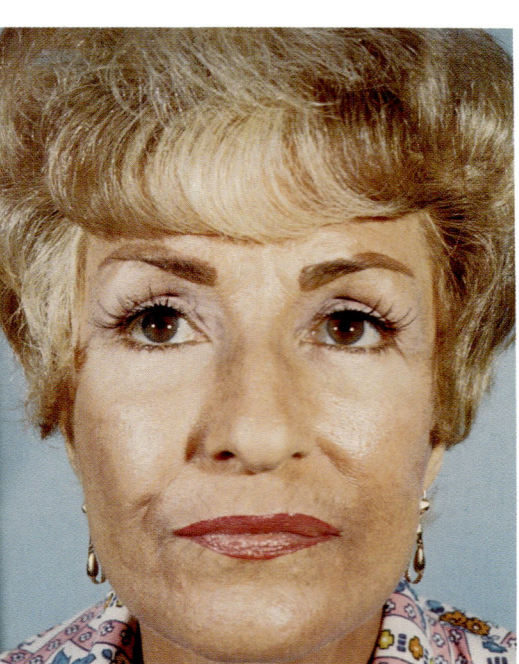

H, The appearance of the matured scar at 1 year. In our opinion, if a skin graft had been used a less acceptable result would have been obtained. **I**, In the frontal view at 1 year, no distortion of the cheek is noted. The probable cause of this problem were the hot lights that were used to film this operation. A review of the videotape revealed no flaws in the surgical technique but did show that the surgeon complained of the heat from the lights.

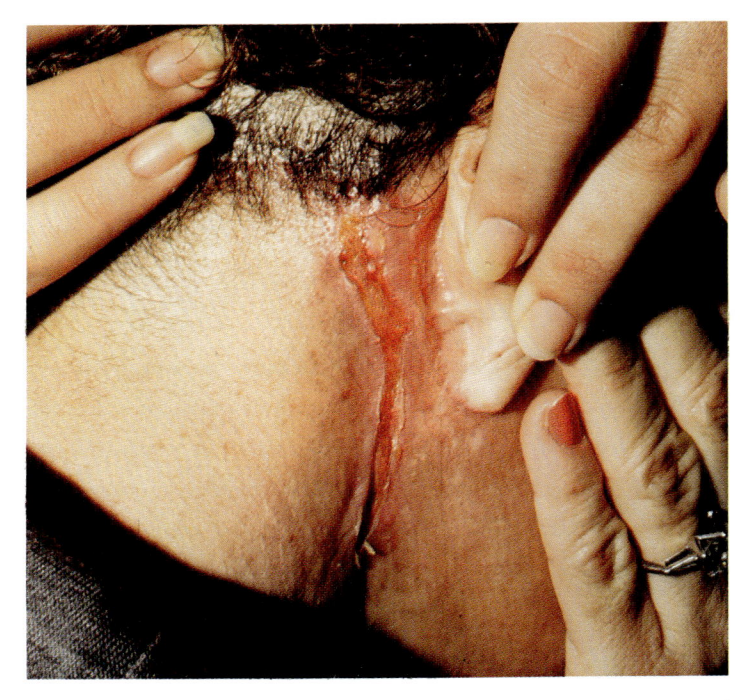

A superficial linear slough in the deep flexion crease of the neck. It is probably a result of the positioning of the head during the first 24 to 48 hours after surgery. If there has been a through-and-through dissection in the neck, and if the head remains in a flexed position, then the stage is set for necrosis along the line of skin flexion. The head should be kept elevated but not on a pillow. This prevents the neck flexion from "creasing" the cervical flap and thus prevents necrosis.

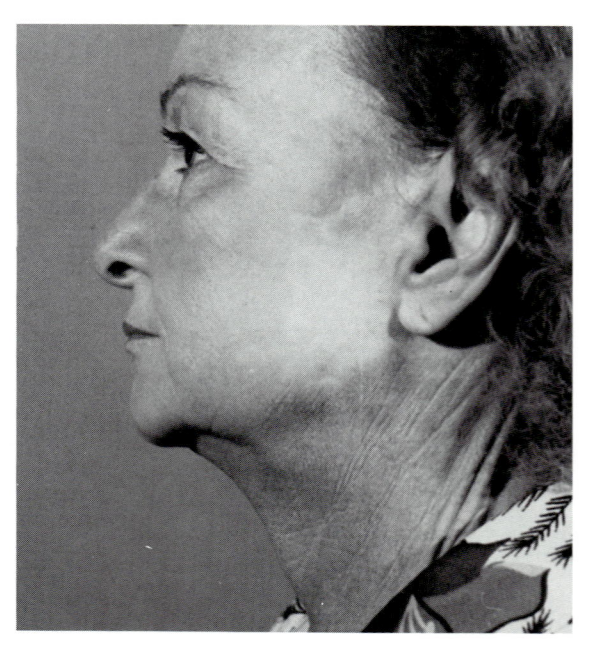

This is an example of what not to do if a slough occurs. This patient was seen in consultation requesting that the depigmented area be removed. The history was that a slough had occurred after a rhytidectomy and that the area had been skin-grafted. The color match is poor, and the skin is of a different texture than the surrounding cheek skin. This case would probably have been better managed by allowing the wound to reepithelialize spontaneously rather than resurfacing with a skin graft.

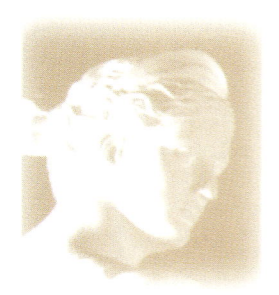

SEROMAS

Serum may collect in small pockets beneath the flaps, most commonly in the cheeks. This should be allowed to reabsorb spontaneously. Reabsorption may take as long as 4 to 6 weeks, but there is less residual wrinkling of the overlying skin in cases where spontaneous reabsorption is allowed to take place than in those where the excess fluid was aspirated.

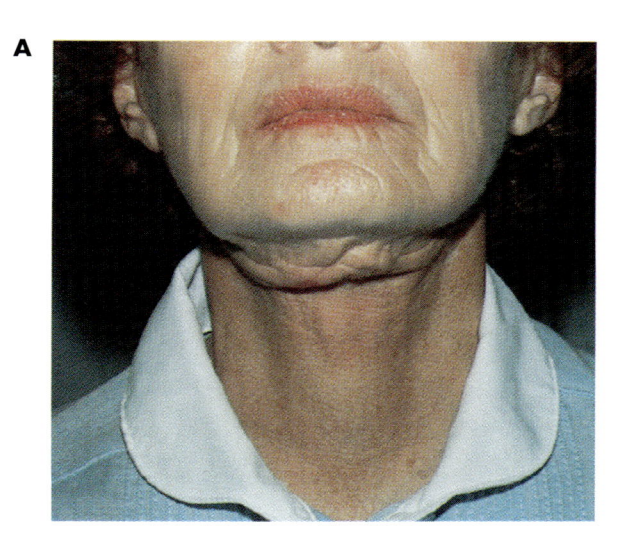

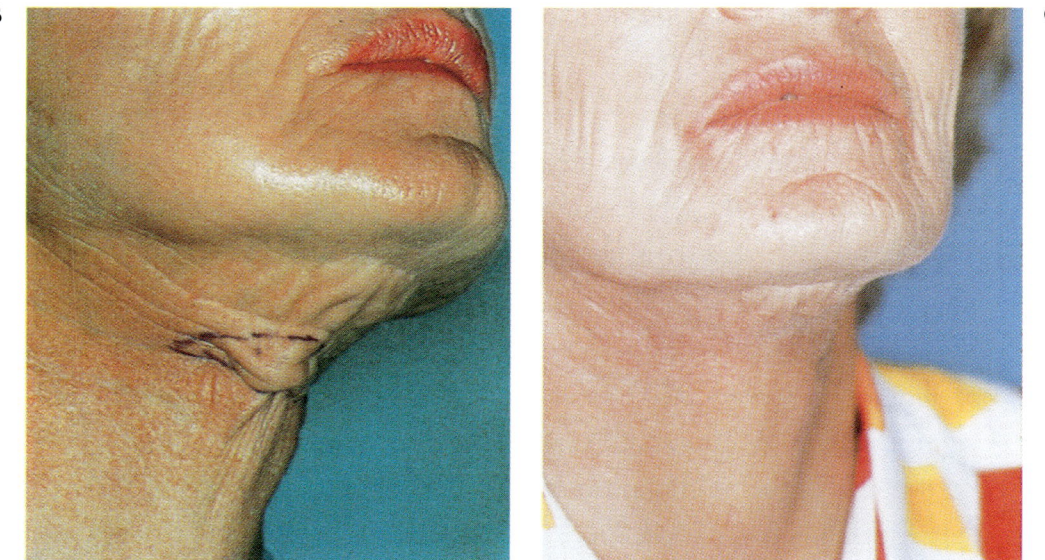

This patient was seen as a referral following the development of a seroma in her neck following a facelift. She was reexplored 6 weeks postoperatively by her original surgeon to evacuate the "fluid" and left with significant cervical irregularity. She was observed for 9 months to allow the wound to mature and later required direct cervical excision to smooth the remaining wrinkling seen in her neck.

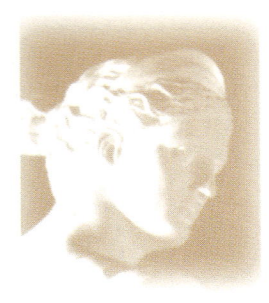

CONTOUR IRREGULARITIES

With the advent of extensive platysma surgery, a higher incidence of surface irregularities has occurred, especially in the neck. Improper defatting may lead to irregularities and asymmetries in the neck. Approximately 5 to 7 mm of fat should be left on the undersurface of the cervical skin flaps. If all of the fat is removed down to or near the dermis, the resultant thin skin flap will adhere closely to the underlying muscle, causing puckering and wrinkling that are apt to be visible after the edema has subsided.

Prolapse of the submaxillary gland has been observed in patients who have had the platysma completely transected, especially when the muscle is divided high in the neck. If it is noted preoperatively that the submaxillary gland is prominent, this is a relative contraindication to completely dividing the platysma, since the gland may be even more prominent following the division.

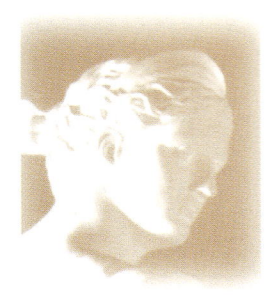

INFECTION

Fortunately, infections following rhytidectomy are rare. The incidence is less than 1%, and severe infections are extremely uncommon. Our own experience leads us to the conclusion that patients having surgery in an outpatient facility, where they are not exposed to hospitalized patients, are less apt to develop infections as compared with those patients who are operated on in a hospital. Infections following facelifting are usually due to *Staphylococcus aureus.*

We use prophylactic antibiotics in all patients undergoing facelifts. Our routine is to give cephalexin 250 mg four times 1 day before surgery and 250 mg four times each day for 4 days following surgery. In our judgment, the wounds look cleaner and healing takes place in a more acceptable manner than it does without antibiotics. We have observed no serious side effects from antibiotic use other than an occasional complaint of nausea or vaginitis in female patients.

RHYTIDECTOMY

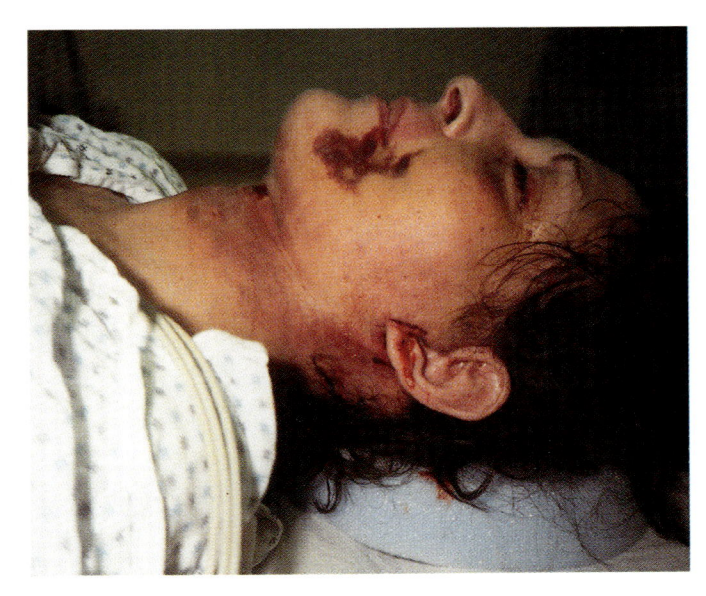

This patient is seen 8 days following primary rhytidectomy. She did not tolerate her perioperative antibiotics because of nausea and therefore did not take them. The causative organism in the infection was Staphylococcus aureus. *The patient required hospitalization, operative drainage, IV antibiotics, and hyperbaric oxygen to resolve the infection.*

SUGGESTED READING

Aston SJ: Platysma-SMAS cervicofacial rhytidoplasty, *Clin Plast Surg* 10:507, 1983.

Baker DC, Conley J: Avoiding facial nerve injuries in rhytidectomy: Anatomical variations and pitfalls, *Plast Reconstr Surg* 64:781, 1979.

Baker TJ, Gordon HL, and Mosienko P: Rhytidectomy, a statistical analysis, *Plast Reconstr Surg* 59:24, 1977.

Baker TJ, Gordon HL: Complications of rhytidectomy, *Plast Reconstr Surg* 40:31, 1967.

Baker TJ, Gordon HL: Rhytidectomy in males, *Plast Reconstr Surg* 44:219, 1969.

Baker TJ, Gordon HL: Adjunctive aids to rhytidectomy, *South Med J* 62:108, 1969.

Baker TJ, Gordon HL, Mosienko P: Rhytidectomy, a statistical analysis, *Plast Reconstr Surg* 59:24, 1977.

Baker TJ: Rhytidectomy in the male patient. In Goulian D, Courtiss EH, editors: *Symposium on surgery of the aging face,* vol. 19, St. Louis, 1978, Mosby, p. 47.

Barton FE, Jr: Rhytidectomy and the nasolabial fold, *Plast Reconstr Surg* 90:601, 1992.

Barton FE, Jr: The SMAS and the nasolabial fold, *Plast Reconstr Surg* 89:1054, 1992.

Bosse JP Pappillon J: Surgical anatomy of the SMAS at the malar region. In *Transactions of the 9th International Congress of Plastic and Reconstructive Surgery,* New York. McGraw-Hill, 1987, p. 348.17.

Cardoso de Castro C: The anatomy of the platysma muscle, *Plast Reconstr Surg* 66:680, 1980.

Connell BF: Contouring the neck in rhytidectomy by lipectomy and a muscle sling, *Plast Reconstr Surg* 61:376, 1978.

Connell BF: Cervical lifts: The value of platysma muscle flaps, *Ann Plast Surg,* 1:34, 1978.

Connell BF, Gaon A: Surgical correction of aesthetic contour problems of the neck, *Clin Plast Surg* 10:491, 1983.

Connell BF: Neck contour deformities: The art, engineering, anatomic diagnosis, architectural planning, and aesthetics of surgical correction, *Clin Plast Surg* 14:683, 1987.

Connell BF, Marten TJ: The male foreheadplasty, *Clin Plast Surg* 18:653, 1991.

Ellenbogen R: Pseudo-paralysis of the mandibular branch of the facial nerve after platysmal face-lift operation, *Plast Reconstr Surg* 63:364, 1979.

Ellenbogen R, Karlin JV: Visual criteria for success in restoring the youthful neck, *Plast Reconstr Surg* 66:826, 1980.

Feldman JJ: Corset platysmaplasty, *Plast Reconstr Surg* 85:333, 1990.

Feldman JJ: Corset platysmaplasty, *Clin Plast Surg* 19:369, 1992.

Freilinger G, Gruber H, Happak W, Pechmann U: Surgical anatomy of the mimic muscle system and the facial nerve: Importance for reconstructive and aesthetic surgery, *Plast Reconstr Surg* 80:686, 1987.

Furnas D: The retaining ligaments of the cheek, *Plast Reconstr Surg* 83:11, 1989.

Guerrero-Santos J: The role of the platysma muscle in rhytidoplasty, *Clin Plast Surg* 5:29, 1978.

Guerrero-Santos J: (Ed.) Neck lift—simplified surgical technique, refinements, and clinical classification, *Clin Plast Surg* 10(3):379-404, 1983.

Hamra ST: The deep plane rhytidectomy, *Plast Reconstr Surg* 86:53, 1990.

Hamra ST: *Composite Rhytidectomy*. Quality Medical Publishing, St. Louis, Mo., 1993.

Jost G, Levet, Y: Parotid fascia and face lifting: A critical evaluation of the SMAS concept, *Plast Reconstr Surg* 74:42, 1984.

Kaye BL: The extended neck lift: the bottom line, *Plast Reconstr Surg* 65:429, 1980.

Lambros V: Personal communication, 1991.

Lawrence WT, Murphy RC, Robson MC, Heggers JP: The detrimental effect of cigarette smoking on flap survival: an experimental study in the rat, *Rr J Plast Surg* 37:216, 1984.

Lemmon M: Superficial fascia rhytidectomy: A restoration of the SMAS with control of the cervicomental angle, *Clin Plast Surg* 10:449, 1983.

Lemmon ML: Color *Atlas of SMAS Rhytidectomy*. Thieme Medical Publishers, New York, 1993.

Letourneau A, Daniel RK: Superficial musculoaponeurotic system of the nose, *Plast Reconstr Surg* 82:48, 1988.

McKinney P, Katrana DJ: Prevention of injury to the great auricular nerve during rhytidectomy, *Plast Reconstr Surg* 66:675, 1980.

Mendelson BC: Extended Sub-SMAS Dissection and Cheek Elevation. *Clin Plast Surg* 22:325, 1995.

Mitz V, Peyronie M: The superficial musculoaponeurotic system (SMAS) in the parotid and cheek area, *Plast Reconstr Surg* 58:80, 1976.

Owsley JQ Jr: SMAS-platysma face lift: A bidirectional cervicofacial rhytidectomy, *Clin Plast Surg* 10:429, 1983.

Owsley JQ Jr: SMAS-platysma face lift, *Plast Reconstr Surg* 71:573, 1983.

Owsley JQ: Lifting the malar fat pad for correction of prominent nasolabial folds, *Plast Reconstr Surg* 91:463, 1993.

Owsley JQ: Aesthetic Facial Surgery. Philadelphia, WB Saunders, 1994.

Pensler JM, Ward JW, and Parry SW: The superficial musculoaponeurotic system in the upper lip: An anatomic study in cadavers, *Plast Reconstr Surg* 75:488, 1985.

Peterson R, Johnston D: Facile identification of the facial nerve branches, *Clin Plast Surg* 14:785, 1987.

Randall P, and Skiles MS: The "SMAS sling": An additional fixation in face lift surgery, *Ann Plast Surg* 12:5, 1984.

Rees TD, Liverett DM, Guy CL: The effect of cigarette smoking on skin-flap survival in the face lift patient, *Plast Reconstr Surg* 73:911, 1984.

Ruess W, Owsley JQ: The anatomy of the skin and fascial layers of the face in aesthetic surgery, *Clin Plast Surg,* 14:677, 1987.

Schwember G, and Rodriguez A: Anatomic surgical dissection of the extraparotid portion of the facial nerve, *Plast Reconstr Surg* 81:183, 1988.

Stuzin JM, Wagstrom L, Kawamoto HK, and Wolfe S: Anatomy of the frontal branch of the facial nerve: The significance of the temporal fat pad, *Plast Reconstr Surg* 83:265, 1989.

Stuzin JM, Baker TJ, and Gordon HL: The extended SMAS flap in the treatment of the nasolabial fold. Presented at the American Society for Aesthetic Plastic Surgery meeting, Chicago, Ill, 1990.

Stuzin JM, Wagstrom L, Kawamoto HK, Baker TJ, and Wolfe SA: The anatomy and clinical applications of the buccal fat pad, *Plast Reconstr Surg* 85:29, 1990.

Stuzin JM, Baker TJ, and Gordon HL: The relationship of the superficial and deep facial fascias: Relevance to rhytidectomy and aging, *Plast Reconstr Surg,* 89:441, 1992.

Stuzin JM, Baker TJ, and Gordon HL: Discussion of Owsley JQ: Lifting the malar fat pad for correction of prominent nasolabial folds, *Plast Reconstr Surg* 91:475, 1993.

Stuzin JM, Baker TJ, Gordon HL: Extended SMAS Dissection as an Approach to Midface Rejuvenation. *Clin Plast Surg* 22:295, 1995.

Vistnes LM, and Souther SG: The anatomical basis for common cosmetic anterior neck deformities, *Ann Plast Surg* 2:381, 1979.

Yousif NJ, Gosain A, Matloub HS, et al: The nasolabial fold: An anatomic and histologic reappraisal, *Plast Reconstr Surg* 93:60, 1994.

Yousif NJ, Gosain A, Sanger JR, et al: The nasolabial fold: A photogrammetric analysis, *Plast Reconstr Surg* 93:70, 1994.

Five

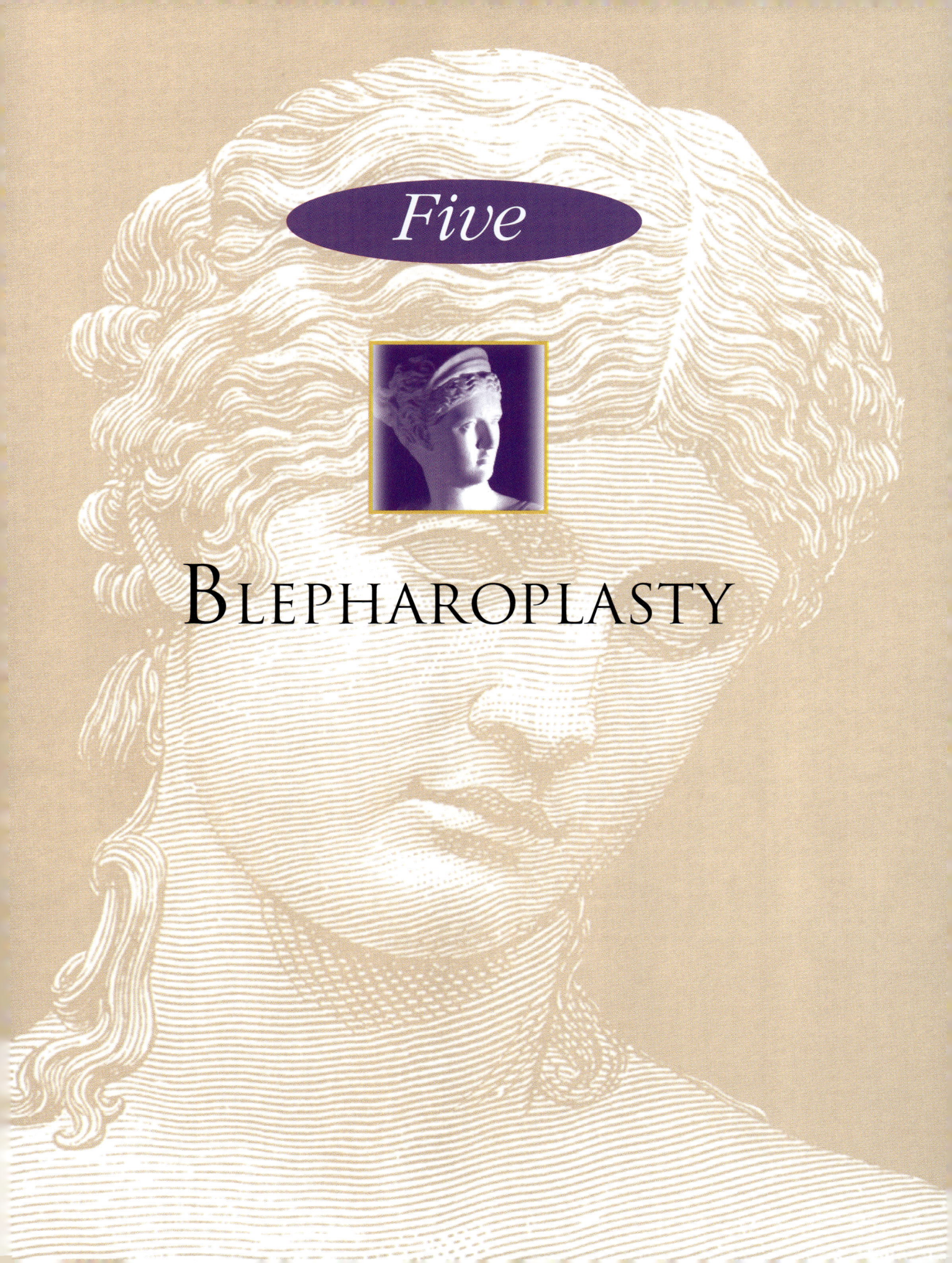

BLEPHAROPLASTY

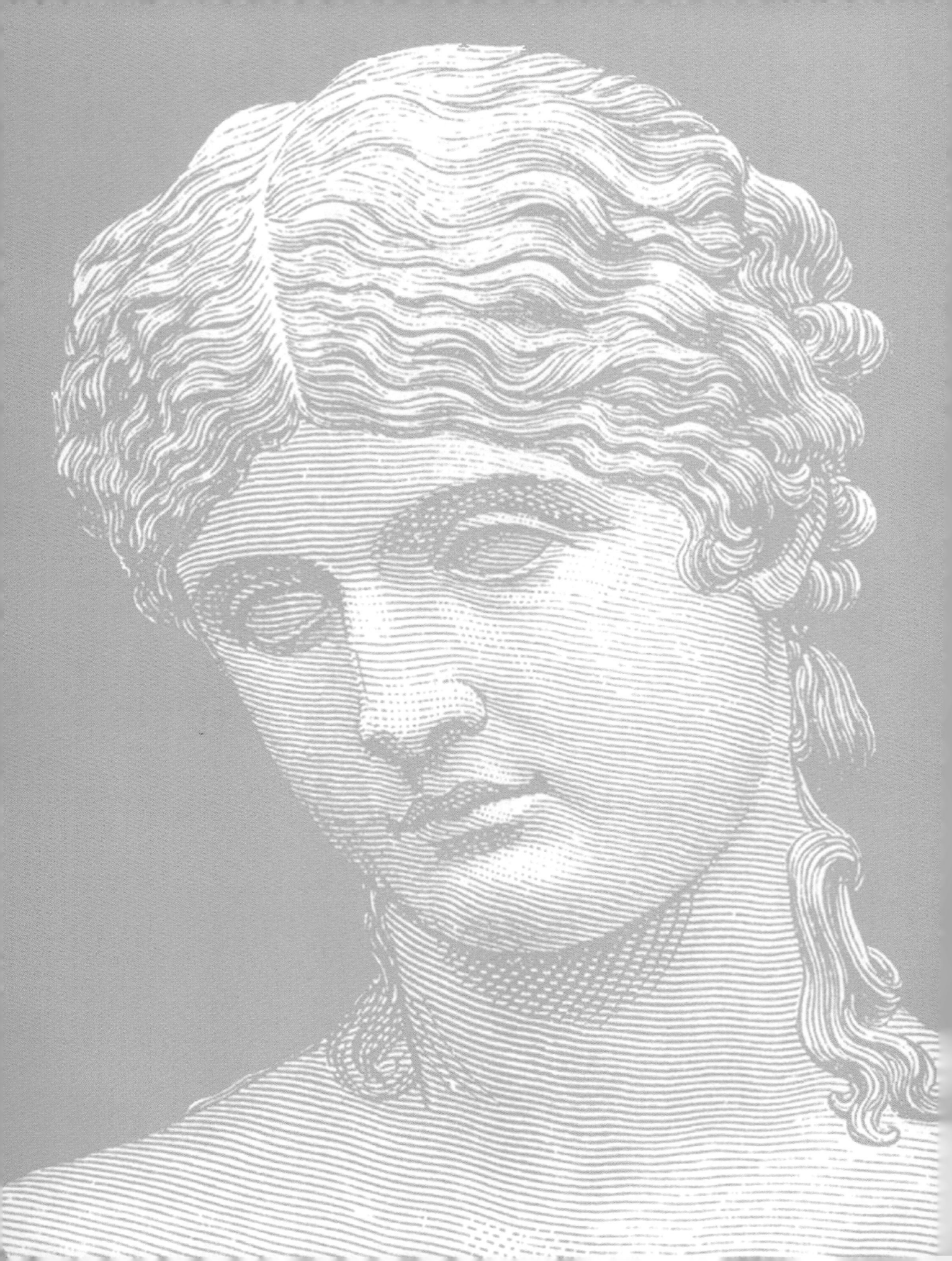

Blepharoplasty, or eyelid surgery, is the operation we most frequently perform, either as an isolated procedure or in combination with rhytidectomy. Few other aesthetic procedures require more skill and finesse; many technical details exist, and the margin for error is millimeters. Conservatism should prevail; it is easier to resect a bit more skin and fat during a secondary procedure than to restore what has been removed. Although there are many medical indications for eyelid surgery, this chapter deals primarily with the non-pathologic indications that result from aging and heredity.

PATIENT SELECTION

The typical patient complains of "baggy eyelids," puffy lower lids, or multiple fine wrinkles in the periorbital region. Suitable candidates for eyelid surgery include individuals with these complaints and those with physical findings that can be improved by surgery.

Excessive upper eyelid skin and crepey eyelid skin can be resected. If the individual has a shallow upper eyelid sulcus (the so-called shallow eye as contrasted to the deep-set), the sulcus can be deepened and accentuated by removing a portion of the underlying fat.

Patients with puffy lower eyelids are excellent candidates for surgery, since proper resection of the lower eyelid fat will significantly improve the puffiness. Often these individuals are young, ranging from 20 to 40 years of age, and need only fat resection, with little or no skin removal.

Other patients, whose lower eyelids have excessive skin or hypertrophied orbicularis muscles, may benefit from this surgery. Relative contraindications for blepharoplasty include the following:

1. Patients with significant orbital pathology
2. Patients with exophthalmos
3. Patients with "dry eye" syndrome
4. Patients with unrealistic expectations; for example, those who ask, "Can you remove all of the lines from around my eyelids?"

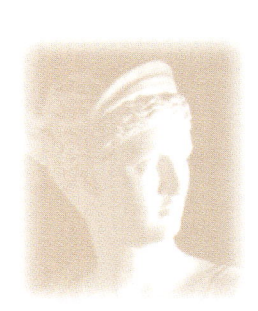

When selecting or rejecting patients for blepharoplasty, the surgeon must be especially alert for the individual who forcibly wrinkles up the orbicularis muscles and demonstrates how the "smile lines" detract from the appearance. This person must be cautioned that surgery cannot eliminate all of the lines. Also the surgeon must beware of the patient who has previously had a successful blepharoplasty performed by another surgeon, but who still wants to correct a "minor" problem. We have observed patients who were displeased with the results from previous surgeons but who could not satisfactorily demonstrate the exact nature of their complaint.

The surgeon must also be cautious of accepting a patient who has had an overly aggressive blepharoplasty performed by another surgeon yet wants more work done around the eyes. The stage may be set for ectropion, dry eye syndrome, or scar contracture. Secondary blepharoplasty can be extremely hazardous if too much eyelid skin or fat has been removed in the first operation.

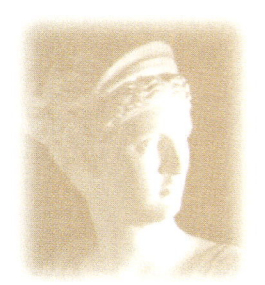

ANATOMIC CONSIDERATIONS

The key to surgery of the eyelid, as in all surgery, is a precise understanding of anatomy. The orbit and eyelid represent an anatomically intricate region with critical structures in close proximity to areas requiring surgical manipulation. Form, function, and appearance of the eyelids are largely a reflection of eyelid and orbital anatomy. A detailed understanding of the structures comprising eyelid and adnexa will allow the surgeon to accurately define the specific problems a patient exhibits on presentation for blepharoplasty and will minimize the possibility of iatrogenic injury during surgery.

◼ Superficial Eyelid Anatomy

The appearance of a patient's eyelids is reflected superficially in topographic form. The palpebral fissure, which is the aperture between the upper and lower eyelid margins, measures vertically between 12 and 14 mm in the adult. In aesthetically pleasing eyes, a common feature is a generous lid aperture associated with limited scleral show. The upper eyelid usually rests between 1.5 and 2 mm below the limbus, with the highest point of the curved upper eyelid slightly nasal to the pupil. The lower eyelid generally lies at the level of the lower limbus, and usually the sclera beneath the limbus is not visible in primary gaze. The lowest point of the lower eyelid is seen slightly temporal, curving superiorly as it travels toward the lateral canthus. The commissures are the junction points where the upper and lower eyelids meet medially and laterally. The horizontal distance between the commissures is between 28 and 30 mm. The lateral commissure rests directly upon the globe, whereas the medial commissure is separated by the intervening caruncle. In the aesthetically pleasing eyelid, the lateral commissure lies slightly superior to the medial commissure.

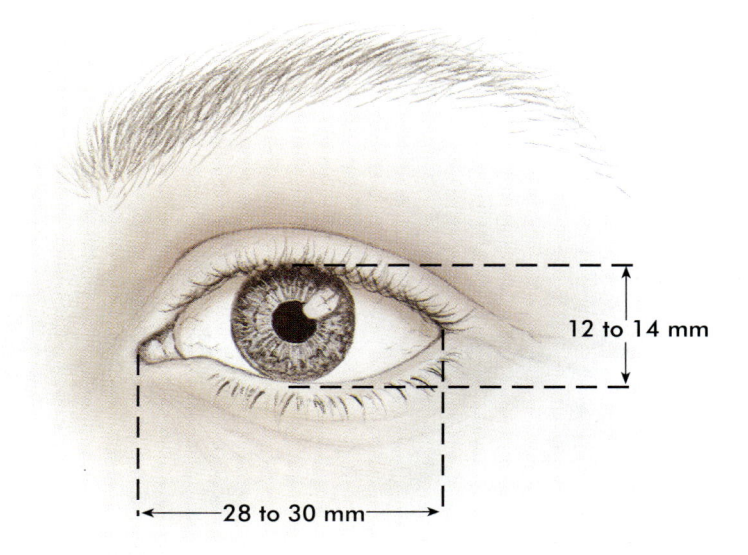

The dimensions of the eyelid aperture. The highest point of the curved upper eyelid is slightly nasal to the pupil, whereas the lowest portion of the curve of the lower eyelid is seen slightly temporal to the limbus. From this point lateral, the lower lid margin curves superiorly toward the lateral canthus. Note that the lateral commissure lies superior to the medial commissure in the aesthetically pleasing lower lid.

SURGICAL REJUVENATION OF THE FACE

The upper eyelid crease is an important structure in eyelid aesthetics. *A crisp and precise upper lid fold, associated with an adequate degree of pretarsal show, is a desirable trait and is synonymous with a youthful appearing eye.* The upper eyelid crease represents an indentation caused by the superficial insertion of fibers from the levator palpebral muscle. This lid crease usually corresponds to the top of the tarsal plate, commonly 10 mm superior to the lash margin. Both medially and laterally, the upper lid crease comes closer to the lid margin; surgical planning in upper lid blepharoplasty must take this into consideration.

The area between the upper eyelid crease and the superior orbital margin is referred to as the superior orbital sulcus. With orbital volume loss, as seen following trauma or with aging, the superior sulcus can appear relatively concave because of lack of support underneath. Focal bulgings or convexity of the superior sulcus usually denotes areas of protruding fat, and this is usually most evident nasally.

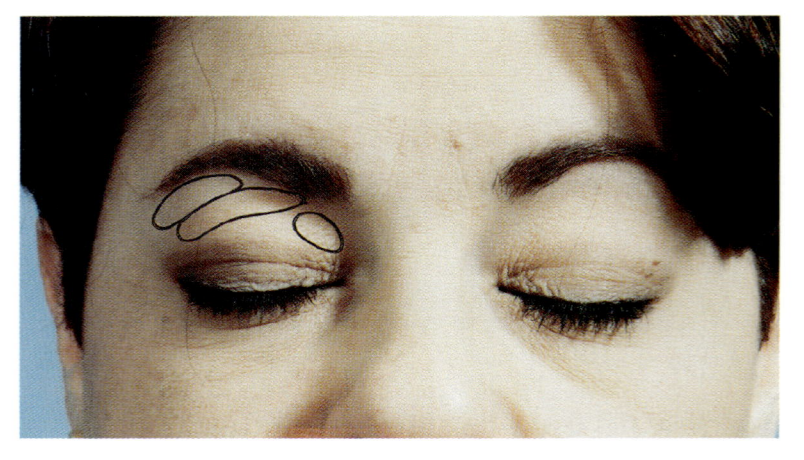

The area between the upper eyelid crease and the superior orbital margin is referred to as the superior orbital sulcus. Much of the definition of the sulcus is related to the prominence of the underlying periorbital fat. The upper eyelid fat is divided into a medial and central compartment. The lateral contour of the orbital sulcus is influenced by descent of the brow fat pad inferiorly, which is a result of brow ptosis and is commonly seen in the aging patient.

The lower eyelid crease begins medially 4 to 5 mm from the eyelid margin and slopes slightly inferiorly as it moves temporally. A less well-defined malar crease is seen below the region of the infraorbital rim, representing the junction between the eyelids and cheek skin. A dense fibrous septum anchors the superior aspect of the nasolabial fold to the maxilla, and its junction with the eyelid forms the nasojugal fold. Fat bagging of the lower eyelids is commonly evident in the region between the inferior orbital crease and the junction of the infraorbital rim. Overcorrection of the protruding fat during lower eyelid blepharoplasty will accentuate the junction between eyelid and cheek skin, producing a hollowed look that is most commonly seen along the nasojugal fold medially.

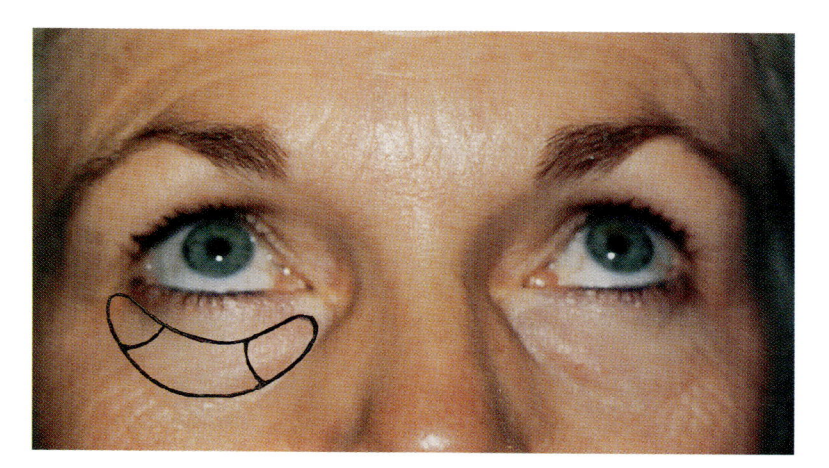

Herniated fat of the lower eyelids is commonly evident in the region between the inferior orbital crease and the junction of the infraorbital rim. The lower eyelid fat has been described as consisting of three compartments: medial, central, and lateral.

The skin of the eyelids is quite thin, with that of the medial upper eyelid being the thinnest found in the body. Transition to the thick skin of the eyebrow above and to the malar region below is rather abrupt. Subcutaneous fat is sparse in the preorbital and preseptal skin and absent in pretarsal skin.

Orbicularis Oculi Muscle

Subjacent and adherent to the eyelid skin lies the orbicularis oculi muscle. The orbicularis oculi represents a muscular sphincter lying superficially within the eyelid, while inserting in a deep and complex fashion along the orbital rim, where it contributes to the formation of the medial and lateral canthal tendons. Topographically, the orbicularis muscle has been described as consisting of defined regions: pretarsal, preseptal, and preorbital. The pretarsal orbicularis is tightly adherent to the tarsus and can be separated only by sharp dissection. The preseptal and orbital component move more freely and are separated from the underlying orbital septum by an areolar plane. Mild eyelid closure is primarily through pretarsal and preseptal function. The orbital portion of the orbicularis oculi is responsible for tight eyelid closure. This segment of the orbicularis oculi extends peripherally into the surrounding forehead and cheek, where it lies superficial to the elevators of the upper lip, as well as superficial to the frontalis, corrugator, and procerus muscles. The orbicularis oculi is supplied by multiple branches of the temporal and zygomatic segments of the facial nerve, which enter along the deep surface of the muscle.

The anatomic insertions of the orbicularis muscle into the medial and lateral canthal tendons are discussed in the following section.

BLEPHAROPLASTY

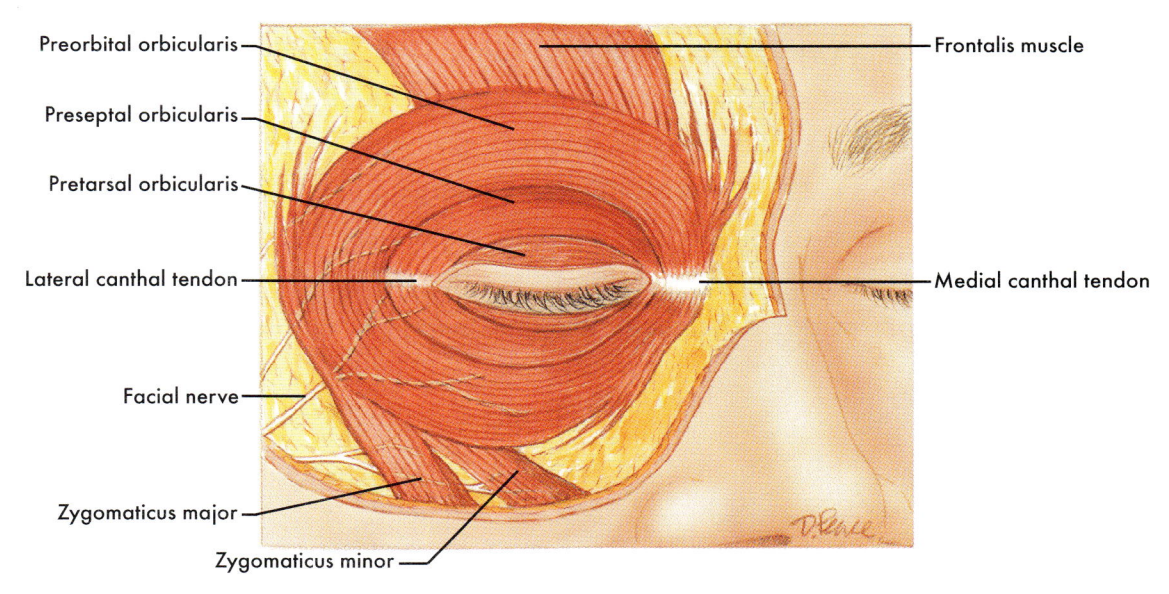

The orbicularis oculi represents a muscular sphincter involved in eyelid closure. The muscle is commonly described as consisting of a pretarsal, preseptal, and preorbital portion. The lateral and medial extents of this muscular sphincter form important contributions to the medial and lateral canthal tendons. The orbicularis oculi muscle is innervated in a segmental fashion along its deep surface via terminal contributions of the temporal and zygomatic branches of the facial nerve.

Orbital Septum

Deep to the orbicularis muscle in both the upper and lower eyelids lies the orbital septum. The orbital septum forms the anterior border of the orbit, confining the orbital fat. The orbital septum represents a continuation of the orbital periosteum anteriorly into the eyelid. Along its junction with the orbital rim, a thickening of the orbital septum becomes firmly attached to bone, forming what has been termed the arcus marginalis. At this junction, periosteum becomes periorbita. In essence, the orbital septum is attached almost exactly to the margin of the orbit. An exception to this conformity to the orbital rim is seen both medially and laterally. Medially, the septum covers the posterior aspect of Horner's muscle, posterior to the lacrimal sac, as it inserts along the posterior lacrimal crest. At the lateral canthus, the orbital septum courses posteriorly to join the lateral canthal tendon, traveling posterior to the orbicularis to insert at Whitnall's tubercle.

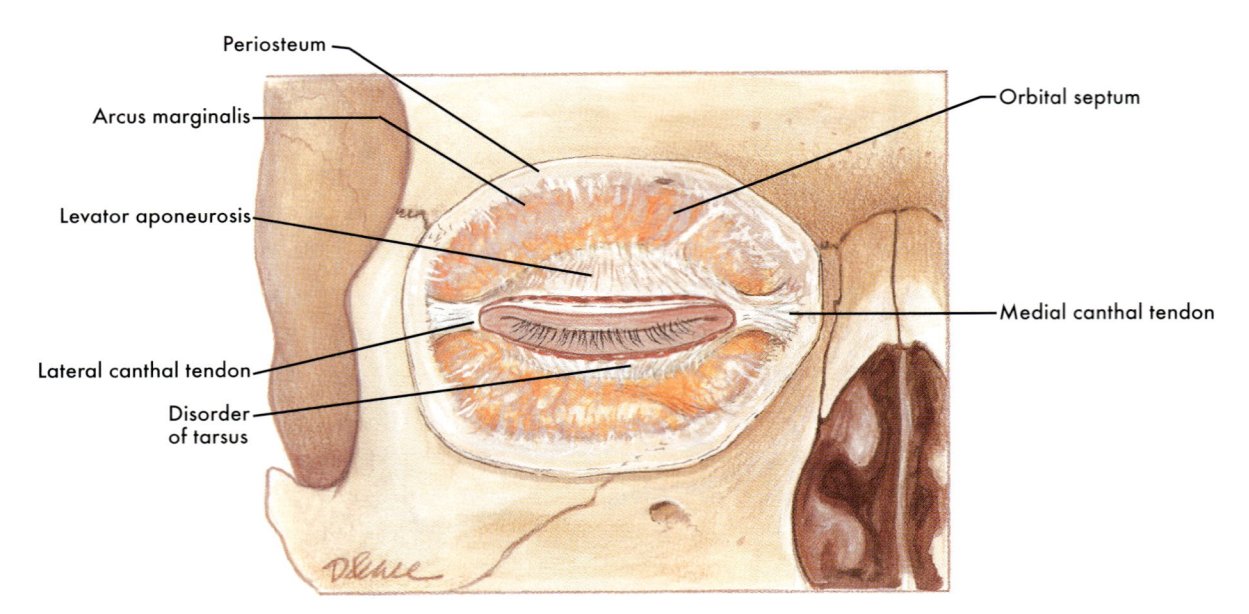

The orbital septum forms the anterior border of the orbit and represents a continuation of the orbital periosteum anteriorly into the eyelid. Medially and laterally, the orbital septum provides contributions to the formation of the medial and lateral canthal tendons, essentially lying directly posterior to the muscular contribution of the orbicularis oculi.

In the lower eyelid, the septum inserts directly along the inferior border of the tarsal plate after joining with the lower eyelid retractors 4 to 5 mm below the inferior tarsus. The superior orbital septum fails to join the superior tarsal margin because of the intervening aponeurosis of the levator muscle. Rather, the orbital septum becomes adherent to the levator aponeurosis approximately 10 mm above the superior eyelid margin and is involved in fibers that extend from the aponeurosis into the dermis of the upper eyelid, responsible for the formation of the upper eyelid crease in Caucasians.

The orbital septum is of great surgical importance, because deep to this structure lies the periorbital fat and orbital adnexae. Individual variation exists in the strength of the orbital septum, and this membrane commonly attenuates with age, allowing orbital fat to herniate anteriorly.

Medial Canthal Tendon

The medial canthal tendon is a well-defined structure lying immediately beneath the skin bridging the area between the medial palpebral fissure and the lateral side of the nose. The medial canthal tendon is formed predominantly from contributions from the orbicularis oculi muscle. As the orbicularis oculi muscle courses medially, it sends superficial and deep fibers along the anterior and posterior surface of the lacrimal sac. The anterior fibers of the medial canthal tendon insert into the anterior lacrimal crest and frontal process of the maxilla. The deeper fibers pass posterior to the lacrimal sac and its fascia to insert into the posterior lacrimal crest and are vital to proper lacrimal pump function. These deep pretarsal fibers of the orbicularis have been termed Horner's muscle. The insertion of the medial canthal tendon along the posterior lacrimal crest provides a strong anchoring position to the medial eyelid, allowing the eyelid to tightly follow and cover the convex globe. This posterior insertion is also responsible for maintaining the depth of the nasoorbital valley.

SURGICAL REJUVENATION OF THE FACE

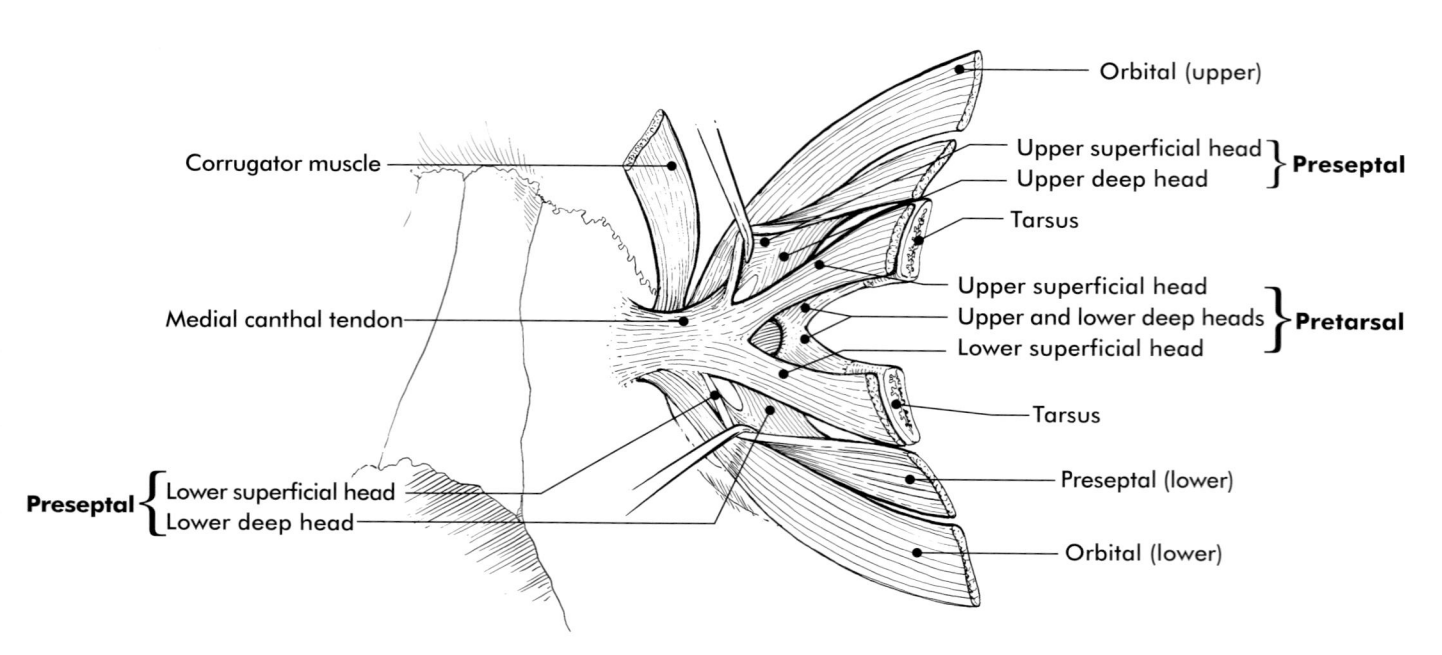

An illustration of medial canthal tendon anatomy, delineating the pretarsal, preseptal, and preorbital portions of the orbicularis contributing to this structure.

Lateral Canthal Tendon

The lateral canthal tendon is an important surgical structure, as attenuation or disinsertion of this ligament is largely responsible for laxity of the lower eyelid seen in the elderly patient. At the lateral canthus the preseptal and orbital orbicularis fibers pass superficially to join at what is termed a "raphe," which is an extension of the orbicularis muscle horizontally along the lateral orbital rim and zygoma. The pretarsal portions of the orbicularis run more deeply and insert 3 to 4 mm posterior to the lateral palpebral raphe at the lateral orbital Whitnall's tubercle. Attaching to the tubercle behind these deep pretarsal fibers are thin, fibrous contributions from the tarsal plates, as well as fibers from the orbital septum, the lateral levator horn, the lacrimal gland fascia, and the lateral rectus check ligament.

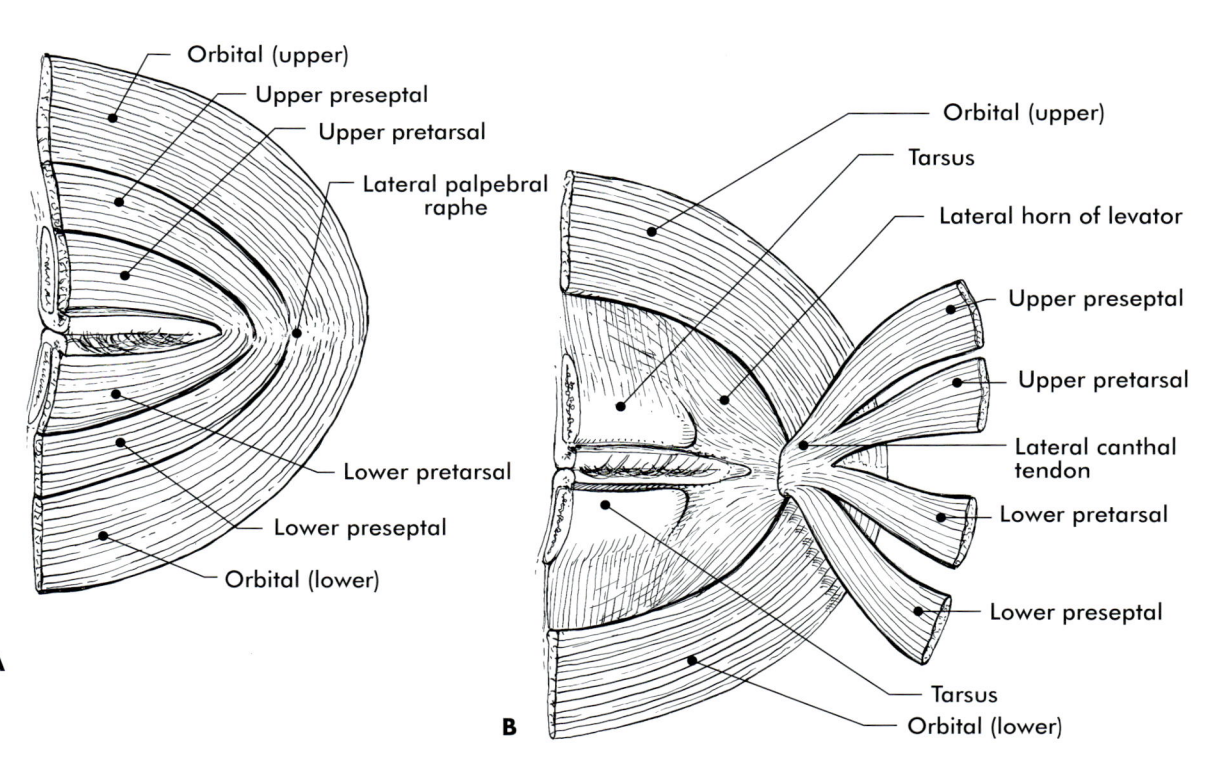

Lateral canthal tendon anatomy seen from an anterior dissection (A) and from a posterior dissection (B) depicting the contributions of the orbicularis oculi.

Levator Palpebrae

The levator palpebrae superioris and its superior tarsal muscle (Muller's) provide vertical mobility to the upper eyelid. Arising from the lesser sphenoid wing, the levator extends anteriorly along the superior orbit with a thin layer of fat, the supraorbital artery, the frontal nerve, and the trochlear nerve separating it from the orbital roof. Deep to the levator lies the superior rectus muscle. As the levator courses toward the superior orbital rim, its diameter increases and the muscle widens. Directly posterior to the rim, between 14 and 20 mm above the superior border of the tarsus, the levator forms a condensation of fascia known as the superior transverse ligament of Whitnall. Whitnall's ligament extends across the length of the superior orbit and terminates medially in fascia surrounding the trochlea of the superior oblique, as well as blending with the fascia surrounding the supraorbital notch. Laterally, the ligament joins with the capsule of the lacrimal gland and frontal bone. This condensed fascial sheath of the levator functions to convert the anterior-posterior pulling force of the levator muscle into a superior-inferior direction, allowing raising and lowering of the upper eyelid. It is analogous to Lockwood's ligament in the lower eyelid. Clinically, the superior transverse ligament represents the transition point where the levator changes from a fleshy, extraocular muscle into a fibrous aponeurotic sheath. The aponeurosis of the levator extends anteriorly into the upper lid, inserting along the anterior surface of the superior tarsal plate.

In addition to its palpebral insertion, the levator aponeurosis becomes a broad fibrous sheath that inserts into the orbital margins behind the medial and lateral commissures of the eyelid. These peripheral insertions are termed the medial and lateral "horns" of the levator. The lateral horn is a strong fibrous band that incompletely divides the lacrimal gland into a posterior-lying orbital lobe and an anterior palpebral lobe. The lateral horn of the levator then continues inferiorly to insert along the lateral orbital tubercle, contributing to the lateral canthal tendon. In contrast, the medial horn becomes filmy as it passes

BLEPHAROPLASTY

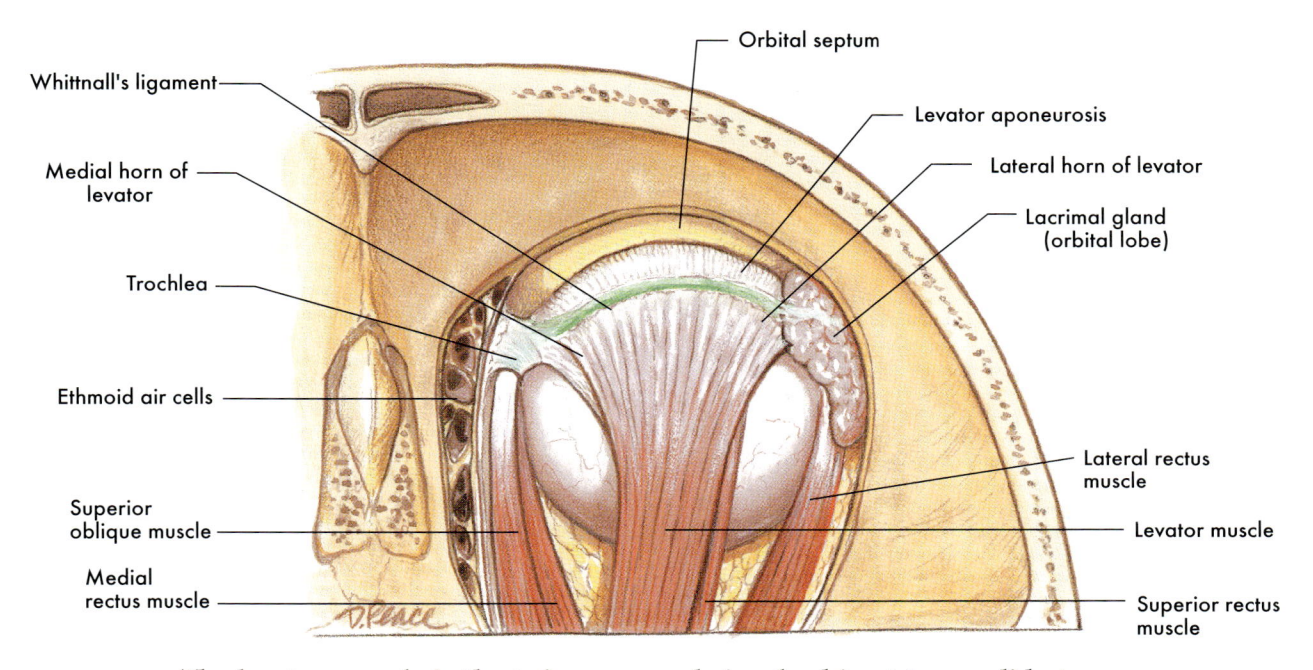

The levator muscle is the primary muscle involved in upper eyelid opening. The transition of the levator from a muscular belly to a fibrous aponeurosis occurs at what is anatomically termed the transverse retinacular ligament of Whitnall, approximately 20 mm above the superior border of the tarsus. The lateral extensions of the levator aponeurosis divide the lacrimal gland into an orbital and palpebral portion and continue laterally to insert along the lateral orbital tubercle, contributing to the formation of the lateral canthal tendon. The medial horn of the levator passes over the superior oblique tendon to insert into the medial canthal tendon and posterior lacrimal crest.

SURGICAL REJUVENATION OF THE FACE

over the superior oblique tendon to insert into the medial canthal tendon and posterior lacrimal crest.

The superficial palpebral insertions of the levator aponeurosis are clinically important. Just cephalad to the superior border of the tarsus, a fusion of the levator aponeurosis with the pretarsal portion of the orbicularis muscle and orbital septum occurs. At this point, the levator aponeurosis sends fibers through the septum and the pretarsal portion of the orbicularis into the overlying dermis. This dermal insertion of the levator aponeurosis is largely responsible for the formation of the upper eyelid crease in Caucasians.

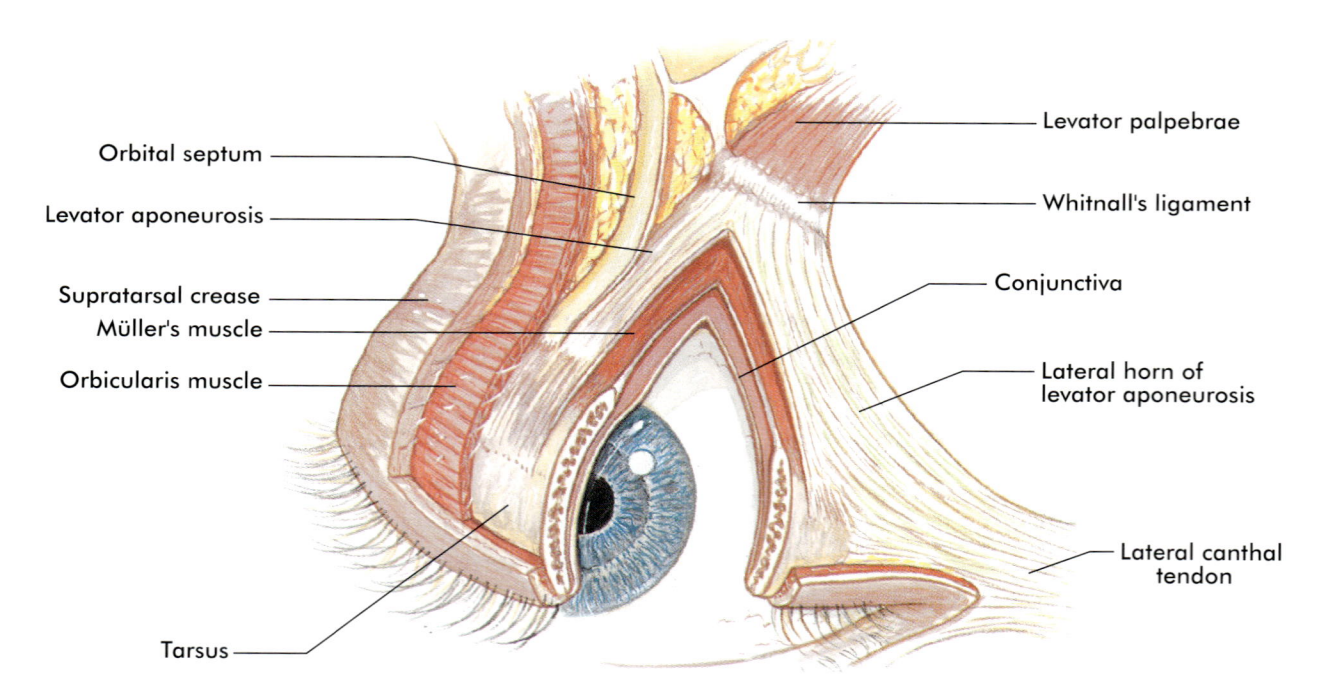

Cross-section anatomy of the upper eyelid. Note that the levator aponeurosis inserts along the anterior surface of the tarsus. At the superior level of the tarsus (approximately 10 mm above the lashline), a fusion of the levator aponeurosis occurs to the orbital septum, orbicularis muscle, and underlying dermis, forming the supratarsal crease in the Caucasian's upper eyelid.

The anatomic fusions that occur between the levator aponeurosis and orbicularis cephalad to the superior border of the tarsus have surgical significance during upper lid blepharoplasty. If the surgical plan simply includes a removal of a strip of orbicularis muscle, we would suggest resection of muscle at a level superior to the tarsus, directly overlying the orbital fat, to minimize the possibility of inadvertently injuring the underlying levator aponeurosis during muscle resection. Resection of a muscle strip at this higher level is quite safe, as both orbital fat and septum lie between the resection and underlying aponeurosis.

Similarly, if supratarsal fixation is to be performed, the pretarsal orbicularis overlying the junction of the levator aponeurosis with the superior tarsal plate must be carefully dissected, so that fixation can be performed precisely at the location desired for the new upper eyelid crease. Sharp and precise dissection is required to separate the pretarsal and lower preseptal orbicularis from the overlying levator without injuring the aponeurosis.

Muller's Muscle

Muller's muscle is a sympathetically innervated smooth muscle that lies immediately beneath the levator aponeurosis and is separated from it by what has been termed the postaponeurotic space. Muller's muscle, also known as the superior tarsal muscle, takes its origin from the underside of the levator muscle and inserts directly along the superior border of the tarsus. A vascular plexus commonly runs along the anterior surface of this muscle. In elderly patients undergoing blepharoplasty, an occasional finding is a partial dehiscence of the levator aponeurosis with the fleshy Muller's muscle seen in its anatomic location directly posterior to the levator.

Orbital Fascia

The fibrous organization within the orbit is divided into three parts: the fascia covering the globe (Tenon's fascia), the fascial sheath surrounding the extraocular muscles, and the intermuscular fascia septa and check ligaments extending from the extraocular muscles into the surrounding bone of the orbit. Tenon's capsule or bulbar fascia is a fibrous membrane that directly surrounds the globe and fuses with the conjunctiva at the cornea-scleral junction. It is closely applied to the globe and is penetrated by both nerves and blood vessels. The extraocular muscles must penetrate this layer of fascia to insert on the globe.

Each extraocular muscle is covered by a fascial network that is thin posteriorly but becomes denser anteriorly. These muscular fascia connect externally to form a fascial network between the muscles known as the intermuscular septum. The medial and lateral condensation of the extraocular fascia to the periorbitum are known respectively as the medial and lateral check ligaments. These are extensions from the sleeves of fascia surrounding the medial and lateral rectus muscles and serve to secure the globe to the periorbita.

Anteriorly, in the lower eyelid, the fascia between the inferior oblique and inferior rectus muscles forms a condensation known as the inferior suspensory ligament of Lockwood. As noted previously, this is analogous to a thickening or condensation of fascia overlying the levator muscle, the superior transverse ligament of Whitnall. Lockwood's ligament is described as a hammocklike structure extending to both medial and lateral orbital walls. This ligament will support the globe following partial maxillectomy with removal of orbital floor, as long as the attachments of this ligament to the medial and lateral retinaculi are not disturbed. Extensions from the extraocular fascia of the inferior oblique and inferior rectus muscle also course anteriorly into the lower eyelid, where they form part of the lower eyelid retractor system as discussed in the following section.

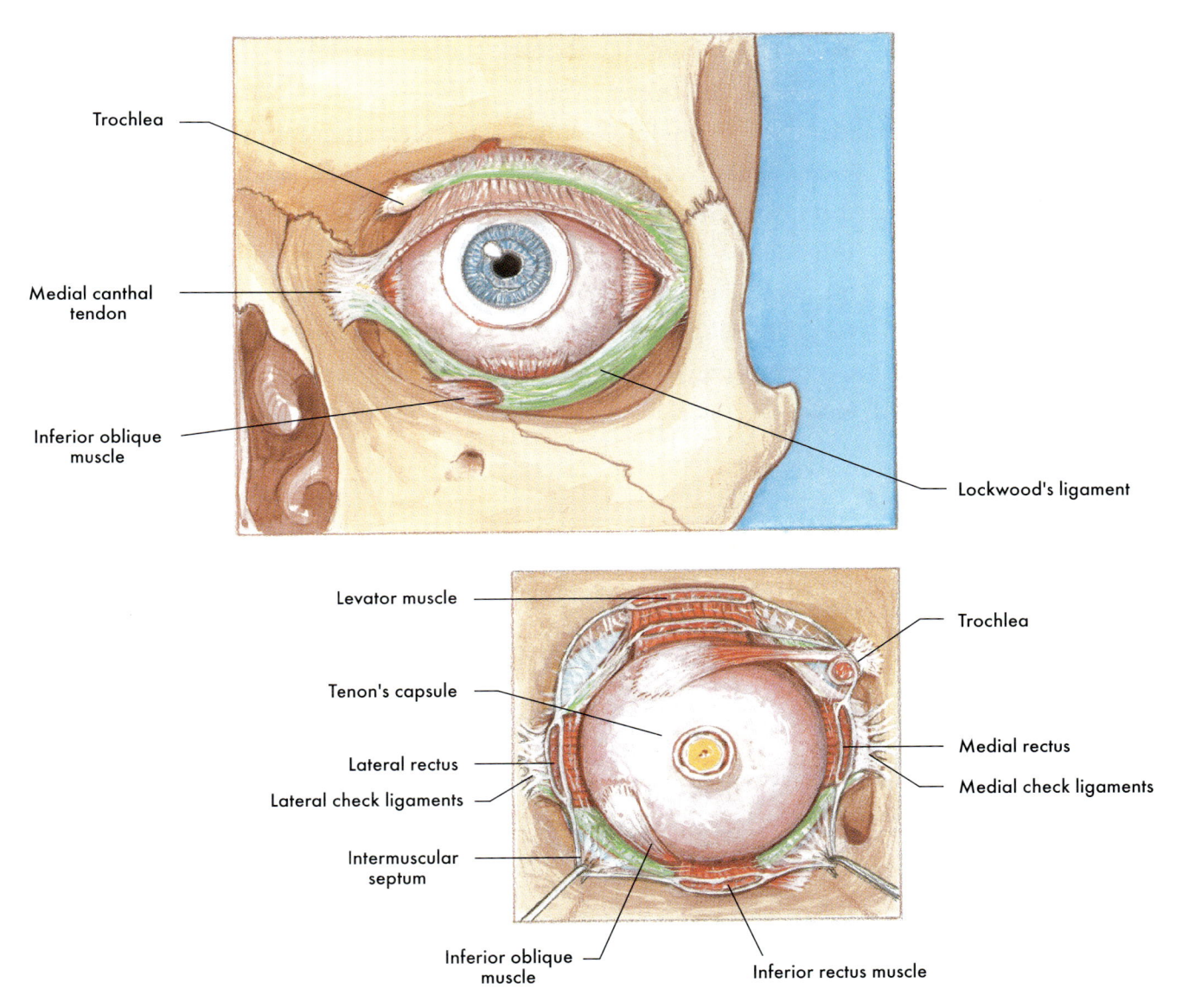

Each extraocular muscle is covered by a fascial network that becomes dense anteriorly along bony insertions and insertions into the lower eyelid. The medial and lateral condensations of this extraocular fascia to the periorbitum are known as the medial and lateral check ligaments. The extensions from the inferior oblique and inferior rectus muscle form a condensation along the inferior aspect of the globe known as the inferior suspensory ligament of Lockwood. This condensation of fascia forms a hammocklike structure extending to both the medial and lateral orbital walls and is important in supporting the globe in its normal anatomic position. Extensions of the fascia of the inferior oblique and inferior rectus muscle course anteriorly to insert into the lower eyelid, forming what is known as the lower eyelid retractor system.

Lower Eyelid Retractors

Unlike the upper eyelid, the lower eyelid has little vertical movement and is predominantly a static structure. On downward gaze the lower eyelid will retract approximately 2 mm, secondary to action of the lower eyelid retractors. The lower eyelid retractors are formed from fascia derived from the inferior rectus and inferior oblique muscles. This fascial extension courses anterior to Lockwood's ligament, forming what is termed the capsulopalpebral ligament. This fascia then courses posterior to the orbital septum and inserts directly along the inferior margin of the tarsus. It is analogous to the levator

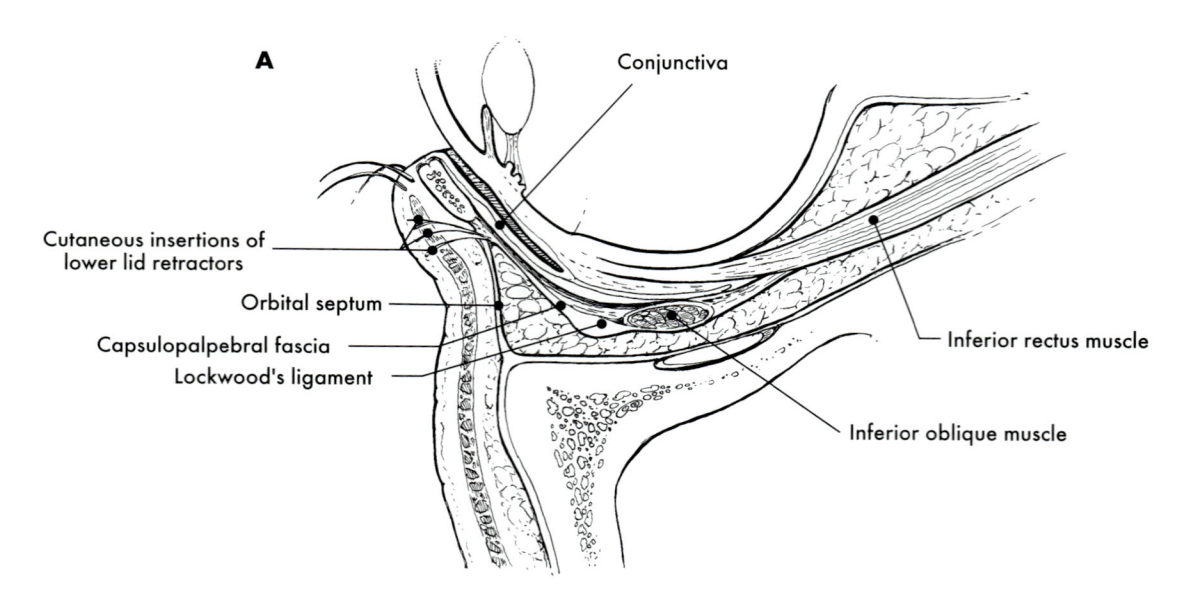

A, The lower eyelid retractor system is formed by extensions of the fascia derived from the inferior rectus and inferior oblique muscles. These fascial extensions course anteriorly to Lockwood's ligament, forming what is termed the capsulopalpebral fascia. The capsulopalpebral fascia is noted to be interposed between the conjunctiva posteriorly and the periorbital fat anteriorly. Approximately 3 mm below the inferior tarsal border the capsulopalpebral ligament fuses with the orbital septum and sends fibrous extensions into the orbicularis muscle and overlying skin, forming the lower eyelid crease.

aponeurosis of the upper eyelid. As the inferior rectus contracts to produce downward gaze, the effects of its muscular action are transmitted to the capsulopalpebral fascia, which in turn produces synchronous depression of the inferior tarsus.

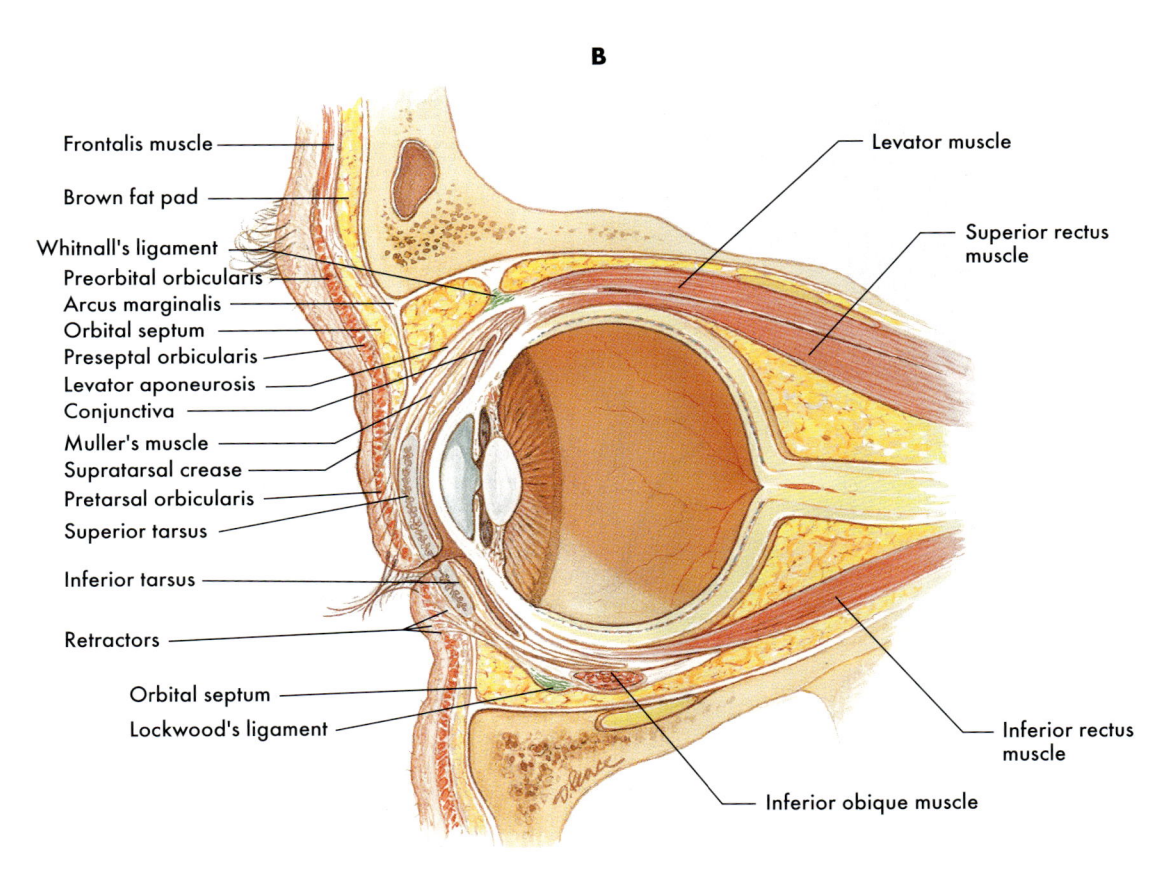

B, Cross-sectional diagram of the upper and lower eyelids illustrating the analogous fascial extensions from both the levator palpebra muscle and the extensions from the inferior oblique and inferior rectus muscles forming a retractor system for the upper and lower eyelids. These systems work in tandem to coordinate eyelid opening with deviations of the globe from primary gaze.

SURGICAL REJUVENATION OF THE FACE

Posteriorly, the capsulopalpebral fascia lies deeply within the lower eyelid, is posterior to the orbital septum and orbital fat, and is just anterior to the conjunctiva. Anteriorly, the capsulopalpebral ligament fuses with orbital septum approximately 3 mm below the inferior tarsal border and at this point sends fibrous extensions into the orbicularis muscle and overlying skin, forming the lower eyelid crease.

The clinical significance of the capsulopalpebral fascia and its fusion with orbital septum is of great importance when performing transconjunctival blepharoplasty. In this procedure, the conjunctiva and capsulopalpebral fascia can be incised superior to the fusion of

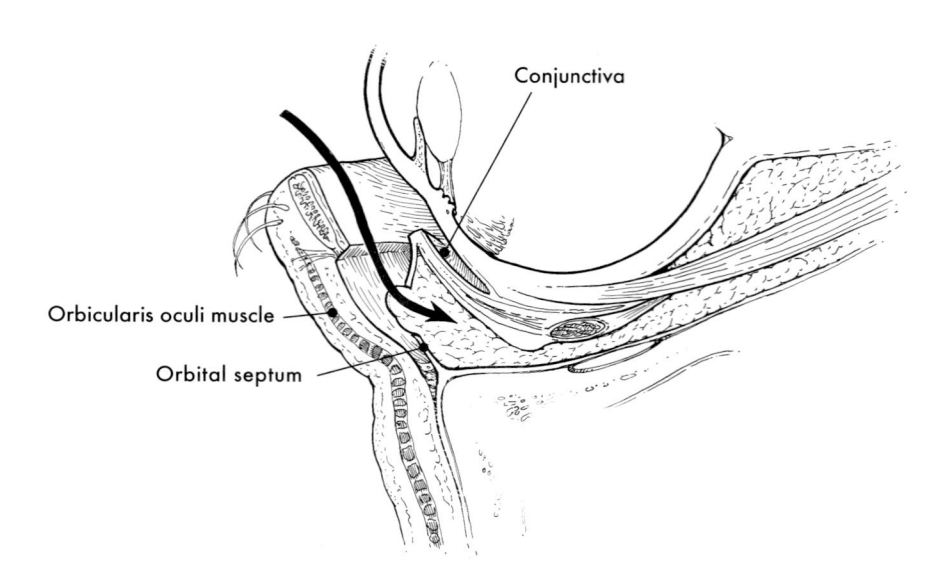

Transconjunctival blepharoplasty via a preseptal approach is performed through an incision just inferior to the tarsal margin. This incises the conjunctiva and capsulopalpebral fascia in the region where they are fused with the orbital septum and allows the surgeon to enter into the preseptal space just posterior to the orbicularis oculi muscle (the plane typically used in transcutaneous blepharoplasty). The surgeon then visualizes the orbital fat through the septum orbitale. This procedure requires opening the septum orbitale to contour the periorbital fat.

The lateral third of the eyelid will commonly contain a lateral fat pad that lies superficial to the orbital septum and directly deep to the orbicularis muscle, termed retroorbicularis oculi fat (ROOF). This fat pad is in reality an extension of the brow fat pad that lies along the superior orbital rim and aids in the smooth sliding of the eyebrow with animation. In patients seeking upper eyelid blepharoplasty who also have ptosis of the eyebrows, the lateral brow fat pad can be contoured to help in highlighting the lateral aspect of the superior orbital rim.

In the lateral third of the eyelid the lacrimal gland should not be confused with the lateral fat pad. The lacrimal gland is divided into the orbital and palpebral portions by the lateral horn of the levator aponeurosis. The orbital lobe conforms to the space between the orbital wall and the globe and rests upon the levator aponeurosis. Anteriorly, it is covered by the orbital septum and central fat pad. The palpebral lobe lies deep to the levator aponeurosis, lying in the subaponeurotic space between aponeurosis and conjunctiva. Clinically, the treatment of a ptotic lacrimal gland can be approached during blepharoplasty, as will be discussed later.

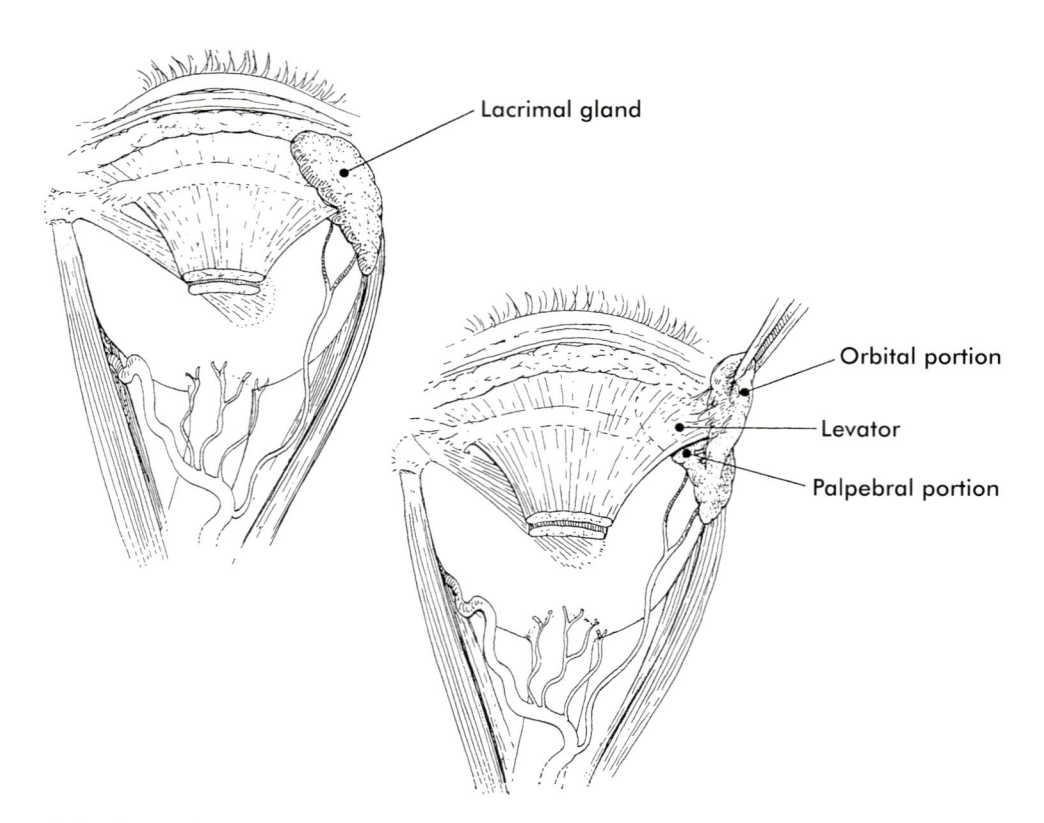

The lateral extension of the levator palpebrae divide the orbital and palpebral portions of the lacrimal gland. The palpebral portion of the lacrimal gland lies just superficial to the conjunctiva. Usually four to six excretory ductules pass from the orbital portion of the gland to the palpebral lobe. From the palpebral lobe, six to eight excretory ductules empty into the temporal conjunctival sac 4 to 5 mm cephalad to the tarsus.

Lower Eyelid Anatomy: The Lower Eyelid Fat Pad

The fat of the lower eyelid is divided into three compartments: medial, central, and lateral. The medial and central compartments are separated from each other by fascial attachments that run from the inferior oblique muscle; dissection between these two compartments, deep to the orbital septum, will reveal the inferior oblique muscle itself. In general, the medial compartment contains fat of a whiter or a lighter coloration. The central compartment fat tends to be more elongated and usually is yellow.

The lateral fat compartment is divided from the more central compartment by fascial attachments derived from the more lateral aspect of the inferior oblique muscle. The lateral fat compartment is situated more superior than the central compartment, and the lateral fat pad tends to be infiltrated with numerous small vessels. The fascial attachments that run from the inferior oblique tend to percolate through the lateral pad and make this pad quite fibrous in its appearance and, therefore, often more difficult to deliver in the operative field.

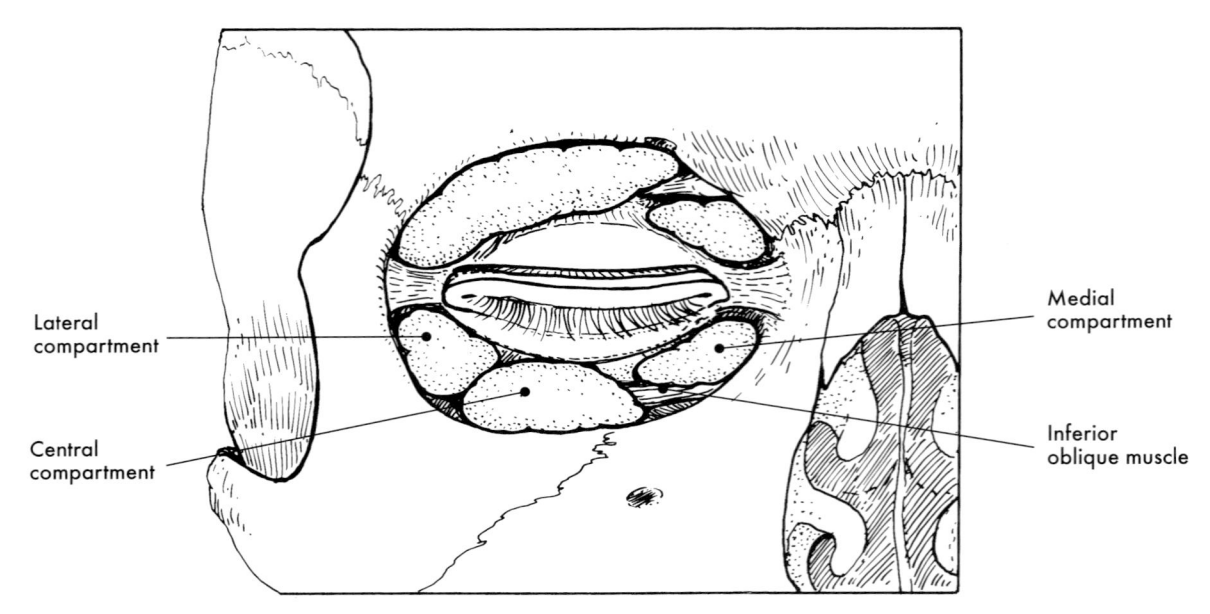

The lower eyelid fat is divided into three compartments: medial, central, and lateral. The medial and central compartments are separated from each other by the inferior oblique muscle and its fascial attachments. The lateral fat compartment is situated more superior than the central compartment and is separated from the central compartment by fascial attachments that extend from the inferior oblique muscle and percolate through the lateral pad.

PREOPERATIVE VISIT AND PATIENT EDUCATION

Patients requesting blepharoplasty tend to be "eyelid conscious." Sometimes this eyelid awareness is emphasized when the individual requesting the initial examination appears in the office wearing dark glasses. Careful screening and refusing to perform surgery on the patient with unrealistic expectations helps to ensure patient and surgeon satisfaction. Many individuals requesting blepharoplasty are not realistic about what can be achieved. Therefore the surgeon should invest time in determining the patient's needs and desires.

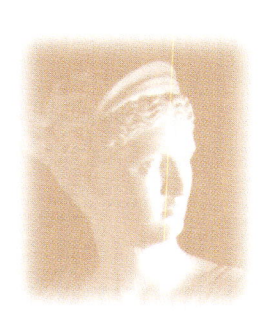

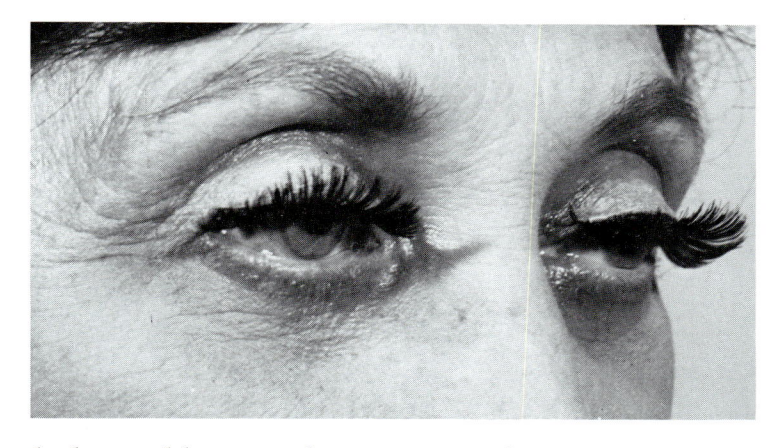

False eyelashes and heavy makeup are worn by many patients. Eyelashes normally are not as long or as thick as those being worn by this individual, but they illustrate the focus that some patients place on the orbital region.

The first and most obvious question for the surgeon to ask the prospective patient is, "What do you wish to achieve by having eyelid surgery?" The surgeon should be wary of the patient who squints and says, "Look at all of these tiny lines around my eyes that appear whenever I smile or squint."

The blepharoplasty patient often expects all the "crow's feet" to disappear after surgery, which is not the case. The surgeon should outline the surgical objectives and explain to the patient that although some of the periorbital lines will be eliminated, others will remain. If the altered eyelids are acceptable in repose, a satisfactory result has been achieved. The final appearance should not be judged during squinting or smiling.

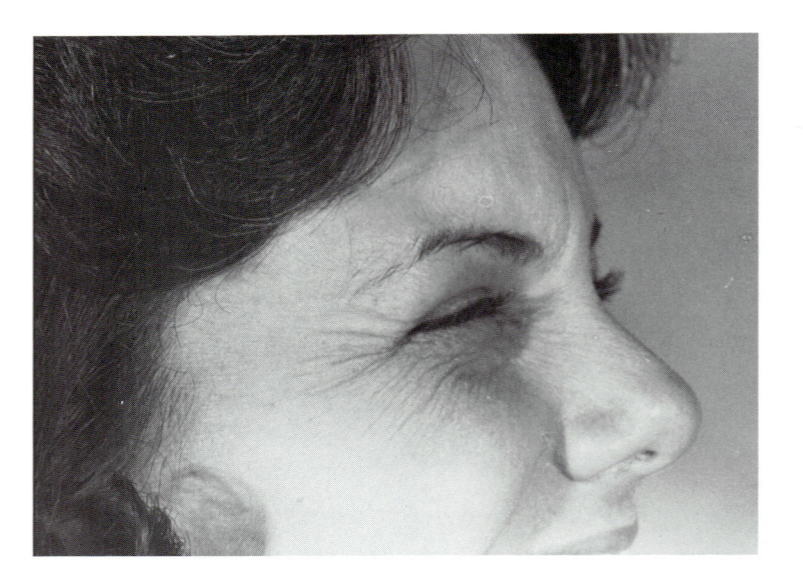

Patients often complain that many lines and wrinkles are present around their eyes when they squint. This is a normal phenomenon that occurs in everyone. A blepharoplasty will not remove the lines caused by squinting. The results of a blepharoplasty must be judged with the face in repose, not forcibly animated.

If the patient holds his or her finger just above the eyebrow while it is elevated and says, "This is how I want my upper lids to look," the surgeon should note that a browlift may be indicated in addition to or instead of a blepharoplasty.

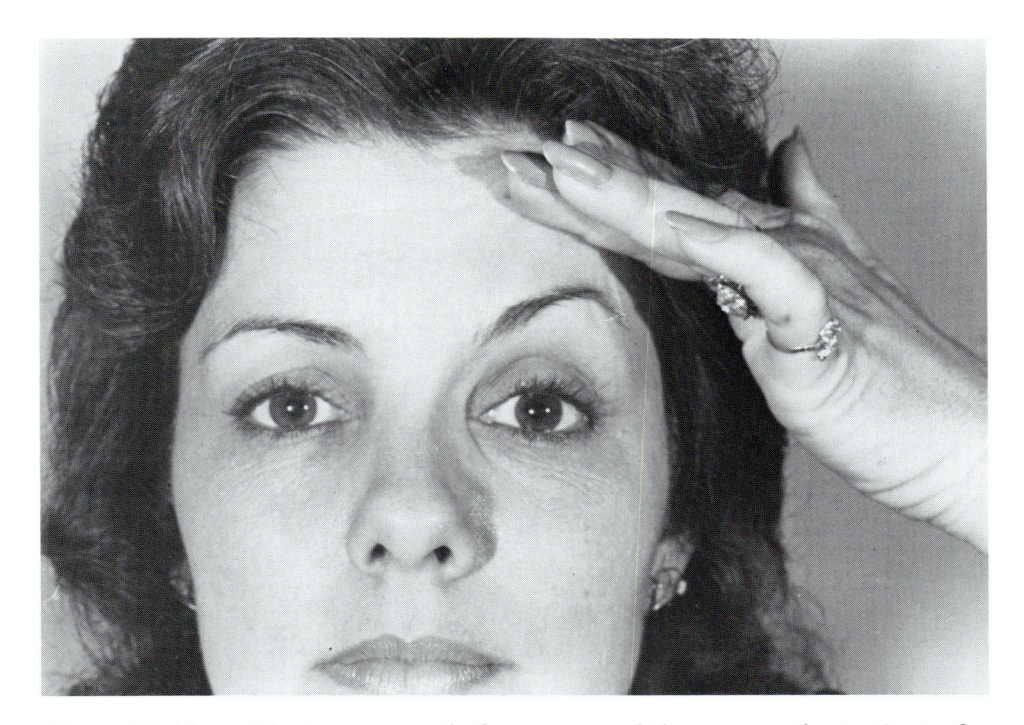

After a blepharoplasty, or even before any eyelid surgery, the patient often holds up her eyebrow and requests that the eyelid and orbital area have this appearance. If this is the case, proceed with caution; the procedure of choice is apt to be a brow elevation rather than a blepharoplasty.

SURGICAL REJUVENATION OF THE FACE

The patient's eyelids and brows should be examined and their positions documented photographically. If a patient has drooping eyebrows, this should be noted. For these individuals, a browlift may be the procedure of choice and should be combined with blepharoplasty.

The surgeon should also evaluate the patient for other eyelid and orbital conditions such as asymmetry, any tendency toward exophthalmos, ptosis, or any preoperative scleral show.

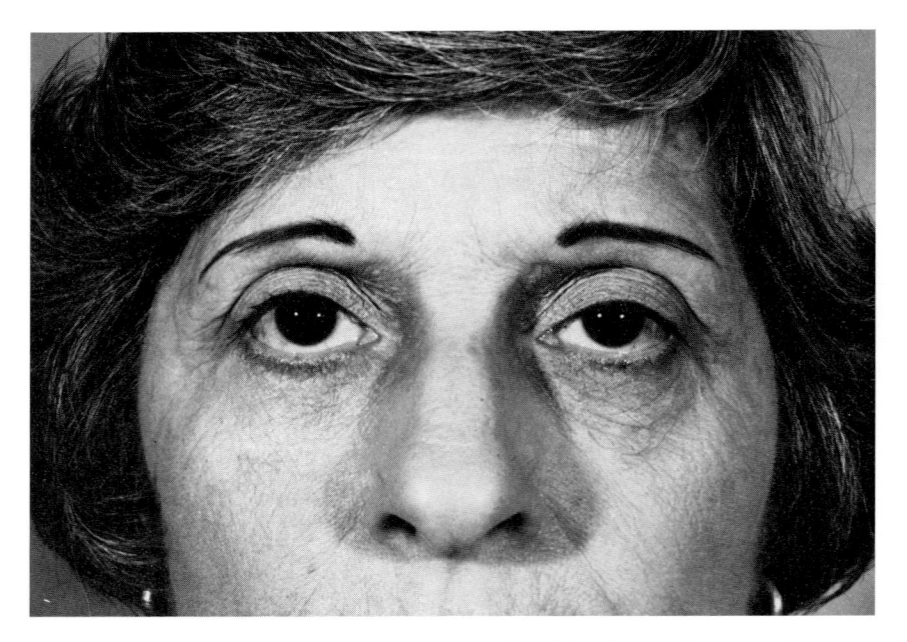

When preoperatively evaluating patients for blepharoplasty, it is a good practice to carefully examine preoperative photographs. Many patients, such as this one, exhibit a slight ptosis of one eye (left) and may not be aware of the deformity. If this is not brought to the patient's attention before surgery, it may cause a misunderstanding postoperatively and the patient will assume that the ptosis was a result of the surgery.

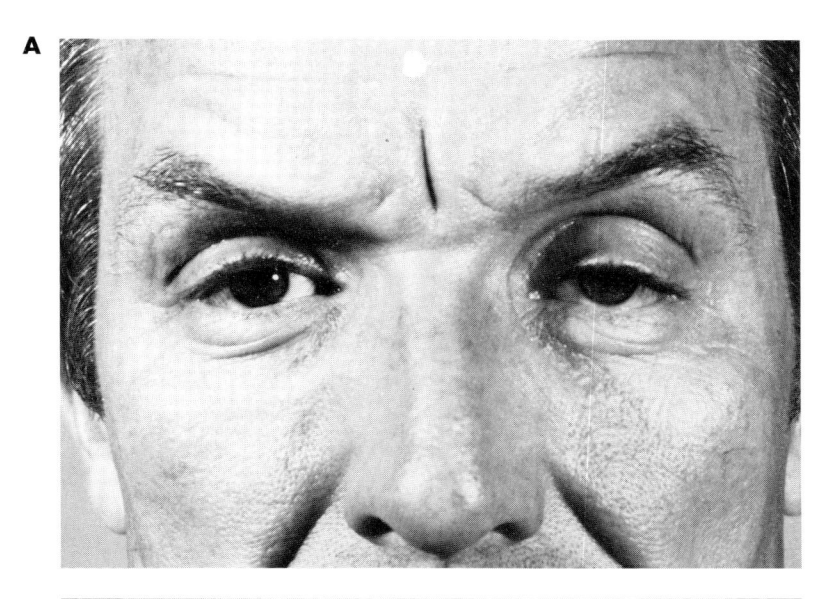

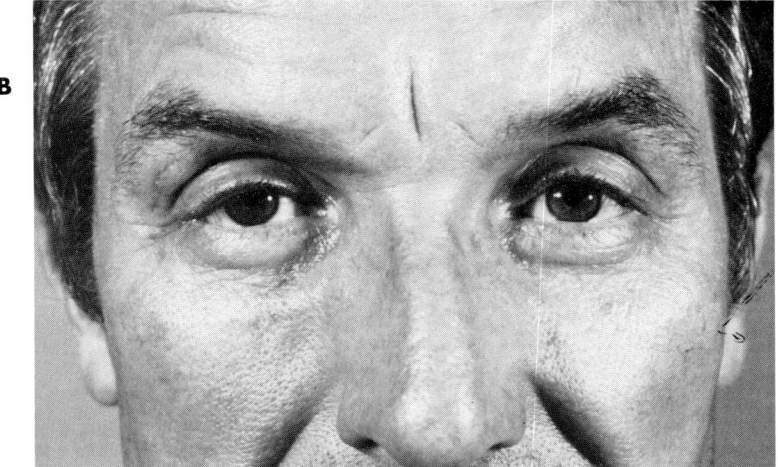

A, This patient requested blepharoplasty for eyelid asymmetry. The problem also involved unilateral ptosis affecting the left upper eyelid. Patients often are unaware of a slight ptosis and may think the surgeon caused the droopy eyelid during the blepharoplasty. It is imperative to check for symmetry preoperatively. B, The left upper eyelid ptosis was corrected, along with lower eyelid blepharoplasty. A skin flap was used on the lower eyelids.

If a female patient has cyclic eyelid and periorbital edema, it should be observed and recorded. This situation should be discussed with the patient, because blepharoplasty will not eliminate allergies and cyclic edema.

The surgeon should note whether other eyelid pathology exists, such as xanthoma, lymphangioma, a benign or malignant tumor, or an injection of a foreign material such as collagen, paraffin, or silicone.

When the surgeon is compiling the patient's medical history, the patient should be asked whether there is a history of any visual disturbances and whether he or she wears glasses. The name of the patient's eye physician should be included in his or her records. Records of visual acuity and other preexisting ophthalmic conditions can then be obtained from the patient's ophthalmologist. When in doubt about any patient who has a history of eye problems, a current ophthalmologic examination is imperative. Preoperatively, the patient should be given a simple eye examination for acuity and gross visual fields. This test can be conveniently given when the preoperative photographs are being taken. Each eye is tested individually. Sometimes an individual is nearly blind in one eye and does not mention this condition. Any unusual impairment should be documented before surgery. Potential dry eye syndrome may be discovered when taking the history, and if there is a suggestion or history of keratitis sicca, a Schirmer's test and an ophthalmological examination should be required. In general, we routinely perform a Schirmer's test and visual acuity on all patients undergoing blepharoplasty.

A small percentage of patients requesting blepharoplasty have glaucoma. Although this condition is not a contraindication to surgery, it should be recorded and the treating ophthalmologist should be contacted for clearance. If the patient is taking ophthalmic medications, the drugs are continued on the usual time schedule.

Common complications are discussed at the initial preoperative visit. These complications include delayed healing, prolonged redness of scars, postoperative edema, eyelid lag, scleral show, patient dissatisfaction, asymmetry, dark circles and lines that will remain, and contour irregularities.

Extremely rare complications such as loss or diminution of vision and extraocular paresis are mentioned for completeness, but in our opinion these should not be dwelled on because the complications occur infrequently and their discussion will only alarm the patient. The most common complications and problems are included in our consent form.

SPECIAL CONSENT TO OPERATION
OR OTHER PROCEDURE

PATIENT: _____

DATE: _____ TIME: _____

1. I hereby authorize Dr. _____ and/or associates to perform a surgical operation known as blepharoplasty, or commonly called plastic surgical operation on the eyelids and surrounding structures, on

   _____
   (Name of patient) or (Myself)

2. The procedure listed in Paragraph 1 has been explained to me by the above doctors, and I completely understand the nature and consequences of the procedure. The following points have been specifically made clear:

   a. Incisions are used in and about the eyelids, and that incisions heal with scar tissue.

   b. That there will be discoloration about the eyes for several days, and that in some cases this can persist for considerably longer.

   c. Due to the nature of the procedure, an exact end-result cannot be predicted, and I have not been given any guarantee of specific results.

   d. That the incision lines usually are conspicuous early postoperatively and for an indefinite period of time.

   e. No assurance is given that the eyelids will be perfectly symmetrical.

3. I recognize that, during the course of the operation, unforeseen conditions may necessitate additional or different procedures than those set forth above. I therefore further authorize and request that the above-named surgeon, his assistants, or his designees perform such procedures as are, in his professional judgment, necessary and desirable, including, but not limited to, procedures involving pathology and radiology. The authority granted under this Paragraph 3 shall extend to remedying conditions that are not known to the above doctors at the time the operation is commenced.

4. I consent to the administration of anesthesia to be applied by or under the direction and supervision of the above doctors or such anesthesiologists as they shall select and to the use of such anesthetics as they may deem advisable, with the exception of

   _____
   (None or a particular one)

5. I am aware that the practice of medicine and surgery is not an exact science, and I acknowledge that no guarantees have been made to me as to the results of the operation or procedure.

6. I consent to be photographed before, during and after the treatment; that these photographs shall be the property of the above doctors and may be published in scientific journals and/or shown for scientific reasons.

7. I agree to keep the above doctors informed of any change of address so that he can notify me of any late findings, and I agree to cooperate with the above doctors in my care after surgery until completely discharged.

8. I have read the above consent and fully understand the same and do authorize the above doctors to perform this surgical procedure on me.

9. I am not known to be allergic to anything except: (list) _____

_____

Witness _____

Witness _____   _____
                                                    (Patient)

IF PATIENT IS A MINOR, COMPLETE THE FOLLOWING:

Patient is a minor _____ years of age, and we, the undersigned, are the parents or guardian of the patient and do hereby consent for the patient.

Witness _____

                                                    _____
                                                    (Parent or legal guardian)

Witness _____

                                                    _____
                                                    (Parent or legal guardian)

Sample consent form.

The surgeon must not hesitate to refuse a prospective patient whose needs cannot be met. If the patient's psychologic problems outweigh the potential advantages of the procedure, a refusal is a sure way to avoid a disappointed patient and possibly a potential medical-legal problem.

PREOPERATIVE EVALUATION

Upper Eyelids

Skin

Most patients undergoing upper eyelid blepharoplasty complain about excess skin present within the upper eyelid, obliterating a sharp supratarsal crease. There is a large degree of variability in terms of the amount of excess eyelid skin present from patient to patient. This can range from a slight amount of excess skin to severe hooding of upper eyelid skin associated with lash ptosis and visual field obstruction in superotemporal gaze.

Patients presenting with concomitant brow ptosis make the evaluation of redundancy of excess upper eyelid skin more complicated. Poor supratarsal crease definition secondary to the ptotic eyebrow skin is most apparent along the lateral third of the upper eyelid. It is important to accurately define in these patients the degree of excess upper lid skin as opposed to the redundancy present secondary to eyebrow ptosis. Although it sounds obvious, it is impossible to correct eyebrow ptosis via an upper eyelid blepharoplasty. The skin resection on an upper eyelid blepharoplasty should only remove redundant upper eyelid skin. The treatment of the ptotic eyebrow, causing obliteration of the supratarsal crease, is a coronal browlift. An over-aggressive resection during upper lid blepharoplasty in an attempt to treat brow ptosis will serve only to further the descent of the eyebrow inferiorly and will not correct the aesthetic problem of the ptotic brow. An aggressive upper eyelid blepharoplasty will also preclude the possibility of coronal browlifting at a later date because of the paucity of eyelid skin remaining following the initial procedure.

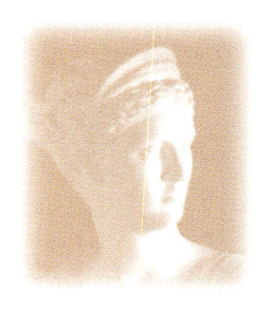

It is perhaps easiest to define the degree of skin redundancy when the patient is evaluated in the sitting position. The surgeon should visualize the upper eyelid crease and then gauge the amount of skin redundancy obscuring this fold. Unequal eyebrow levels and asymmetry in skin redundancy must be taken into consideration when deciding on the amount of skin to remove.

The most common mistake made in upper eyelid blepharoplasty is the overresection of eyelid skin. We feel that this is caused by an incomplete understanding of the purpose of upper eyelid skin resection. Often the attitude is that if a little is good, then more is better. Nothing could be further from the truth. Although skin resection is an important aspect of defining the upper lid crease, other aspects of eyelid surgery similarly help in sharpening this fold, including orbicularis muscle resection, opening of the orbital septum, fat contouring, and supratarsal fixation. All that is accomplished by over-aggressive resection of upper eyelid skin is lag ophthalmos, an inferior migration of the eyebrow, and possibly a superior migration of the upper blepharoplasty scar. This does not lead to an aesthetically pleasing appearance and usually ends in an unnatural and severe look to the upper eyelids.

A

B

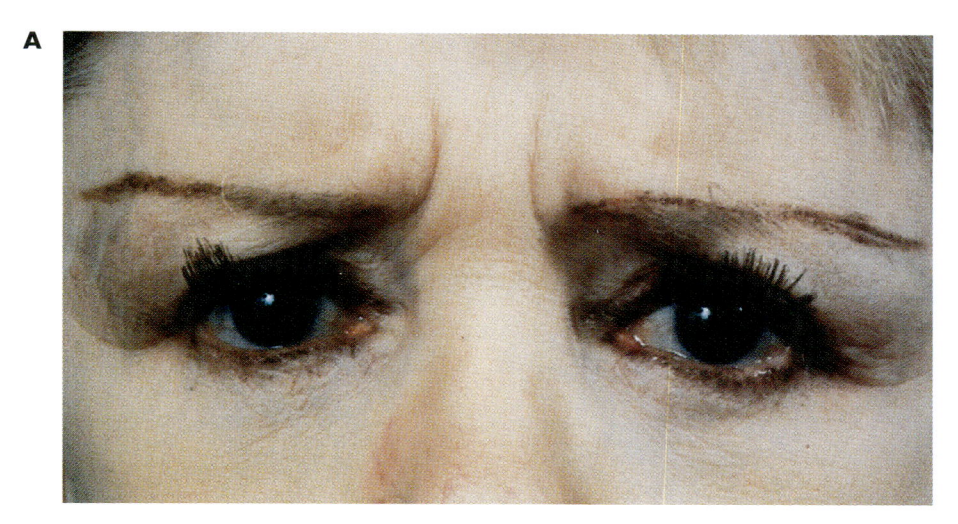

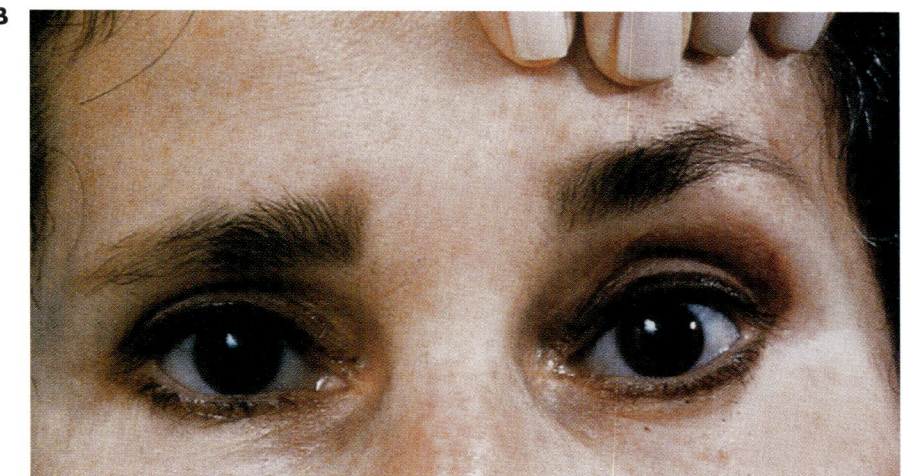

This patient is seen after having undergone two upper lid blepharoplasties performed in another office. Note the very low position of her eyebrows associated with a significant amount of temporal hooding. When the brow is placed to its normal position above the supraorbital rim, this patient no longer has enough skin to close her eyes. A result such as this typically occurs in patients whose main aesthetic problem is brow ptosis, but in which only an upper lid blepharoplasty has been performed. The end result of an aggressive resection of upper eyelid skin is to bring the brows to a more inferior position, which worsens the appearance of the upper eyelids and precludes a browlift being performed at a later date. B, This patient illustrates the outcome of an over-aggressive upper lid blepharoplasty. When the brow is placed above the level of the orbital rim, note that the blepharoplasty scar is visible and lies well above the supratarsal fold. She also lacks sufficient upper lid skin, and when her brow is elevated to a more natural level, she is unable to close her eyes, precluding the possibility of a browlifting procedure. Note also on the contralateral side, the effect of an aggressive removal of upper lid skin. This has brought her lateral brow to lie at a level inferior to her medial brow, which produced a sad and tired aesthetic appearance.

Evaluation of the supratarsal crease

The aging of the upper eyelid region is a complex process. It involves several factions, including descent of the position of the eyebrow below the superior orbital rim, excess upper lid skin, and an attenuation of the connections of the levator aponeurosis influencing skin invagination. The loss of a sharp supratarsal crease adds to the appearance of greater skin redundancy and lessens the show of pretarsal skin. Many of the aesthetic goals in blepharoplasty can be achieved not only by skin and fat excision but also by upper lid invagination procedures that define the supratarsal crease, improve pretarsal show, and minimize the need for excessive skin excision.

The location of the supratarsal crease will vary from patient to patient. In most patients the supratarsal crease will measure between 8 and 12 mm above the ciliary margin. The ideal level of the lid crease in the female is approximately 10 mm above the ciliary margin, whereas 8 to 9 mm is perhaps preferable in males, so as not to feminize the upper eyelids. It is important to analyze the level of the crease that exists preoperatively; in general, the inferior limb of the skin excision is placed adjacent to the naturally occurring supratarsal fold. In some patients with a very low upper eyelid crease, this can be raised to perhaps a more aesthetically pleasing level (10 mm) if desired. Some patients will present with ill-defined or asymmetric supratarsal creases. In patients with significant asymmetries or poorly defined creases, supratarsal fixation to invaginate the redundant skin is a useful procedure to sharpen and define this fold.

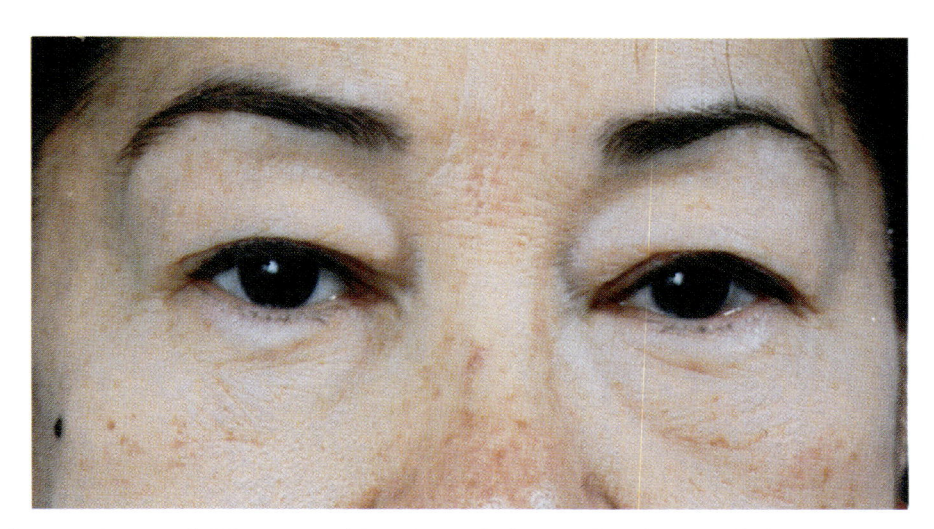

This patient exhibits a combination of skin redundancy of the upper eyelid, a significant amount of preaponeurotic fat, and a poorly defined supratarsal fold associated with hooding of the upper eyelid. Note the complete lack of pretarsal show. In approaching patients such as this, attention should be given to creation of a sharp supratarsal fold through a lid invagination procedure such as supratarsal fixation. This will allow the surgeon to create a crisp supratarsal fold with adequate pretarsal show, without the need to aggressively resect upper eyelid skin.

SURGICAL REJUVENATION OF THE FACE

Fat

The amount of fat to excise is an important part of upper eyelid blepharoplasty. Perhaps even more than on the lower eyelid, excessive resection of upper eyelid fat (usually medial aspect of the central compartment) can produce a hollowed-out, cadaveric look, which is essen-

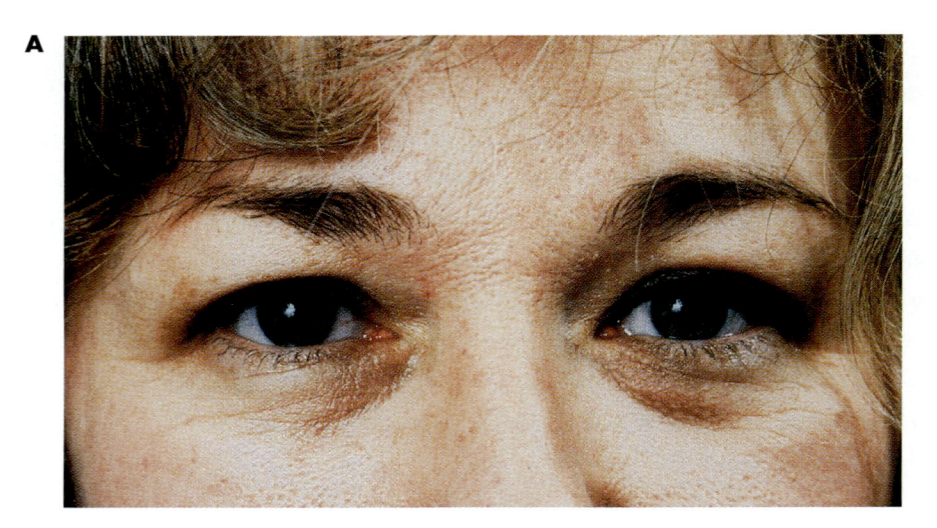

A, Patient with loss of supratarsal crease definition secondary to an attenuation of the connections of levator aponeurosis. This has led to essentially vertical appearing upper eyelids with lack of well-defined orbitopalpebral sulcus and minimal pretarsal skin show. This type of patient often will benefit not only from skin excision but also from contouring of the medial and central fat pads, as well as supratarsal fixation.

tially impossible to correct at a later date. In all patients, the amount of fat to be resected at the time of blepharoplasty should be decided on through careful preoperative evaluation. In patients with well-defined orbitopalpebral sulcus with a somewhat concave upper eyelid and deep set eyes, very little fat must resected from the central com-

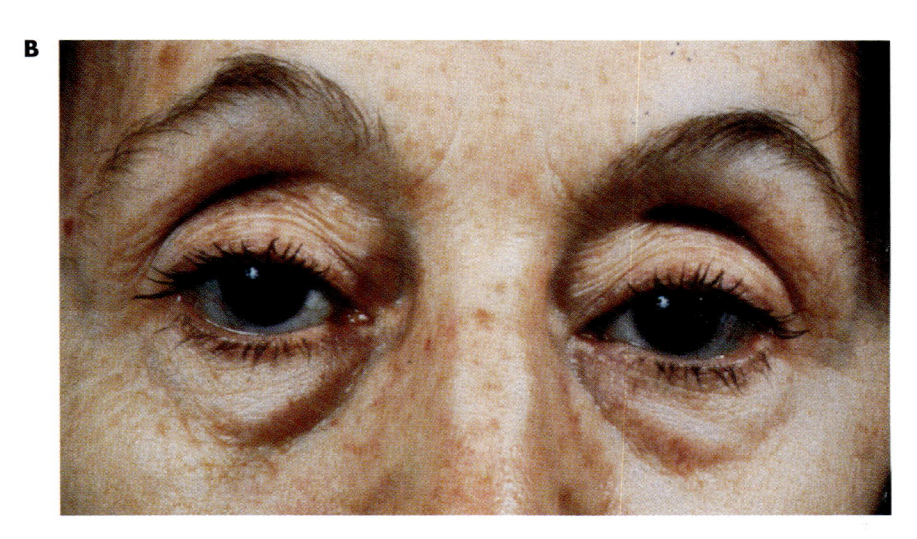

B, This patient has deep-set upper eyelids with a lack of central eyelid fat and moderate prolapse of medial eyelid fat. She has mild skin redundancy with a poorly defined supratarsal fold that is present high in the orbit associated with excess pretarsal skin show. A patient such as this requires minimal skin excision, and absolutely no central fat removal should be performed, since this will only worsen the cadaveric appearance of her upper lids.

partment. Conversely, in patients with convexity present in the orbitopalpebral sulcus associated with poorly defined or obliterated upper eyelid fold, contouring of the central fat pads will help to define the sulcus, as well as recreate a crisp and precise upper eyelid fold. It is much easier to overresect fat from the central compartment than the medial one, and a common complaint following blepharoplasty is an underresection of medial fat. As less skin is usually resected medially than centrally, resection of the medial fat often is helpful in eliminating the fullness that is commonly apparent in this portion of the eyelid and allowing the apparently redundant skin to settle posteriorly into the nasoorbital valley.

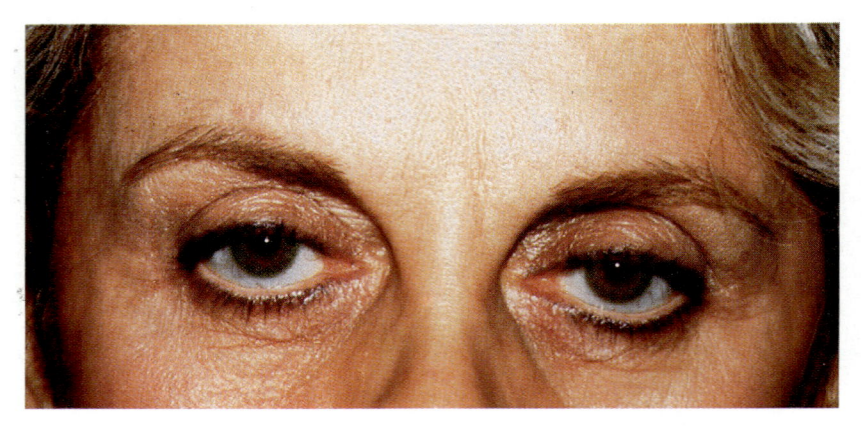

This patient is seen following an upper and lower blepharoplasty in another office. Too much fat has been removed from both the upper and lower eyelids. Note that the upper eyelids appear to be deeply set, especially on the left upper lid, where too much fat was removed from the medial portion of the central pad, an all-too-common scenario following upper eyelid blepharoplasty. These effects become even more noticeable when the patient's brows are elevated to their proper level, which accentuates the hollowness from overresection of upper eyelid fat. In the lower eyelid, an overly aggressive fat removal likewise accentuates the nasojugal groove, highlighting the outline of the bony infraorbital rim. Also note that an overresection of lower eyelid skin has led to significant scleral show in this patient and an obliteration of the normal S-shaped configuration of the lower lid. The lateral commissure now lies at a level inferior to the medial commissure.

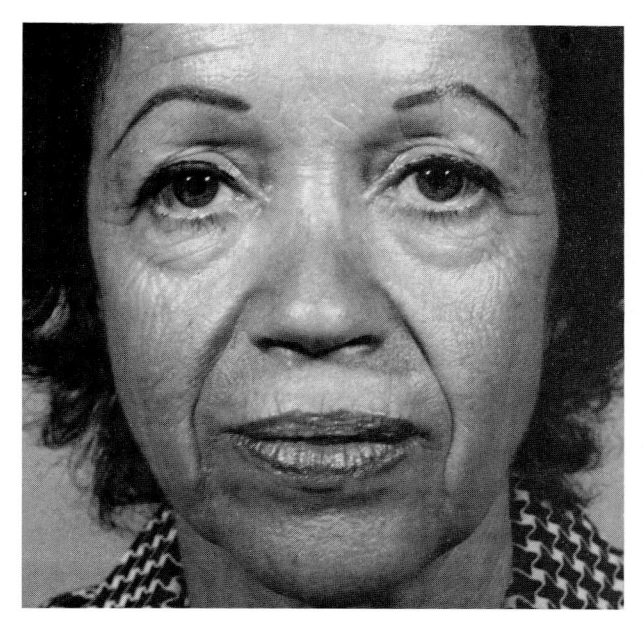

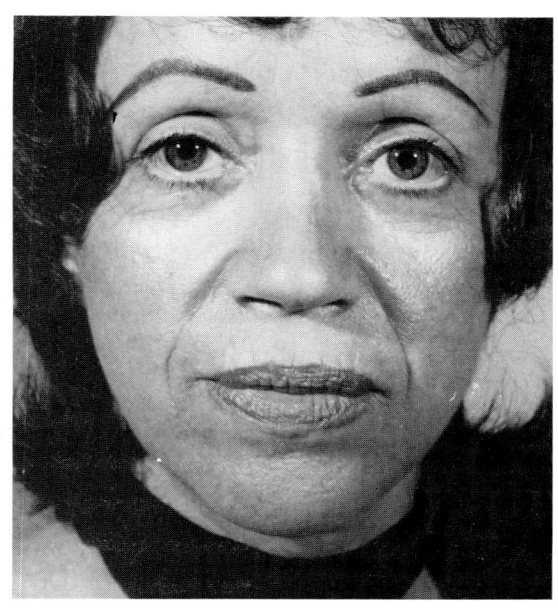

This patient requested greater definition to her upper eyelids. She is seen postoperatively following resection of redundant skin and orbicularis muscle and contouring of the upper eyelid fat. Perhaps too much fat was removed from the medial portion of the central fat pad, which has resulted in the superior palpebral sulcus appearing a bit too deep. Because the orbital septum runs cephalad along its medial extent, the medial portion of the central pad lies more posterior than the lateral portion of the central pad. For this reason it is quite easy to overresect the medial portion of the central pad; thus great care must be used contouring this portion of the fat pad to prevent overresection.

Lower Eyelids

Many elderly patients undergoing upper eyelid blepharoplasty have redundant skin within the lower eyelid, associated with wrinkling of both pretarsal and preseptal skin. Animation, squinting, or smiling often accentuates these lines; although blepharoplasty will improve this effect, it certainly will not remove all rhytides in the lower eyelid. Although skin redundancy is commonly a problem within the lower eyelid, conservatism should be the rule when performing lower eyelid resection. Many cases of scleral show or a frank ectropion have been produced by an overly aggressive resection of lower eyelid skin. Resection of skin is dictated not only by degree of skin redundancy but also by tonicity present within the lower eyelid. In patients with poor eyelid tone, preoperative scleral show, or preoperative dry eye, virtually no skin should be resected at the time of blepharoplasty. Concomitant lid tightening procedures are usually necessary in these patients.

Again, the dictum of if a little resection is good, then more resection is better seems to be an all-too-common scenario in lower lid blepharoplasty. Besides the more obvious problems of scleral show or frank ectropion, if too much skin is resected, a subtle change in lower eyelid shape commonly results. The aesthetically pleasing lower eyelid has an S-shape, high nasally, dipping lower just temporal to the limbus before swinging superiorly toward the lateral canthus. The lateral canthal angle should lie at a level slightly superior to the medial canthal angle. In lower eyelids where skin resection has been aggressively

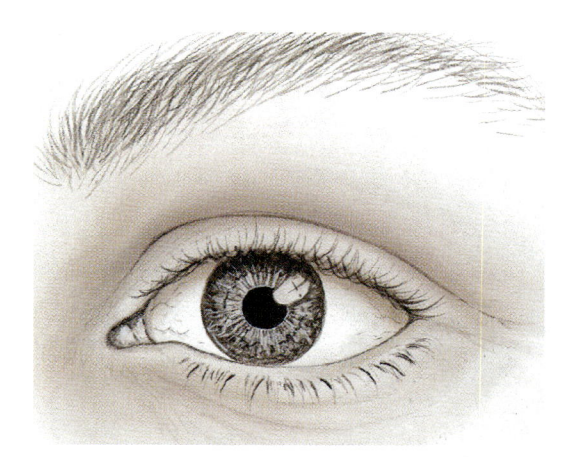

The normal configuration of the lower eyelid is essentially S-shaped. The S-shape of the lower lid begins at the medial canthus and dips down to its lowest point along the lateral aspect of the limbus before sweeping upward toward the lateral canthus. Of note, the lateral canthal insertion should be approximately 2 mm higher than the level of the medial canthus. Whether the patient exhibits scleral show in primary gaze is less important than the maintenance of a normal S-shaped curvature to the lower lid.

SURGICAL REJUVENATION OF THE FACE

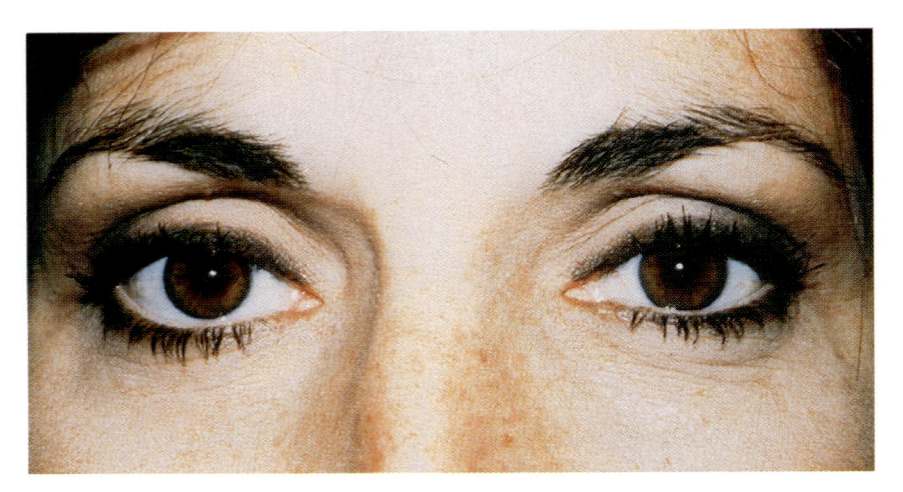

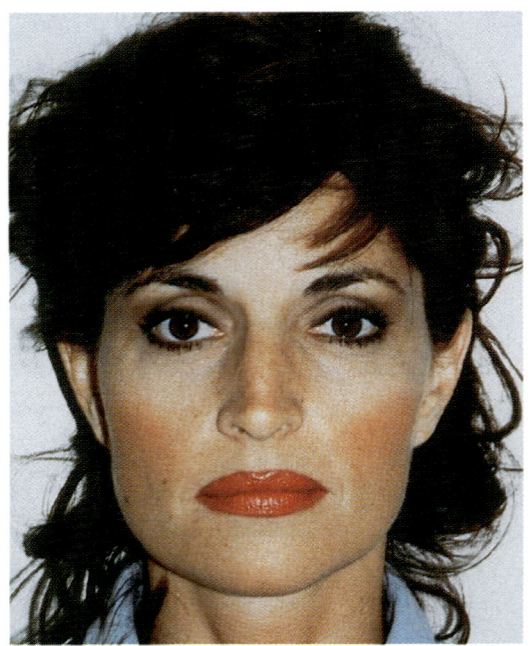

This patient is a 40-year-old model with significant asymmetries between the two sides of her face. The right brow is higher than the left brow, the right eye is larger than the left eye, and in general the right side of her face appears to be larger than the left side of her face. Note the scleral show present in primary gaze in the right eye as compared with the left eye. Nonetheless, her face is attractive and photogenic. Despite the presence of scleral show on the right side, the lower lid maintains its S-shaped configuration. Most beautiful faces are not symmetric, and the purpose of aesthetic surgery is not to restore symmetry to the face, but rather to maintain and restore natural beauty.

performed, this natural S-shape often has been changed to a U-shape, which is not aesthetically pleasing even if scleral show is not evident.

The amount of fat to be resected from each compartment is an important preoperative consideration. Having the patient gaze superiorly with the head in a neutral position will define the degree of excess fat present within the lower eyelids, as well as delineate the com-

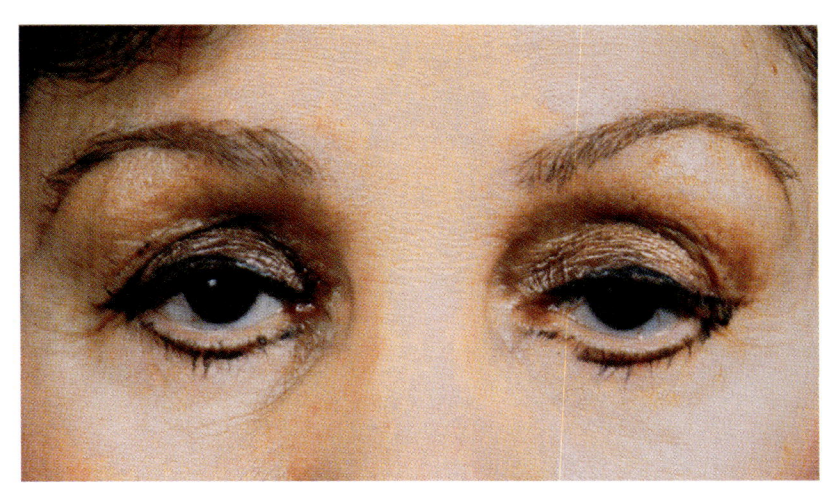

This patient is seen following an upper and lower blepharoplasty performed in another office. Note the position of the lower eyelid. In primary gaze, 2 mm of scleral show is evident. The normal S-shaped configuration of the lower lid is absent, and now the lateral canthal angle lies at or below the level of the medial canthal angle with lid retraction most noted on the left side. Note also an overresection of fat present in the upper eyelids, especially in view of the prominence of her supraorbital rims. She also exhibits a moderate degree of upper lid ptosis associated with a high supratarsal crease.

partments where the extra fat is present. Although it is important to resect and contour the fat of the lower eyelid, it is equally important not to overly remove the fat and produce a hollowed-out or cadaveric look to the lower eyelid. This is most commonly seen medially along the nasal jugal fold in the lower eyelids. The most common fat pad missed in lower blepharoplasty is the lateral pad. This is usually secondary not only to its superior temporal location but also to the fact that the fat present in the lateral fat pad often is quite fibrous and can be difficult to deliver into the operative field. Preoperatively, the surgeon should have a good idea how much fat will be removed from each compartment. If on preoperative examination a large amount of fat is present laterally, and this amount is not found at the time of exploration, perhaps a bit more time should be spent ensuring that an accurate exploration of this area is performed before closure.

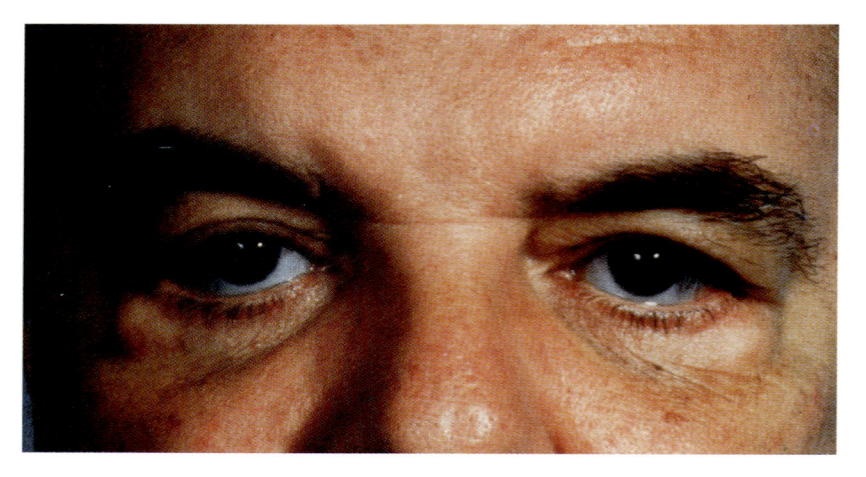

This patient is seen following upper and lower blepharoplasty performed in another office, during which both lateral pads were underresected. Also note the significant amount of scleral show present in the lower eyelid and the loss of the normal S-shaped configuration of the lower eyelid secondary to poor lid tonicity associated with excessive skin removal.

Laxity of the lower eyelid

Laxity of the lower eyelid is common as people age. This phenomenon is secondary to either dehiscence or attenuation of the lateral canthal tendon and usually is associated with a round appearance of the lateral canthal angle. The evaluation and treatment of the lax lid will be discussed later in this chapter. Suffice it to say that recognition of poor eyelid tone is extremely important when planning lower eyelid blepharoplasty. Both the degree of skin resection and the need to restore tone to the lower eyelid must be addressed at the time of blepharoplasty.

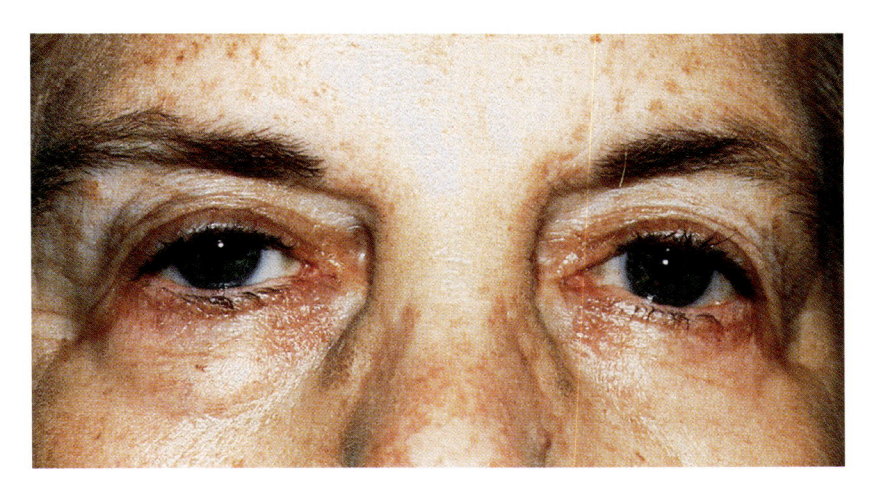

Patient seen with the typical stigmata of lateral canthal disinsertion, which is more obvious in the left lower eyelid. Note the significant descent of the lateral commissure in relation to the medial commissure and loss of the S-shaped curvature to the lower lid. Also note that the lateral canthal angle lies several millimeters medial to the lateral orbital rim denoting the degree of lateral canthal tendon disinsertion. This type of patient requires formal reattachment of the lateral canthal tendon to the periosteum to both improve the position of the lower eyelid and prevent worsening of scleral show in the postoperative period.

Considerations of the Exophthalmic Eye

Patients with a mild to moderate degree of proptosis of the globe deserve certain considerations. These patients will exhibit bulging of the globe associated with a fullness of the superopalpebral crease and an increase in scleral show, especially laterally.

The possibility of thyroid disease should be considered and appropriately evaluated. The proptotic-appearing globe is commonly a normal variation and can be associated with myopia. In these patients blepharoplasty must be performed very cautiously. Removal of fat both in the upper and lower eyelid must be performed conservatively or these patients will commonly look hollowed-out postoperatively, aggravating the appearance of their proptosis. In a similar fashion, resection of skin in the lower eyelid should be kept at a minimum, since any lid retraction that occurs postoperatively will magnify the degree of proptosis apparent preoperatively.

In patients with exophthalmus, consideration should also be given to lateral canthopexy. These patients commonly exhibit a lateral canthus that is posteriorly and inferiorly positioned relative to the globe. A blepharoplasty that results in worsening scleral show on these types of individuals can be improved by repositioning the lateral canthus, restoring lateral canthal support.

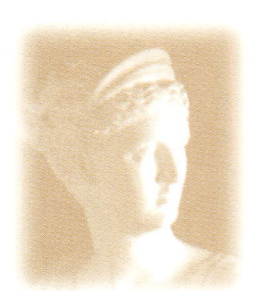

SUMMARY

Goals of Upper Eyelid Blepharoplasty

The planning of the upper eyelid blepharoplasty involves the following objectives:

1. Removal of sufficient redundant upper eyelid skin.
2. Production of an area of well-defined pretarsal skin with a defined supratarsal fold.
3. Creation of symmetric, inconspicuous scars, a clearly defined orbitopalpebral sulcus, and symmetrical upper eyelids.

Goals of Lower Eyelid Blepharoplasty

Surgery of the lower eyelid with appropriate resection of skin and muscle leaves very little margin for error. Overresection is unforgiving. The preoperative plan should consider the following:

1. Amount of skin to be removed.
2. Amount of fat to be resected.
3. Which compartments require resection and how much.
4. Necessity for some form of lid tightening procedure or consideration for lower lid support in the perioperative period.

OPERATIVE TECHNIQUE: UPPER BLEPHAROPLASTY

Preoperative Preparation

The patient is instructed to remove all eye and facial makeup before coming to the operating suite and to wash his or her face thoroughly on the morning of surgery.

The patient is placed in a comfortable position on the operating table and is adequately premedicated. After the intravenous route has been established and the monitoring equipment is in place, the surgical preparation is performed. This consists of applying Betadine solution to the entire face and eyelids, carefully avoiding the conjunctival surface. No medications are instilled onto the surface of the globe.

Anesthesia

Adequate premedication is essential. An intravenous route is always established, and the patient is monitored carefully. A suggested routine is to give the patient diazepam by mouth 45 minutes preoperatively and fentanyl (Sublimaze) intravenously 5 to 10 minutes before surgery. Approximately 5 to 7.5 mg of midazolam (Versed) and 2 ml or 0.1 mg of fentanyl is suggested for a 50 kg, 50-year-old woman, titrated over a period of time. Ketamine may also be used.

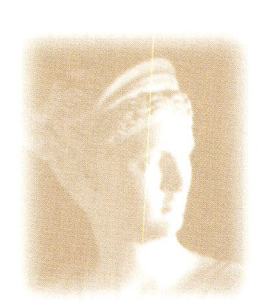

We prefer to use local anesthesia for this procedure, since general anesthesia carries additional risks and unnecessary costs. The local anesthetic agent of choice is lidocaine 1% with epinephrine 1:100,000 administered through a 27-gauge needle, using dental Carpules and syringes. By using small amounts of anesthetic solution injected with fine needles, the volume of injected solution is kept to a minimum, thereby obliterating fewer landmarks because of unnecessary distortion.

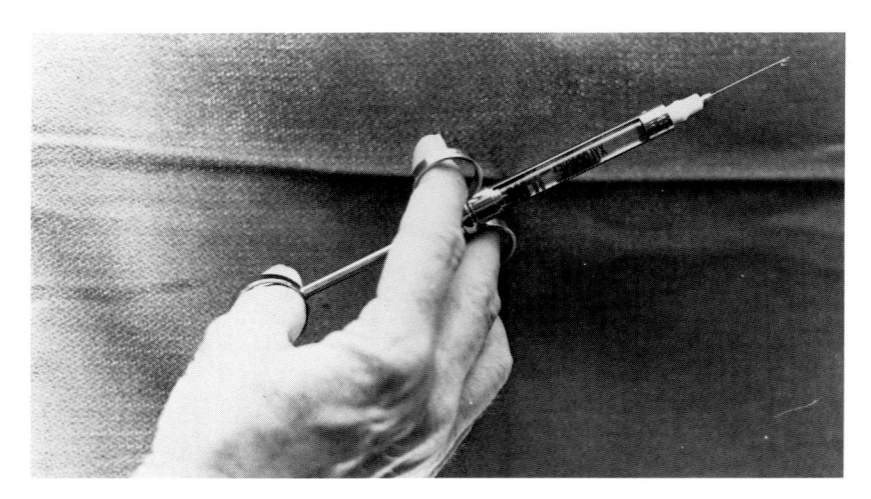

This dental syringe is well suited for local anesthesia when small volumes of the anesthetic agent are indicated, such as in blepharoplasty. The 27-gauge needle and 1.8 ml volume in the disposable Carpule also aid in keeping the volume injected to a minimum, thus reducing tissue distortion.

Incision Placement

The inferior limb of the elliptical incision performed in the upper eyelid is usually placed adjacent to the supratarsal crease. As stated earlier, the level of the crease varies between 8 and 12 mm superior to the lid margin, and although it is well defined in most patients, it is poorly defined in others. Having patients slowly open and close their eyes as they are being marked is helpful in determining their supratarsal fold. If the upper lid crease is poorly defined or abnormally low, the lower limb of the incision can be placed 10 mm superior to the eyelid margin. This placement enables the surgeon to obtain a well-defined segment of visible pretarsal skin. The placement of this incision should be accurately measured with calipers or a ruler. If it is elected to form a new supratarsal crease rather than use the patient's original crease, consideration should be given to supratarsal fixation to define the new crease, at the termination of the procedure.

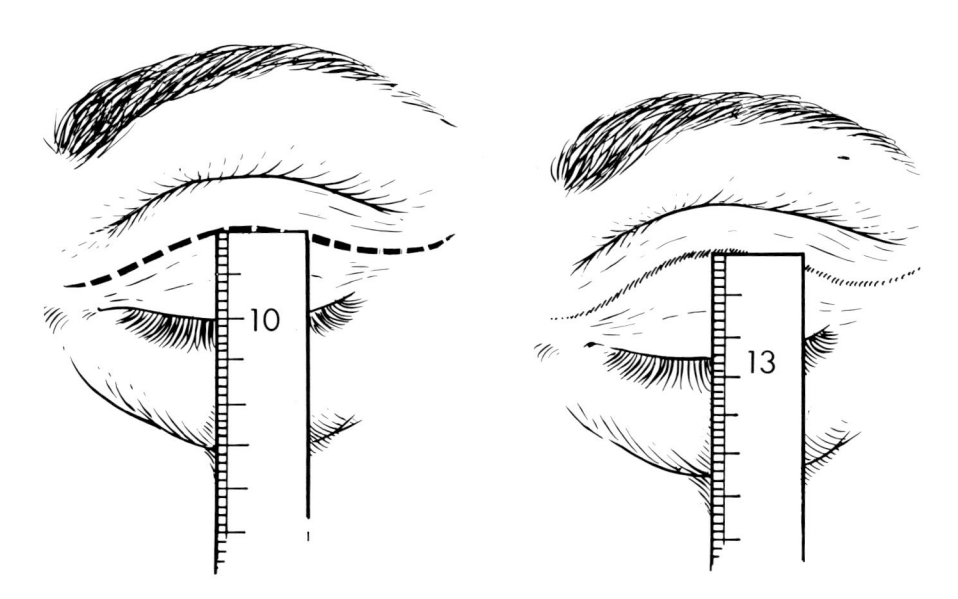

Placement of the lower limb of the incision is usually at the level of the naturally occurring supratarsal fold, approximately 10 mm above the lid margin. Note that over time the incision appears to migrate superiorly, which is related to the tension of the skin closure. It is important that the final incision lie within the naturally occurring supratarsal fold, so that when the patient's eyes are open in primary gaze the incision is well concealed.

The medial extension of the incision is usually the medial extension of the naturally occurring upper eyelid fold. More medial excision is possible if significant redundancy exists.

The major disadvantage of extending skin resection medial to the caruncle is that the incision will be visible in this region when the eyelid is open. Under no circumstances should the incision extend onto nasal skin along the nasoorbital valley, as not only will a noticeable scar occur, but transverse scar contraction or webbing will commonly also result.

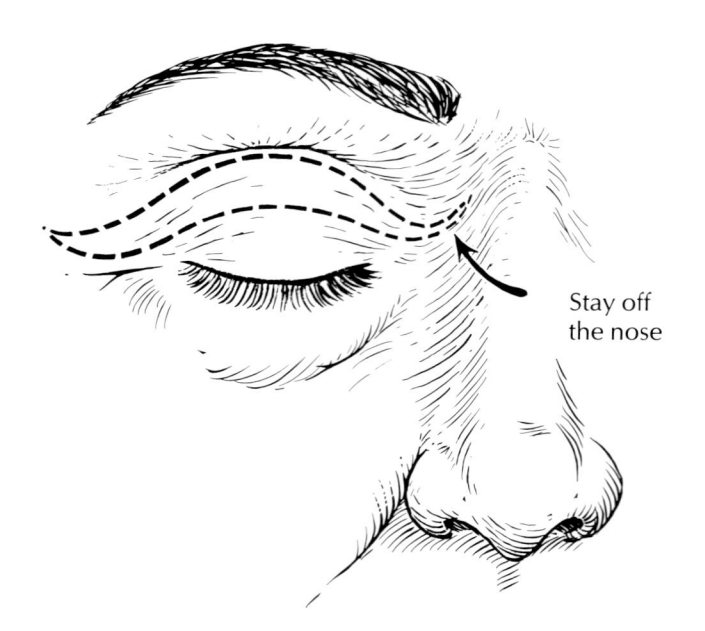

If the upper eyelid incision is extended onto nasal skin, a transverse scar contracture or webbing will occur.

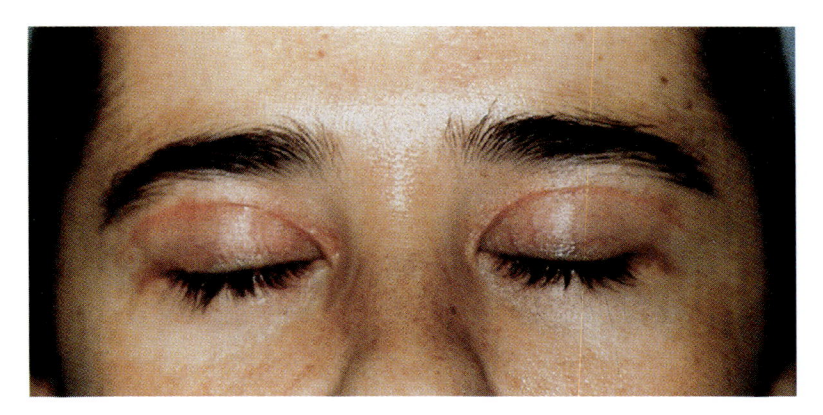

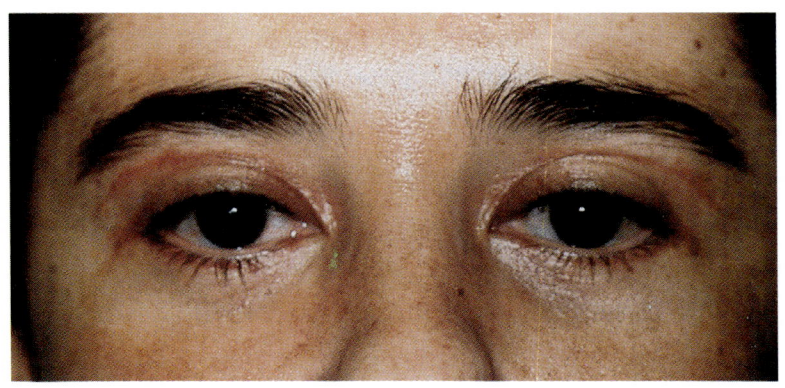

Patient is seen approximately 1 month following upper lid blepharoplasty performed in another office. Note that the incision has been placed well above the supratarsal fold, extending medially into the nasoorbital valley, and a large amount of upper eyelid skin has apparently been resected. In primary gaze, the incision now lies well above the naturally occurring supratarsal fold, which makes it visible. Because of the large amount of upper eyelid skin resected, notice that the lateral portion of the brow has been pulled inferiorly, producing a sad expression to her face. Note also that the incision extending medially into the nasoorbital valley has produced an apparent epicanthal fold or webbing in this region, which can be difficult to correct.

The temporal extension of the incision should correspond to the degree of redundancy present laterally. This can be ascertained when the patient is sitting and staring straight ahead. When marking the patient who is on the operating room table, it is simple after marking the lateral extent of the supratarsal crease to just extend the lateral excision toward one of the normally occurring crow's feet. Having the patient then look superiorly will commonly delineate the excess skin present laterally. This usually measures between 12 and 15 mm from the lateral canthus and should be measured to ensure symmetry in lateral skin resection. The lateral incision should not cross the lateral orbital rim.

In marking the superior aspect of the elliptical incision, the surgeon should try to accurately determine the degree of redundancy present in upper eyelid skin. Careful inspection of upper eyelid skin will commonly demarcate the darker wrinkled redundant skin of the upper eyelid (to be excised) from the preorbital and brow skin that should not be resected. Another useful method is to gently approximate the redundant eyelid skin with forceps, lifting the eyelid skin in a superior fashion and noting where the excess tissues meet. The upper incision should be designed so that pinching of eyelid skin between upper and lower limbs of the ellipses produces only slight movement of the upper lid eyelashes, but not a superior retraction of the upper eyelid. This will ensure a conservative removal of upper lid skin, avoiding the consequence of overresection. It is much easier to remove a bit more skin as a secondary procedure than it is to correct an aggressive resection of upper eyelid skin.

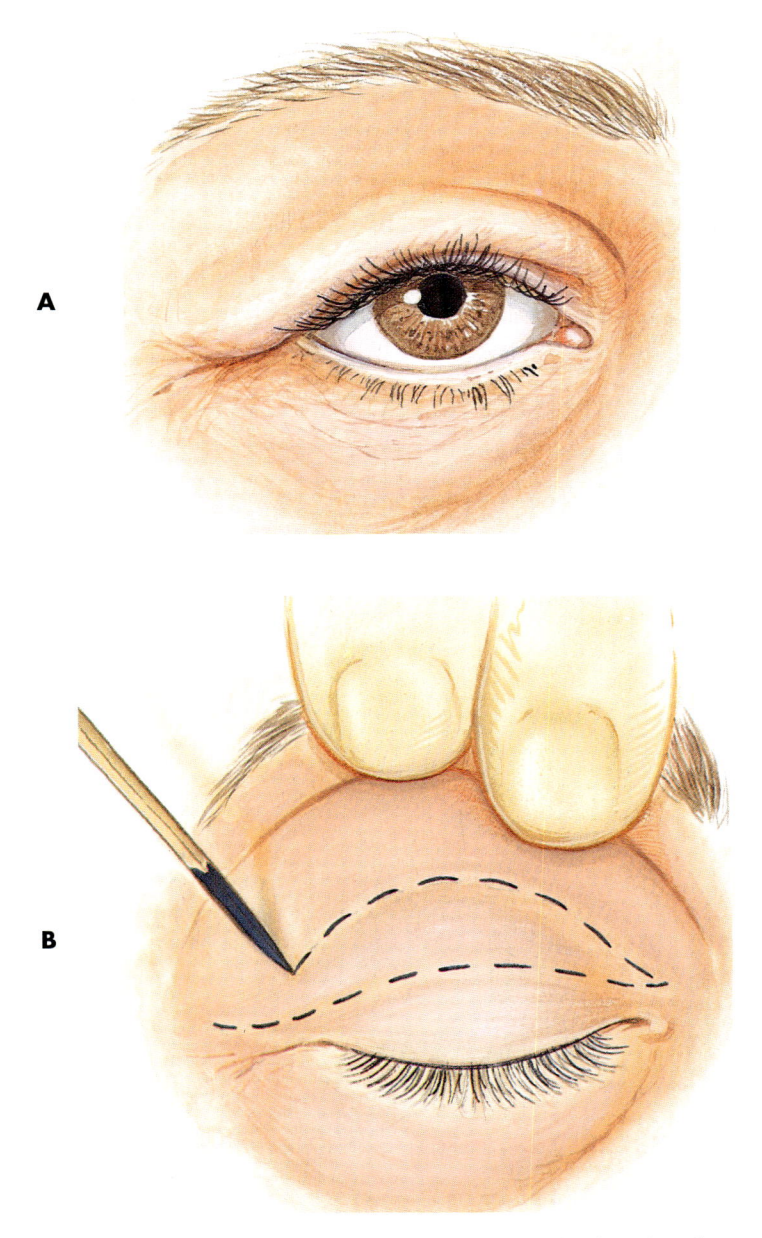

A, *On inspecting the upper eyelid, there is a marked redundancy of the skin, a protrusion of intraorbital fat.* **B,** *The usual incision is made 10 mm from the eyelid margin, corresponding to the superior edge of the tarsal plate.*

SURGICAL REJUVENATION OF THE FACE

■ Muscle and Fat Resection

A resection of orbicularis muscle, averaging 3 mm in width, is then performed. This excised muscle strip extends along the entire width of the upper eyelid and parallels the superior margin of the tarsus. Great care is used when resecting muscle in the region of the supratarsal fold because of the fusion that occurs between the orbicularis and the levator aponeurosis in this region. When resecting orbicularis muscle, it is important to prevent injury to the underlying levator aponeurosis. The removal of this muscle strip commonly will help to define the supratarsal fold. It also provides good visualization of the underlying orbital septum and upper eyelid fat.

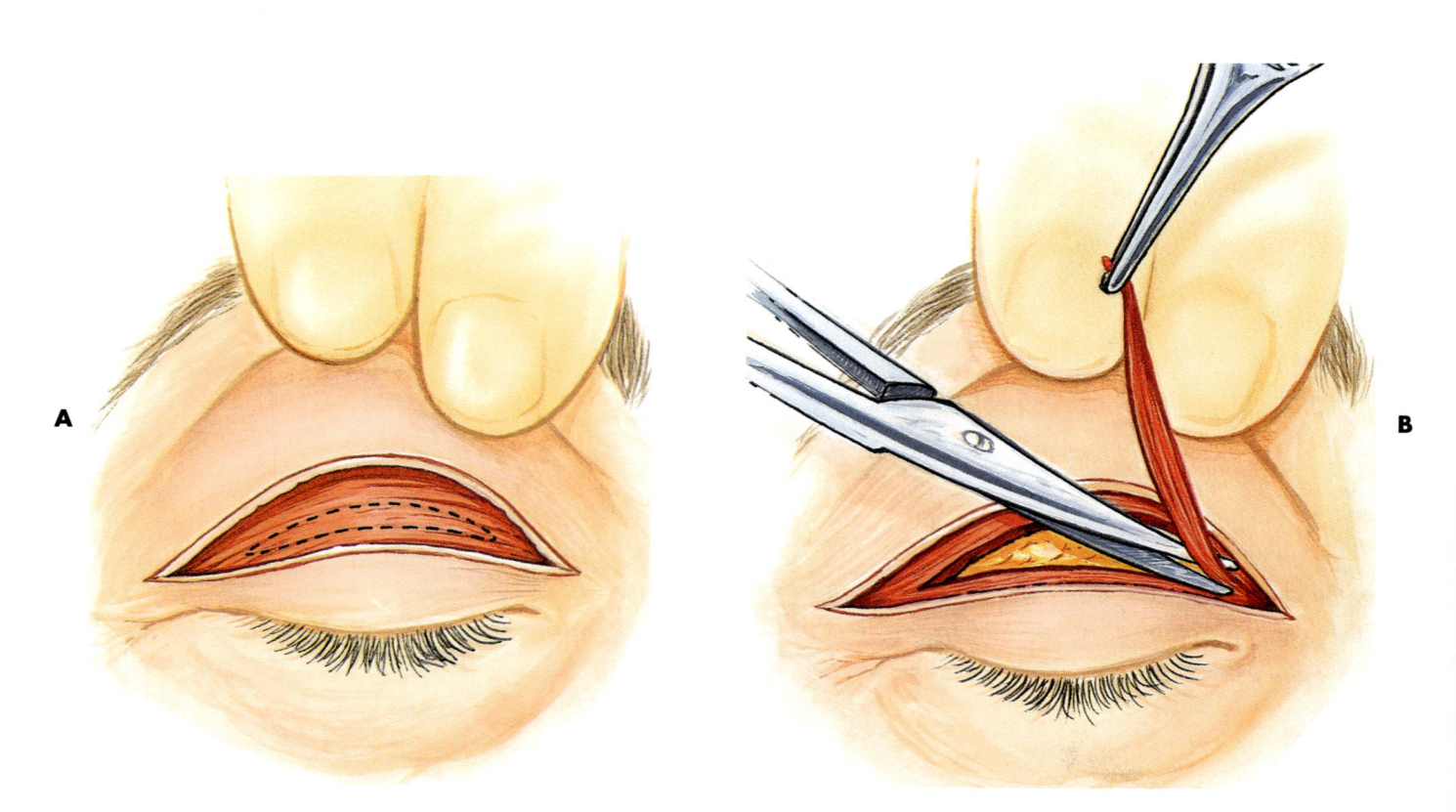

A, After the skin has been excised, the orbicularis muscle is inspected and approximately 3 mm of muscle will be excised. B, After the skin has been removed, a strip of orbicularis muscle is excised. This exposes the septum orbitale with the underlying fat pads in their respective pockets.

In most blepharoplasties the orbital septum is opened along its entire length. The orbital septum should be opened directly anterior to the orbital fat and well superior to the area where the septum merges with the levator aponeurosis. Opening the orbital septum along its entirety exposes the central preaponeurotic fat pad and allows access to the medial fat pad.

Central fat resection is performed along preoperative guidelines for contouring of the fat. Commonly, the sausage-shaped central fat pad is removed beginning along its lateral extent. Conservatism is the hallmark of contouring the medial portion of the central pad, with emphasis on prevention of overresection.

The medial fat pad is then opened through a puncture of the orbital septum. In a similar fashion, excess fat present within the compartment is delivered, clamped, and secured with the use of electrocautery.

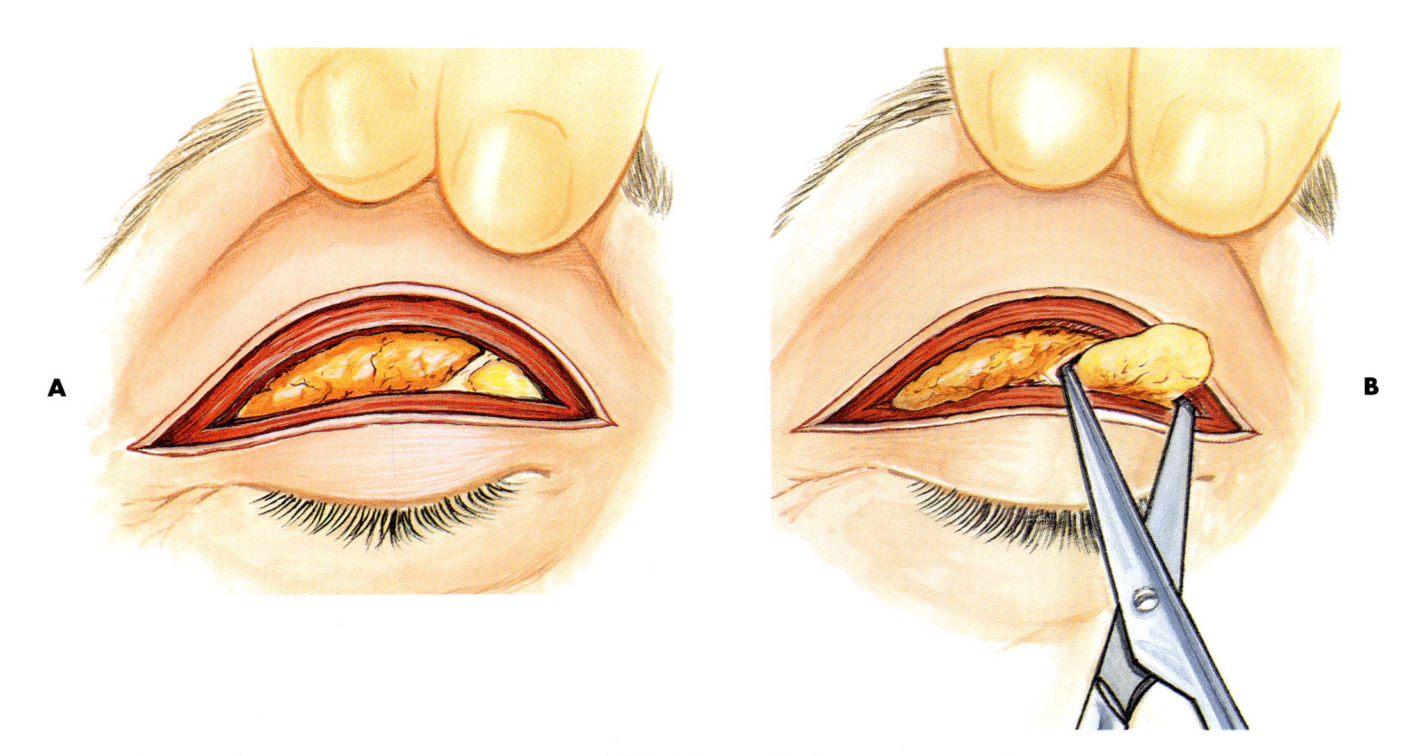

A, The two fat compartments are now visible. The medial compartment is usually smaller and the fat has a lighter yellow color than the fat in the larger lateral compartment. B, The fat pads are gently eased partially into the wound.

Continued.

SURGICAL REJUVENATION OF THE FACE

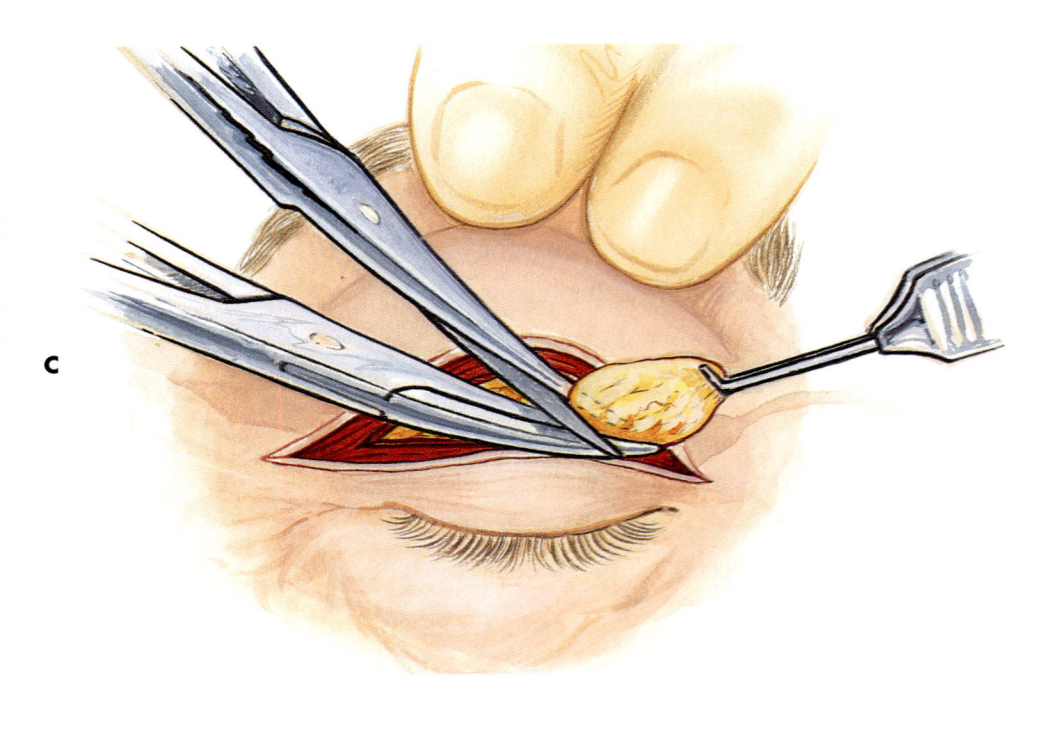

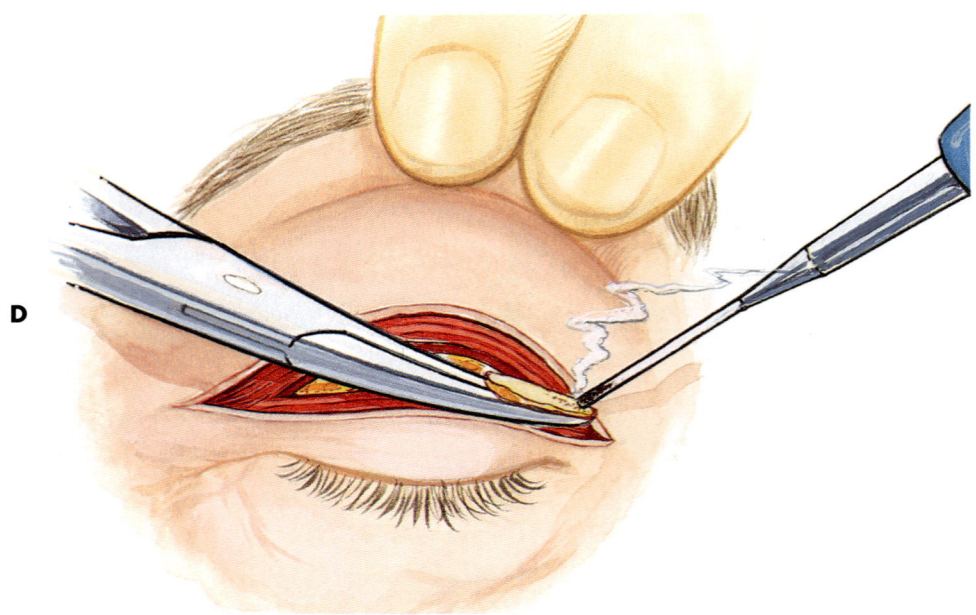

C, The fat pads are clamped and the excess is removed. D, The fatty stumps are electrocoagulated.

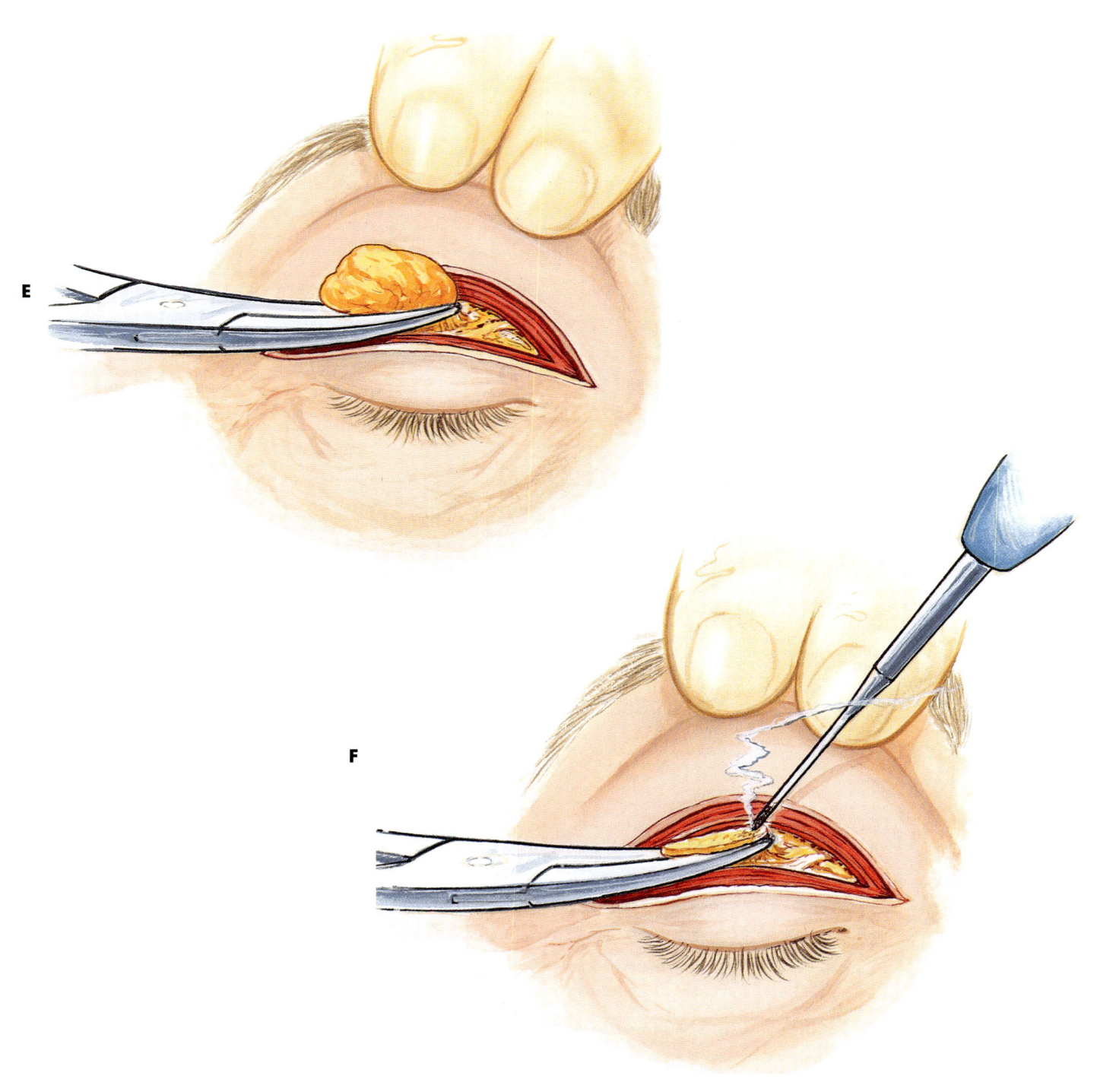

E, *The central fat pad usually is larger than the medial fat pad and has a deeper, yellow color.* ***F,*** *The central fat pad stump is electrocoagulated.*

SURGICAL REJUVENATION OF THE FACE

Before closing the upper eyelid wound, the lateral aspect of the upper rim of the incision is usually inspected for protruding fat from the brow fat pad. This fat, as noted previously, sits in a location deep to the orbicularis oculi muscle and superficial to the orbital septum. This retroorbicularis fat is commonly abundant in patients who are undergoing upper eyelid blepharoplasty with concomitant brow ptosis. A judicious contouring of this fat, usually done with an electrocautery, will serve to reduce fullness in the lateral upper lid and help to delineate the lateral supraorbital rim in the postoperative period.

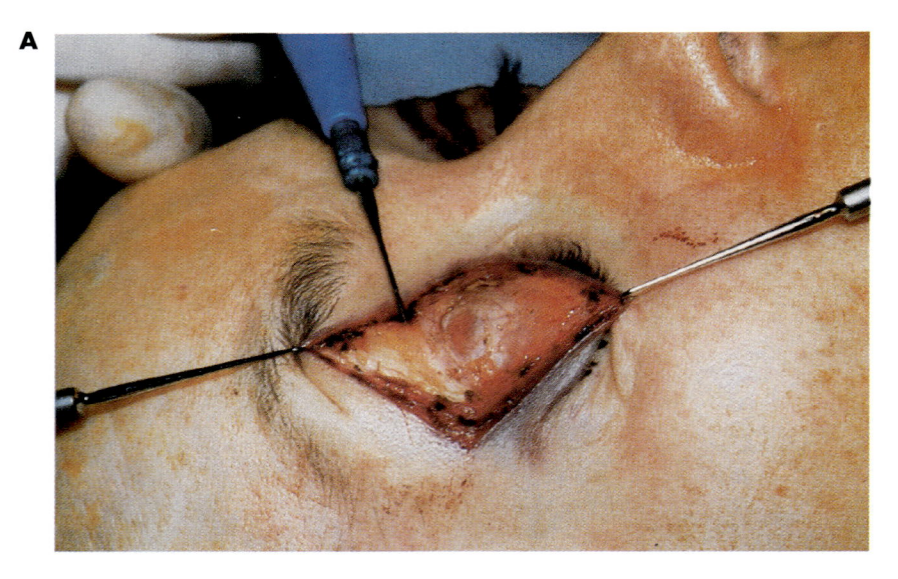

A, *Judicious contouring of the caudal aspect of the brow pad (ROOF) will help contour the lateral orbital rim and remove some of the bulk present in patients who have concomitant ptosis of the brow pad associated with blepharochalasis. This fat is identified along the lateral orbital rim sitting directly posterior to the orbicularis muscle and lying superficial to both orbital septum and orbital fat.*

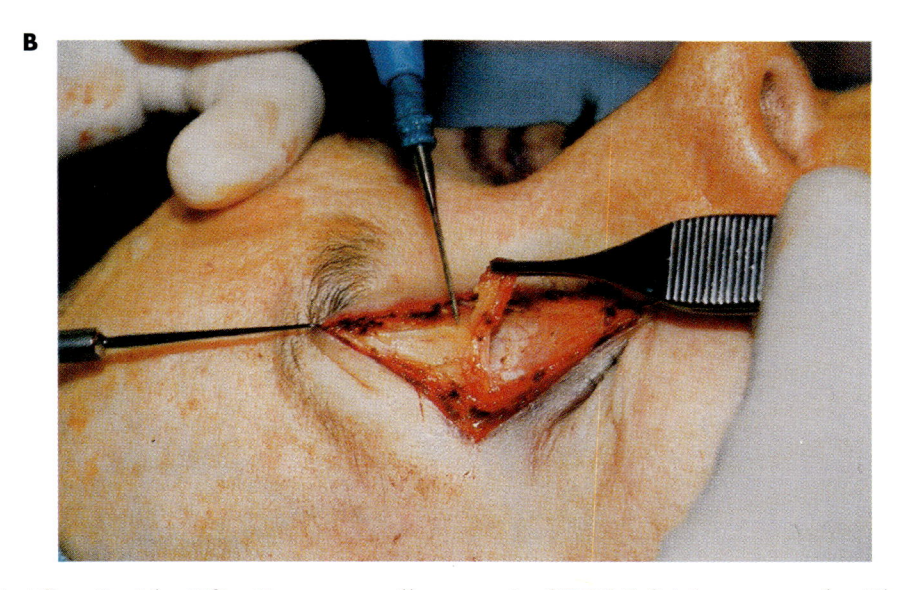

B, After its identification, a small amount of ROOF fat is removed with the use of electrocautery to help define the lateral orbital rim. Conservatism in resection of ROOF fat is important; whereas the lateral orbital rim remains a bit more defined, its appearance remains soft rather than harsh, which can result from an overresection of brow fat.

◼ Closure

The skin edges are approximated with a subcuticular pull-out suture of 5-0 nylon or a running suture of 6-0 or 7-0 monofilament nylon; either works well.

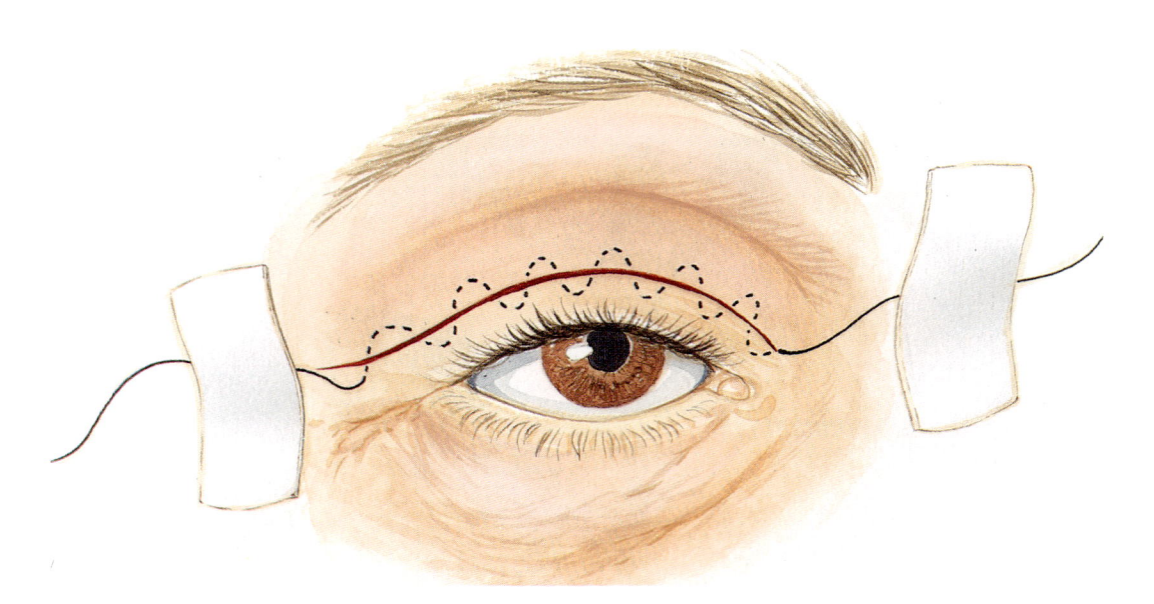

The skin edges are approximated with a 5-0 monofilament nylon pull-out suture.

Supratarsal Fixation

Supratarsal fixation is a technique used to restore and define a crisp eyelid crease. As we have gained more experience with this technique, we have found lid invagination procedures to be helpful in obtaining a crisp, well-defined, lasting supratarsal crease, which enhances pretarsal skin show. In those individuals who do not have a well-defined crease preoperatively, supratarsal fixation serves as an alternative to the overresection of skin and muscle. Supratarsal fixation is an anatomic procedure in that the upper lid crease can be reconstructed in a precise and controlled fashion following upper lid blepharoplasty.

Although many techniques have been described to reconstruct the upper eyelid crease, the technique that we use is quite simple and is performed just before closure. The most common problem with supratarsal fixation is the possibility of creating the upper eyelid crease at asymmetrical levels. For this reason it is imperative that the lower limb of the skin excision be at exactly the same level bilaterally. In performing the procedure it is necessary to remove the orbicularis that is present directly along the length of the inferior incision, exposing the cephalad margin of the tarsus. This must be performed carefully, as it is in this location that the orbicularis muscle is in close proximity with the levator aponeurosis. With sharp dissection, the orbicularis muscle is removed so that the muscle does not intervene between the overlying dermis, tarsal border, and underlying levator aponeurosis. Three 6-0 nylon sutures are then placed (central, medial, and lateral), securing skin along the superior border of the tarsus inferiorly to the underlying levator aponeurosis. The fixation is completed by suturing a full thickness bit of skin along the superior limb of the elliptical skin excision. These three sutures are then tied bilaterally and the patient is asked to open his or her eyes to ensure the presence of a symmetrical lid crease. Closure is then performed as described previously.

SURGICAL REJUVENATION OF THE FACE

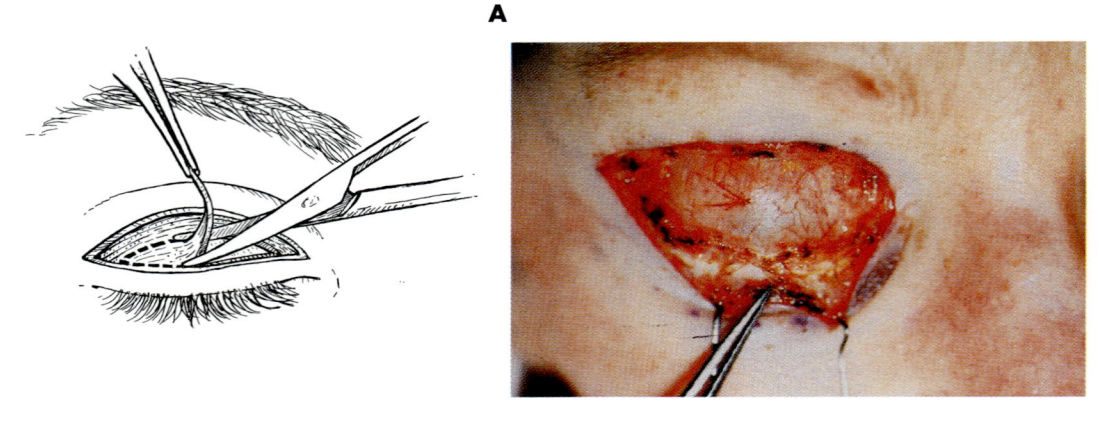

A, In performing supratarsal fixation, it is necessary to remove the orbicularis muscle situated between the inferior limb of the skin incision and the underlying levator aponeurosis. This will expose the superior border of the tarsal plate (forceps).

BLEPHAROPLASTY

B

C

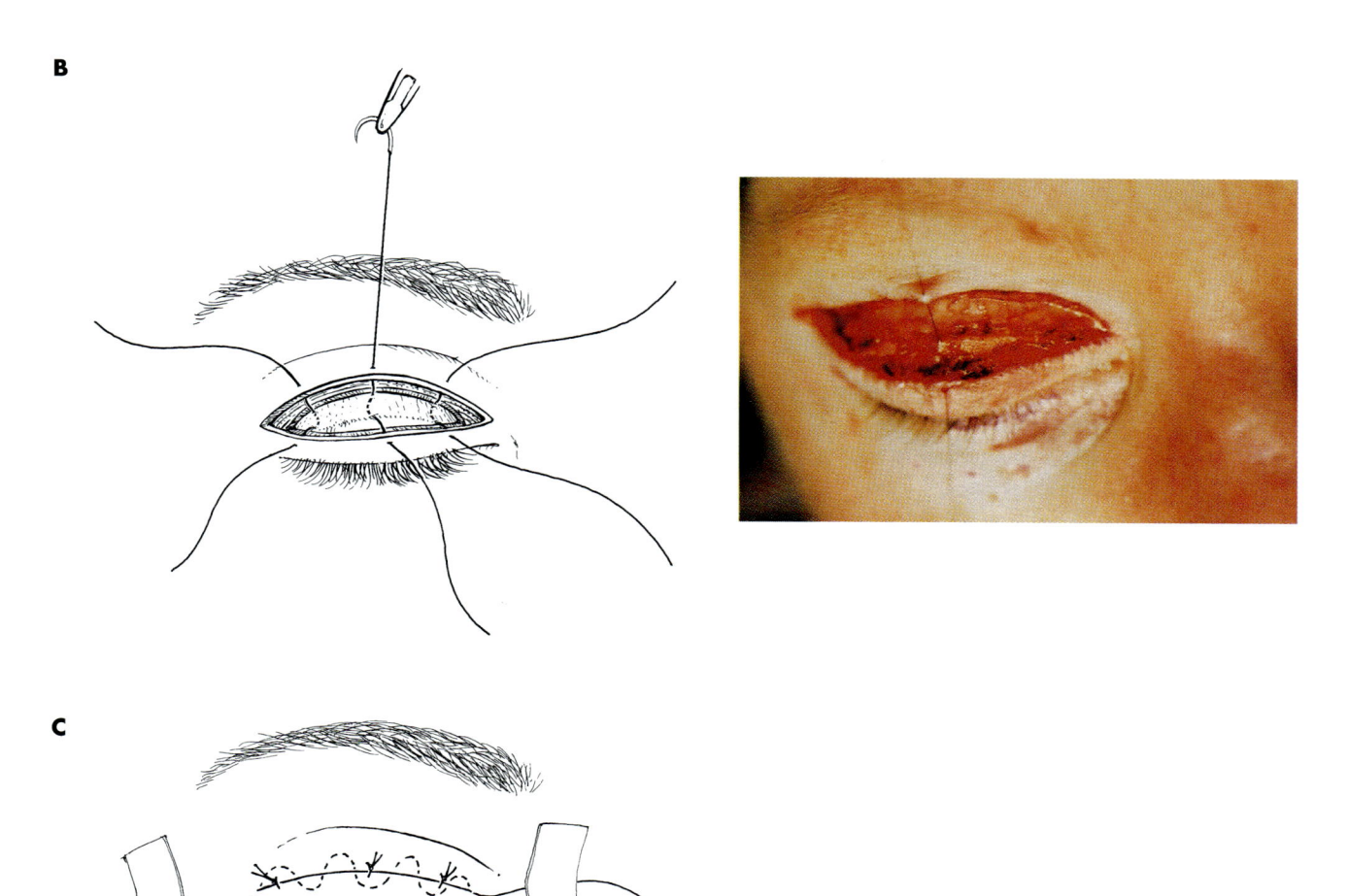

B and C, An interrupted suture is then placed along the center of the incision, going from skin through the levator aponeurosis just superior to the tarsal plate and then extending into the skin of the upper limb of the incision. To complete the supratarsal fixation, similar sutures are placed both medially and laterally, securing the margin of the skin excision to the levator aponeurosis just superior to the tarsus. These sutures are then ligated to create an adhesion between the superior aspect of the pretarsal skin and the underlying levator aponeurosis. When the patient then opens the eyes, there is a well-defined supratarsal fold. Eyelid closure is then performed in the standard fashion.

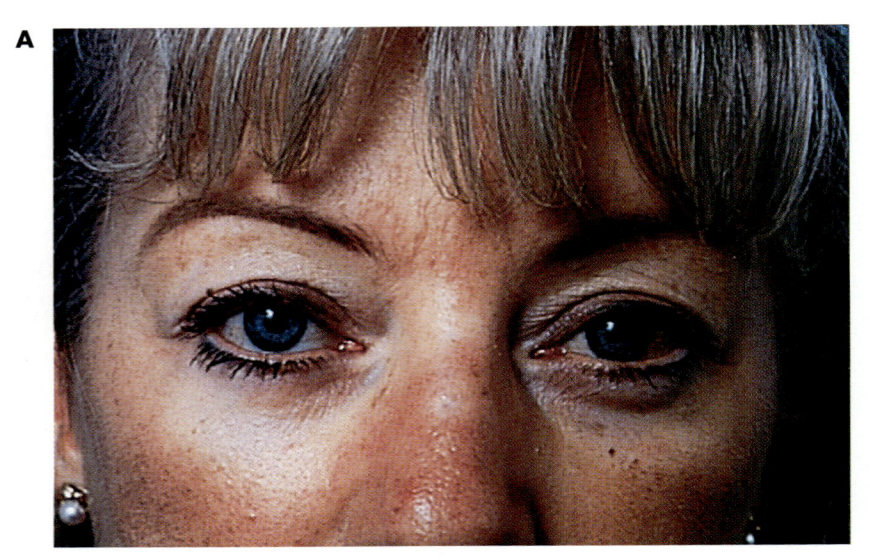

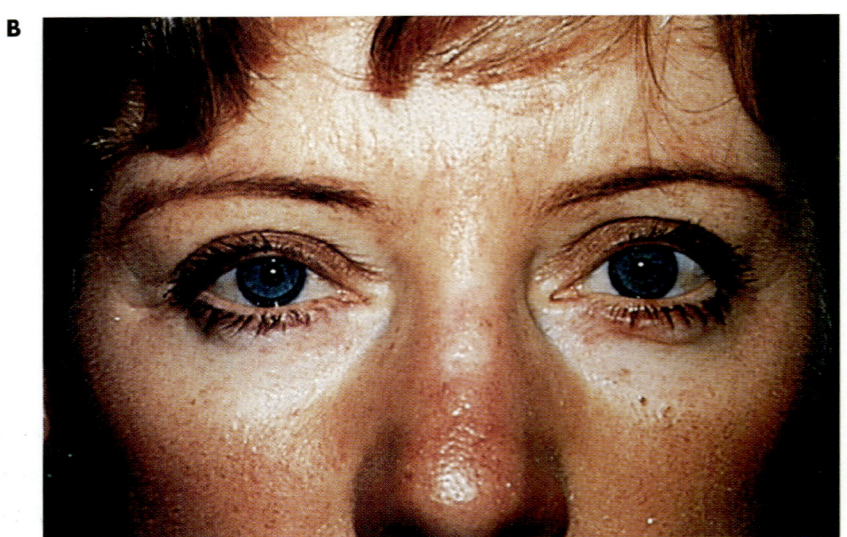

A, Patient is seen preoperatively following a previous upper lid blepharoplasty performed in another office. Note the significant amount of upper eyelid hooding associated with the poorly-defined supratarsal fold. B, Postoperative result following a limited skin excision of the upper eyelid associated with supratarsal fixation.

LOWER EYELID BLEPHAROPLASTY

The skin flap and the skin-muscle flap are the two basic operative procedures commonly used for lower eyelid surgery.

■ Placement of Incisions

With either procedure, the skin incision is placed approximately 2 mm below the ciliary margin of the lower eyelid, extending it into one of the natural creases laterally. We try to leave approximately 7 to 10 mm between the lateral aspect of the upper and lower blepharoplasty incisions and limit the extension of the lateral incision.

■ Skin Flap

If a skin flap is used, the skin is carefully separated from the underlying orbicularis muscle. The subdermal plane is relatively avascular, especially when the epinephrine effect is pronounced. Hemostasis is obtained with the electrocautery unit, but this should be used conservatively to avoid damaging the overlying skin. We do not apply a topical anesthetic to the eye surface to avoid anesthetizing the cornea and exposing it to possible irritation during surgery.

SURGICAL REJUVENATION OF THE FACE

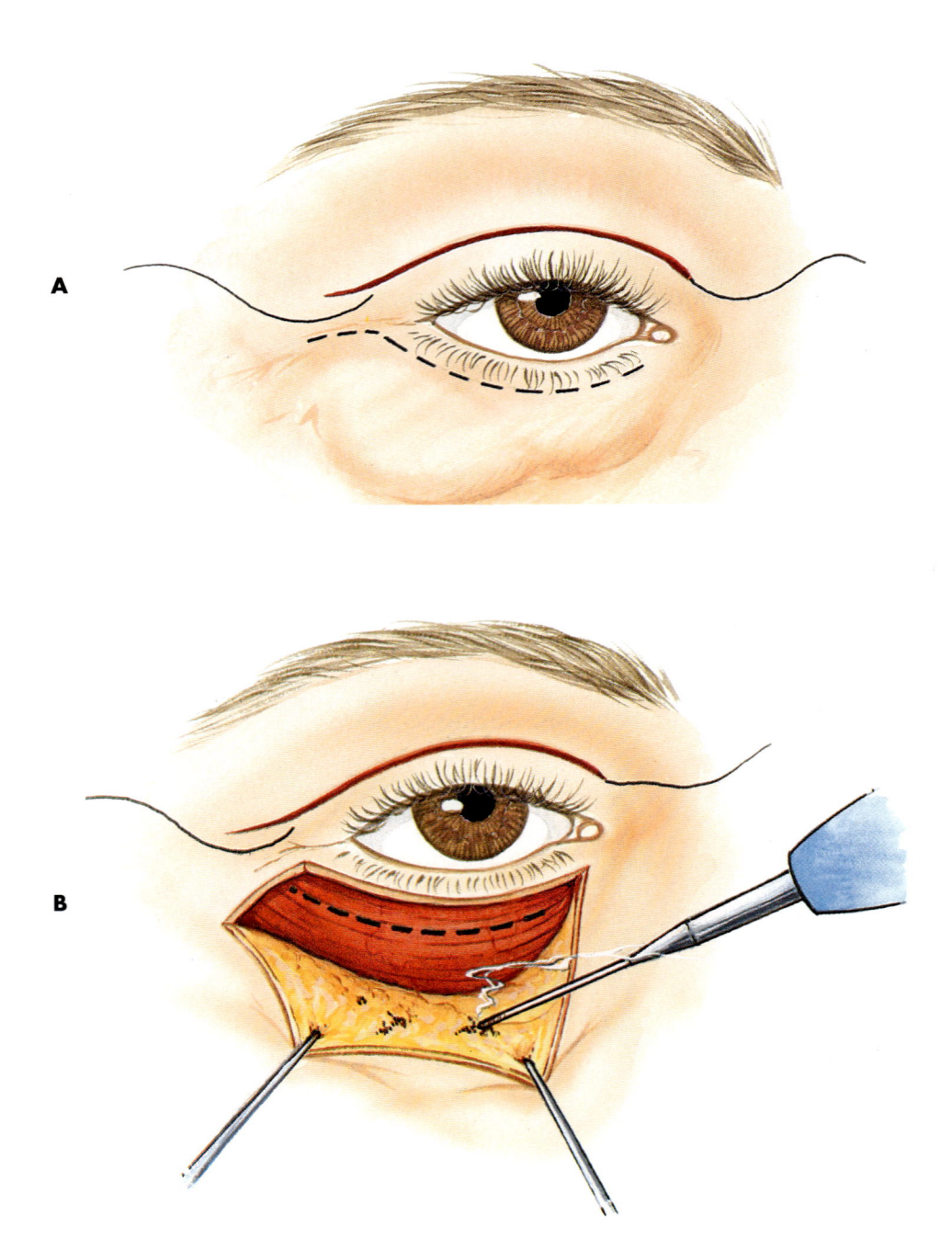

A, The usual lower eyelid incision. *B,* The skin flap is elevated, and bleeding is controlled with the electrocautery. The dotted line indicates where the muscle is divided by blunt dissection to expose underlying fat compartments.

BLEPHAROPLASTY

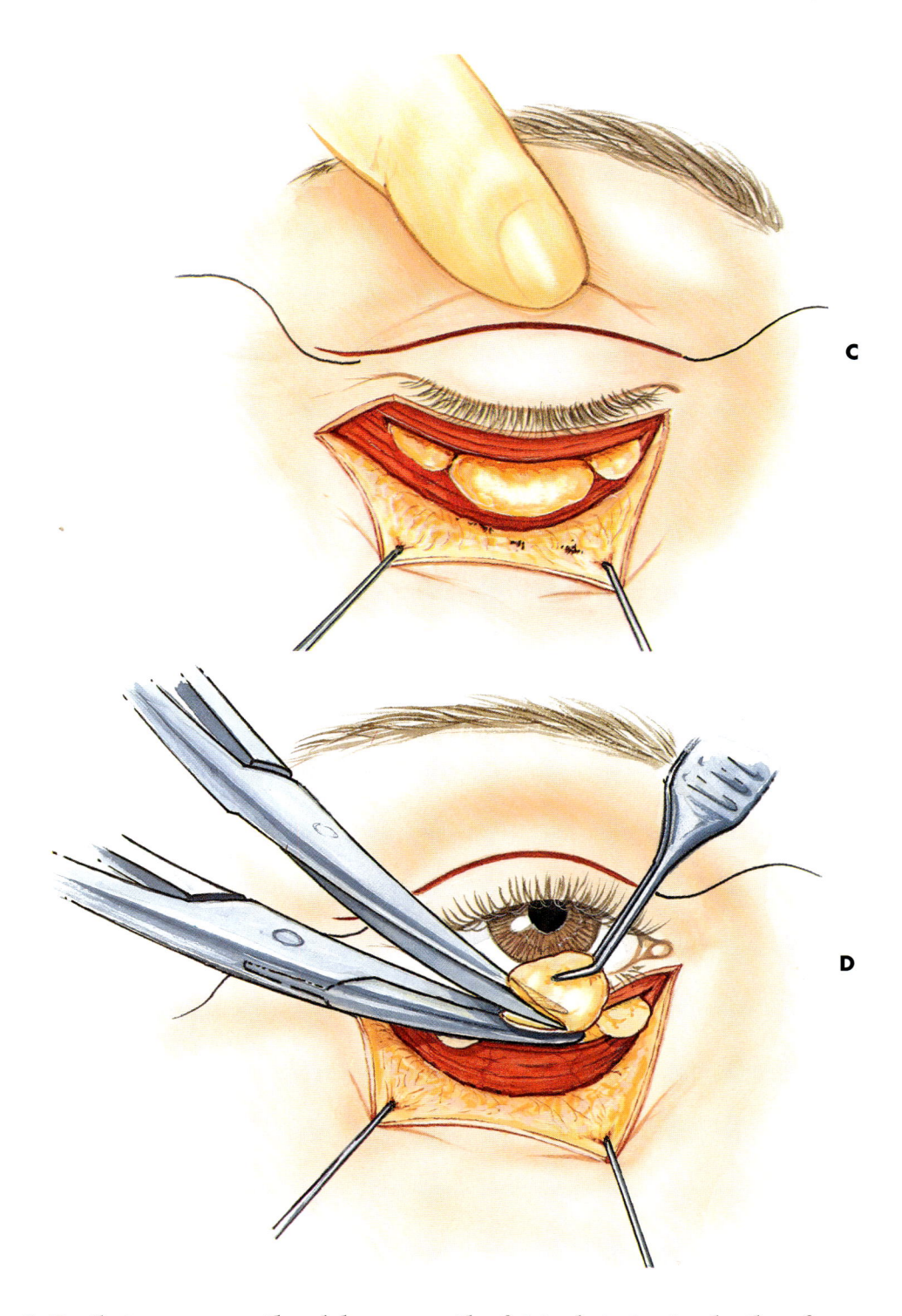

C, Gentle pressure on the globe causes the fat pads to protrude, thus facilitating excision. D, The bulging fat is clamped and excised, and the stump is electrocoagulated.

Continued.

SURGICAL REJUVENATION OF THE FACE

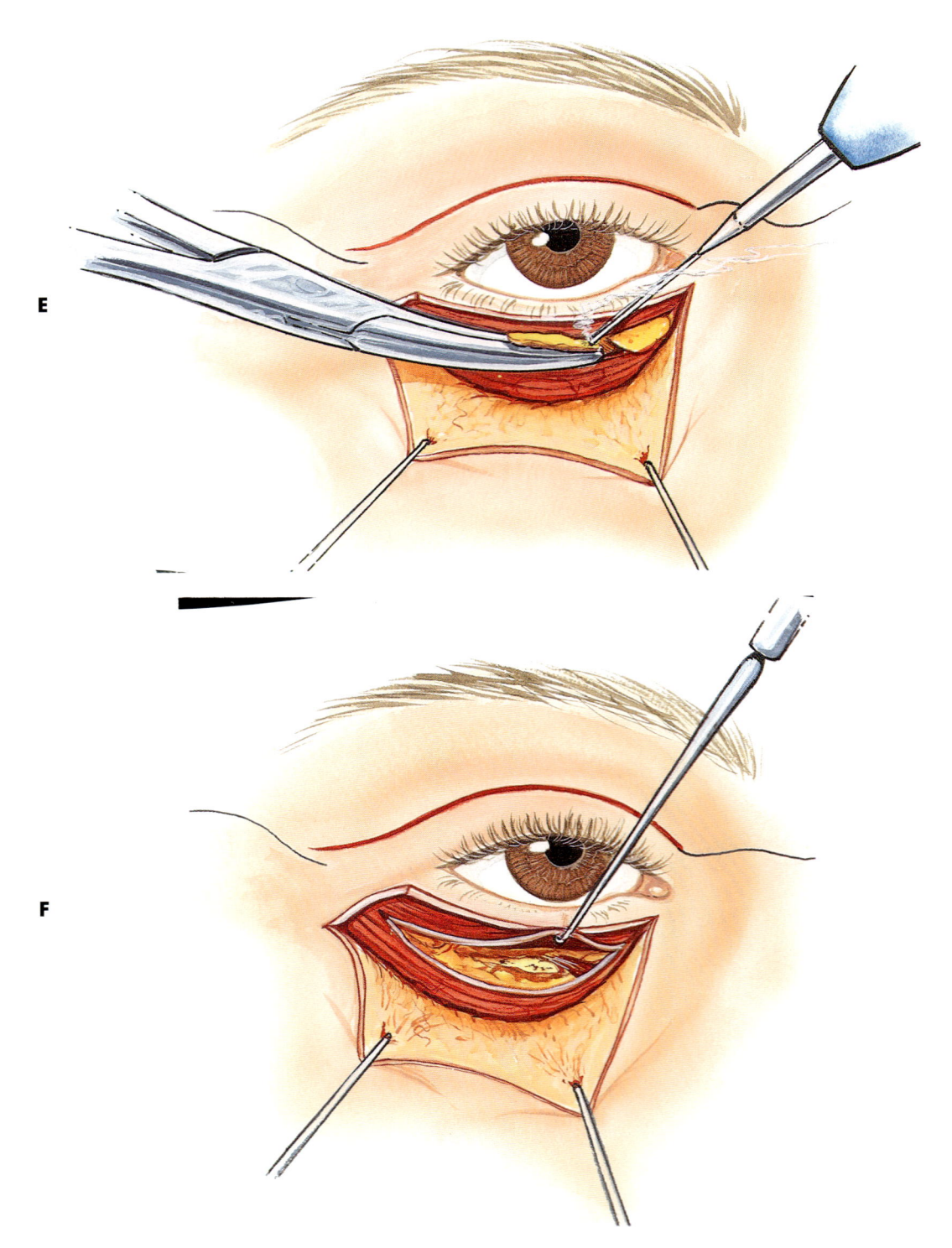

E

F

E, The other compartments are inspected, and an appropriate amount of fat is removed. F, This illustrates the coagulated stumps after the fat has been removed.

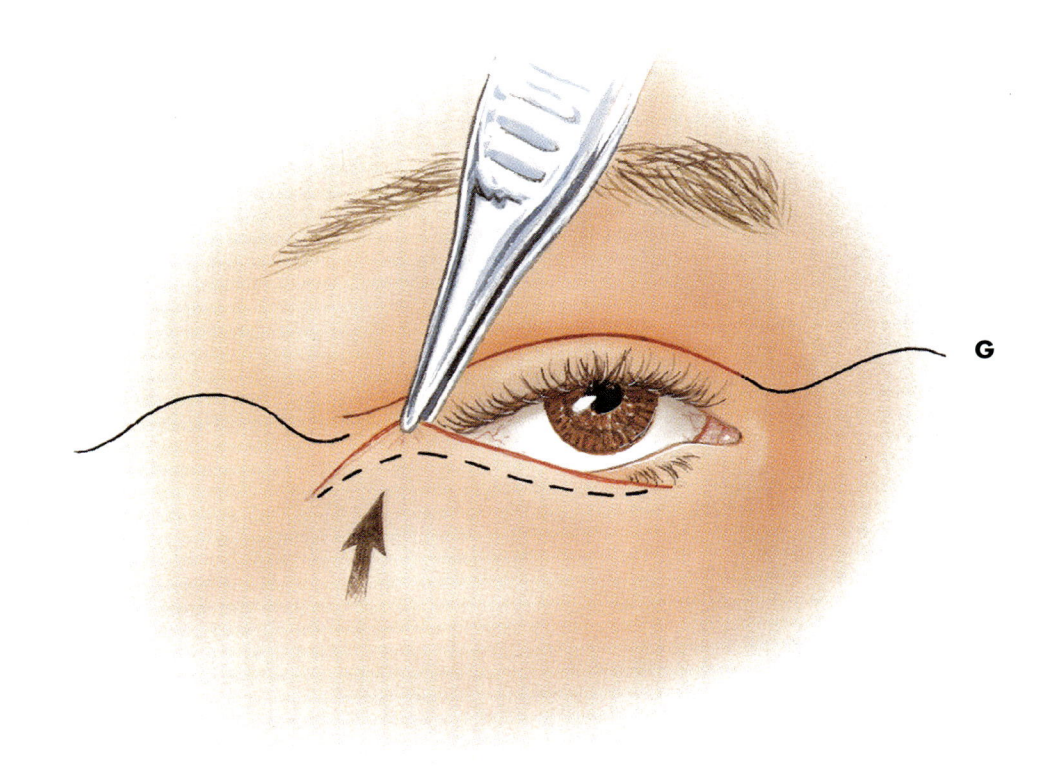

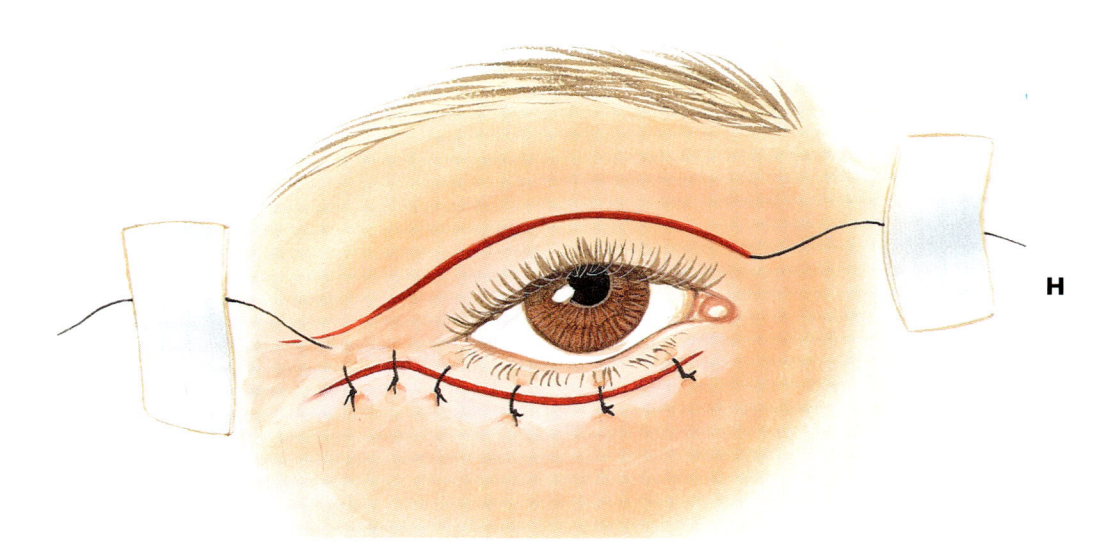

G, The skin flap is advanced superiorly, and the redundancy is excised.
H, Interrupted 6-0 nylon sutures are used for closure.

SURGICAL REJUVENATION OF THE FACE

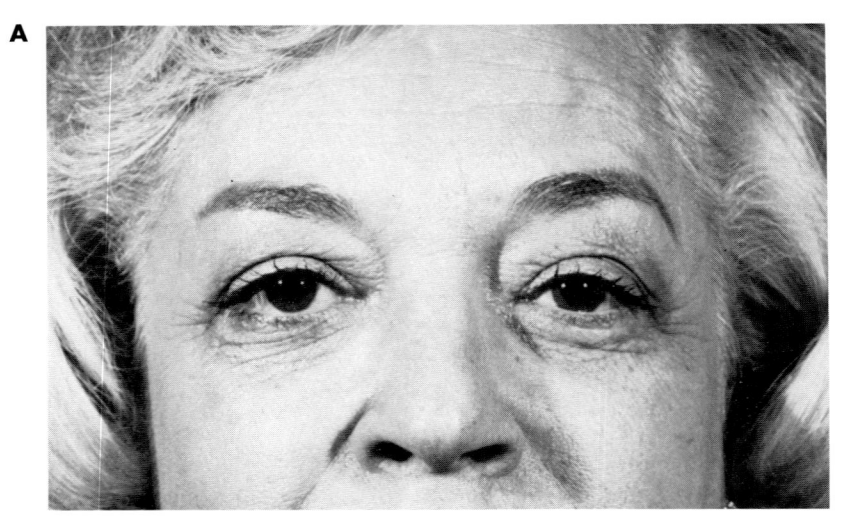

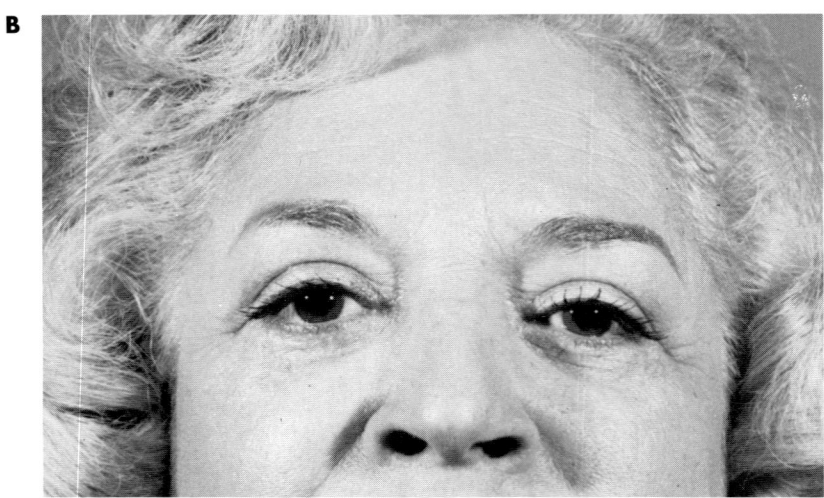

A, This woman was an ideal candidate for a skin flap of the lower eyelid instead of a skin-muscle flap. When there is excessive skin extending over the orbital rim and many fine mosaic lines, the skin flap is preferred, since there appears to be a smoother redraping of skin over the underlying orbicularis muscle. B, This postoperative view demonstrates the redraping of the skin that has occurred.

Skin-Muscle Flap

If a skin-muscle flap is used, the skin incision is the same. To elevate the muscle with the flap, the incision is extended deep into the orbicularis muscle. The tip of the scissors is inserted through the orbicularis muscle, and the areolar plane between the orbicularis and the orbital septum is defined with blunt dissection. An important point is to *leave at least 5 mm of pretarsal orbicularis intact over the tarsus* to aid in lid closure and lid support.

The skin-muscle flap is raised easily in a nearly avascular plane. As it is elevated, the orbital fat becomes readily visible.

The skin-muscle flap is useful for most clinical situations. If there is excessive fine wrinkling of the lower eyelid skin, then a skin flap is perhaps a better solution.

SURGICAL REJUVENATION OF THE FACE

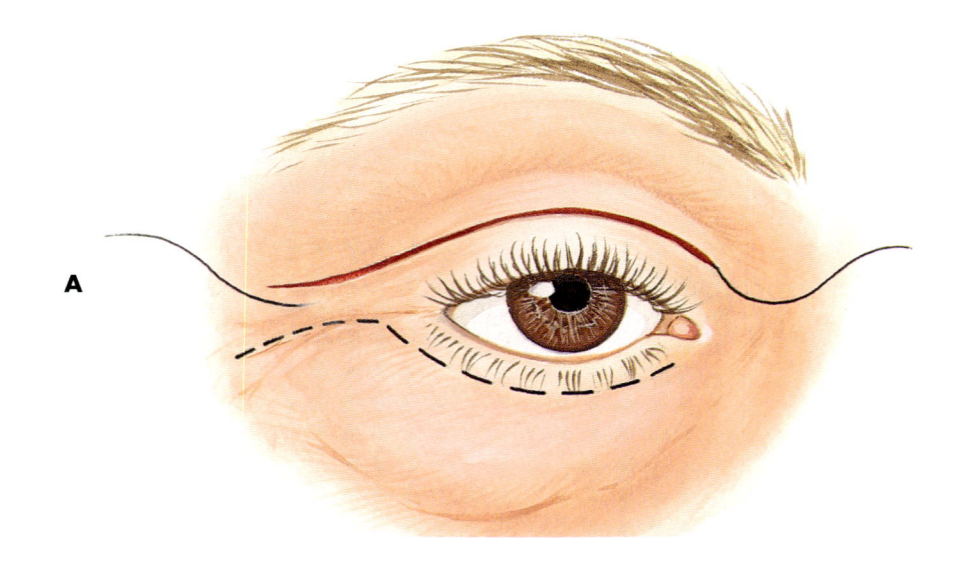

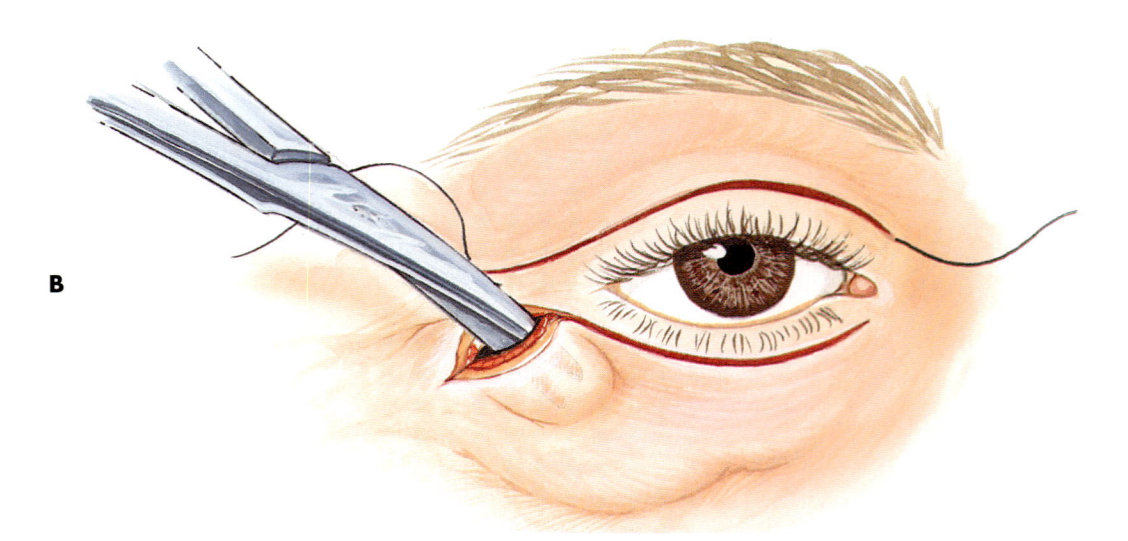

A, The line of incision is the same for either a skin flap or a skin-muscle flap. B, It is easier to undermine the muscle from the lateral incision before completing the incision along the eyelid margin. Gentle opening and closing of the scissors in the submuscular plane facilitates elevation of the flap.

BLEPHAROPLASTY

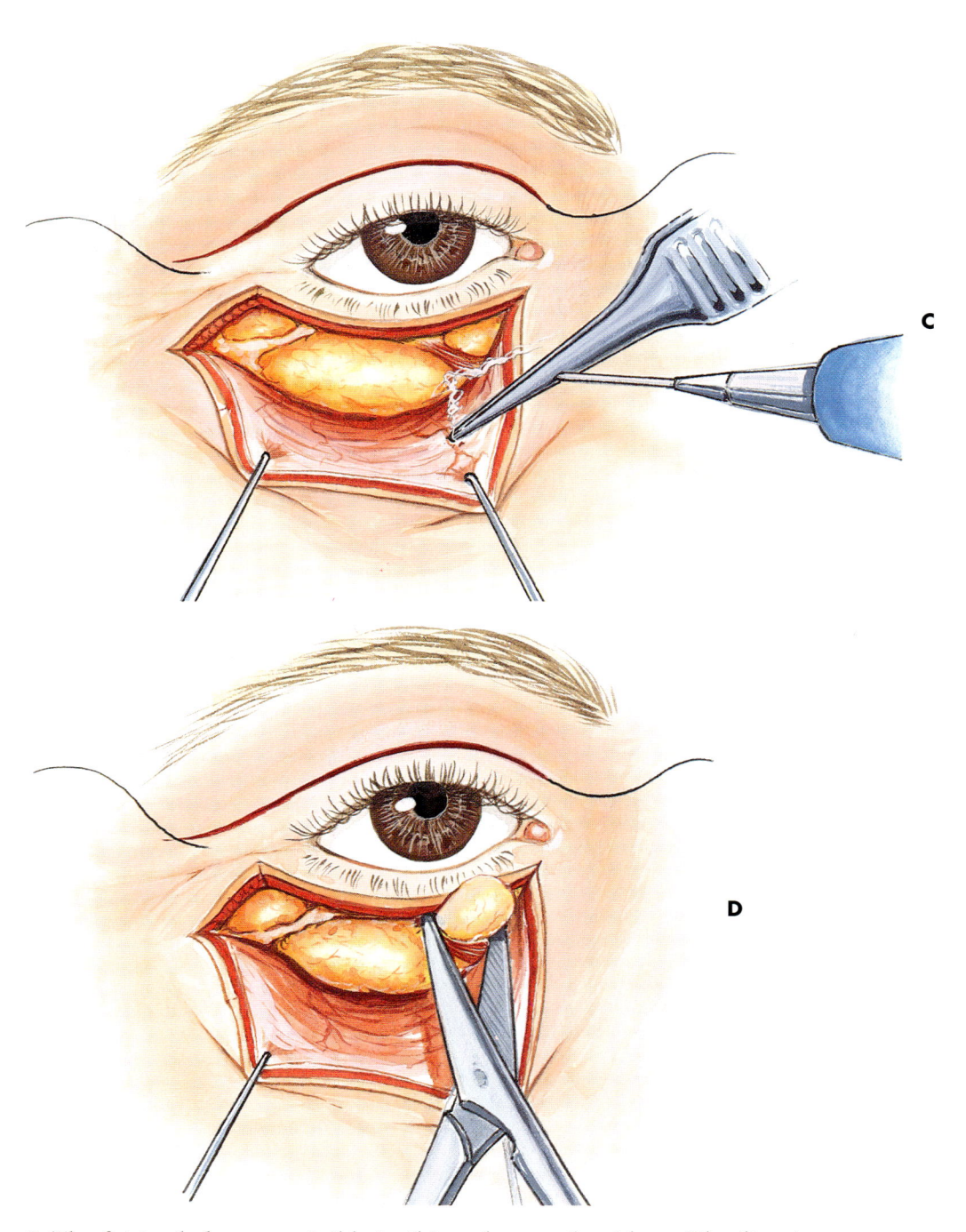

C, The fat pads become visible in this submuscular plane. Bleeding is controlled with the electrocautery. D, The fat from the three compartments is easily dissected

Continued.

SURGICAL REJUVENATION OF THE FACE

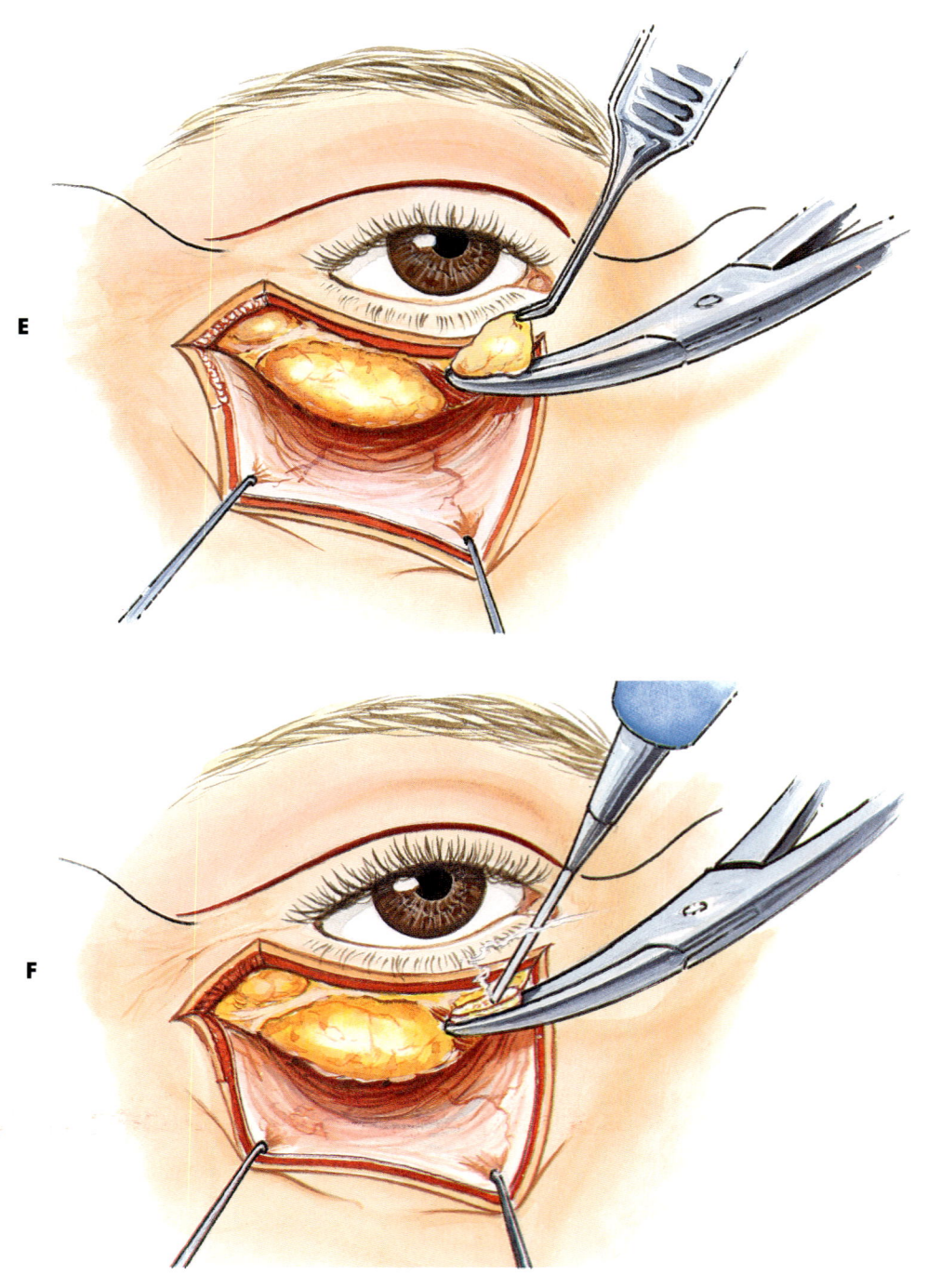

E, Each fat pad is gently eased from its pocket, clamped and severed, and the base electrocoagulated. F, Take caution to prevent the hemostat from inadvertently touching the skin when coagulating. The medial fat pad may not be completely anesthetized from the original injections, and the patient may require a small quantity of local anesthetic solution directly into the fat pad to prevent pain.

BLEPHAROPLASTY

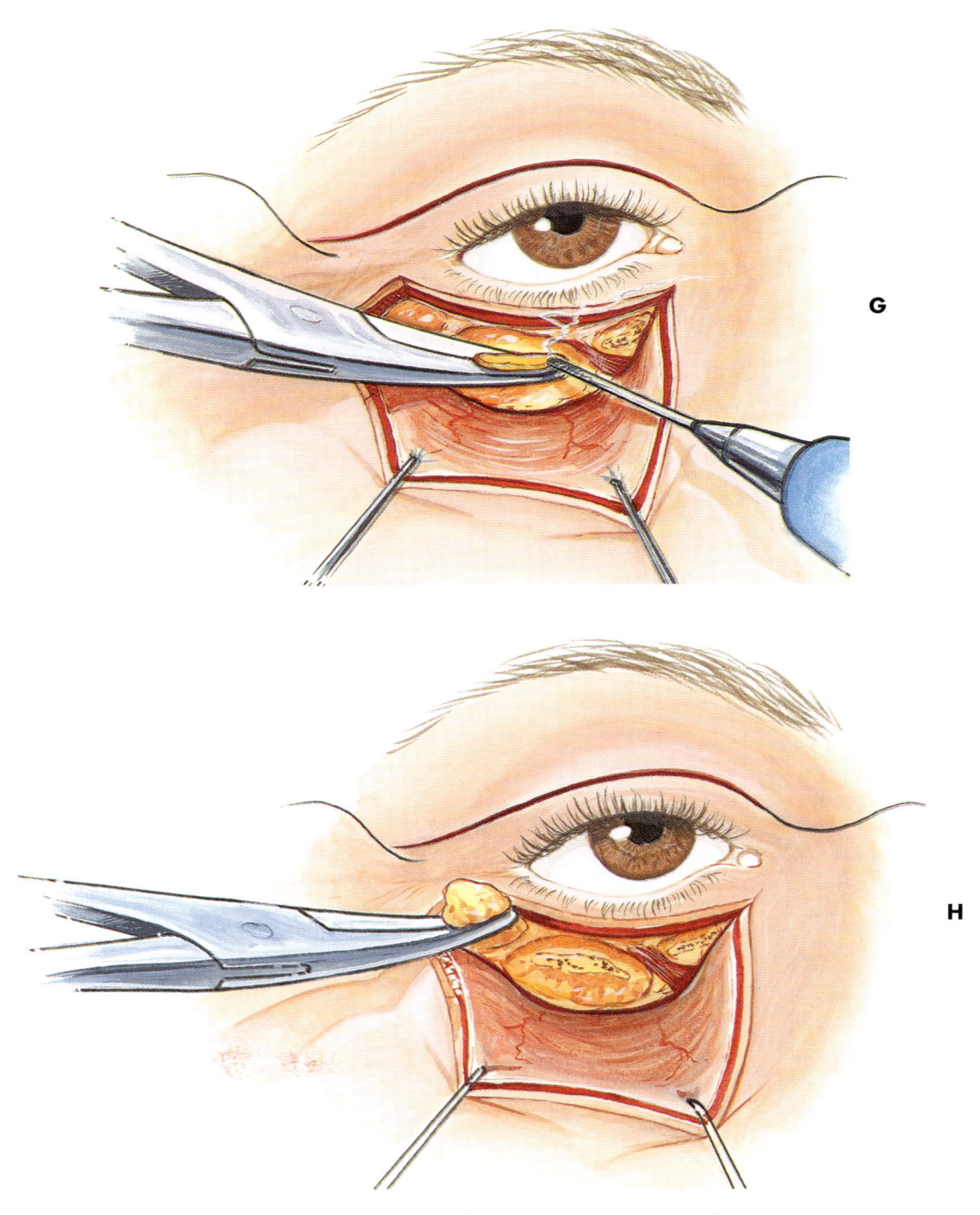

G, The other fat pads are managed in the same manner. *H,* The lateral fat pad is usually smaller than the other two fat pads.

Continued.

SURGICAL REJUVENATION OF THE FACE

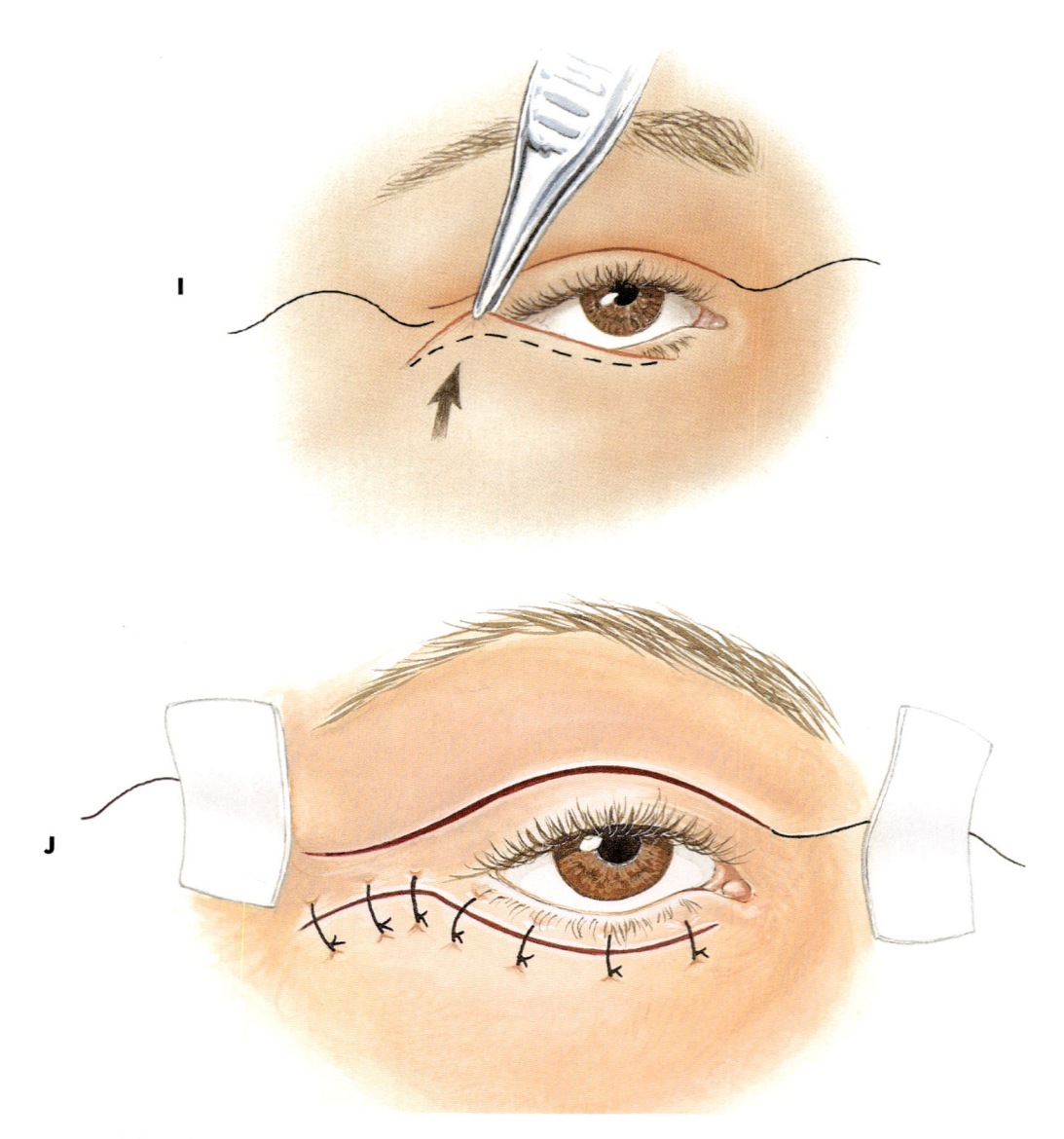

I, The skin-muscle flap is advanced superiorly and the appropriate amount is resected. The resection includes skin and muscle. Recheck the superior margin of the skin-muscle flap before closure, because small vessels may begin bleeding after the flap has been trimmed. J, Close the incision with interrupted 6-0 nylon sutures.

BLEPHAROPLASTY

■ Fat Removal

If a skin flap has been used, the orbicularis muscle is punctured above each fat compartment, parallel to its fibers. After exposure, each fat compartment is approached separately through these small stab wounds extended within the orbital septum. After the compartment has been entered, gentle pressure is used on the globe to allow the fat to protrude external to the orbital septum. The excess fat is clamped with the use of a hemostat, resected, and the base of the fat pad meticulously cauterized. All three fat compartments of the lower eyelid are inspected to determine the amount of resection needed. In terms of the proper contouring of fat, in general the fat should be resected so that it lies just within the infraorbital rim. With gentle pressure on the globe, the fat pads should then rest at the level of the infraorbital rim; this simulates the natural gravitational effect that would occur if the patient were upright. Over-contouring of fat to well within the in-

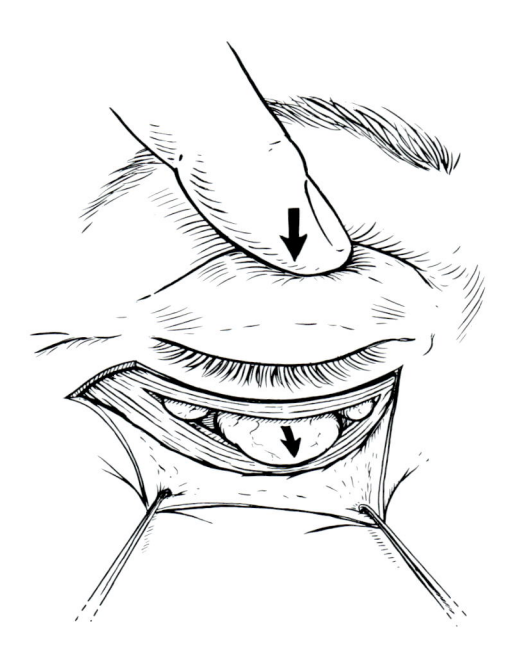

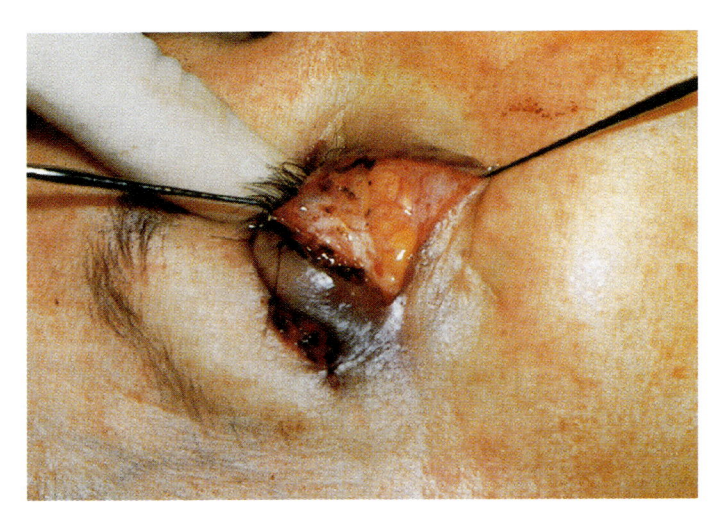

Gentle finger pressure on the globe facilitates removal of the infraorbital fat pads. Exercise care not to remove an excessive amount of fat, since this will cause the lower eyelid to have a sunken appearance postoperatively. Also do not tug at the fat pads, since this could disrupt a blood vessel in the orbit and cause a retrobulbar hematoma.

fraorbital rim should be avoided as this will accentuate the appearance of the rim externally, producing a hollowed-out, cadaveric look to the lower eyelids.

The muscle fibers of the interior oblique are occasionally visualized separating the medial and central compartments and obviously should be avoided at the time of fat pad resection. Since the inferior oblique lies posterior to the orbital septum, its visualization is not mandatory as long as fat pad resection is always performed anterior to the orbital septum. Proper delineation of orbital fat from the septum and fibers that extend from the lower lid retractors should always be performed so that only fat is resected at the time of blepharoplasty. This will avoid incidental injury to adnexal structures. Sometimes the fat is a bit difficult to deliver. Resection of a small portion of the superficial-lying fat will commonly allow the surgeon to expose the deeper-lying bulk of the fat pad.

The lateral fat pad is the fat pad most commonly undercorrected and should always be carefully explored to ensure its proper contouring. Its location, superior and lateral to the central compartment, can be easily overlooked and may be responsible for the recalcitrant bulging commonly seen from underresection. Gentle pressure on the globe will usually delineate the location of the lateral fat pad. The lateral fat pad can be fibrous and difficult to deliver into the operative field. If preoperative evaluation shows that a large amount of fat is present laterally, then patience in ensuring that the lateral fat pad has been properly contoured is necessary to avoid postoperative dissatisfaction and secondary revision.

Lower Skin Excision

Some surgeons prefer to mark preoperatively the amount of skin and muscle to be excised; however, it is more practical to do this after the flaps have been elevated. There are various ways to determine how much skin to excise. One technique is to estimate the amount of skin to be removed by having an assistant place his or her fingertips below the malar eminence in the middle of the cheek and pull down the soft tissues of the cheek, placing tension on the lower lid in a caudal direction. As the lid is being pulled down, the skin flap is laid over the open wound with no tension. From this position the excess skin is easily visualized and excised. Some sources suggest having the patient open his or her mouth widely, as if yawning, and gaze upward. We have found this maneuver to be imprecise in judging excess lower lid skin. We suggest simply redraping the eyelid skin in a superior medial direction, with the lower lid in normal position. The amount of resection is then carefully marked, and should be uniform in its design and remove only enough skin so that the lower eyelid skin loosely approximates the initial lower eyelid incision. It is essential to understand that the lower eyelid flap, whether it is a skin-muscle flap or a skin flap, is a superior advancement flap and not a lateral rotation flap. It is important to redrape the skin in a predominantly superior-medial direction to accurately define the degree of laxity present within lower eyelid skin. Too many lid retraction syndromes following lower lid blepharoplasty have been caused by failure to understand the vector of aging seen in the lower eyelid. Excess resection of lateral eyelid skin is uniformly followed by a change in eyelid shape leading to scleral show or frank ectropion.

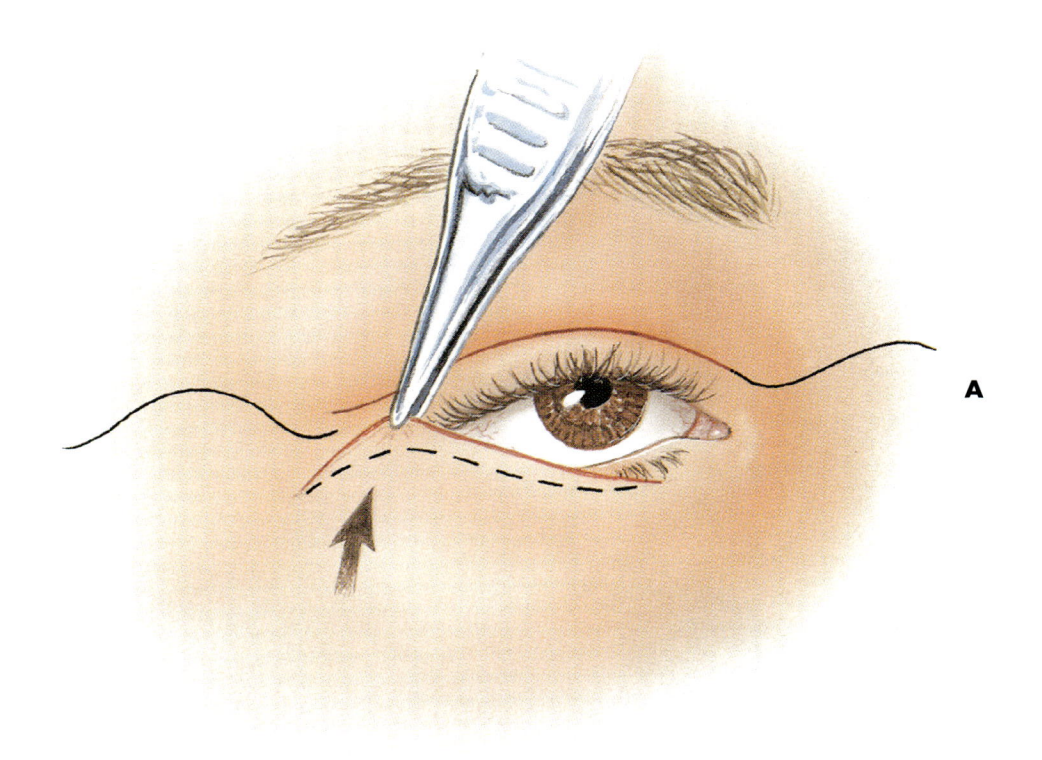

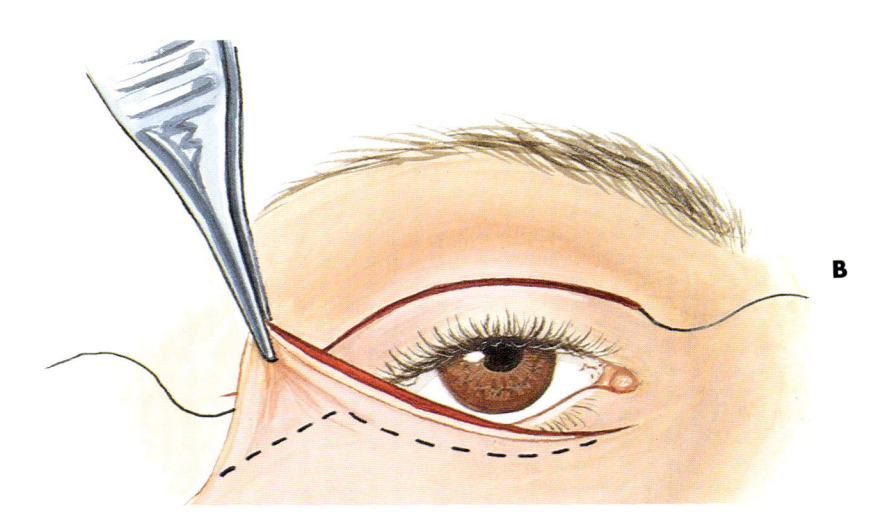

A, Illustration delineating the amount of lower eyelid to be resected. Note that the lower eyelid skin has been redraped in a superomedial direction and that the planned excision is essentially uniform in its design. *B,* If the lower eyelid is redraped in a superotemporal direction, note the apparent excess skin that would be removed temporally. This all-too-common scenario in planning lower lid resection is the most common mechanisms for producing lower lid retraction symptoms and temporal scleral show following lower lid blepharoplasty.

After the lower eyelid flap is trimmed, the wound is closed with interrupted 6-0 monofilament nylon sutures.

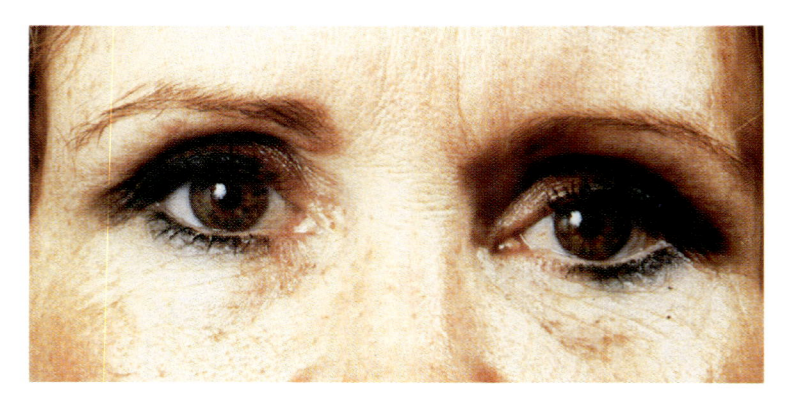

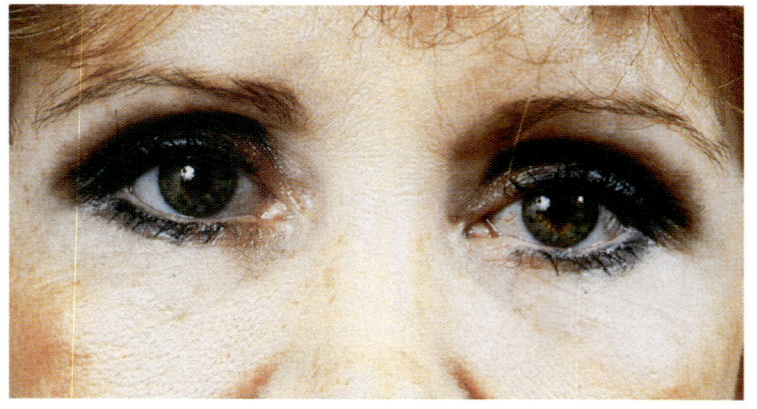

Pre- and postoperative result in a young patient following upper and lower blepharoplasty.

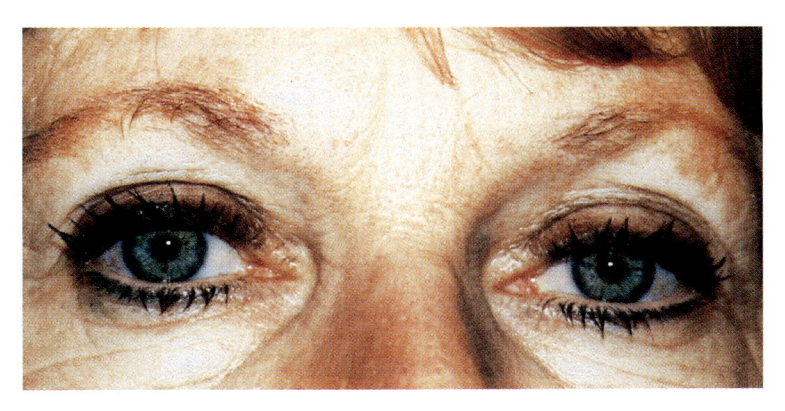

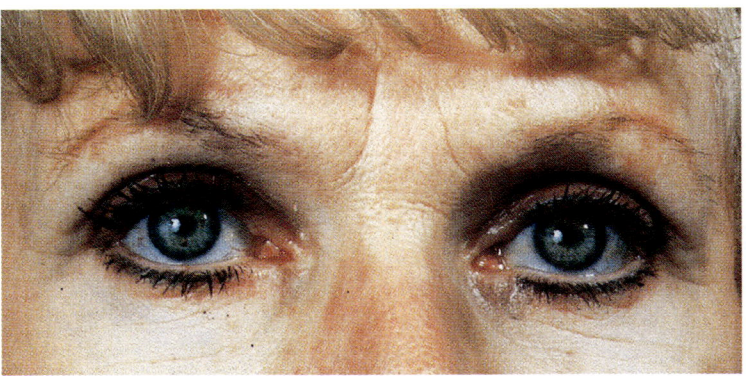

Pre- and postoperative result in 65-year-old patient following upper and lower lid blepharoplasty. Patient is seen before undergoing TCA peeling for remaining lower eyelid rhytides.

SURGICAL REJUVENATION OF THE FACE

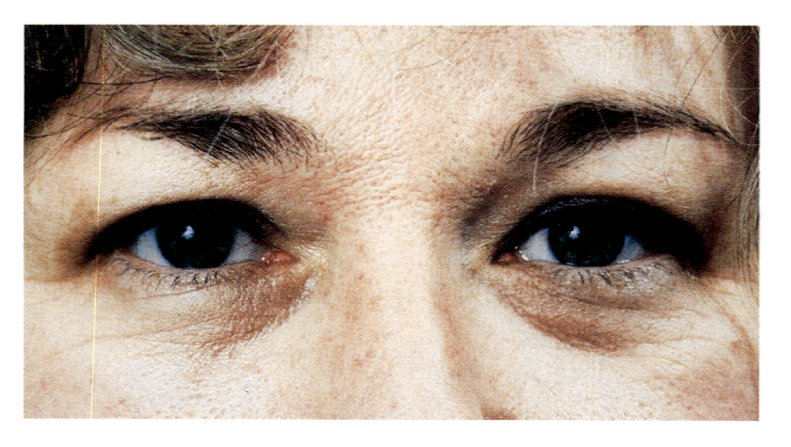

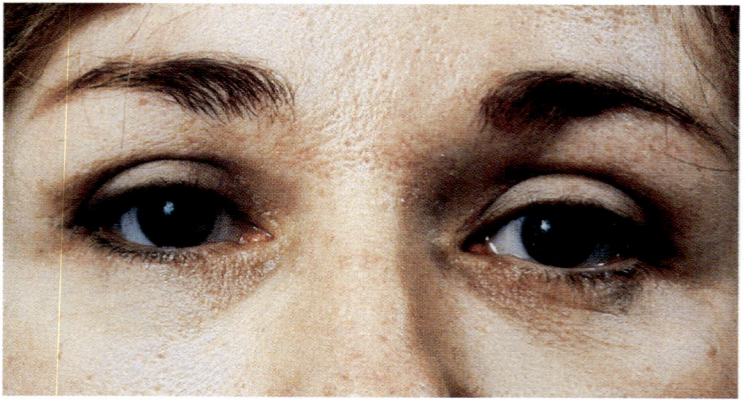

Pre- and postoperative upper and lower blepharoplasty with enhancing of the upper eyelid crease via supratarsal fixation.

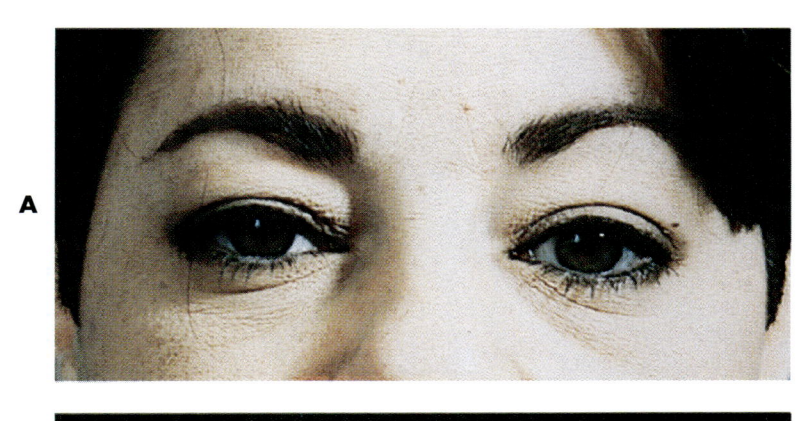

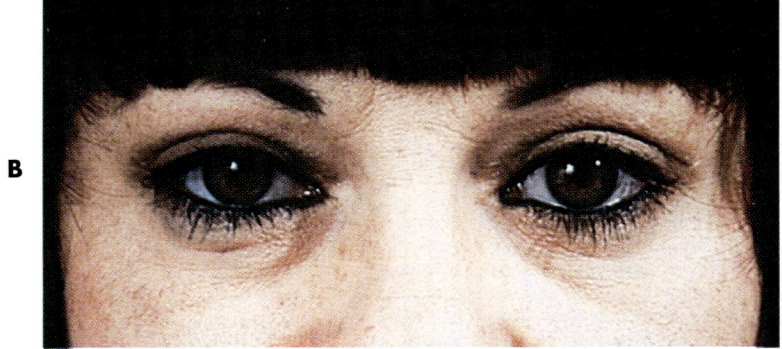

A and B, *Pre- and postoperative result of upper lid blepharoplasty with supratarsal fixation.*

Continued.

SURGICAL REJUVENATION OF THE FACE

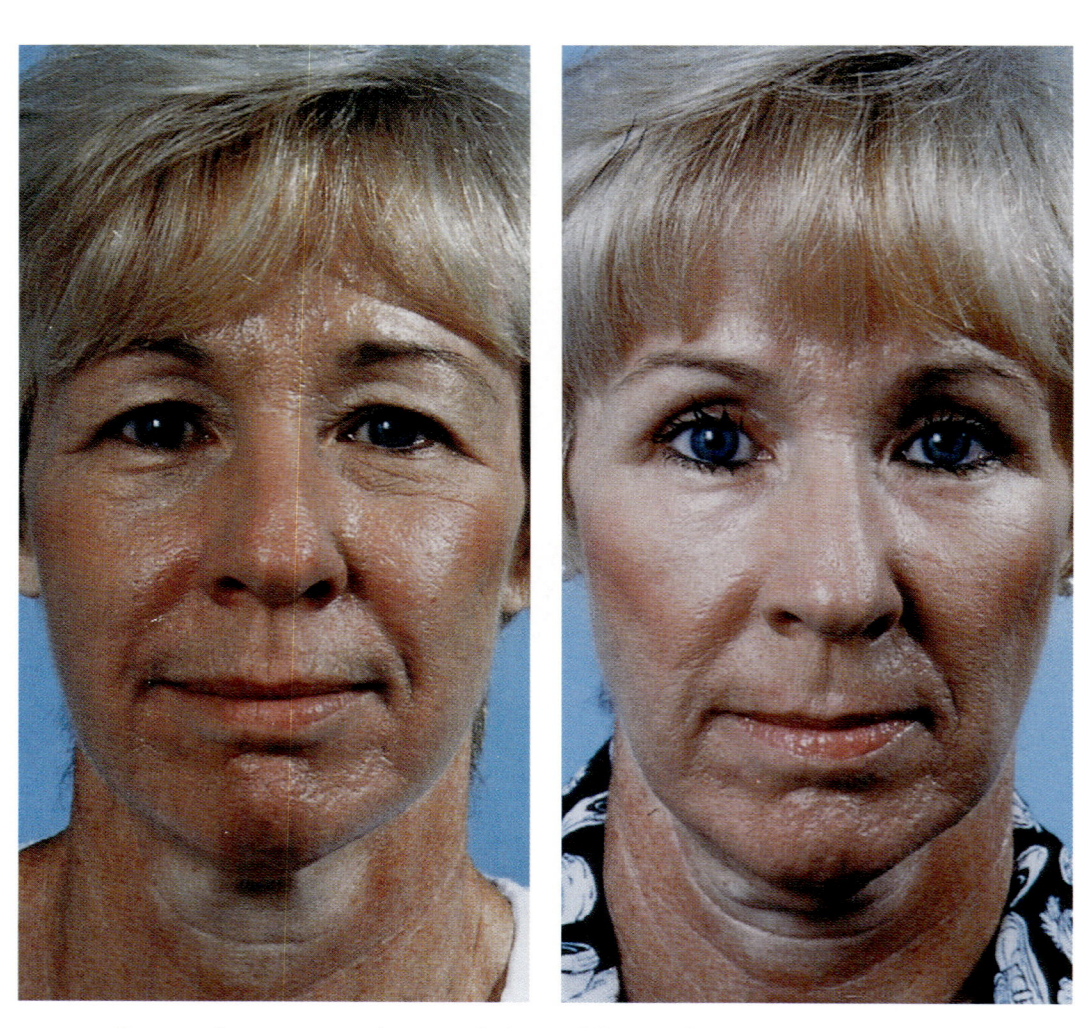

Pre- and postoperative result in middle-aged patient following upper blepharoplasty with supratarsal fixation.

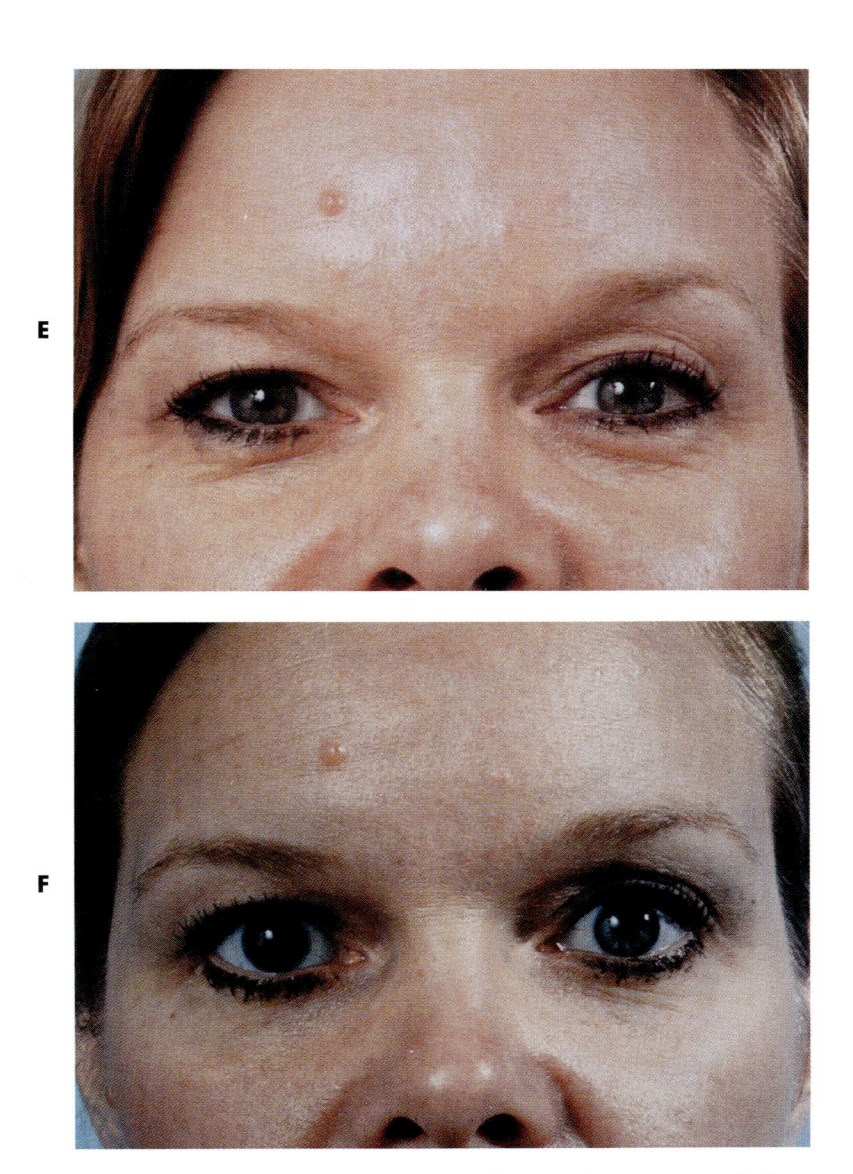

E, Preoperative appearance in patient whose primary complaint was that her infraorbital rim was prominent, making her lower lids appear harsh. F, Postoperative appearance following lower lid blepharoplasty in which the medial and central fat pads were mobilized and transposed across the infraorbital rim and fixated in a subperiosteal pocket. The transposition of lower eyelid fat across the infraorbital rim serves to both blunt the rim and provide a smooth transition between the lower lid and the infraorbital region.

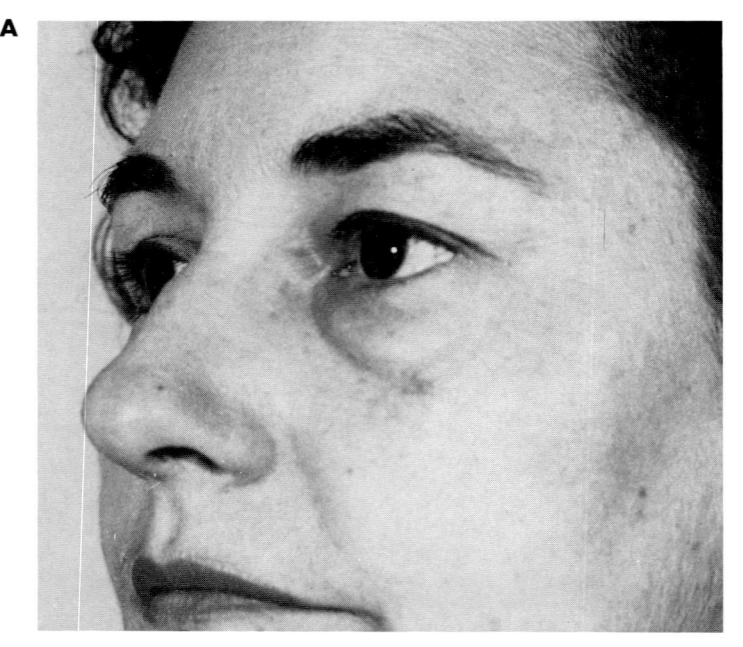

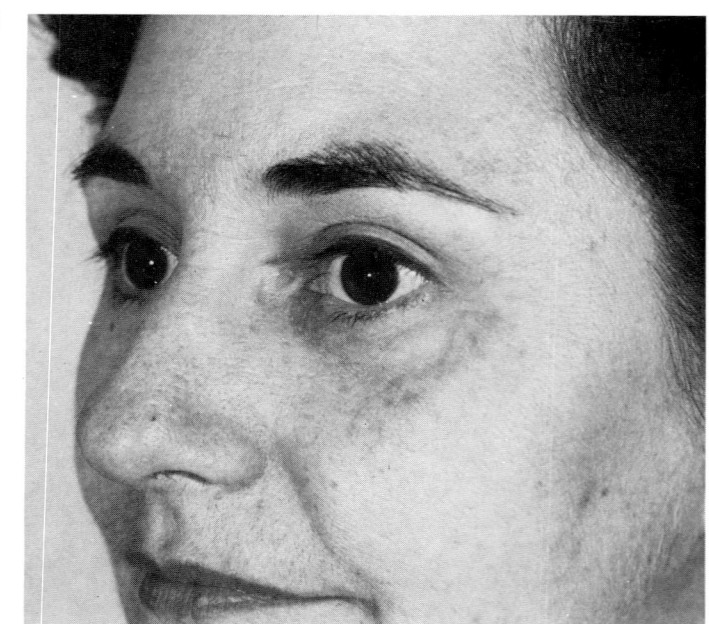

A, This patient demonstrates large infraorbital fat bulges and moderate upper eyelid redundancy. B, After removal of the infraorbital fat and a modest upper eyelid blepharoplasty, there is a "softer" look about the eyes. More pretarsal upper eyelid skin is visible, and the lower eyelid correction has given a smoother look beneath the eyes.

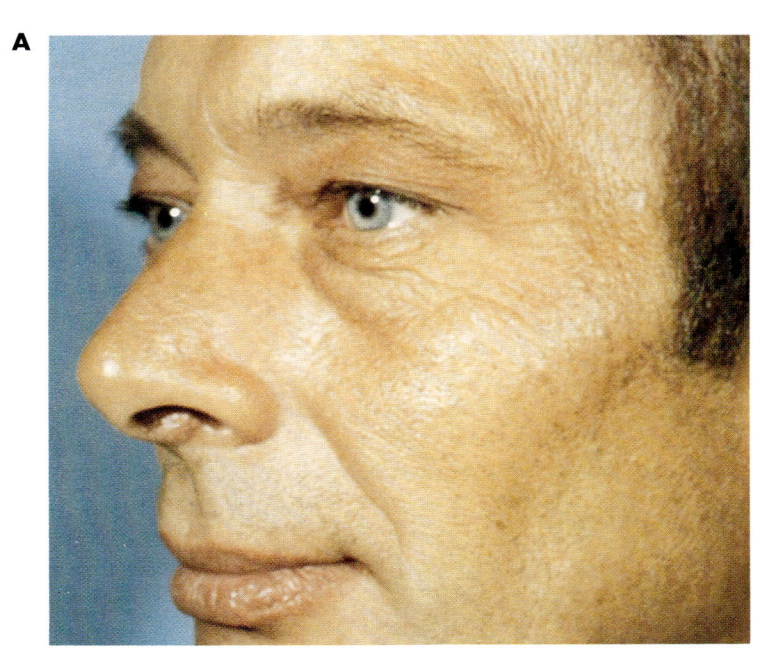

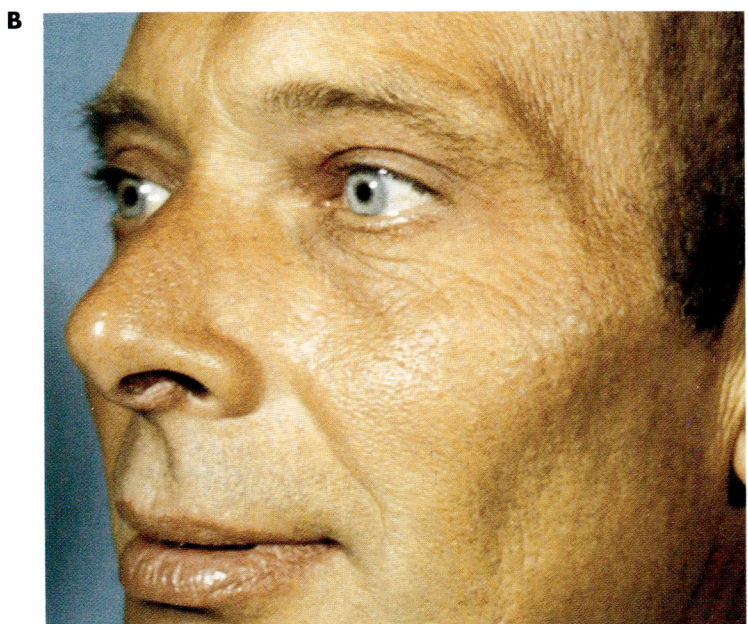

A, In the male patient the objectives are similar, but the procedures can be modified to produce less dramatic results. B, Postoperatively, there is more visible pretarsal skin but not as much as would be desirable in a female eyelid. The fat pads have been partially resected. The scars are inconspicuous, and the eyelids are symmetrical. The objectives have been achieved.

Transconjunctival Lower Eyelid Blepharoplasty

The transconjunctival approach to lower eyelid blepharoplasty is gradually gaining popularity. This operation is useful in younger patients who have fat bagging associated with very little excess of lower eyelid skin. The advantage of this procedure is that it avoids an external incision, and when performed in a retroseptal fashion, avoids opening of the orbital septum and thereby diminishing the possibility of postoperative lid retraction.

Anatomic considerations

In performing transconjunctival blepharoplasty, topical anesthetic drops are placed into the conjunctival sac and a corneal protector is placed. A slight amount of local anesthetic is injected at the outer orbital rim, extending from the medial to the lateral canthus. The conjunctival surface is then slightly infiltrated after the lid is everted.

The incision is made approximately 7 to 8 mm below the lid margin and approximately 3 to 4 mm below the inferior tarsal plate. Medially, the incision must be at or well below the inferior punctum. This places the incision halfway between the inferior border of the tarsus and the inferior fornix. The use of electrocautery to make the transconjunctival excision simplifies this procedure. After the conjunctiva is incised, traction sutures are placed and the lid everted over a Desmorres retractor. The capsulopalpebral fascia is then incised and blunt scissor dissection is performed, directing the scissor toward the inferior orbital rim. As the dissection extends through the capsulopalpebral fascia, the periorbital fat is exposed. The first fat pad usually visualized is the central fat pad. After it is identified, the incision is extended nasally and temporally until both the medial and lateral fat pads are identified. Care is used to identify and preserve the inferior oblique muscle. The temporal fat pad is usually the most difficult fat pad to identify through the transconjunctival approach. Adequate exposure usually can be obtained with the use of a small retractor, which is inserted inside the cut edge of the capsulopalpebral fascia, then incising a fascial band that commonly overlies the lateral fat pad. We prefer to excise fat with the use of an insulated electrocautery (Denver tip) in an incremental fashion.

The infraorbital rim is not readily available as a landmark for the contouring of fat in transconjunctival blepharoplasty. This makes the proper contouring of the fat pads a bit more difficult than in the transcutaneous approach to blepharoplasty. After resecting orbital fat, a good guide is to remove the corneal protector and look at the lower eyelid externally while gently pressing on the globe. Any focal areas of fat bulging will usually be evident externally. Further resection within individual compartments should allow a smooth, even contour from medially to laterally across the lower eyelid. In general our impression is that slightly more fat must be removed via transconjunctival blepharoplasty than in transcutaneous blepharoplasty to obtain the same result in fat contouring.

After the fat pads have been excised and hemostasis obtained, closure is accomplished with a single 6-0 chromic suture that approximates the capsulopalpebral fascia and conjunctiva.

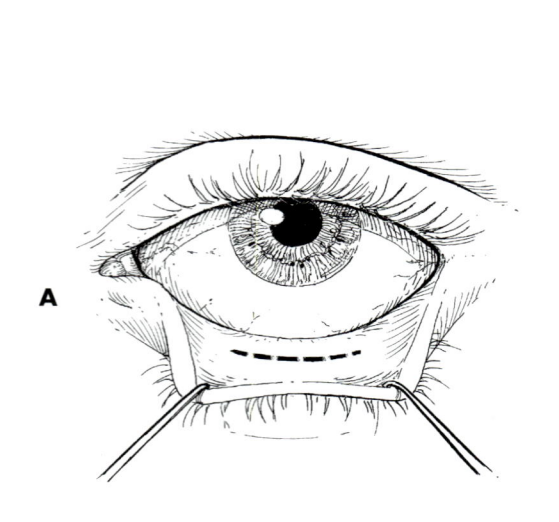

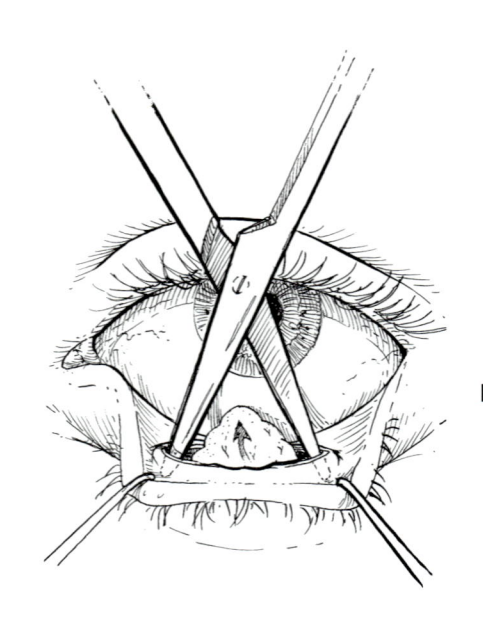

C

Conjunctiva
Capsulopalpebral fascia
Orbital septum

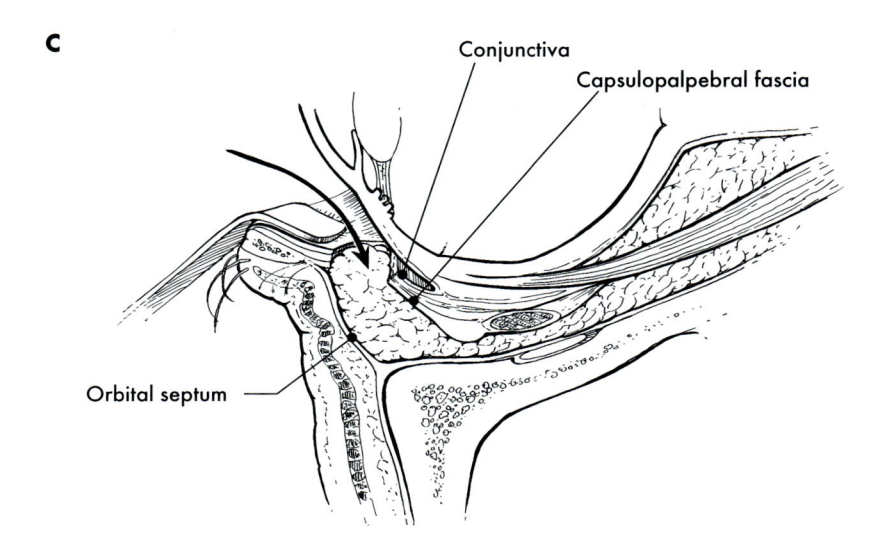

A, The transconjunctival incision is usually made 7 to 8 mm below the lid margin, approximately 4 mm below the inferior tarsal plates with the use of electrocautery. This places the incision approximately halfway between the inferior border of the tarsus and the inferior fornix. The incision usually is made centrally and extended nasally and temporally as needed, with care taken to not injure the inferior punctum or inferior canaliculi. Of note, this procedure should be performed with the use of a corneal protector in place (not shown). B, Following incision of the capsulopalpebral fascia, the scissors is inserted in the retroseptal space and the central fat pad is identified. Note that the eyelid is everted, and the scissors is placed in a direction tangential to the lateral orbital rim. It is important not to place the scissors angling posteriorly toward the globe. After the central fat is contoured, the medial and lateral fat pads are identified and resected with the use of an insulated electrocautery tip. C, Sagittal section illustrating the approach to lower lid fat through a transconjunctival retroseptal approach, which involves incision of only conjunctiva and capsulopalpebral fascia. The orbital septum and anterior lamella are not traumatized in this procedure, thereby preventing lower lid retraction.

SURGICAL REJUVENATION OF THE FACE

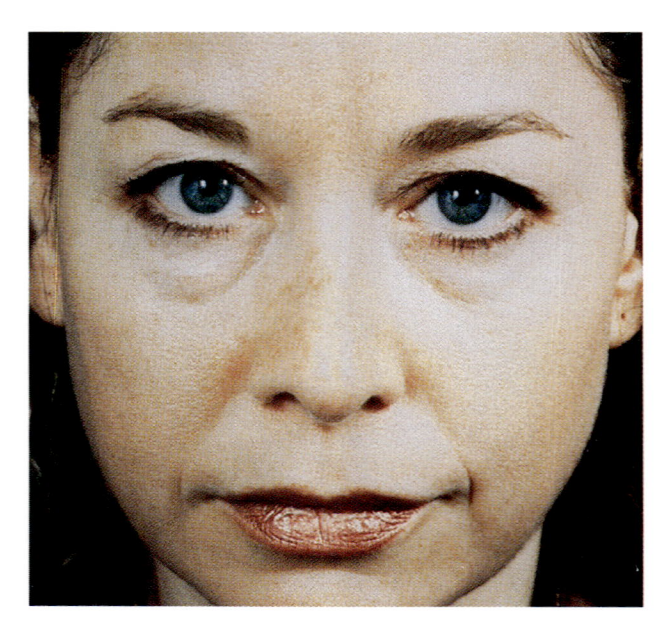

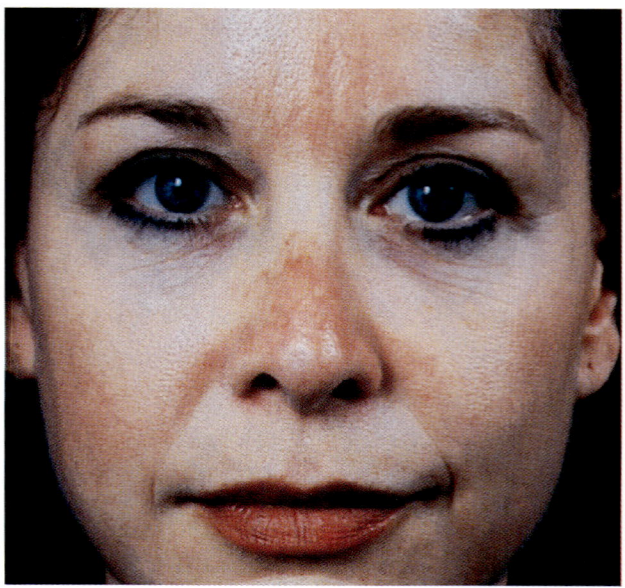

Pre- and postoperative result following transconjunctival lower blepharoplasty.

POSTOPERATIVE CARE

Some patients' eyelids may ooze along the lines of incision postoperatively, and temporary bandaging with a minimum of pressure is occasionally used. The amount of postoperative edema after 72 to 96 hours is not significantly altered by using bandages.

If bandages are used, all personnel must be alert for any patient complaint of eye pain, especially if it is experienced unilaterally. If the patient has pain, the bandages are removed immediately and the eyelids are inspected to see if there is any problem that requires attention. A significant number of patients feel claustrophobic when their eyes are bandaged. If the patient cannot tolerate them, the bandages should be removed immediately. These bandages should always be removed before the patient leaves the outpatient unit.

If there is no significant oozing, ice compresses are applied directly to the eyelids. We usually use iced 4×4 in compresses, changing them at 20- to 30-minute intervals, three or four times a day. This routine is continued for several days, mostly for the soothing effect of the cold. Ice compresses are helpful in preventing excessive edema and have the added advantage of keeping the patient occupied and not focused on any discomfort he or she may be experiencing.

The sutures are removed on the fourth or fifth postoperative day. Patients are instructed to gently cleanse the suture lines with hydrogen peroxide and apply a topical antibiotic ointment to the suture lines. This treatment will soften any remaining crusts and make the patient more comfortable. Eye makeup is permitted in 9 or 10 days, but artificial lashes are discouraged for 3 weeks postoperatively. Contact lenses may be worn at the end of the second week. (See frequently asked questions on p. 515.)

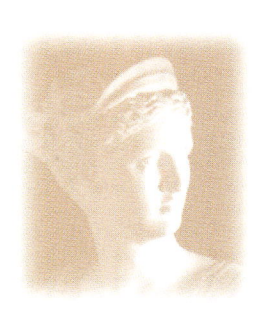

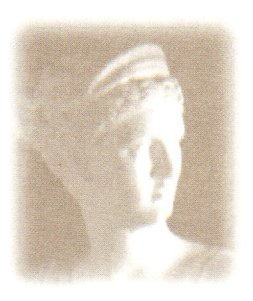

COMPLICATIONS

■ Dry Eye Syndrome

As discussed earlier, the patient with preoperative dry eye syndrome may still undergo blepharoplasty, but it must be a more conservative procedure and should be performed only after a consultation and with the endorsement of the patient's ophthalmologist. Care is taken to keep this patient's eyes well-lubricated both during and after surgery. When this troubling condition occurs postoperatively, it is imperative that the surface of the patient's eye be kept lubricated. Several commercial lubricating products are available for treatment. Bland ointments such as lacri-lube can be applied and are especially beneficial during sleep, when the most severe drying occurs. The patient may sleep with partially separated eyelids and further aggravate the condition. In this situation, taping the eyelids shut at bedtime can be a helpful therapeutic maneuver. It is rare for this condition to persist for more than a few weeks. If it does, consultation with an ophthalmologist is indicated.

■ Hypertrophied Scars and Keloids

Scars and keloids are rare complications, and true keloids have not been observed. Occasionally, a patient may exhibit a slight scar contracture near the medial canthus of the upper eyelid, especially if a significant amount of skin has been removed. For the first few postoperative days the patient may observe a slight irregularity or elevation of the lower eyelid where the "hockey stick" incision angles laterally and becomes an extension into a natural line at the lateral canthus. In 6 to 8 weeks this irregularity will usually smooth out spontaneously. In some individuals the scar may remain red or pink for several weeks. Most of these situations will subside spontaneously if given sufficient time. The surgeon should not hastily recommend corrective Z-plasties, scar revision, or other procedures in the early weeks following eyelid surgery.

Epiphora and Chemosis

A small percentage of patients experience excessive tearing during the immediate postoperative phase because of a mechanical alteration in the tear-collecting mechanism or an obstruction in the ductal system. However, this condition usually subsides in a matter of days. When the patient has severe lateral chemosis following surgery, the eyelid may be retracted downward, causing the punctum to be out of alignment with the eyelid. This situation prevents natural drainage of tears. Chemosis, which is presumably secondary to an interference with lower eyelid lymphatics, usually spontaneously resolves over a period of 2 to 6 weeks. As it resolves, the lower lid returns to its normal position relative to the globe, and the epiphora is resolved. In patients without tendency toward high extraocular pressure, a flourinated steroid solution (Flarex), 2 drops applied 4 times a day, is useful in helping to resolve the troublesome symptom.

Prolonged Discoloration

In a small percentage of cases, prolonged discoloration occurs. This condition is probably caused by extensive bruising that occurs during the initial procedure, along with the subsequent deposit of blood pigments such as hemosiderin into the skin itself. It is more common when a skin flap has been used and is rare following skin-muscle procedures to the lower lid. The discoloration usually subsides within several weeks, but in some individuals it may take 1 to 2 years, and rarely may be permanent. For those cases that are persistent, the surgeon might want to recommend a chemical peel to bleach the skin. Treatment with topical retinoic acid and hydroquinone is also useful.

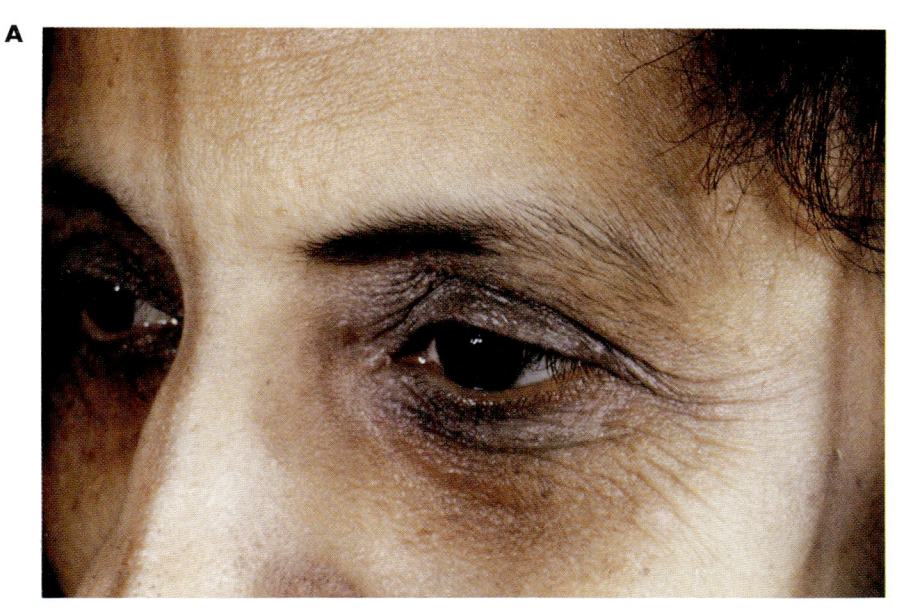

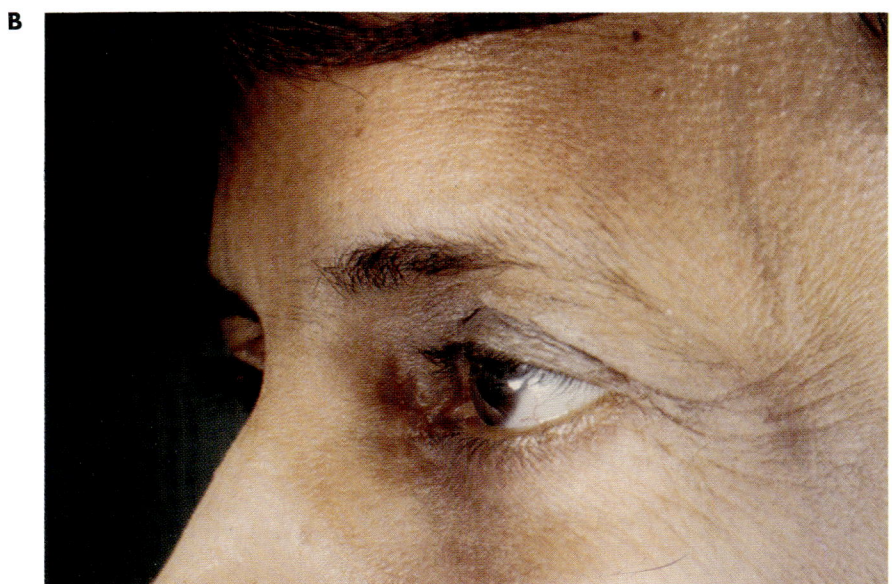

A, This patient has periorbital hyperpigmentation. B, Following a periorbital chemical peel, the pigmentation has been reduced. The patient is not wearing makeup.

Postoperative Bleeding

If bleeding occurs while the patient is still on the operating table or within the first 24 hours postoperatively, the incision should be reopened, the point of bleeding located, the clots evacuated, and the incisions resutured. If a small hematoma is observed later, it is advisable to wait several days until liquification occurs. Then the small amount of blood is removed through a small stab wound made directly over the most prominently distorted area. These small hematomas are troublesome and often cause the area to be indurated for several weeks. Healing seems to be extremely slow. The injection of steroids is not beneficial and offers more potential dangers than benefits.

Atrophy Resulting from Steroid Injections

Steroid injections can cause serious problems. Atrophy can occur even with minute amounts of steroids, and the atrophic area may be difficult to correct. The injection of malar bags with steroids has been universally unsuccessful, and if the malar bags cannot be significantly improved by a blepharoplasty or temporal rhytidectomy, then perhaps direct excision is indicated.

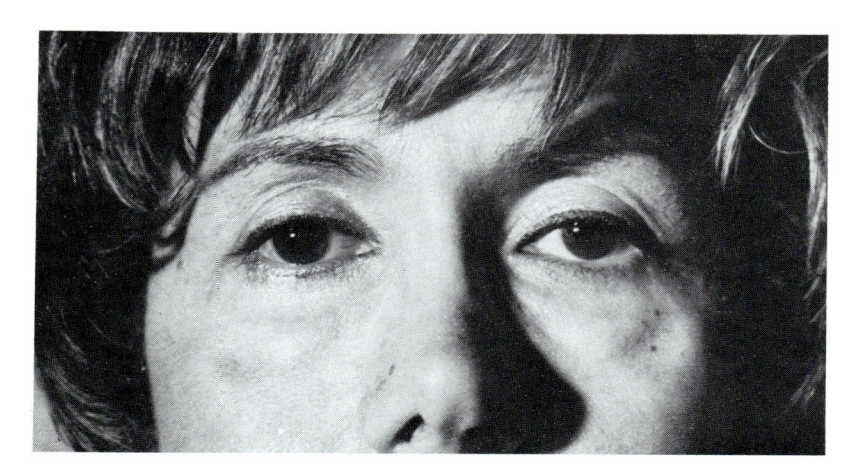

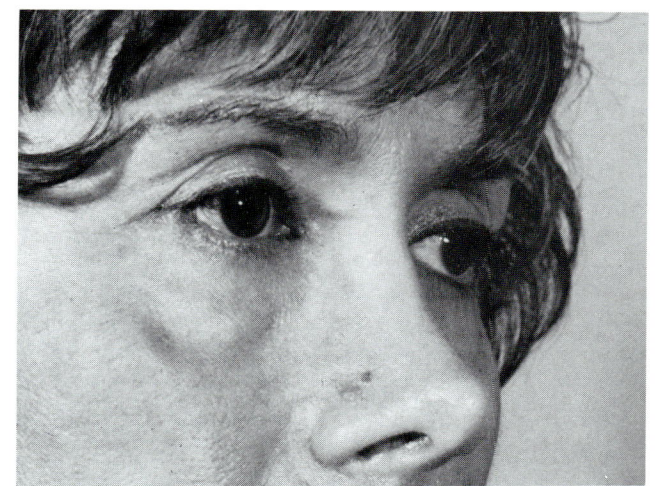

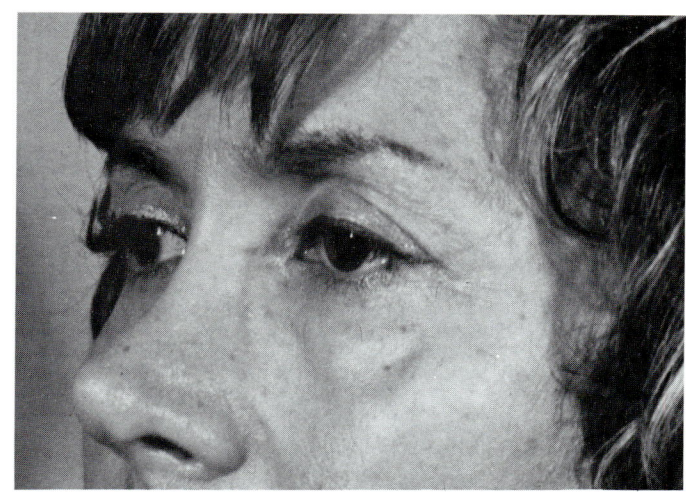

Note the severe depressions in the infraorbital areas bilaterally. The patient stated that "something was injected" into these areas to reduce the swelling. It is believed that steroids were used and that the injections produced atrophy of these areas.

Retrobulbar Hematoma

Retrobulbar hematoma is an accumulation of extravasated blood behind the eyeball, and may be caused during surgery by tugging on the fat pads or before surgery through a "blind" or percutaneous injection of the fat pads in preoperative preparation. Symptoms of this condition are proptosis or protrusion of the eyeball, globe induration, inadequate eyelid coverage of the globe surface, dilated pupils, pain, and possible loss of vision. Ophthalmologists sometimes encounter this condition when administering retrobulbar injections for cataract surgery. Because the central and lateral fat pads are relatively insensitive, no injection of anesthetic solution is usually necessary during excision. The medial fat pads are more sensitive to dissection and excision, but after exposure they can be safely injected under direct vision.

If this condition does occur, the incisions are reopened and any collection of blood around the eye or in the spaces where the fat pockets are resected is relieved. The orbital septum is then widely opened. An ophthalmologist should always be consulted. If possible, the partially resected fat pads should be visualized and the source of the bleeding determined. Additional treatment includes elevating the head of the bed, ice compresses, controlling blood pressure, and using diuretics. We have encountered only two cases of retrobulbar hematoma in more than 10,000 blepharoplasties; both cases subsided spontaneously with no residual effects. Because we no longer inject fat pads percutaneously, but only under direct vision, we have not seen any cases of retrobulbar hematoma in the past decade.

Loss of Vision

The most feared complication of blepharoplasty is loss of vision, which is rare. In some cases this condition was present preoperatively. In some isolated instances, retinal artery occlusion associated with retrobulbar hematoma was felt to be responsible. In Moser's classic article, an international survey reported only seven cases of unilateral blindness. This study established no causal relationship between blindness and blepharoplasty. Obviously, uncontrolled retrobulbar hemmorrhage is the intraoperative event most likely to lead to this disastrous complication. Hemostasis in blepharoplasty cannot be overemphasized.

Overresection of Fat Pads

In cases where the eye appears to be deep-set or even borderline, the appearance of the eyes can be made worse by overly aggressive resection of the fat pads. Minimum fat resection or, in some cases, no fat resection is advised in these individuals.

In cases of routine blepharoplasty, we have found it rarely necessary to excise bony prominences of the infraorbital or supraorbital rims.

Ptosis

Ptosis should be diagnosed preoperatively. At that time, many cases of minimum ptosis or "lazy eye" will be discovered. If a true ptosis exists, it can be corrected in conjunction with the blepharoplasty.

Patients should be informed of these problems, because they may not be aware that their eyelids are asymmetric or that ptosis exists. These conditions must be documented photographically and demonstrated to the patient before surgery. Most plastic surgeons have had the unpleasant experience of having a blepharoplasty patient return and complain that the eyelids are not level in relation to the pupils, suggesting that the resultant ptosis was caused by the operation. Careful examination of the preoperative photographs usually reveals that the ptosis or asymmetry was present preoperatively and that neither the physician nor the patient was aware of this condition.

Persistent Small Wrinkles

Some patients return to say, "Look at me when I smile. Look at these lines on my lower eyelids and look at my crow's feet," complaining that surgery has not corrected these lines. In some individuals, a chemical peel performed 3 to 6 months postoperatively may be beneficial. (See Chapter 3 for more information on this technique.) In the past, phenol was our preferred peeling agent; however, we currently favor TCA peeling for residual lower lid rhytides following blepharoplasty.

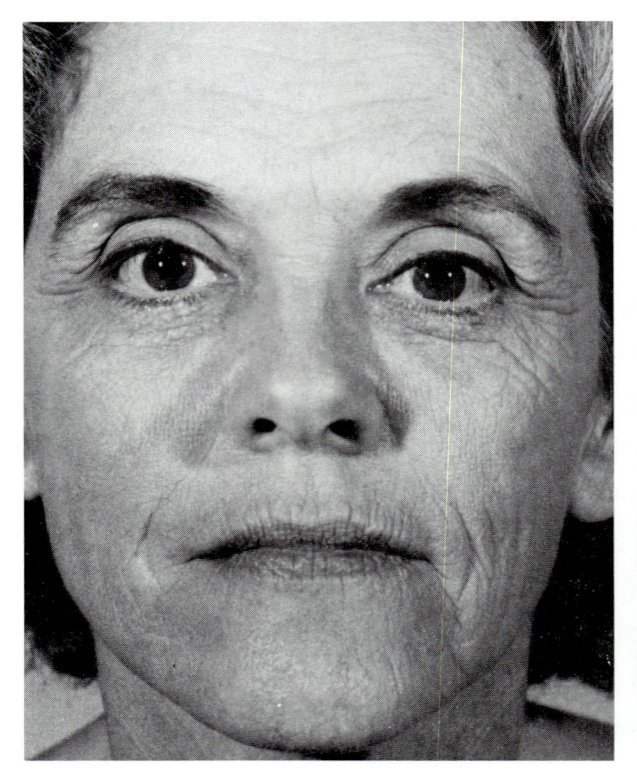

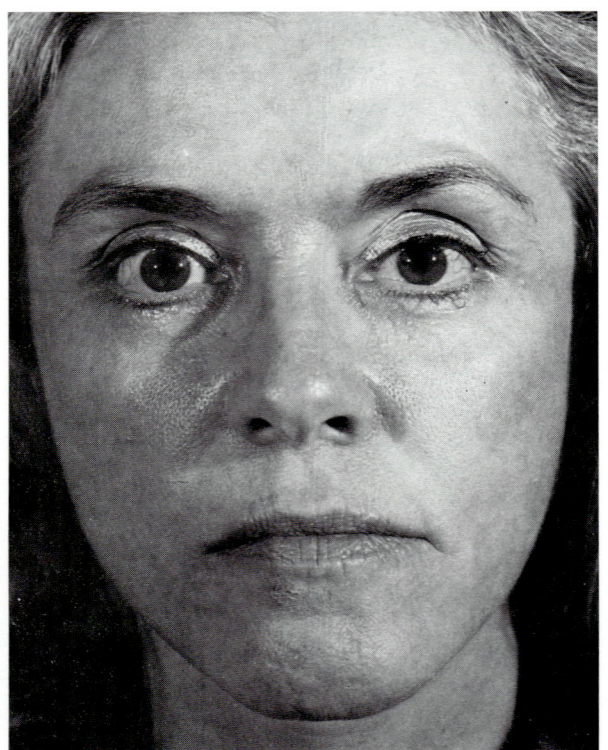

This patient requested elimination of the fine lines of her face, especially the periorbital lines. She strongly objected to the "crows-feet" overlying the malar prominences. The patient is shown in the photograph on the right 2 years after a total chemical face peel. The "crows's-feet" are gone, as are the other fine mosaic lines in the periorbital area (see technique in Chapter 3).

Temporary Paresis of the Lower Lid

Partial interruption of the seventh nerve may cause temporary paresis of the lower lid. We have not seen this problem in our series of cases. Spontaneous correction has been reported to occur within a few days.

Damage to the Inferior Oblique Muscle

Although damage to the inferior oblique muscle is extremely rare, it is certainly possible. Since the inferior oblique muscle separates the medial and central fat compartments in the lower eyelid, care must be taken during their dissection not to injure the muscle. Persistent diplopia is an obvious symptom of injury. Treatment should include an ophthalmologic consultation and possible exploration if the condition persists.

Wound Dehiscence

Wound dehiscence can occur accidentally if the patient collides with a blunt object or inadvertently scratches the lines of incision in the early postoperative period. Wound dehiscence is usually seen in the first 2 or 3 days after suture removal and can be adequately managed by simple resuturing.

Infection

Infection following blepharoplasty is extremely rare. We have encountered one case of this troublesome problem; the organism was *Staphylococcus aureus,* coagulase positive. Treatment consisted of reopening the wound, securing a culture, determining organism sensitivity, and administering the appropriate antibiotics. The value of prophylactic antibiotics in preventing infection is questionable and is left to the discretion of the individual surgeon. Small pustules rarely occur around the suture lines but have been observed if the sutures are left in too long. This situation is treated by removing the sutures and applying warm compresses and topical antibiotics.

Blepharitis

Blepharitis marginalis, or inflammation of the eyelid margins, is a rare complication occasionally noted along the base of the lashes. It has been observed when the incision has been made too close to the lash margin, thereby irritating the follicles and the dermal appendages in this area. If the incisions are made approximately 2 mm below the margin of the lower eyelid, this condition will probably not be encountered.

Inability to Close the Eyes

It may be difficult for the patient to close his or her eyes during the early postoperative period, especially while the swelling persists. Drying of the corneal surface can be prevented by using ointments and lubricating drops. Dark glasses should be worn in case of possible photophobia. If upper eyelid skin shortage is severe, then a graft similar to the lower eyelid graft may be necessary. Split-thickness skin grafts are better for upper eyelid replacement because full-thickness grafts are too thick for adaptation to the necessary mechanics of upper eyelid excursion.

Secondary Blepharoplasty

A word of caution to the inexperienced surgeon attempting secondary procedures: The patient who has had a previous blepharoplasty and who is unhappy with the results may have unrealistic expectations and must be treated accordingly. Careful screening is necessary for this individual. A secondary operation is frequently unnecessary. We have encountered patients who think their eyelid appearance is unacceptable, yet no significant deformity is detected upon examination and photographic documentation. Others complain that their "incisions are not equally distanced from the eyelash margin." This problem can occur even in experienced hands; however, after several weeks, when the redness in the incisions has faded out, the scars are far less apparent. If possible, the patient should be urged to wait to allow the scars to heal and fade. As previously observed, many of these patients are extremely eyelid conscious and no degree of surgical expertise will satisfy their desires.

Some patients complain of bulges that remain after their first operation. This problem could be caused by fat pockets that were overlooked or improperly resected. If there is a bulging of the muscle or orbital fat, this can be treated appropriately. However, the surgeon must not be too anxious to reoperate on these individuals until 6 to 12 months have passed. Surprisingly, most of these conditions improve and the patients do not return for additional surgery.

■ Too Much Upper Eyelid Skin Remains

The patient may hold his or her fingers above the eyebrow, pull the brow upward slightly, and say, "You should have taken out more eyelid skin." The situation here is usually a drooping eyebrow. The novice surgeon may be duped into removing more eyelid skin, actually creating a shortage of upper eyelid skin, and possibly accentuating the problem. If a browlift is indicated, then this becomes the procedure of choice. Additional surgery on the eyelid will only complicate the existing situation. Trite as it sounds, a blepharoplasty will not correct a drooping brow.

Occasionally, a slight trim of upper eyelid skin is performed as a secondary procedure if the problem truly results from excess skin remaining in the upper eyelids.

■ Irregular or Unsightly Scars

Scars often self-correct in a few weeks or months; therefore procrastination is in order. Slight bulges and irregularities, especially at the outer canthus in the area of the lower eyelid incision, seem to improve dramatically over an 8- to 10-week period. Z-plasties and scar revisions are rarely necessary and should be reserved for defects that persist after a few months have passed.

It must be remembered that very little skin and muscle can be sacrificed in a secondary procedure, and conservatism must be emphasized.

SURGICAL REJUVENATION OF THE FACE

■ Persisting Malar Pouches

A standard blepharoplasty usually will not significantly improve the malar pouch. If a combination of lower eyelid blepharoplasty and elevation of the temple does not adequately correct the problem, then direct excision may be the only answer.

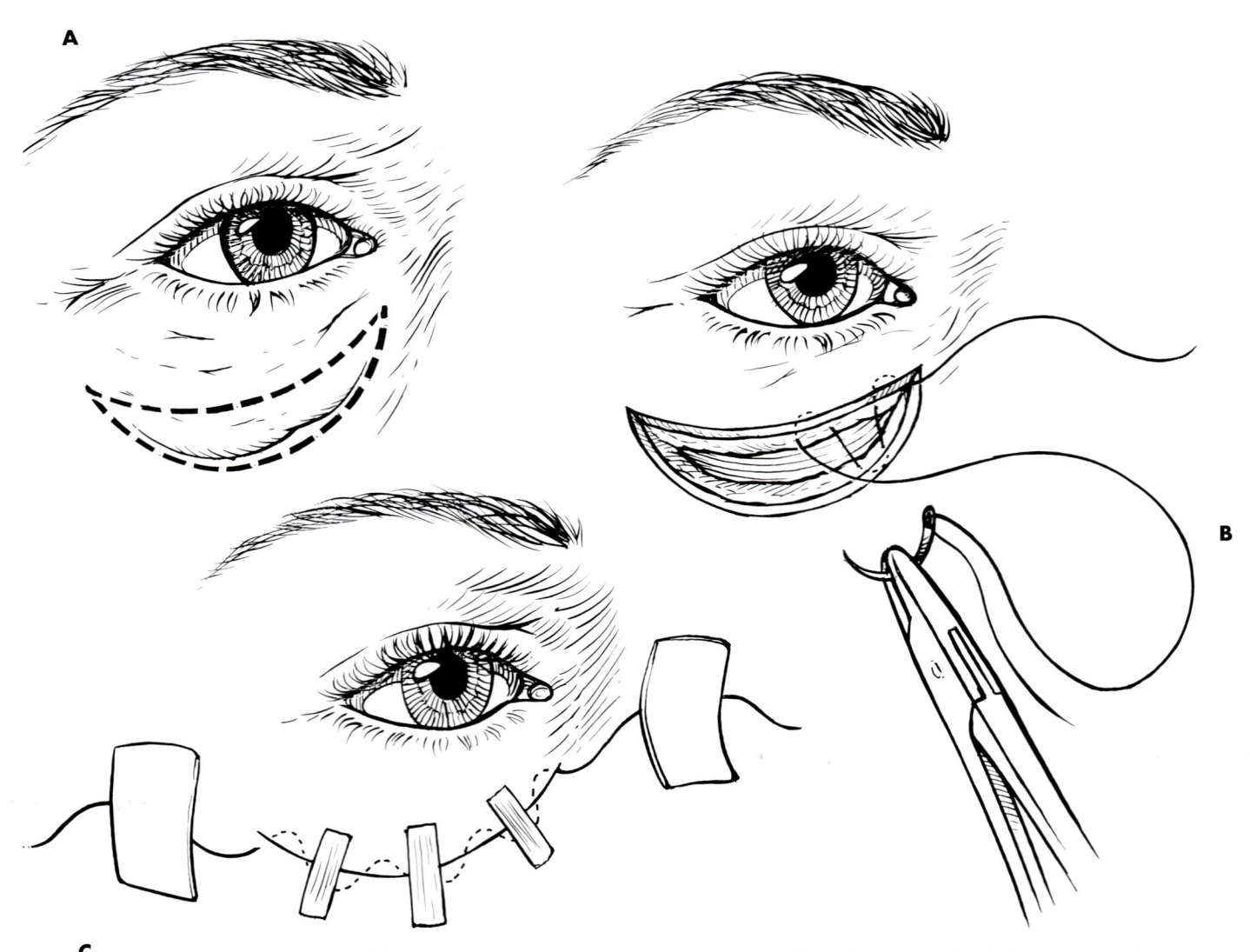

A

B

C

The malar or secondary bags can be directly excised. If the excess skin redundancy in this area cannot be completely removed by a lower eyelid blepharoplasty or if residual laxity remains, then the direct excision is an option. The area to be excised is marked (A), the ellipse is removed (B), and the wound is closed with a subcuticular pull-out suture (C).

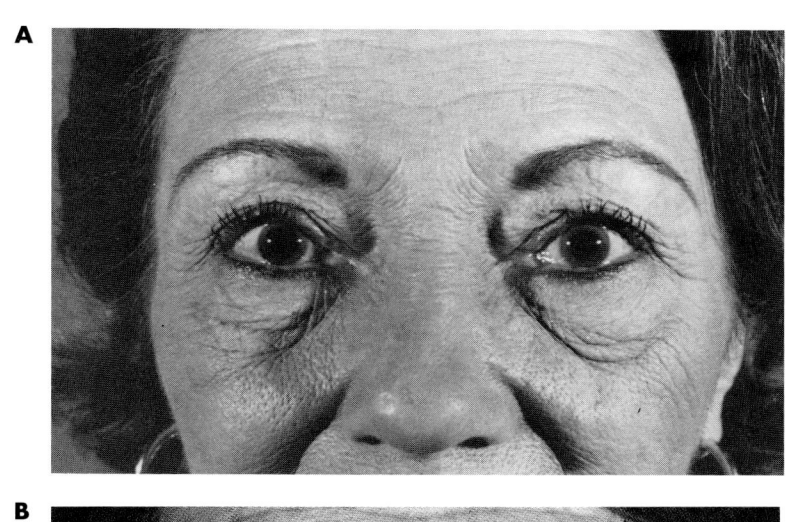

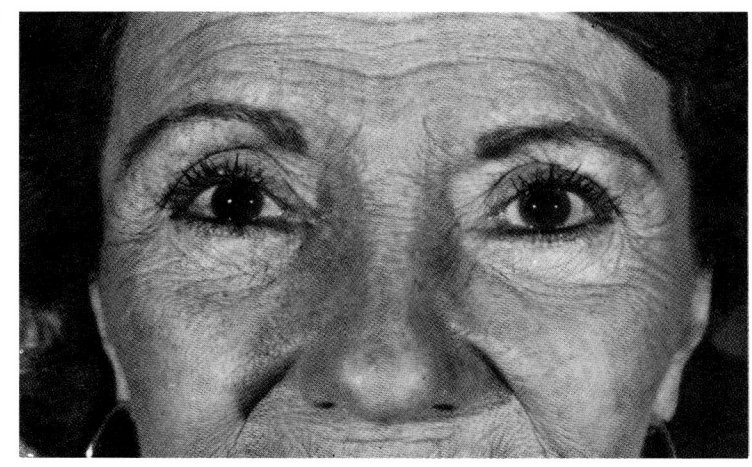

A, This patient has large secondary bags of the lower eyelids to be corrected by direct excision. This is occasionally indicated when a standard lower eyelid blepharoplasty will not correct the problem. B, Postoperatively the scars of the incisions used for the direct excision are well concealed. The upper eyelids also had a blepharoplasty. This patient would further benefit from a coronal browlift and a total chemical face peel.

■ Lower Eyelid Laxity

The examination of every patient considering lower eyelid blepharoplasty should include the evaluation of eyelid tone. Loss of tone is commonly seen in the aging patient, and failure to recognize and correct this problem places the patient at high risk for developing postoperative scleral show or ectropion. Lower eyelid laxity is most commonly secondary to attenuation and disinsertion of the lateral canthal tendon. Preoperative evaluation of lower eyelid tone will allow the sur-

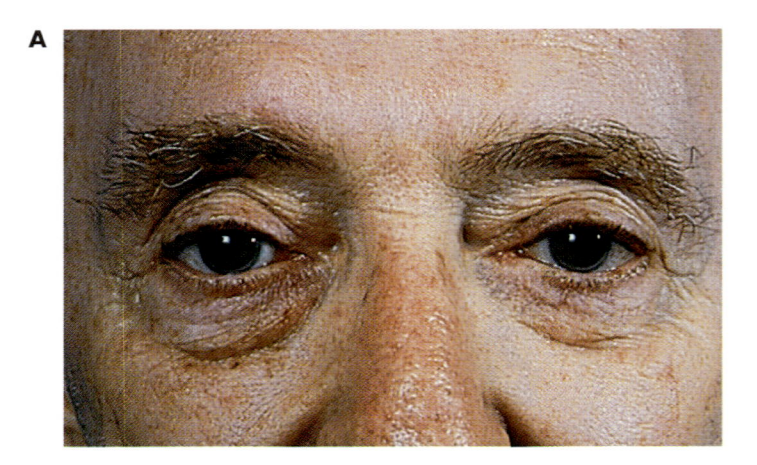

A, This patient exhibits the typical stigmata of lateral canthal disinsertion. Note the scleral show present at the temporal limbus, along with a loss of the normal S-shaped curve of the lower lid, which now appears U-shaped. The angle of the lateral commissure is indistinct and lies several millimeters medial to the lateral orbital rim. The lateral commissure lies at a level equal to the medial commissure in primary gaze, again suggesting poor lid tone secondary to lateral canthal disinsertion.

geon to recognize the possible need for treatment at the time of blepharoplasty, thereby preventing untoward sequela following surgery. The most effective test for evaluation of the lower eyelid is the "snap-back test." This test is performed simply by pulling the lower eyelid inferiorly toward the infraorbital rim and instructing the patient not to blink. If the lower eyelid remains suspended away from the globe and only returns to its normal position with blinking, then significant laxity of the lower lid exists and should be corrected during blepharoplasty.

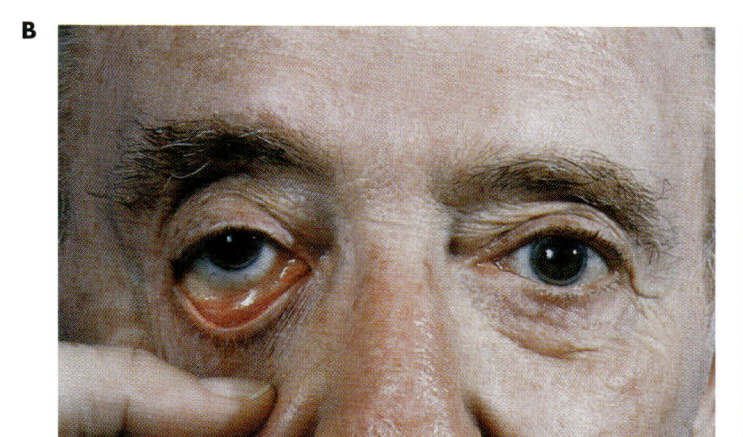

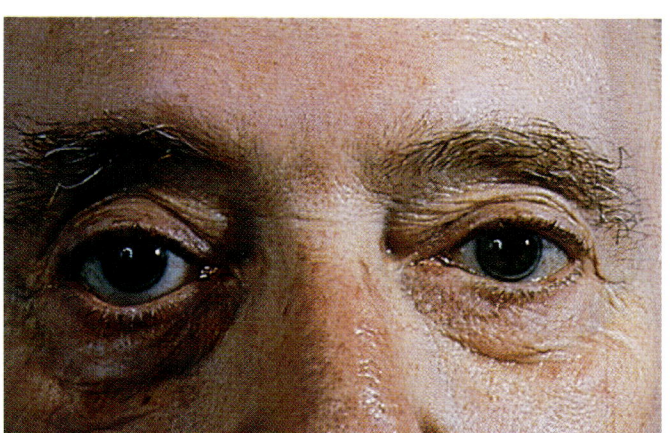

B, The patient is asked to pull the lower lid inferiorly. Note that because of the lateral canthal disinsertion and poor support to the lower lid, the base of the fornix is visible. C, Following release of the lower eyelid, note that it does not return to its normal resting position against the globe without blinking. This again confirms the diagnosis of poor lower lid support secondary to lateral canthal disinsertion. A patient such as this often requires some form of lower lid support, such as lateral canthopexy to prevent further lid retraction following lower lid blepharoplasty.

The eyelid distraction test is another simple method of evaluating lid tone. If the eyelid can be pulled away from the globe a distance greater than 7 to 8 mm, this again suggests lower eyelid laxity and requires lower eyelid tightening during surgery.

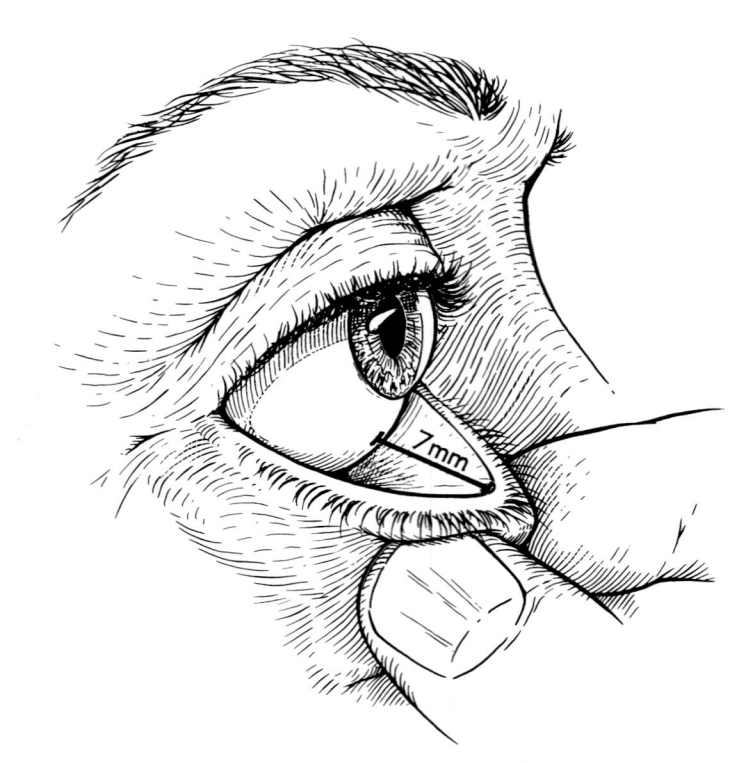

The eyelid distraction test is a simple method of evaluating lower lid tone. The eyelid is simply pulled away from the globe. If a distance of greater than 7 to 8 mm is present following lower lid distraction, this confirms a diagnosis of lower eyelid laxity and suggests that some form of lid tightening procedure should be incorporated in the blepharoplasty plan.

Detachment or attenuation of the lateral canthal tendon is commonly responsible for lower eyelid laxity. Simple observation of the morphology of the patient's lower eyelid will commonly reveal a problem in this region. Under normal circumstances the lateral canthal angle is sharp and well defined. In disinsertion of the lateral canthal tendon, there commonly will be a blunting or roundness of the lateral canthal angle, which is obvious on physical examination. Under normal circumstances the distance between the lateral orbital rim and the lateral end of the eyelid is negligible and usually corresponds to within 1 to 2 mm of the lateral orbital wall. With lateral canthal disinsertion, the distance between the lateral commissure of the eyelid and the lateral orbital rim is increased and often there is several millimeters of distance between the lateral commissure and the lateral orbital rim. This increase in distance from the lateral canthal angle to the lateral orbital wall is associated with rounding of the lateral commissure associated with scleral show and a downward displacement of the temporal portion of the lower eyelid. Our surgical approach to the lax lower lid includes (1) suture support to the lateral canthus and taping of the lower lid, (2) wedge excision lateral to the limbus, and (3) tarsal strip procedure.

Suture support to the lateral canthal tendon

A simple procedure that is useful in the patient with mild lower lid laxity is simply a suture support to the lateral canthal tendon. This procedure involves suturing the lateral aspect of the lateral tarsal plate and lateral canthal tendon superiorly to the orbital periosteum without formal cantholysis. The advantage of this procedure is that it is rapid to perform and is associated with minimal morbidity. The disadvantage of this procedure is that it is useful only in patients with mild lower eyelid laxity and should in no way substitute for a formal tarsal strip procedure if lateral canthal disinsertion is advanced.

The technique for suture support is quite simple and involves placing a fine suture from the lateral canthal tendon or lateral tarsus superiorly to the medial aspect of the lateral orbital rim. It is important when placing the suture that not too much of the lower lid margin be gathered, or buckling of the lateral aspect of the lower lid will occur. We suggest that if persistent buckling occurs upon suture placement, suggesting a significant degree of disinsertion of the lateral canthal tendon, consideration should be given to a formal lateral tarsal strip procedure.

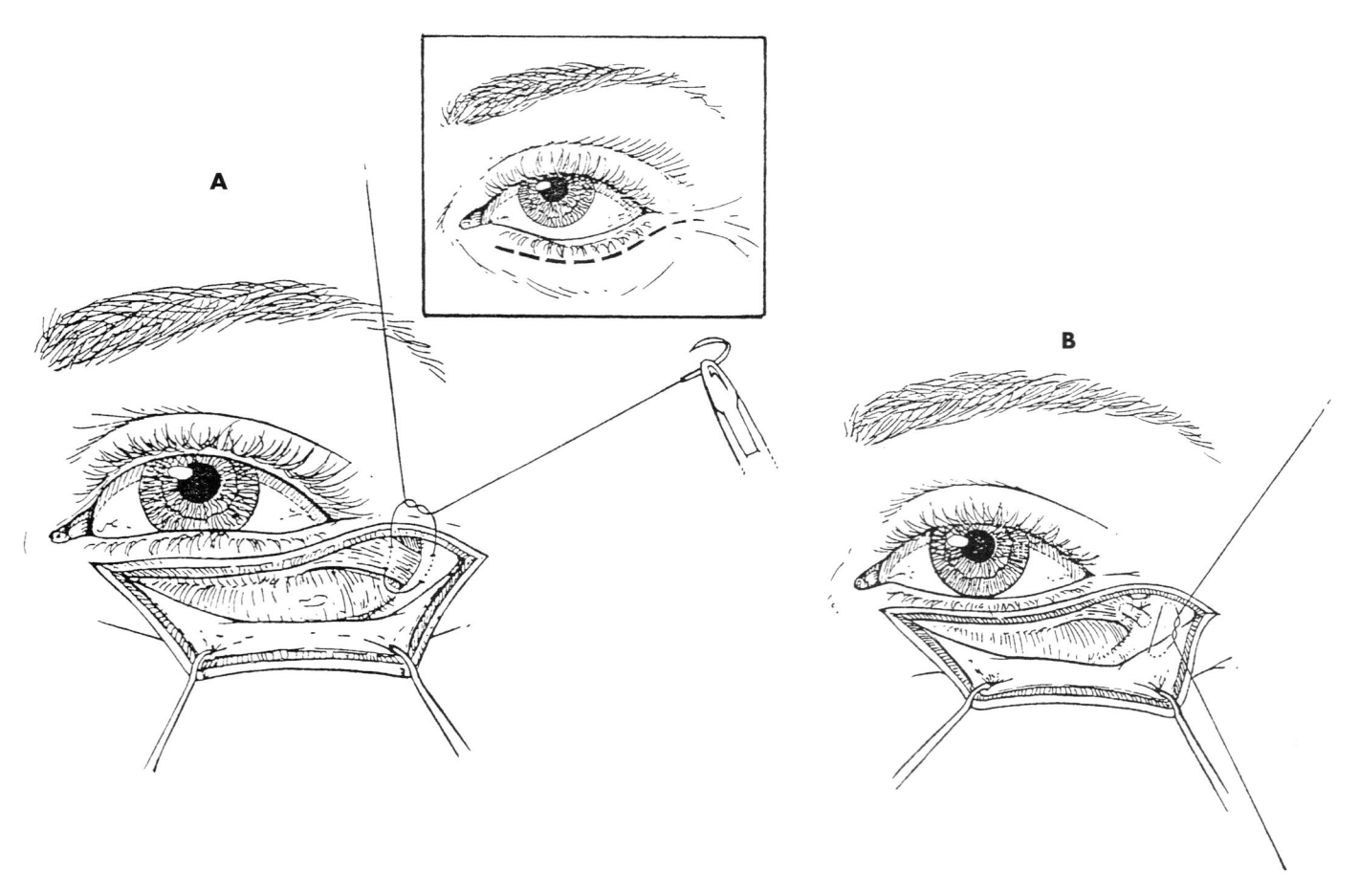

A, Suture support to the lateral canthal tendon. We prefer to use a fine absorbable suture (5-0 Vicryl), which is placed between the lateral canthal tendon and the medial aspect of the orbital periosteum. It is important that when this suture is tied it not produce a buckling of the lower lid. If this occurs, the suture should be either replaced or consideration given to a formal lateral tarsal strip procedure. B, The skin-muscle flap is similarly supported laterally via a suture placed from the orbicularis to the lateral orbital rim periosteum.

In patients requiring suture support of the lower lid, we commonly will perform taping as an additive measure to maintain lower lid position in the early postoperative period.

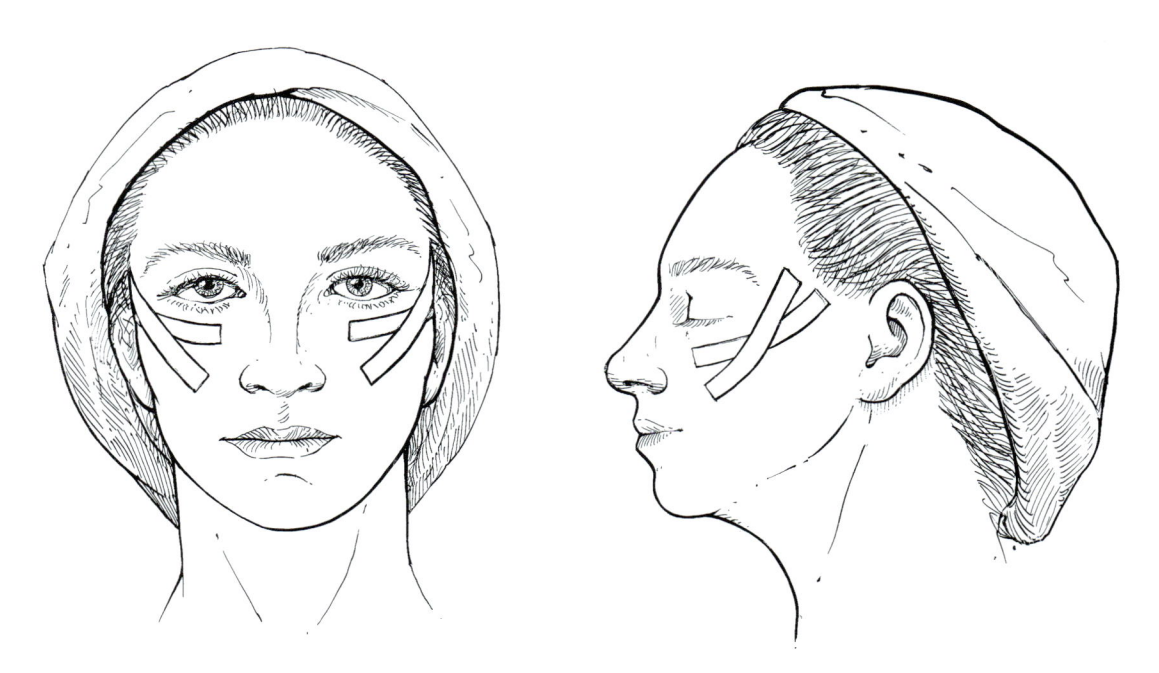

Perioperative taping is also a useful adjunct to preventing postoperative lid retraction. These tapes are placed in the malar area directly below the lower eyelid and extend in a superotemporal direction to the temporal area. We usually leave them in place for approximately 4 to 7 days following lower lid blepharoplasty.

Wedge excision lateral to the limbus

The oldest procedure described in the treatment of the lax lid is wedge partial excision somewhere in the region of the mideyelid. We have used a modification of the Kuhnt-Szymanowski procedure for many years with very good success. This procedure is usually performed just lateral to the limbus of the globe and is performed before closure in blepharoplasty. To remove a wedge from the lower eyelid, the skin (or skin muscle) flap is turned down in the routine fashion and the orbital fat contoured. Before closure, a full thickness resection of tarsus, including conjunctiva, is performed along the eyelid margin. The size of resection varies but is usually no more than 4 to 5 mm in width. The excision is always made lateral to the limbus. The wound is then repaired with 6-0 silk sutures. Usually three sutures are adequate. The first suture is placed to realign the skin at the junction along the subciliary incision. The second suture is then placed to realign the eyelashes. The third suture is placed just posterior to the gray line at the junction of conjunctiva with lid margin. A 6-0 Vicryl suture can be placed within the lower portion of the tarsus but should not be placed through the conjunctiva. There is no need to suture the conjunctiva, since this heals spontaneously without problem as long as the tarsus and lid margin are carefully reapproximated. The silk sutures are then left long and are removed 1 week postoperatively.

Of note, at this time we rarely use wedge resection procedures and prefer to reconstruct the lax lower lid through some form of lateral canthopexy.

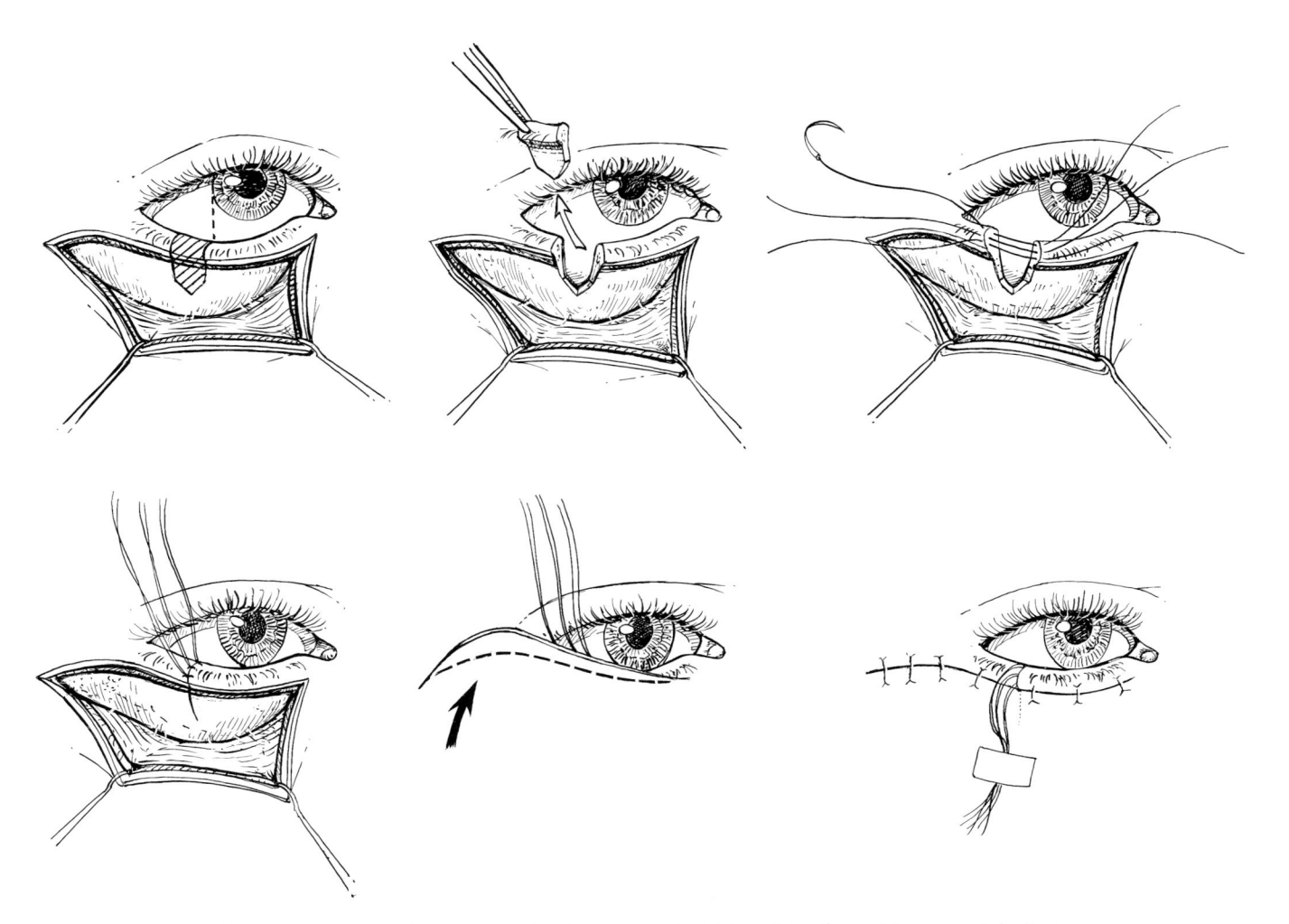

To remove a wedge from the lower eyelid, the skin (or skin-muscle) flap is turned down in a routine fashion. A wedge including conjunctiva through the eyelid margin is then removed. The size varies but is usually 4 to 5 mm in width. The excision is always made lateral to the limbus. The wedge is excised, including all layers. The wound is approximated with 6-0 silk sutures. Usually three sutures are adequate. The sutures should not go through to the conjunctiva. There is no need to suture the conjunctiva, since this heals well spontaneously without approximation. The sutures are in place and left long.

■ Lateral Canthopexy (Tarsal Strip Procedure)

Lower lid laxity is commonly secondary to lateral canthal disinsertion. The anatomic solution to this problem is to reattach the lateral canthal tendon to the lateral orbital periosteum in the region of Whitnall's tubercle. For this reason lateral canthopexy procedures such as the tarsal strip anatomically restore tone to the lax lower lid. Although a bit more technically demanding than wedge-excision procedures (Kuhnt-Szymanowski), tarsal-strip procedures offer the advantage of being an anatomic reconstruction to the problem, elevating the temporal aspect of the lower eyelid and avoiding any webbing or notching that can occur with wedge resection procedures. In general, the aesthetic results of lateral canthopexy are superior to those obtained with wedge excision procedures.

Tightening of the lateral canthal tendon can be performed at the termination of the blepharoplasty procedure just before trimming of the lower lid skin. The procedure is begun by an incision made in the inferior limb of the lateral canthus. Following a cantholysis of the inferior limb of the lateral canthal tendon, mobilization of the lateral eyelid is performed by using sharp scissor dissection to separate and free the attachments of the orbital septum to the underlying lateral orbital rim. The freed lower tarsus and lateral canthal tendon is then stretched tight against the lateral orbital wall to determine the amount of lateral tarsus available to perform the tarsal strip. Usually a 3 mm resection of the lateral canthal tendon is all that is required. A mattress suture is then placed through the tarsal strip, which is then secured to the medial aspect of the lateral orbital wall, usually 2 to 3 mm cephalad to Whitnall's tubercle (a bony landmark that is easily palpable in most patients). We prefer to use a 4-0 permanent mattress suture, using double-armed needles. Before securing this suture it is important to realign the gray line of the upper and lower eyelid to reform the lateral commissure. After reformation of the lateral commissure, the tarsal strip is secured to the lateral orbital rim such that the lateral canthal tendon and lateral commissure lie at least 2 mm above the medial canthal tendon. The level of the midpupil serves as a useful guide for the proper level of reattachment of the tarsal strip to lateral orbital periosteum.

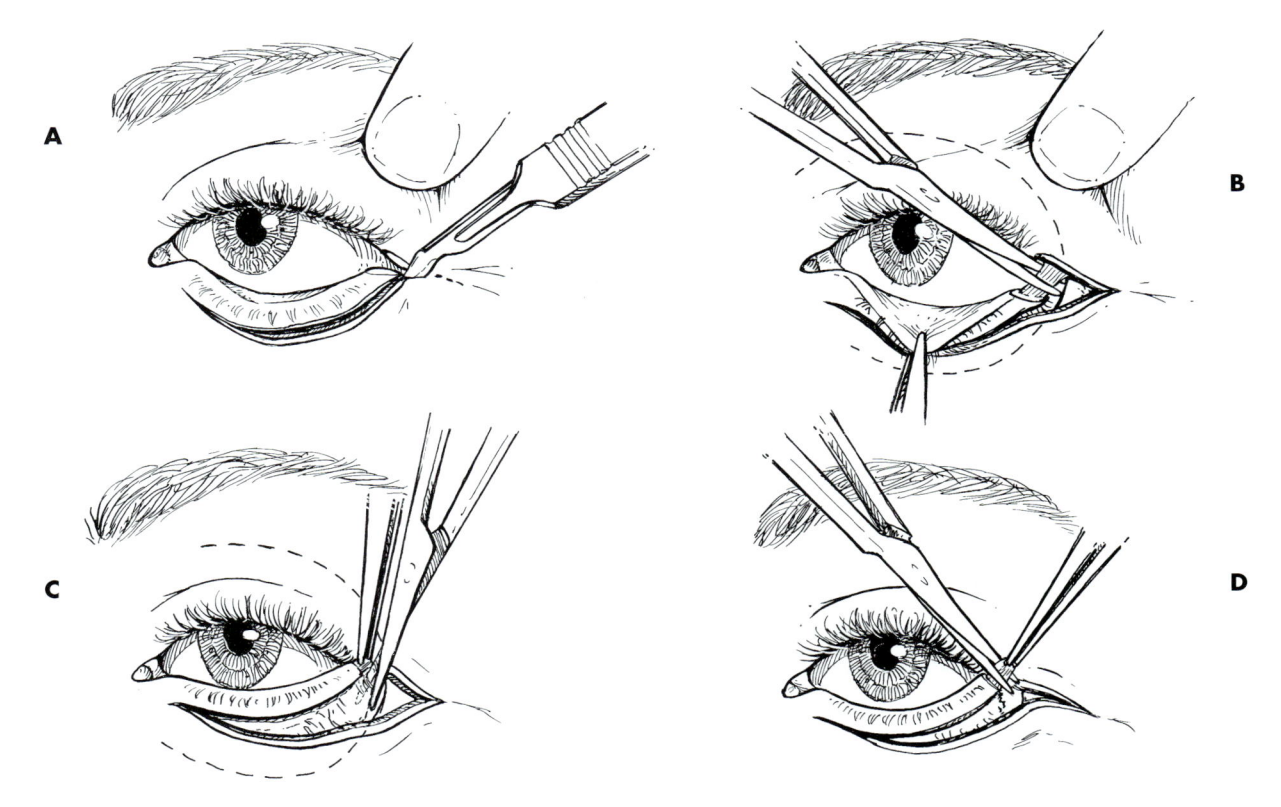

A and B, The first step in a lateral canthopexy is to perform a canthotomy of the inferior limb of the lateral canthal tendon. This is performed by designing the canthotomy to correspond with the lateral aspect of the subciliary incision. C, Following canthotomy, cantholysis is necessary to free the lateral canthal tendon and lateral aspect of the tarsus from its attachments to the orbital septum and the lateral orbital rim. This procedure is performed with sharp scissor dissection, incising the lateral aspects of the orbital septum until the eyelid margin can move freely toward the lateral orbital rim. D, A conservative trim of the lateral canthal tendon is then performed in a full-thickness manner after judging the degree of resection required so that the lower lid will fit against the lateral orbital rim without undue tension. Usually a 2 to 4 mm resection is all that is required.

Continued.

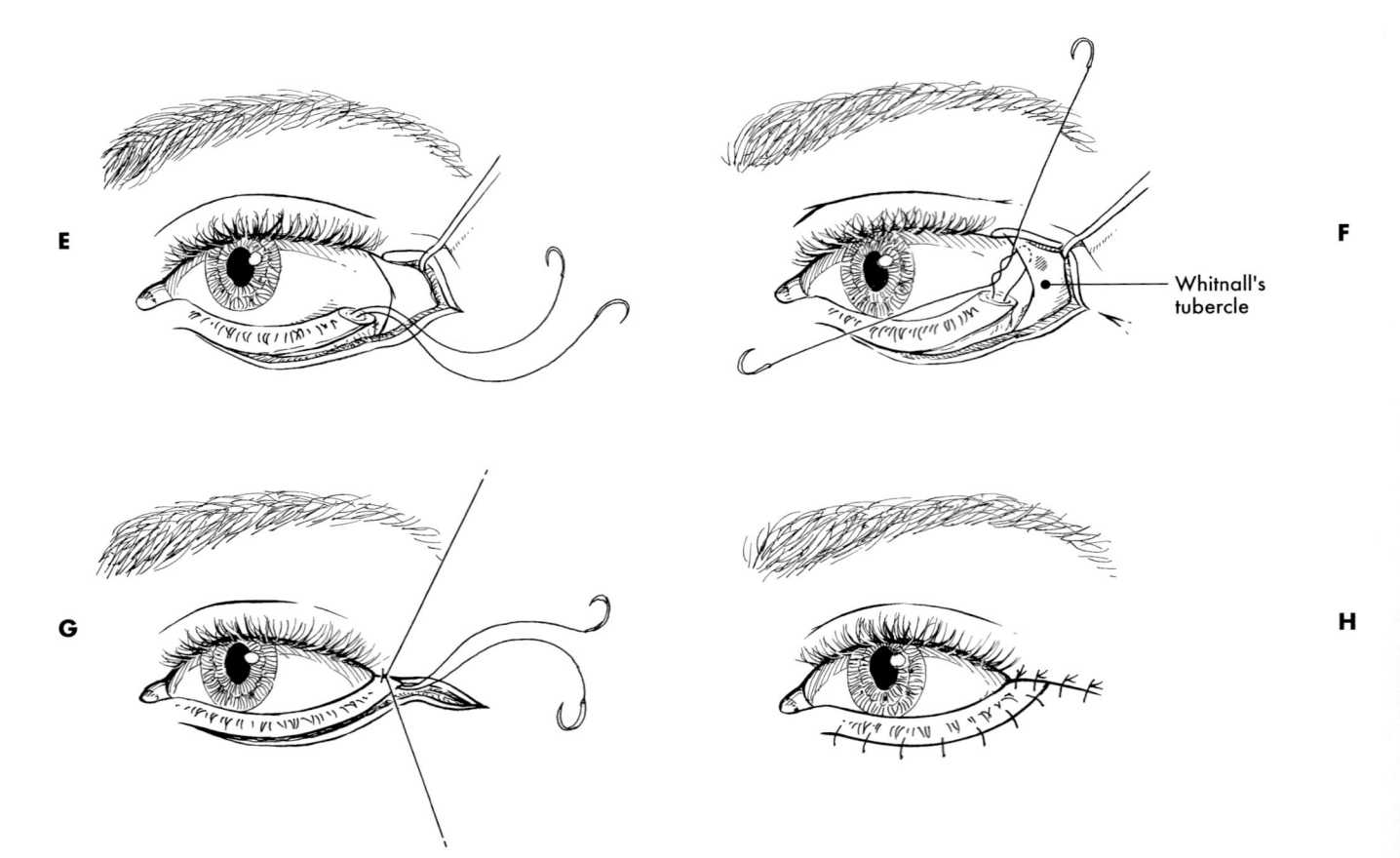

E, A double-armed mattress suture is placed into the stump of the lateral canthal tendon. **F,** This suture is then placed to the periosteum along the medial aspect of the lateral orbital rim. In placing this suture, Whitnall's tubercle, which is easily palpable, serves as a useful landmark. We usually place this suture 2 to 3 mm cephalad to Whitnall's tubercle. This region represents the deepest portion of the lateral orbital rim, and from this junction cephalad, the lateral orbital rim travels more anteriorly toward the lacrimal fossae. **G,** Before ligation of the lateral canthal tendon suture, the lateral commissure is restored by placing a skin suture into the gray line of the upper and lower lid. Following commissure restoration, the suture from the lateral canthal tendon to the lateral orbital rim is ligated, serving to secure the lateral canthopexy. **H,** Skin closure is then performed, suturing the lateral canthotomy before securing the skin-muscle flap in proper position.

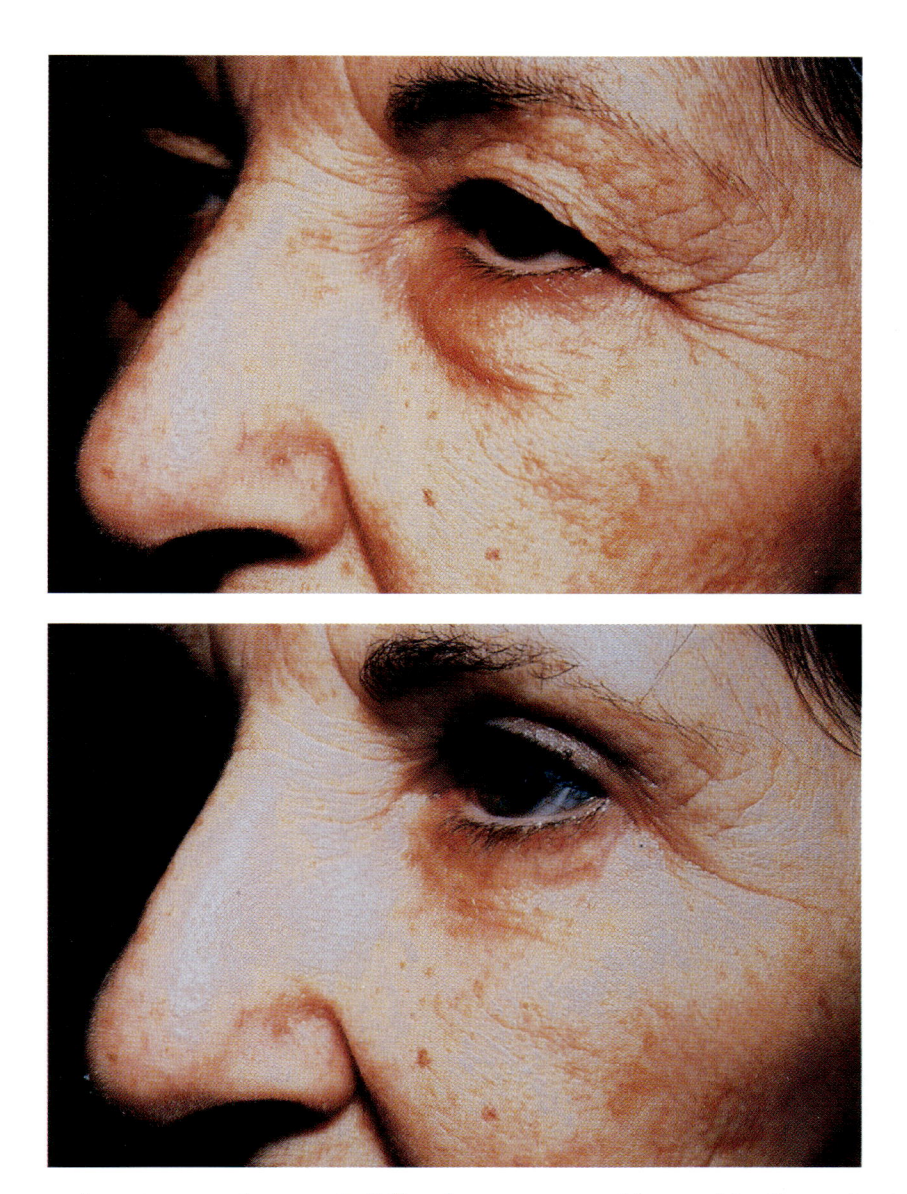

Pre- and postoperative result following upper and lower blepharoplasty with lateral canthopexy.

Ectropion

Severe eyelid ectropion following blepharoplasty is commonly associated with an overresection of skin. This produces a shortened anterior lamella of the eyelid and has been termed a cicatricial ectropion. Concomitant laxity of the lower eyelid is usually seen. Lower lid ectropion is most severe along the temporal aspect of the lower lid and often corresponds to where the majority of skin is resected in blepharoplasty, as well as to the coexistence of laxity in this region secondary to attenuation of support from the lateral canthal tendon. In evaluating the patient with postoperative ectropion, if too much skin resection is responsible for the lid retraction, the surgeon will be unable to elevate the lower eyelid above the level of the limbus.

Severe ectropion resulting from too much skin resection will rarely correct itself spontaneously; surgical intervention is indicated. To treat this condition, the incision is reopened along the lower eyelid margin, all the surrounding tissue is freed, and a full-thickness skin graft is used to replace the missing skin. The opposite upper eyelid skin with its similarity in color and texture provides an ideal donor site. However, if the upper eyelid has been resected following a four-eyelid blepharoplasty, sufficient skin may no longer be available. In that case, retroauricular or preauricular skin is the next choice. These donor sites give adequate color match. A stent dressing is applied and usually left in position for 7 days. If an attenuation of lateral canthal support also exists, then lateral canthopexy should also be performed at the time of skin graft placement.

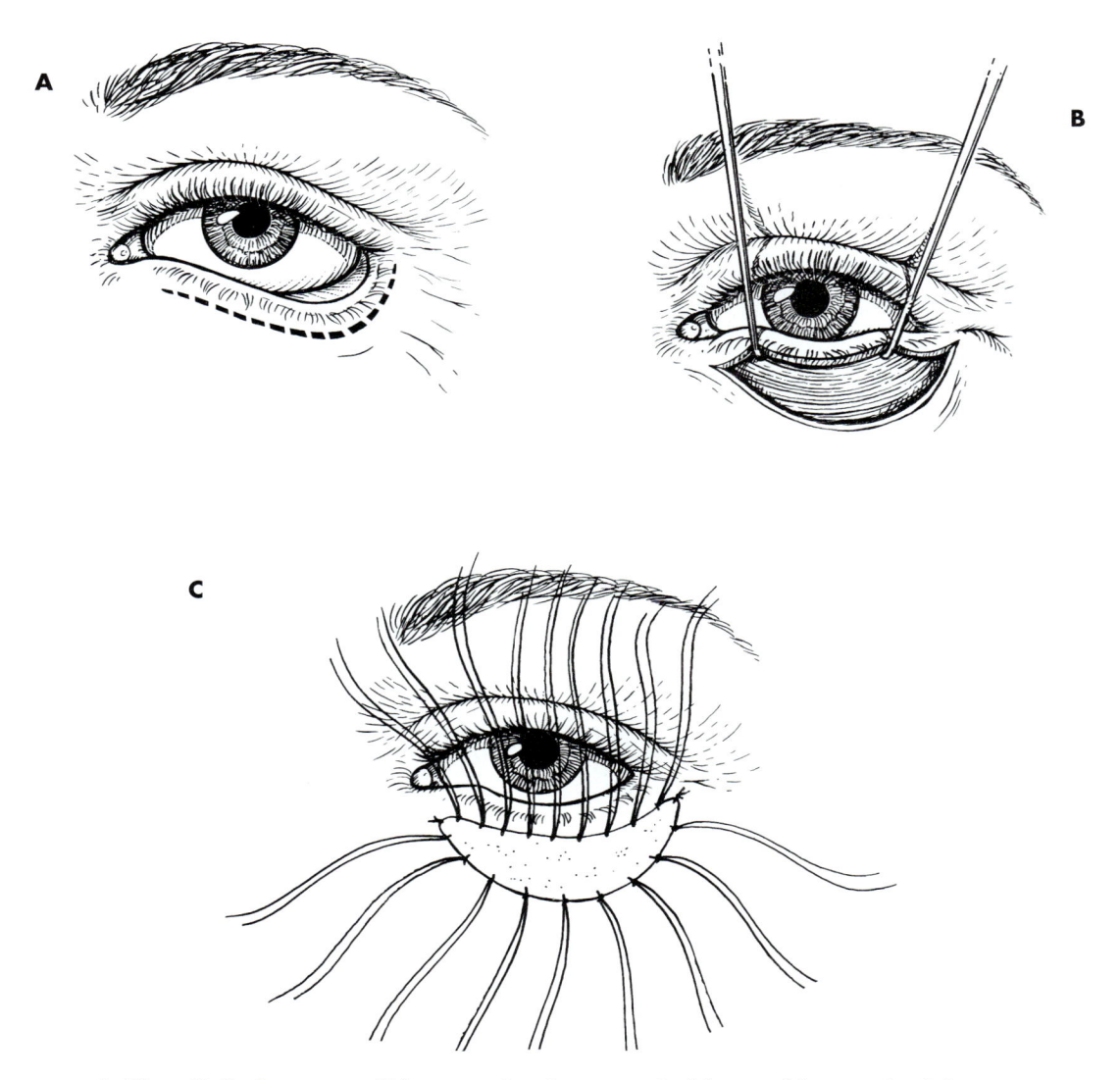

A, The slight lower eyelid ectropion is corrected by making an incision just beneath the ciliary margin, usually opening the original incision. **B,** The eyelid is allowed to move up to its original position after the incision is opened. **C,** A full-thickness skin graft is sutured into position to correct the ectropion. The sutures are tied over a bolster dressing. The graft is left undisturbed for 7 days.

SURGICAL REJUVENATION OF THE FACE

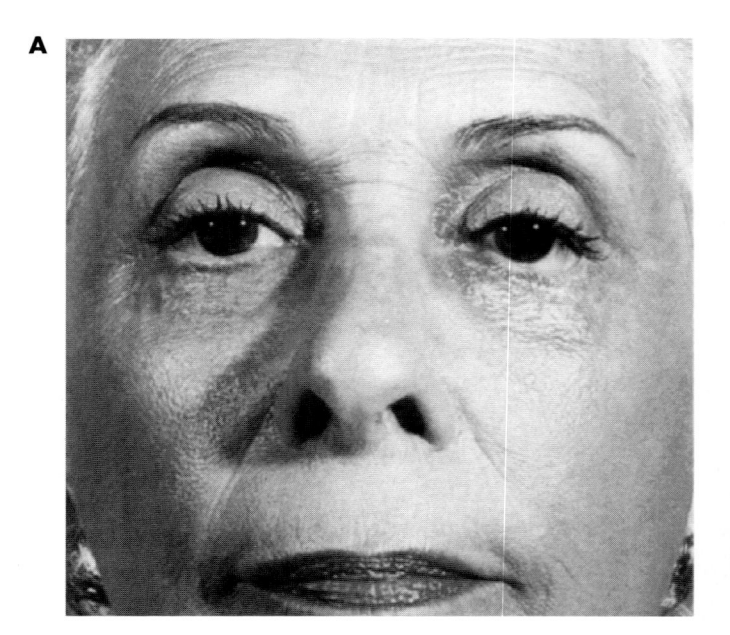

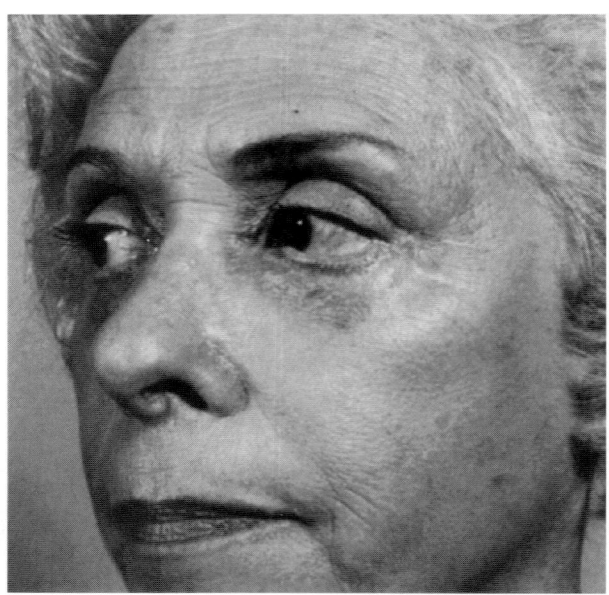

A, *This patient has a left lower eyelid ectropion that has persisted for 1 year after a four-lid blepharoplasty. The oblique view shows the retraction of the eyelid as evidenced by the obvious asymmetry. The patient was acutely aware of the deformity. She was unwilling to return to her original plastic surgeon for correction.*

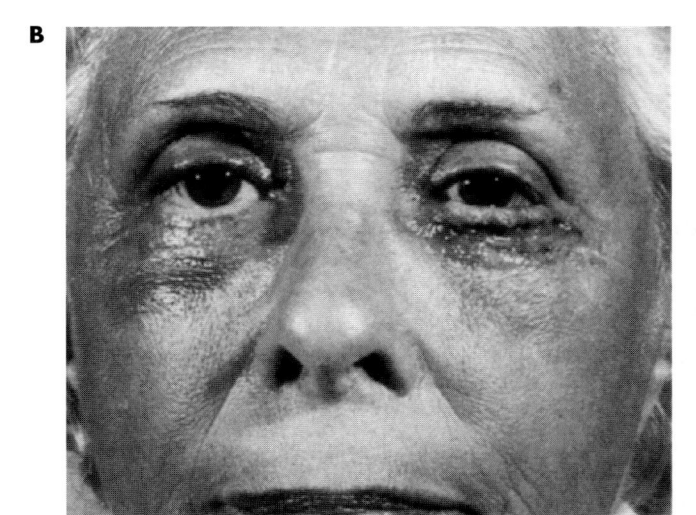

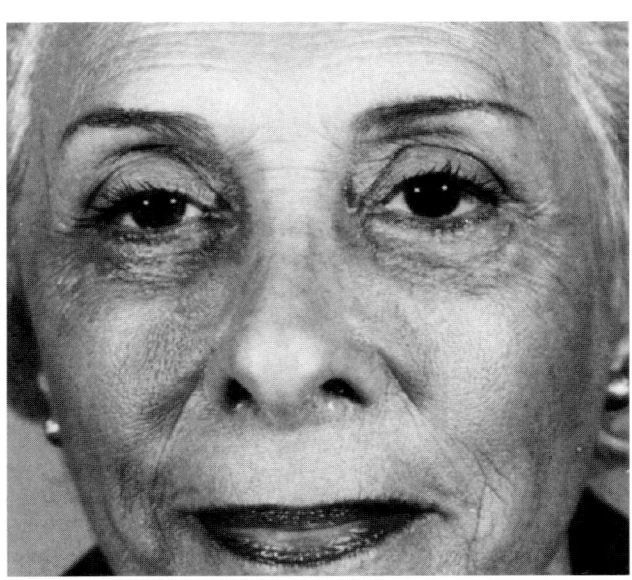

B, The ectropion was released by incising approximately 2 mm beneath the lash margin. The wound was allowed to open wide, and the missing skin was replaced with a full-thickness skin graft taken from the retroauricular area. The patient is shown 7 days postoperatively. C, This is the patient's appearance 6 months postoperatively. The graft has a good color match, and the ectropion has been corrected.

Management of Prolapsed Lacrimal Glands

With aging, the suspensory ligaments that support the lacrimal gland in its position within the lateral orbit often become attenuated and the lacrimal gland prolapses. The orbital globe of the lacrimal gland is usually responsible for this protrusion, and palpation with a forefinger along the lateral orbit will usually reveal a freely movable mass that can be repositioned within the lacrimal fossa. When the palpebral lobe prolapses, a pink mass is present beneath the conjunctiva within the lateral fornix. A prolapse of the lacrimal gland should not be confused with a prominent lower lid fat pad, and the treatment of the prolapsed gland should not involve resection. Partial resection of the orbital portion of the lacrimal gland can interrupt some of the excretory ducts that pass into the palpebral lobe and interfere with lacrimal gland function.

The surgical correction of lacrimal gland herniation involves repositioning the gland into its normal anatomic location within the lacrimal fossa. This can be done at the time of upper eyelid blepharoplasty. The orbital septum should be incised along its entire length to expose the underlying lacrimal gland within the lateral orbit. A 5-0 suture is then placed in a mattress fashion along the protruding edge of the lacrimal gland. Dissection is then continued superiorly between lacrimal gland and periosteum to expose the orbital roof. The suture is then passed through the periosteum of the orbital roof and superior rim. The orbital septum is then closed laterally if this is desired. Skin closure then proceeds as normally performed in blepharoplasty.

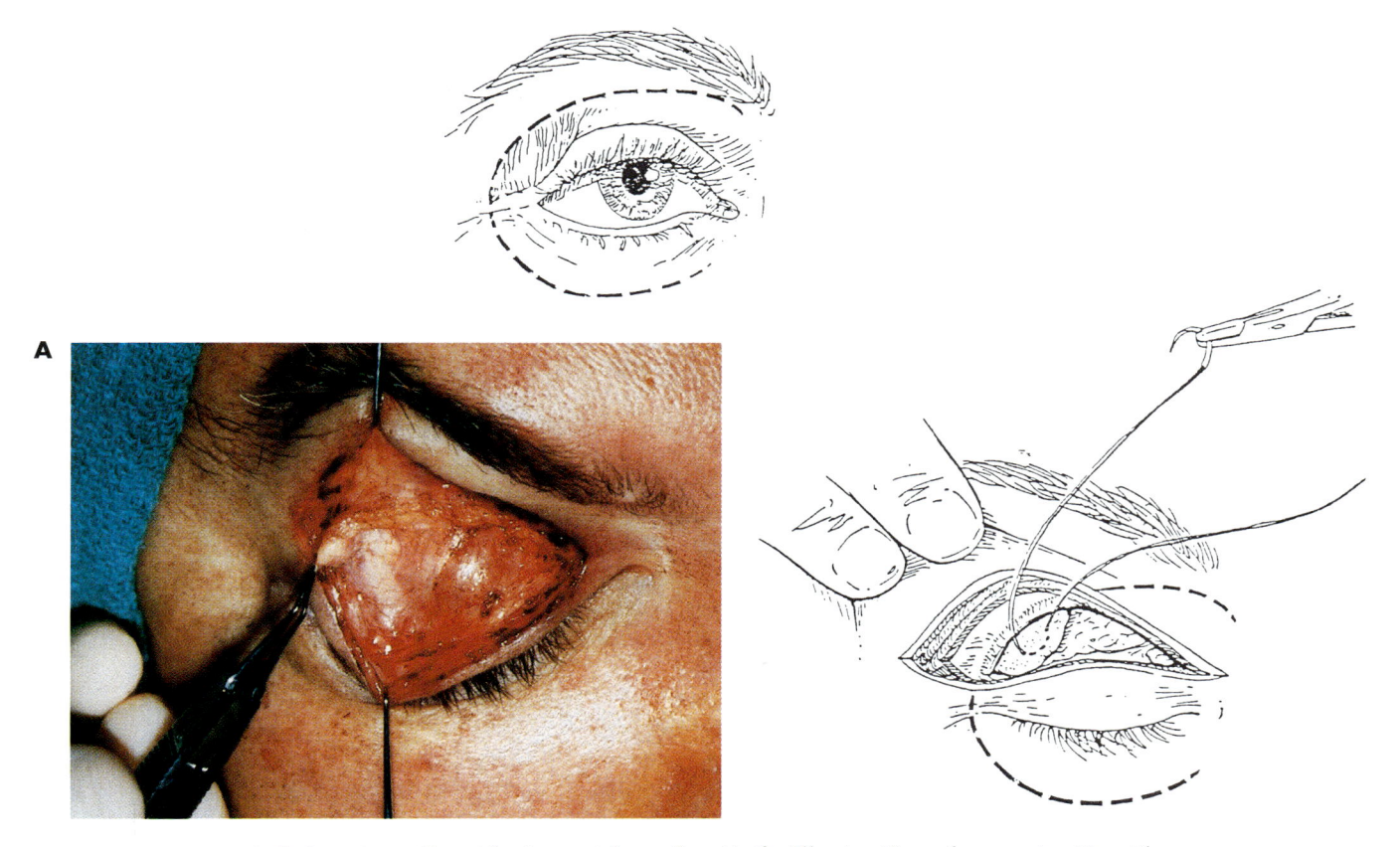

A, Intraoperative photograph and artist's illustration demonstrating the treatment of prolapse of the orbital portion of the lacrimal gland. This is most commonly noted following resection of the lateral aspect of the central fat pad of the upper lid.

Continued.

SURGICAL REJUVENATION OF THE FACE

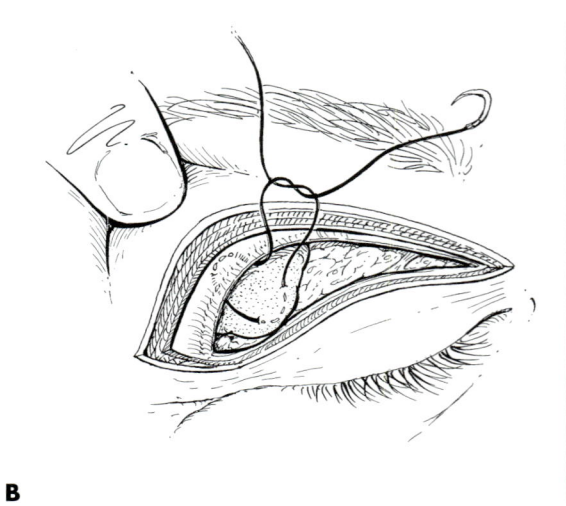

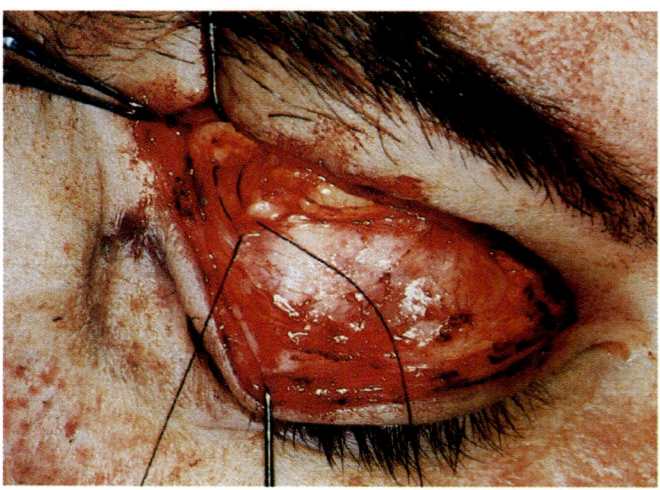

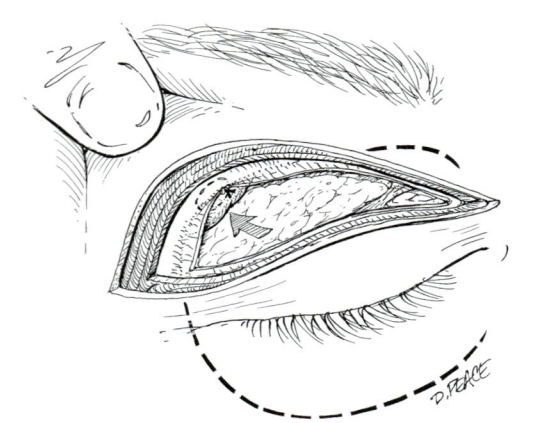

B, A horizontal mattress suture is then placed from the periosteum of the lacrimal fossa along the superior orbital rim through the outer pole of the lacrimal gland. Following ligation of this suture, the lacrimal gland is restored to its normal position within the lacrimal fossa.

Q&A FREQUENTLY ASKED QUESTIONS

"How long should I sleep with my head elevated?"
Elevating the head aids in diminishing the swelling around the eyes and is advised for the first few days after surgery but can be discontinued after a week.

"When can I return to my social life?"
Since the patient is not ill after this procedure, it is a matter of determining when the individual wishes to go out in public. Many patients will return to their business or social life wearing dark glasses for the first few days after surgery, but an average of 2 to 3 weeks pass before discarding the glasses and eliminating makeup.

"When can I go into the sun?"
The sun is destructive to the skin, and a sunscreen should be worn to protect the skin from solar damage. Although the sun will not affect the results of the operation, sundamaged skin will wrinkle more rapidly than skin that has not been exposed to chronic solar radiation.

"When can I wear my glasses or contact lenses?"
Glasses may be worn immediately after surgery, and the patient may resume wearing contact lenses 3 weeks postoperatively.

"When can I drive?"
Since a slight blurring of vision is likely to occur during the first 2 or 3 postoperative days while the periorbital region is swollen, it is advisable not to allow the patient to drive a car during that time. As soon as the blurring has disappeared, usually in 2 to 3 days, the patient can use his or her judgment as to whether driving is safe.

"When can I travel by air?"
There is no restriction on this activity.

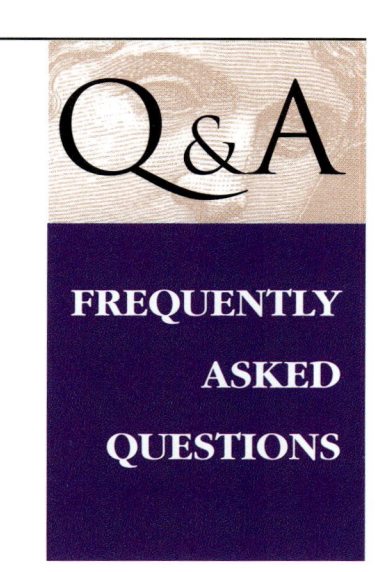

"How many postoperative visits are involved?"
There are usually two or three visits, provided there are no postoperative problems. The typical patient is discharged within 3 weeks.

"How do I clean my lashes during the early postoperative period?"
Cotton swabs moistened with clear tap water or hydrogen peroxide work well.

"Will the eyelid surgery remove all of these little crinkly lines when I squint?"
Some of the lines will be improved, but they will not be totally eliminated by the blepharoplasty. Some natural lines around the crow's feet are normal, and the patient must understand that they will not be totally eliminated.

SUGGESTED READING

Anderson RL, Gordy DD: The tarsal strip procedure, *Arch Ophthalmol* 97:2192-2196, 1979.

Aston SJ: Skin muscle flap lower lid blepharoplasty, *Clin Plast Surg* 15:305, 1988.

Baylis HI, Long JA, Groth MJ: Transconjunctival lower eyelid blepharoplasty: technique and complications, *Ophthalmology* 96:1027, 1989.

Carraway JH: Surgical anatomy of the eyelids, *Clin Plast Surg* 14:693, 1987.

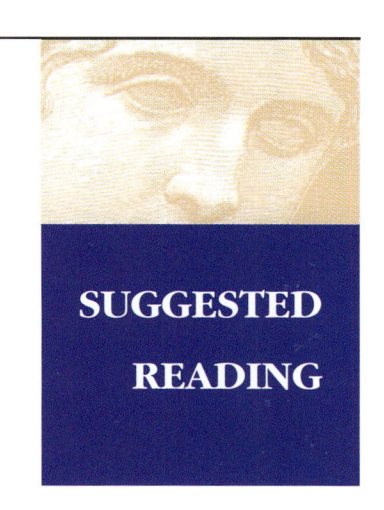

Carraway JH, Mellow CG: The prevention and treatment of lower lid ectropion following blepharoplasty, *Plast Reconstr Surg* 85:971, 1990.

Casson P, Siebert J: Lower lid blepharoplasty with skin flap and muscle split, *Clin Plast Surg* 15:299, 1988.

Castanares S: Blepharoplasty for herniated intraorbital fat: an anatomical basis for a new approach, *Plast Reconstr Surg* 8:46, 1951.

De la Plaza R, Arroya JM: A new technique for the treatment of palpebral bags, *Plast Reconstr Surg* 81:677, 1988.

Fernandez LR: Double eyelid operation in the Oriental in Hawaii, *Plast Reconstr Surg* 25:257, 1960.

Flowers RS: The art of eyelid and orbital aesthetics: multiracial surgical considerations, *Clin Plast Surg* 14:716, 1987.

Flowers RS: Periorbital aesthetic surgery for men, eyelid and related structures, *Clin Plast Surg* 18:689, 1991.

Flowers RS, Caputy GG, Flowers SS: The biomechanics of brow and frontalis function and its effect on blepharoplasty, *Clin Plast Surg* 20:255, 1993.

Flowers RS: Upper blepharoplasty by eyelid invagination: anchor blepharoplasty, *Clin Plast Surg* 20:193, 1993.

Flowers RS, Flowers SS: Precision planning in blepharoplasty, *Clin Plast Surg* 20:303, 1993.

Flowers RS: Canthopexy as a routine blepharoplasty component, *Clin Plast Surg* 20:351, 1993.

Furnas DW: Festoons of orbicularis muscle as a cause of baggy eyelids, *Plast Reconstr Surg* 61:540, 1978.

Gradinger GP: Cosmetic upper blepharoplasty, *Clin Plast Surg* 15:289, 1988.

Hartley JH, Lester JC, Schatten WE: Acute retrobulbar hemorrhage during elective blepharoplasty, *Plast Reconstr Surg* 52:8, 1973.

Jelks GW, McCord CD Jr: Dry eye syndrome and other tear film abnormalities, *Clin Plast Surg* 8:81, 1981.

Jelks GW, Jelks EB: The influence of orbital and eyelid anatomy on the palpebral aperture, *Clin Plast Surg* 18:183, 1991.

Jelks GW, Jelks EB: Preoperative evaluation of the blepharoplasty patient, *Clin Plast Surg* 20:213, 1993.

Jelks GW, Jelks EB: Repair of lower lid deformities, *Clin Plast Surg* 20:417, 1993.

Lisman RD, Rees T, Baker D, et al: Experience with tarsal suspension as a factor in lower lid blepharoplasty, *Plast Reconstr Surg* 79:897, 1987.

Loeb R: Fat pad sliding and fat grafting for leveling lid depressions, *Clin Plast Surg* 8:4, 1981.

McCord CD Jr, Shore JW: Avoidance of complications in lower lid blepharoplasty, *Ophthalmology* 90:1039, 1983.

May JW, Fearon J, Zingarelli P: Retro-orbicularis oculus fat (ROOF) resection in aesthetic blepharoplasty: a 6-year study in 63 patients, *Plast Reconstr Surg* 86:682, 1990.

Mendelson BC: Herniated fat and the orbital septum of the lower lid, *Clin Plast Surg* 20:323, 1993.

Ousterhout DK, Weil RB: The role of the lateral canthal tendon in lower eyelid laxity, *Plast Reconstr Surg* 59:620, 1982.

Owsley JQ Jr: Restoration of the prominent lateral fat pad during upper lid blepharoplasty, *Plast Reconstr Surg* 65:4, 1980.

Rafety FM: Transient total blindness during cosmetic blepharoplasty, *Ann Plast Surg* 3:373, 1979.

Rees TD: Dry eye complications after blepharoplasty, *Plast Reconstr Surg* 56:375, 1975.

Rees TD: Prevention of ectropion by horizontal shortening of the lower lid during blepharoplasty, *Ann Plast Surg* 11:17, 1983.

Rees TD, Jelks GW: Blepharoplasty and the dry eye syndrome: guidelines for surgery, *Plast Reconstr Surg* 68:249, 1981.

Rees TD, LaTrenta GS: The role of the Schirmer's test and orbital morphology in predicting dry eye syndrome after blepharoplasty, *Plast Reconstr Surg* 82:619, 1988.

Sheen JH: Supratarsal fixation in upper blepharoplasty, *Plast Reconstr Surg* 54:424, 1974.

Tenzel RR: Complications of blepharoplasty, orbital hematoma, ectropion and scleral show, *Clin Plast Surg* 7:797, 1981.

Tenzel RR: Surgical treatment of complications of cosmetic blepharoplasty, *Clin Plast Surg* 5:517, 1978.

Zarem HA, Resnick JI: Expanded applications for transconjunctival lower lid blepharoplasty, *Plast Reconstr Surg* 88:215, 1991.

Zarem HA, Resnick JI: Operative technique for transconjunctival lower lid blepharoplasty, *Clin Plast Surg* 19:351, 1992.

Zide BM: Anatomy of the eyelids, *Clin Plast Surg* 8:623, 1981.

Zide BM, Jelks GW: *Surgical anatomy of the orbit,* New York, 1985, Raven Press.

Six

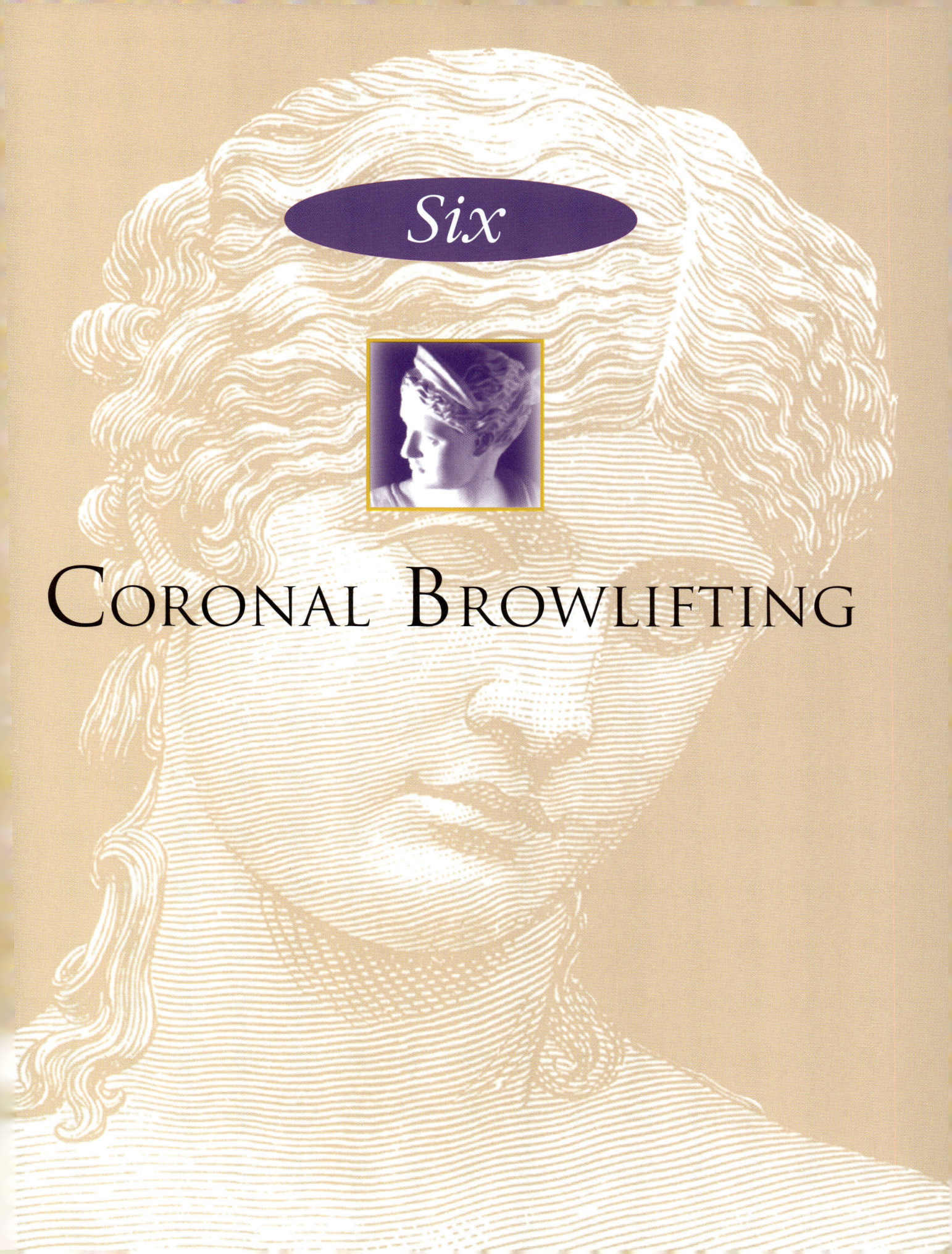

Coronal Browlifting

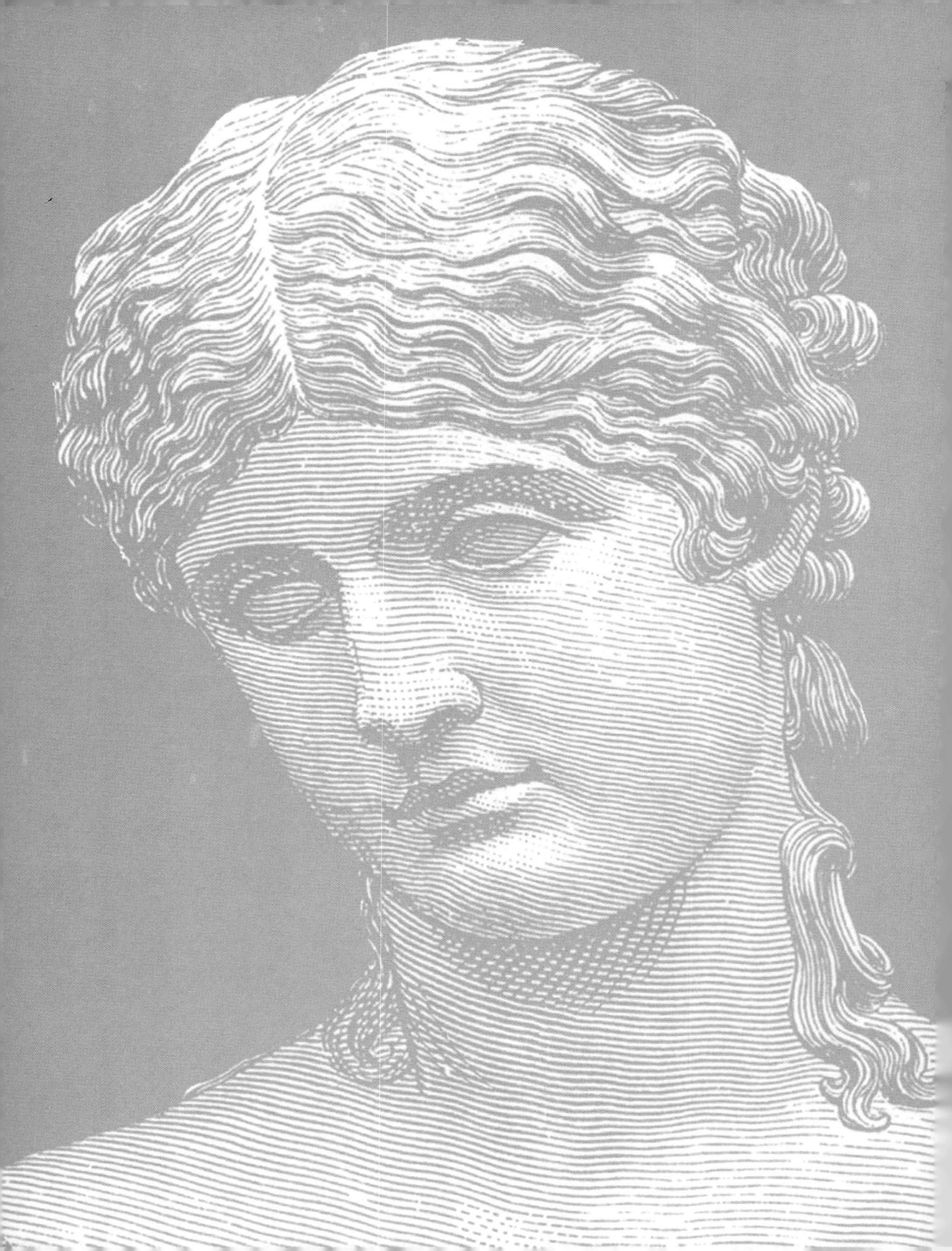

Plastic surgeons commonly perform rhytidectomy of the lower two-thirds of the face to correct gravitational and degenerative defects of that area but they often do not advise their patients about the aging process that has affected the upper third of the face. Gravity and degenerative changes of aging also take their toll on the forehead and on the remainder of the face. In our opinion, many individuals' appearances can be dramatically improved by panfacial rejuvenation rather than rejuvenation surgery, which affects only the lower part of the face. Coronal browlifting in association with rhytidectomy has produced some of the most dramatic results we have seen in our practice. It is associated with a high incidence of patient satisfaction and generally produces long-lasting results with a few complications.

The most common difficulty we encounter when suggesting coronal browlifting to patients is that the magnitude of the procedure often seems quite extensive. Many individuals who might find the browlift to be most helpful are discouraged by what they perceive as being extensive surgery. Their fears might be reflected in questions such as "Are you going to cut me from ear to ear?" Although a detailed description of the procedure might induce them to elect not to have the surgery, it is important to carefully explain the surgical procedure to them. Although the surgery appears to be extensive it is no more extensive than routine rhytidectomy. To allow the patient to understand the proposed operative procedure, it suffices for the surgeon to explain that the incisions will already have been made in the temple for the standard rhytidectomy. The surgeon can further explain that if the coronal browlift is performed, these incisions will merely extend toward the midline. This does not sound as crude or barbaric to the patient as a description of cutting the scalp from ear to ear. In our opinion, stressing the significant improvement of facial appearance associated with brow elevation and removal of glabellar and forehead rhytides commonly assuages patients' doubts, which form from what many of them perceive as a formidable procedure.

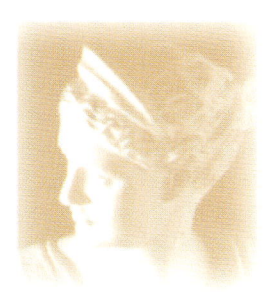

EARLIER APPROACHES

Injury to the frontal branch, which paralyzes the frontalis muscles, was at one time necessary to remove forehead rhytides. Early on, denervation of the forehead was performed on several occasions because of its associated improvement in forehead wrinkling. Although division of the frontal branch of the facial nerve will eliminate forehead wrinkles, the brow will subsequently droop from the lack of muscular support needed to resist gravitational forces. Loss of forehead animation is also a communicative disaster, since the forehead is perhaps the most animated portion of the face and is involved in most forms of facial communication.

Surgeons using earlier approaches to browlifting lacked a thorough understanding of the importance of proper contouring of the forehead musculature. Similarly, the amount of dissection required to adequately mobilize the eyebrow was imperfectly understood, leading to unsatisfactory results that were also only temporary in longevity. Those who criticized coronal browlifting as not being worthwhile were most likely performing the procedure improperly. In our experience the results following browlifting are at least as permanent as those from a routine facelift and are perhaps longer lasting. Perhaps the reason for the longevity of the browlift is that the foundation on which the browlift takes place and adheres to postoperatively is formed from a hard tissue framework with essentially no elasticity.

As we have gained experience with this procedure and our technical expertise has improved, we have found patient satisfaction to be high following a successful coronal browlift. Proper brow elevation, when associated with improvements in the contour of the upper eyelid, removal of forehead and glabella wrinkles, and overall smoothing of the forehead, significantly improves the appearance of the aging face. Remarks such as, "My eyes seem more open," and "I don't appear angry or sad anymore," are typically heard following this procedure.

We believe that many surgeons who condemn coronal browlifting fail to understand some of its indications, limitations, and technical points. Although we let all patients judge for themselves whether they wish to undergo this procedure, we always try to point out the presence of brow ptosis and associated forehead wrinkling during preoperative evaluation. A properly informed patient can then decide whether he or she desires this form of surgery. Many patients who refuse browlifting at the time of upper and lower blepharoplasty and rhytidectomy can later have a browlift performed as a secondary procedure as long as skin resection during upper blepharoplasty remains conservative.

ANATOMY OF THE TEMPORAL REGION

As in other areas of the face, the forehead region is comprised of concentric layers; skin, subcutaneous fat, mimetic muscle invested in the superficial fascia (galea, SMAS), pericranium, and underlying calvarial bone. In general the skin of the forehead is thicker than that of the eyelids or lower face and usually is paler in complexion. Musculature of the forehead includes the frontalis, procerus, corrugator superciliaris, and orbicularis oculi.

The frontalis muscle inserts into the skin of the forehead via the fibrous investiture of the superficial facial fascia (SMAS). The frontalis is responsible for eyebrow elevation; since it is a vertically oriented muscle, its chronic muscular activity is associated with horizontal forehead rhytides.

The procerus is continuous with the frontalis medially along the nasal root and originates directly from the nasal bones. Through its dermal attachments via the superficial fascia, action of the procerus acts to pull the glabella skin inferiorly and is responsible for horizontal wrinkle lines seen along the nasal root.

The corrugator superciliaris is an obliquely oriented muscle extending from the nasal root approximately 3 cm superolaterally to blend with the orbicularis oculi and frontalis muscle. The action of the corrugator serves to translocate the eyebrows medially and is responsible for the formation of vertical glabellar furrows.

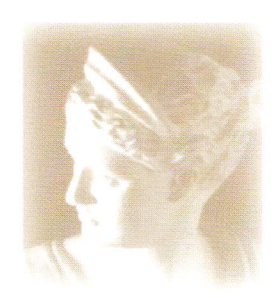

SURGICAL REJUVENATION OF THE FACE

In general the sensory nerves, arteries, and veins that supply the forehead region and scalp run in the subcutaneous layer just superficial to the mimetic muscles. The supraorbital nerve is a large bundle that exits through the midportion of the superior orbit, commonly through its own foramina or bony notch. After it exits the orbit, the supraorbital nerve and its accompanying artery initially lie deep and are easily visualized adjacent to the pericranium. The neurovascular bundle then pierces the frontalis muscle 2 to 3 cm above the supraorbital rim and thereafter travels in a subcutaneous position through the forehead and scalp.

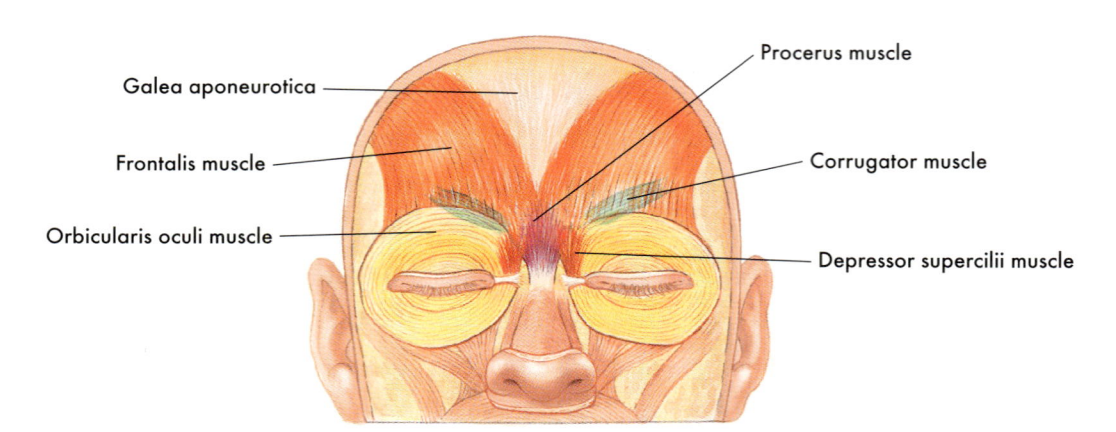

Muscular anatomy of the forehead and the glabella. Note that the frontalis muscles are predominantly vertical and act as the primary elevators of the brow. Their muscular activity is responsible for horizontally oriented forehead rhytides. The corrugator superciliaris muscles lie deep to the frontalis, extending from the supraorbital nerves medially toward the glabella. Their activity brings the brow medial, and it is this movement that is largely responsible for the development of vertically oriented glabellar creases. The procerus muscle is essentially a vertically oriented muscle, beginning along the nasal root and extending superiorly into the glabella. Muscular activity of the procerus is responsible for horizontally oriented wrinkles noted along the nasal root.

CORONAL BROWLIFTING

The supratrochlear nerve and artery exit the orbit medially, just cephalad to the trochlea of the superior oblique muscle, usually leaving the orbit as multiple small nerve branches that ascend into the glabella. A transition occurs between its deep orbital location and its subcutaneous location as these nerves traverse through the corrugator muscles. A series of twigs of the supratrochlear nerve, lying within the superficial portion of the corrugator muscle, are commonly visualized during coronal browlifting.

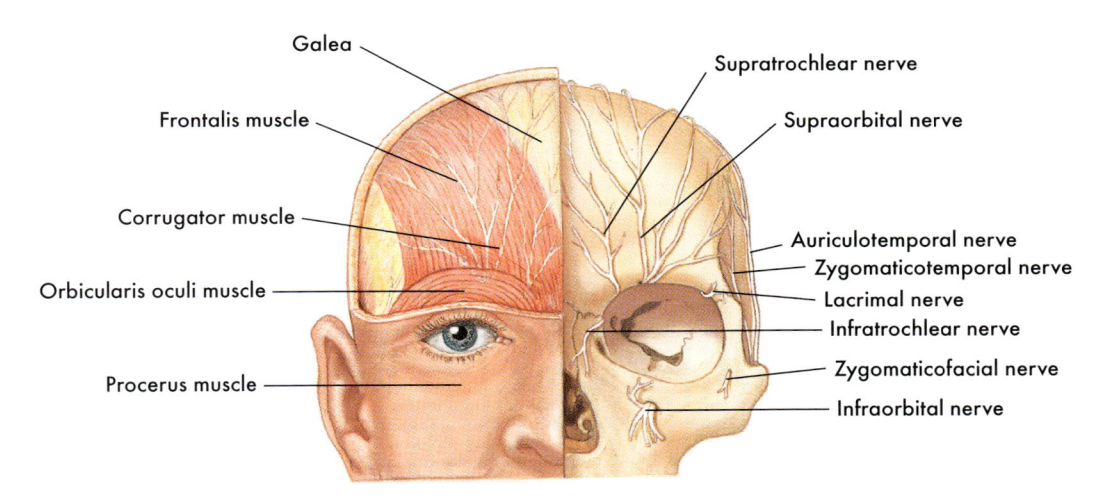

The sensory nerves of the forehead include the branches of the supratrochlear and supraorbital nerves, which are terminal branches of the upper division of the trigeminal nerve. These nerves exit the orbit inferiorly and penetrate the corrugator and frontalis muscles 2 to 3 cm above the supraorbital rim. From this point cephalad these nerves travel in a subcutaneous position throughout the forehead and scalp, though deeper branches to galea and pericranium also exist.

The forehead musculature is innervated by the frontal branch of the facial nerve. One of the dangers of coronal browlifting involves frontal branch injury. To protect the frontal branch, an accurate understanding of its location as it traverses the temporal region is required.

After leaving the parotid, the frontal branch of the facial nerve crosses the zygomatic arch where it traverses the temporal region along the undersurface of the temporoparietal fascia. In this location the frontal branch is invested in sub-SMAS fat. The frontal branch lies within this sub-SMAS fat until it reaches the lateral aspect of the frontalis muscle, where it penetrates the undersurface of the temporoparietal fascia to innervate the frontalis along its deep surface.

The key to preventing frontal branch injury during coronal browlifting is to understand the proper plane of dissection from the coronal incision caudal to the supraorbital rim. In general the preferred plane of dissection is in the subgaleal (or subaponeurotic) plane, which is identified immediately following the initial scalp incision and incision of the galea. The surgeon must understand that this subgaleal or subaponeurotic plane contains a thickness of soft tissue, which has been termed the subgaleal fascia. Dissection should always be carried along the deep surface of the subgaleal fascia, coursing directly along the superficial surface of the pericranium and deep temporal fascia. As long as the dissection is carried deep to the subgaleal fascia (that is, the subgaleal fascia is left intact up on the coronal flap), the frontal branch will be protected, since this nerve branch lies superficial to the subgaleal fascia.

Anatomically, the sub-SMAS fat that marks the plane of the frontal branch through the temporal region lies directly superficial to the subgaleal fascia. This sub-SMAS fat can usually be identified approximately 3 to 5 cm cephalad to the superior orbital rim. After this sub-SMAS fat is visualized in an area peripheral to the frontal branch of the facial nerve, the surgeon should keep both this fat pad and the subgaleal fascia directly deep to it up on the flap and carry the dissection deep to these structures. This method of dissection will protect the frontal branch.

CORONAL BROWLIFTING

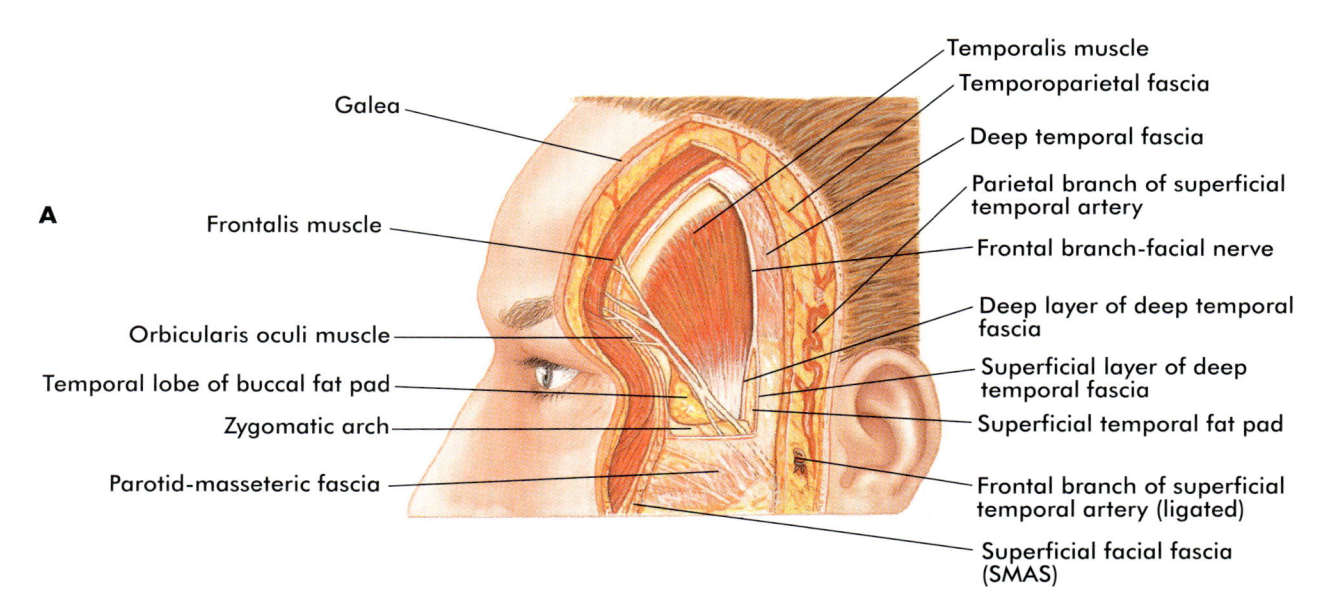

A, *The frontal branch of the facial nerve usually consists of multiple branches and in general travels on a line from the base of the tragus to approximately 1.5 cm above the eyebrow. The key to preventing injury to the frontal branch during coronal browlifting is to understand the plane in which the frontal branch of the facial nerve traverses the temporal region. Once the frontal branch crosses cephalad to the zygomatic arch, it lies directly along the undersurface of the temporoparietal fascia invested in subSMAS fat and superficial to the subgaleal fascia (loose areolar fascia). As it reaches the frontalis muscle along the lateral orbital rim, it then penetrates the temporoparietal fascia to innervate this muscle along its deep surface. In coronal browlifting it is imperative that the surgeon carry the dissection deep to the frontal branch (i.e., carrying the dissection directly along the pericranium and deep temporal fascia), thereby keeping the subgaleal fascia (and the subSMAS fat that lies superficial to the subgaleal fascia) up on the flap.*

Continued.

SURGICAL REJUVENATION OF THE FACE

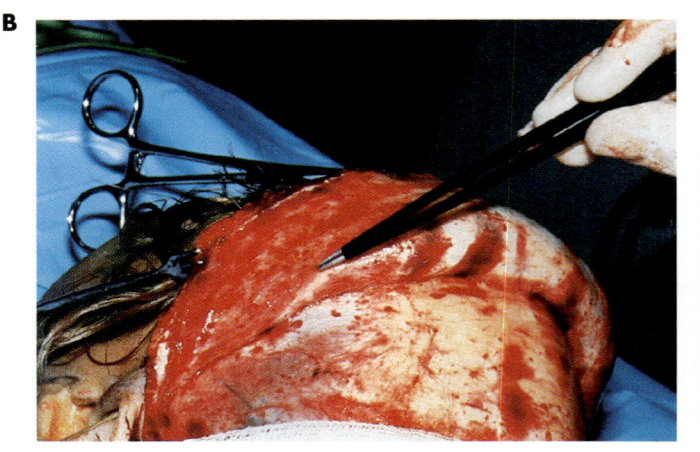

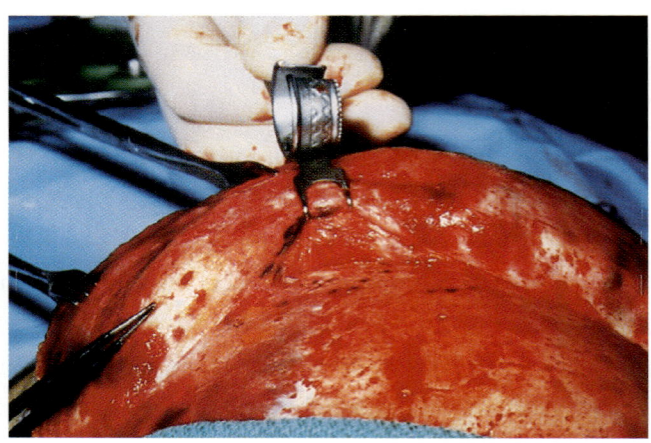

B, Subgaleal fascia. The subgalea or subaponeurotic plane is noted to have a thickness of loose areolar tissue that is filmy in appearance and has been termed subgaleal fascia. The surgeon must recognize this layer and carry the dissection deep to the subgaleal fascia (forceps). C, Completion of the dissection down to the lateral orbital rim, with the periosteum incised along the lateral orbital rim (held by double hook). Laterally, the dissection has been carried directly along the superficial surface of the deep temporal fascia, thereby keeping the subgaleal fascia and the subSMAS fat superficial to the subgaleal fascia (forceps) up in the flap. The frontal branch of the facial nerve lies directly superficial to the subSMAS fat visualized in this photograph.

At the lateral aspect of the superior orbital rim there often is a fibrous adherence where the pericranium, lateral brow pad, and temporal aponeurosis become fused. This usually is the most difficult portion of the dissection. We commonly use a combination of both sharp and blunt dissection in this area, making sure that the dissection is carried directly along pericranium or deep temporal fascia. Since the frontal branch is in close proximity, if the dissection plane becomes obscure in this region it is better to err on keeping the dissection deep to both the pericranium and deep temporal fascia (carrying the dissection within the superficial temporal fat pad) rather than coursing superficially.

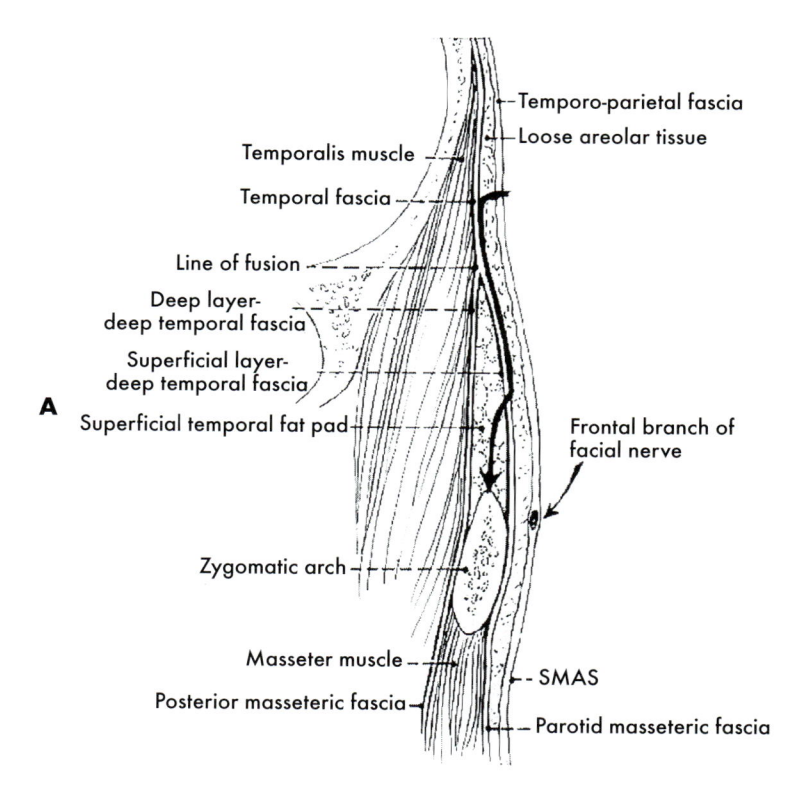

A, A cross-section of the anatomy of the temporal region. Note the generalized fusion between the deep temporal fascia, pericranium, and temporoparietal fascia along the lateral orbital rim. If the plane of dissection becomes obscured in this area, it is quite simple to incise the superficial layer of deep temporal fascia and carry the dissection caudally in the superficial temporal fat pad. In our opinion this is the preferred plane of dissection in procedures requiring exposure of the zygomatic arch.

Continued.

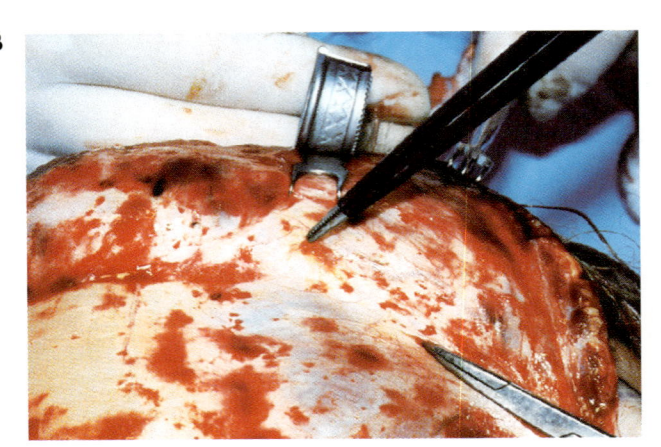

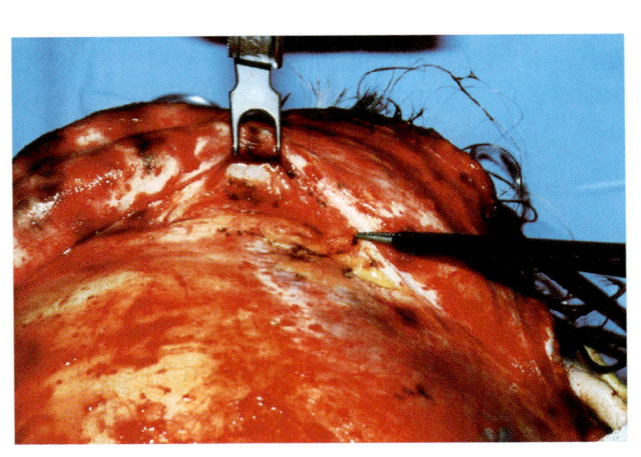

B, *Dissection being carried in the subgaleal plane directly external to the deep temporal fascia, directly deep to the subgaleal fascia (held in pickups). As the dissection is carried caudally toward the supraorbital rim, the superficial temporal fat pad can be identified lying directly deep to the superficial layer of the deep temporal fascia (hemostat).* **C,** *As the lateral orbital rim is approached, there is a general fusion between the pericranium, lateral brow pad, and deep temporal fascia. If the dissection becomes obscure in this area, it is safer to incise the superficial layer of the deep temporal fascia and carry the dissection laterally within the superficial temporal fat pad (held in forceps). This will ensure that the dissection is carried deep to the frontal branch of the facial nerve.*

The SMAS invests both surfaces of the frontalis muscle but is noticeably thinner along the superficial surface of the muscle and is more substantive along its deeper surface. The deep galea, as it traverses toward the supraorbital rim laterally, splits to encompass a fat pad present directly beneath the eyebrow, which has been termed the brow fat pad (ROOF fat). Fibrous septa exist between the fascia, encompassing the brow fat pad and the underlying supraorbital rim. When attempting to elevate the eyebrow, the surgeon must completely divide these dense attachments existing between the eyebrow, the eyebrow fat pad, and the underlying bone. The key to obtaining consistent results in browlifting is obtaining adequate mobilization between the brow fat pad and the underlying bony supraorbital rim.

INDICATIONS

1. Ptosis of the brow
2. Forehead wrinkles
3. Glabellar frown lines

The most common indication for coronal browlifting is brow ptosis. Patients with ptosis of the brow usually have a lateral fullness along the orbital rim, which is commonly associated with upper eyelid blepharochalasis. It is important with these patients for the surgeon to differentiate how much of the problem results from fullness of the upper lid versus the malpositioned brow. The most common mistake we have seen in contouring this region is the substitution of an upper eyelid blepharoplasty for a browlift. It seems obvious to us that an aggressive removal of upper eyelid skin will not improve brow position, but this is commonly performed as a substitute for browlifting. An aggressive removal of eyelid skin will preclude a subsequent browlift because of the possibility of lagophthalmus, and these patients will be doomed to wear an inappropriate, sad expression caused by malposition of the lateral eyebrow. Another problem is that an aggressive removal of upper eyelid skin invariably is associated with a downward migration of the eyebrow, which aggravates an already compromised brow position.

Some patients will complain of an incomplete correction in eyelid appearance after an initial upper eyelid blepharoplasty and will say they desire a secondary blepharoplasty. The surgeon should not be trapped into removing more eyelid skin in these cases. Removal of an additional strip of eyelid skin will pull the brow down even further and compound the problem. The additional skin removal may make it impossible to perform a subsequent browlift. Despite the patient's belief that only a slight skin excision will take care of the problem, the surgeon must carefully explain the need for coronal browlifting to adequately address the problem.

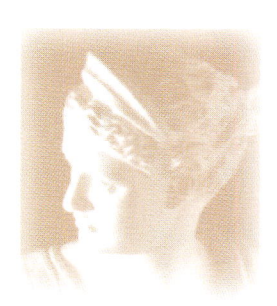

Deep transverse forehead wrinkles, vertical glabellar frown lines, and transverse wrinkles of the root of the nose associated with sagging glabellar skin are secondary indications for browlift. These problems all contribute to an angry or tired appearance of the patient's face and are only incompletely treated with other modalities such as collagen injection or chemical peeling. The ability to eliminate forehead rhytides, remove deep glabellar creases, contour hypertrophic corrugator musculature, and improve the thick, soft tissue present along the upper third of the nose all offer striking improvement to facial aesthetics that can only be accomplished through a browlifting procedure.

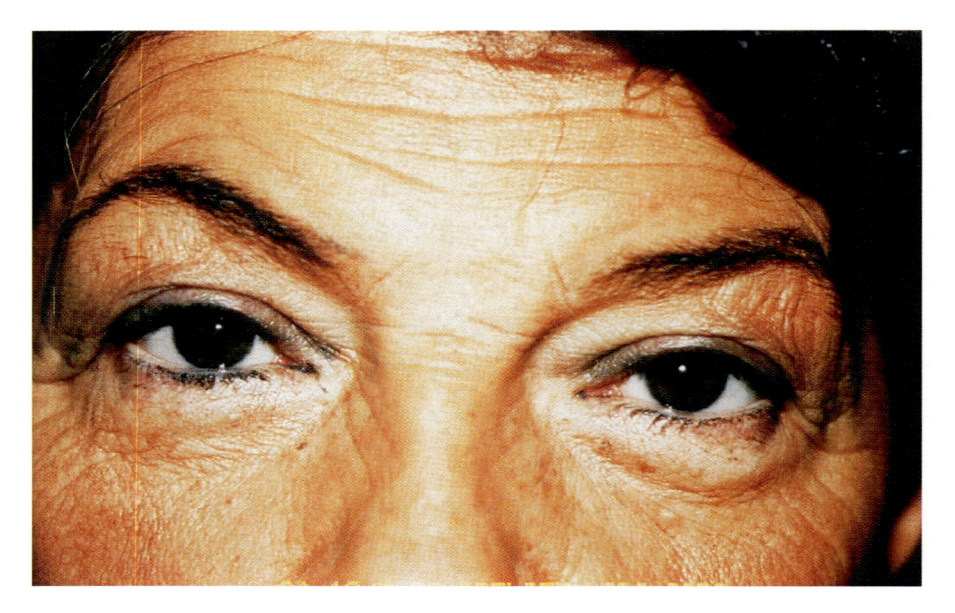

Patient is seen preoperatively with deep forehead rhytides associated with chronic muscular activity related to brow ptosis. As the brows descend inferiorly, this produces crowding of the upper eyelids with a tendency toward limitation of visual field, especially noted in superior temporal gaze. The involuntary reaction to crowding of the upper eyelid is to initiate frontalis activity, which brings the brows to a more superior position. Although this mechanical activity improves visual fields, the chronic hyperactivity of the frontalis muscle is associated with significant forehead rhytides.

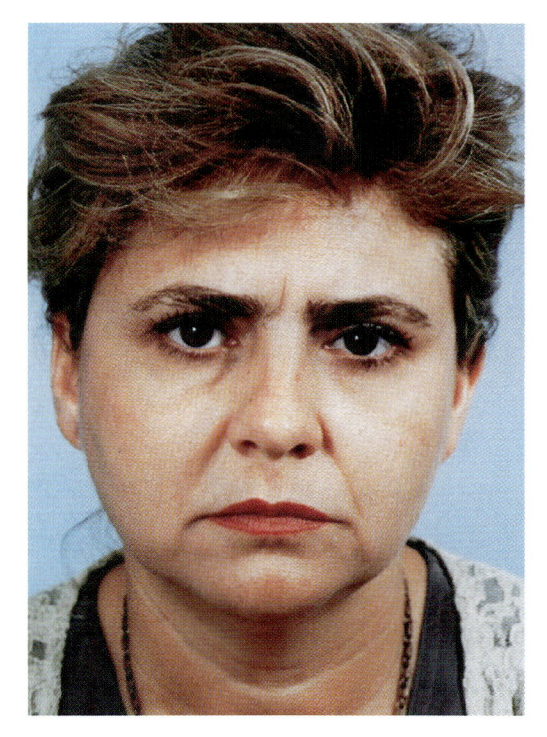

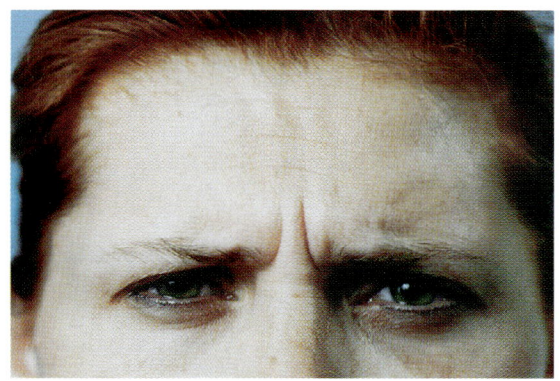

Chronic corrugator hyperactivity is associated not only with deep glabellar creases but also with corrugator hypertrophy. This produces bulkiness in the central portion of the forehead and is associated with a tired, sad, or angry look; the patient appears to be in a perpetual scowl. Smoothing of the glabellar region, a diminishing of the corrugator hypertrophy, and treatment of the deep glabellar frown lines are part of the primary improvement following browlifting procedures.

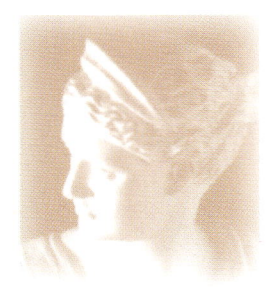

HAIRLINE INCISION

Contraindications to coronal incision include a high forehead with a high hairline and thinning hair. If the individual has a high hairline, the hairline should not be raised further by placing an incision inside it. In this situation an incision placed along the frontal hairline should be considered. Careful discussion with the patient is necessary to avoid postoperative misunderstanding. If an incision will be placed at the hairline, the patient should be informed that a visible scar may be obvious postoperatively and hair styling might be required for concealment.

Although we have seen many surgeons advocate incisions placed at the hairline, we have been displeased with their results because of the visible scars left. Although incisions placed at the hairline can yield satisfactory results, these incisions must be carefully placed and meticulously closed because of the lack of camouflage that exists when incisions are placed at the junction between the forehead and scalp.

If hairline incisions are going to be used in browlifting procedures, they must be artistically designed and meticulously closed, controlling tension to minimize scar detectability. The portion of the incision which runs at the frontal hairline should be designed so that it lies just within the fine hair along the junction between forehead and scalp, and the incision is beveled according to the direction of the hair shafts. Along the junction where the hairline incision swings posteriorly into the frontal and temporal hair, the surgeon must adequately understand the shifts that will be obtained following forehead advancement. This incision should not be placed directly at the junction between the thick and the fine hair of the forehead, as incisions placed in this region will tend to produce a more obvious transition point which will be visible postoperatively. Notching in this area, bringing bare scalp adjacent to thick hair is often quite noticeable. In designing hairline incisions, we prefer to bring the transition point from the hairline into the scalp incision along thinner temporal hair so that following move-

CORONAL BROWLIFTING

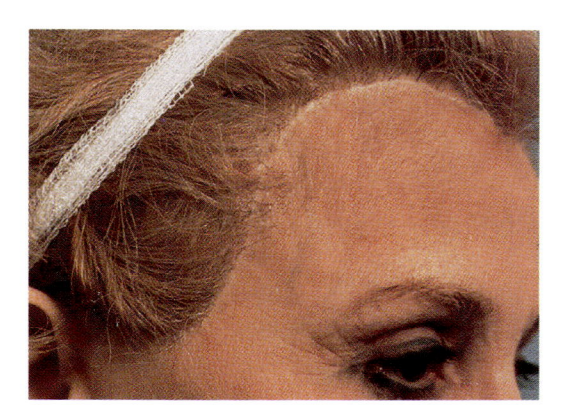

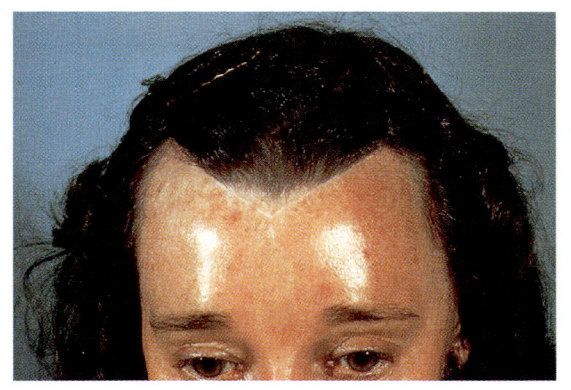

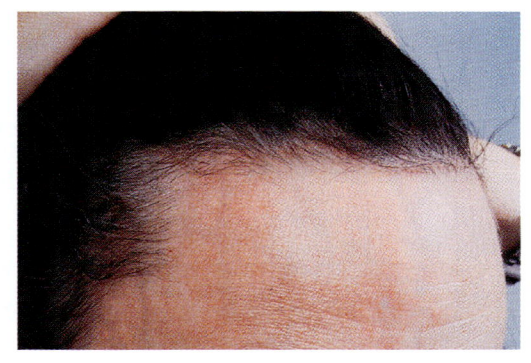

Although hairline scars are appropriate for patients who have high central foreheads and require elevation of the medial brows, when they are poorly performed they produce not only a visible scar but also an unnatural appearance to the forehead and hairline regions. In these two patients an unartistic joining of forehead skin with the scalp leads to an unnatural juxtaposition between hairline and forehead skin, which is difficult to correct postoperatively. Hairline incision performed in our office approximately 3 months following surgery. Note that while the scar is still a bit red, it is well camouflaged because of proper scar design, which has produced a blending between forehead skin and scalp.

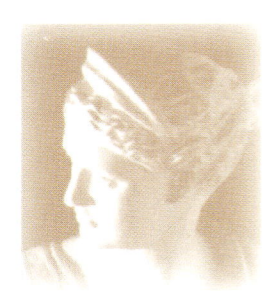

ment from the forehead advancement, the patient is left with an incision in which thin hair is adjacent to thin hair. Again, if the direction of the hair follicles are respected and tension is properly controlled, this usually produces a fine imperceptible scar which will usually not require hair styling for concealment.

PREOPERATIVE PLANNING

A careful discussion with the patient regarding desires and anticipated results of surgery should take place. Observation of the patient both in repose and in animation is important in determining brow position, severity of glabellar and forehead wrinkling, and hypertrophic glabellar musculature. Adequate analysis of that patient's particular problems must precede the plan.

Many patients who suffer from brow ptosis will show hyperactivity of the frontalis muscle. When these patients are in animation, the brow appears to be in an elevated position and is associated with a significant degree of forehead wrinkling. Many of these patients have learned to compensate for their brow ptosis, in conjunction with their upper eyelid blepharochalasis, by using frontalis animation to mechanically elevate the eyebrow. It is important when analyzing brow position to get patients to relax their eyebrows into a position of repose, at which point the degree of brow ptosis is definable.

In ideal positioning of the eyebrow, the medial and lateral end of the brow lie approximately at the same horizontal level; the apex of the brow lies on a vertical line directly above the lateral limbus. In terms of its vertical positioning, the supraorbital ridge serves as an adequate reference point. In general the eyebrow should arch above the supraorbital rim in women and lie approximately at the level of the rim in men.

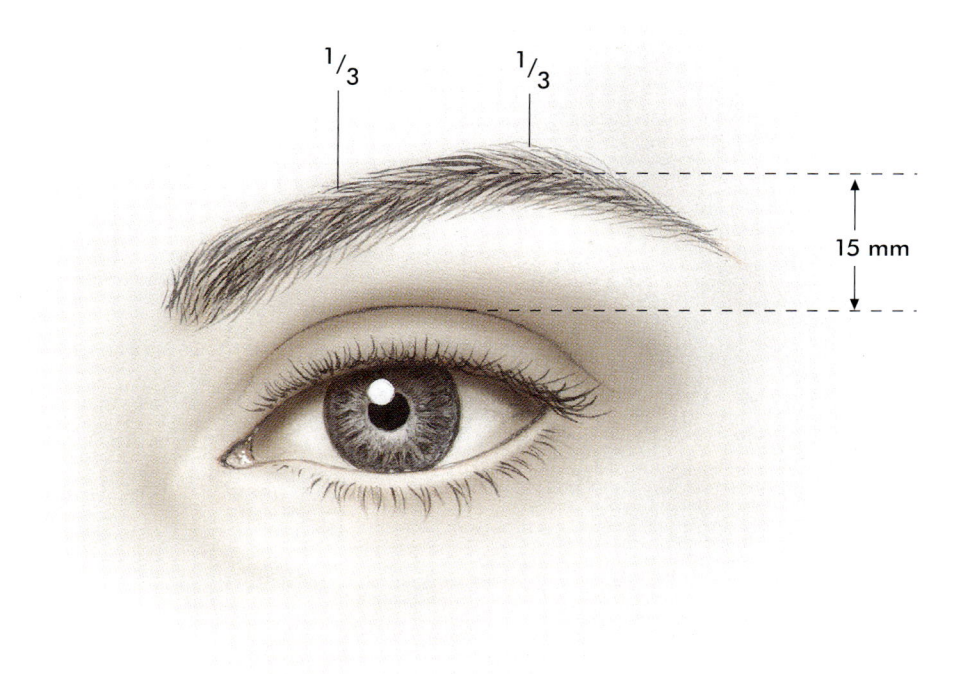

Ideally, the apex of the brow should be at the junction between the middle and lateral third of the eyebrow. The ideal brow position should be at a level superior to the supraorbital rim, and a distance of approximately 15 mm should exist between the lateral brow and the supratarsal fold.

In determining where to place the eyebrow, it is helpful to mark the resting eyebrow in three places with a marking pen while the patient is in the upright position. The brow is then elevated to its ideal aesthetic location while the patient observes that position in the mirror. Upon the patient's agreement, this ideal brow location should be marked and measurements should be taken between the resting position and the ideal location. A useful rule is that for every millimeter of brow elevation desired, approximately 2 cm of hair-bearing scalp must be resected following redraping. Another helpful rule is that in the anesthetically pleasing eyebrow, a distance of approximately 1.5 cm exists between the eyebrow and the supratarsal fold, and approximately 2.5 cm of distance is present between the eyebrow and the pupil in primary gaze. Although these measurements serve as parameters for brow elevation, the individual patient's preference and the surgeon's aesthetic judgment must also be taken into account when deciding on brow position.

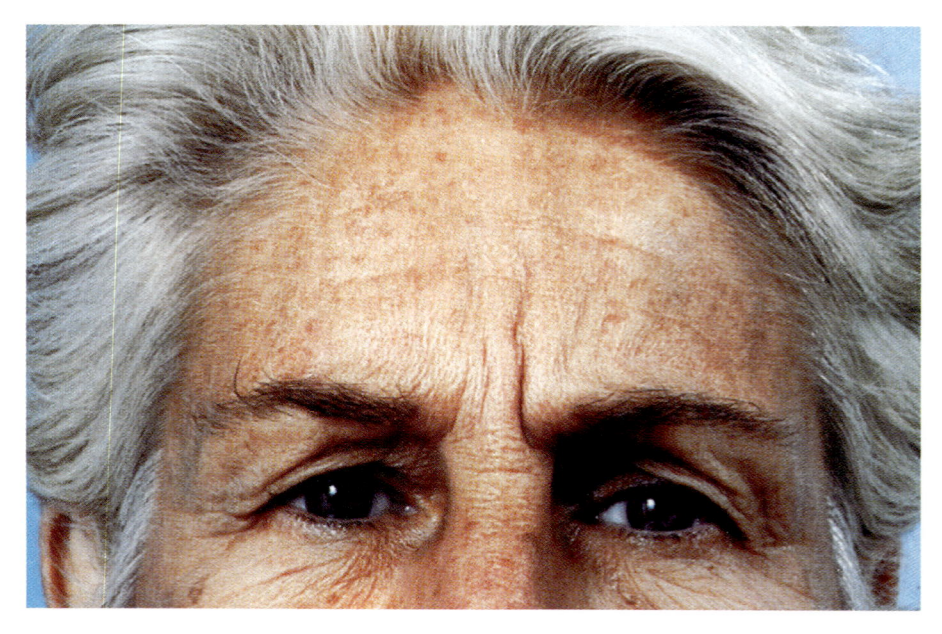

Patient is seen preoperatively with corrugator hypertrophy. Although chronic corrugator activity is usually responsible for the deepening of the glabellar creases, it also produces bulkiness in the central aspect of the forehead. Resection of the hypertrophic corrugator musculature is responsible for smoothing of the central forehead following surgery.

We find it important to topographically map the corrugator muscle contour preoperatively while the patient is scowling. In patients with deep glabellar frown lines these muscles will produce an unattractive bulge above the medial eyebrows and within the glabellar region, and careful sculpting of these muscle bundles will produce a smoother glabellar contour postoperatively. In a similar fashion, heavy glabellar frown lines and forehead lines are marked preoperatively so that the treatment of these coarse rhytides can be precisely performed during the surgery.

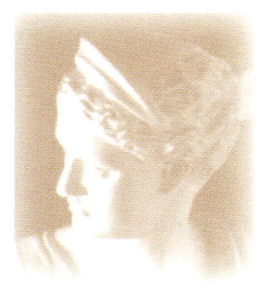

TECHNIQUE

The procedure can be performed on patients who are under either local or general anesthesia. For local anesthesia, a supraorbital and supratrochlear nerve block is performed. The anticipated line of incision is similarly infiltrated with a lidocaine and adrenalin solution. Additional lidocaine is then infiltrated into the anticipated plane of dissection to aid in hemostasis and anesthesia.

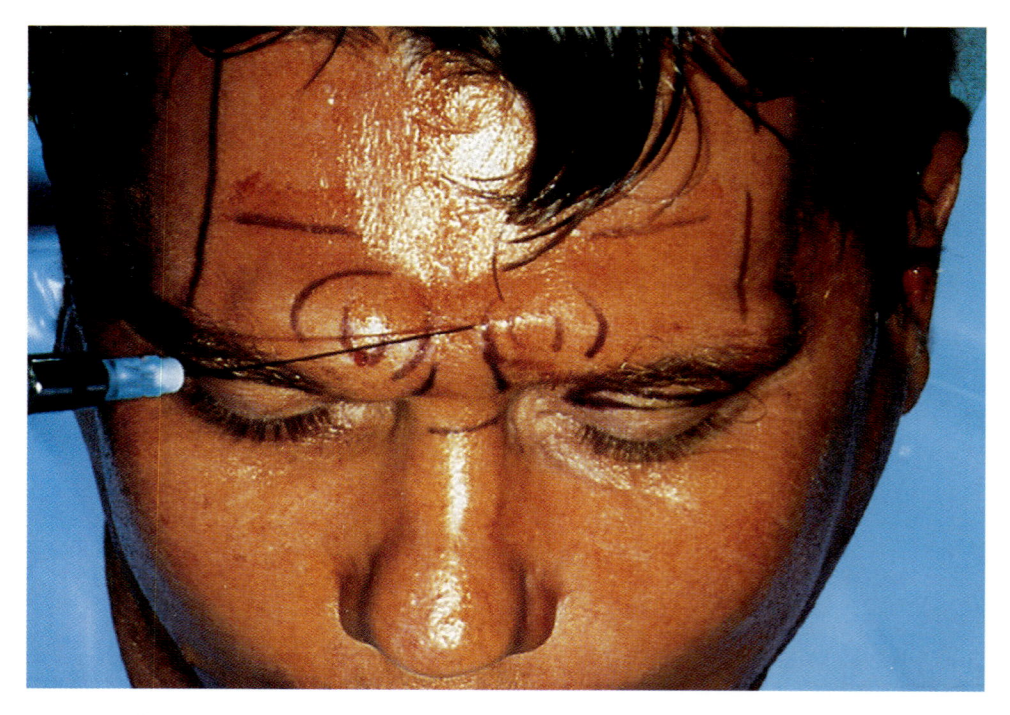

Essentially, all our patients undergoing browlifting procedures are intravenously sedated through local and regional infiltration of lidocaine and adrenaline solution. The first portion of injection is usually infiltrated along the supraorbital rims, where the supraorbital and supratrochlear sensory branches of the trigeminal nerve are blocked.

CORONAL BROWLIFTING

We prefer to use a coronal incision whenever possible, placing this incision approximately 5 cm posterior to the hairline. If a facelift is being performed at the same time (a common situation), the facelift incision is simply extended vertically where it joins a similar incision from the opposite side. We prefer to arc the incision as it approaches the midline to prevent a straight line incision design. We usually simply part the hair and control it with rubber bands; we prefer not to shave the hair, to allow better judgment of the direction of angulation of the individual hair shafts.

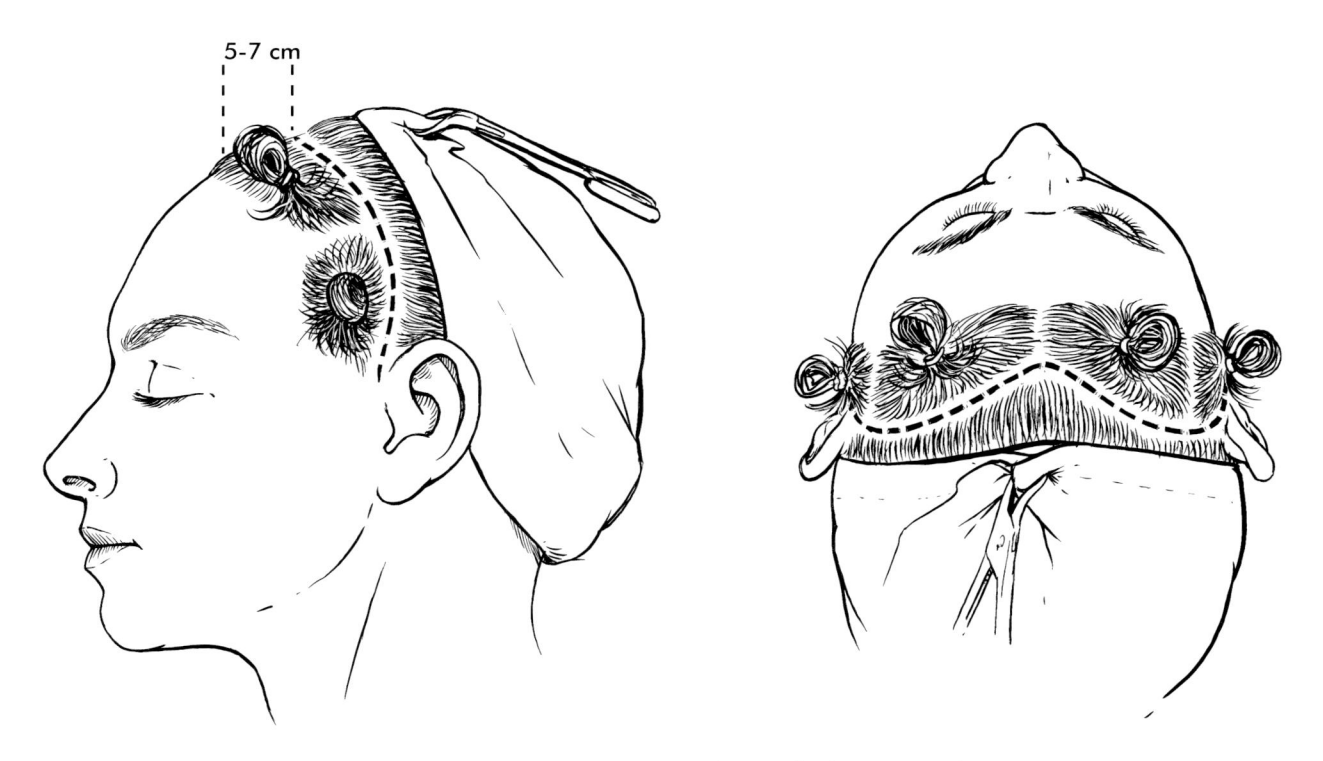

Most of our browlifting procedures are performed through the coronal approach. These procedures are usually between 5 and 7 cm posterior to the hairline. The central portion of the incision design is curved anteriorly.

When making the incision, it is important for the surgeon to bevel the cut in the direction of the hair follicles. The direction of the hair follicles will change several times from the temporal region toward the most cephalad portion of the scalp and should be carefully followed. The incision then goes through the galea, and the dissection plane between the pericranium and galea is encountered.

Since the scalp is undermined beneath the galea and overlies the pericranium, the dissection will usually proceed quite rapidly. As the dissection extends laterally, the proper plane is immediately external to the deep temporal fascia. This areolar plane is thick so it is much safer to dissect directly along the external surface of the deep tempo-

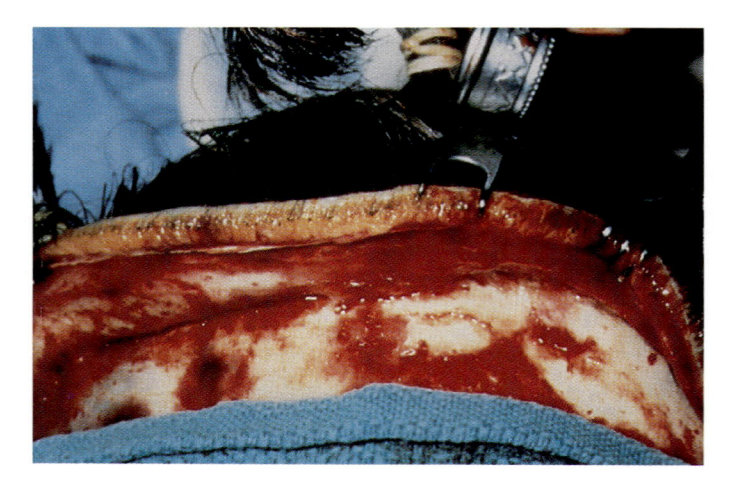

It is important to follow the direction of the hair follicles when making the scalp incision. For this reason we never shave the scalp but instead simply part the hair, which allows us to better judge hair-shaft angulation. As noted in this photograph, if the incision is made along the direction of the shafts of the hair follicle, these follicles will remain intact following completion of the incision.

ral fascia than to dissect directly beneath the galea in order to preserve the frontal branch.

The lateral dissection should extend inferiorly until the eyebrows are adequately freed from their periosteal attachments along the supraorbital rim. This is an essential portion of the procedure. The subgaleal dissection is carried inferiorly down to the level of the supraorbital rim; this is a safe plane as long as the overlying galea is not violated. After the supraorbital rim is identified, the periosteum along the lateral rim can be incised and dissected with a periosteal elevator to ensure adequate brow mobility.

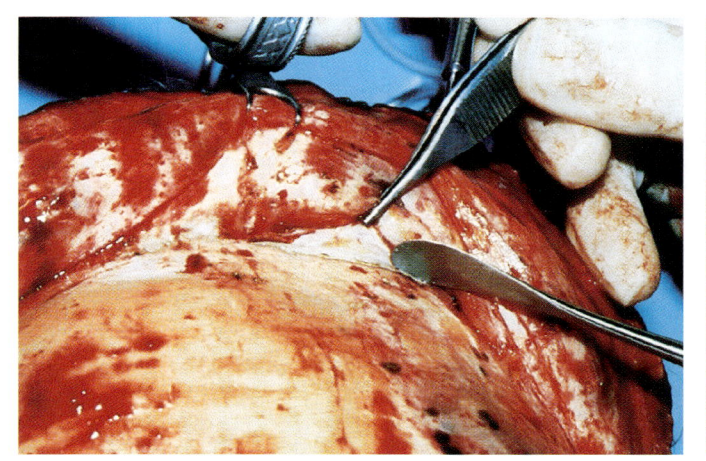

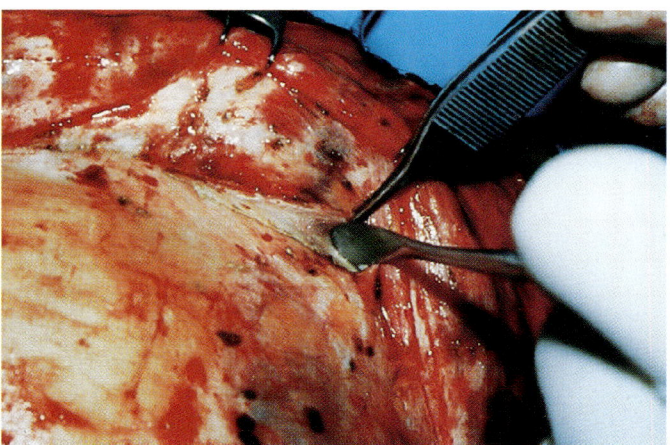

Intraoperative illustration of the amount of dissection required to adequately free the brow pad from the superior orbital rim. Usually the dissection is carried in the subgaleal plane down to the level of the supraorbital rim. The periosteum along the supraorbital rim from the supraorbital nerve laterally to the frontozygomatic suture is then incised. Subperiosteal dissection is then performed to ensure that all of the attachments between the lateral brow pad and periosteum are liberated.

The dissection then proceeds towards the glabellar region in the subgaleal plane. This dissection continues inferiorly to expose the medial portion of the orbital rim and along the superior portion of the nasal bones. We commonly undermine along the nasal dorsum caudal to the nasal tip. As the supraorbital nerves are encountered, they are identified and preserved. An adequate degree of dissection is ensured when all soft tissues have been completely elevated off the supraorbital rims, the eyebrows are free and mobile, and the origins of the corrugator muscles and procerus muscles are well-identified.

Following identification of the corrugator musculature, they are modified in accordance with the preoperative evaluation. The dissection usually begins just medial to the supraorbital neurovascular bundle. The corrugator muscle is identified and exposed with the use of blunt hemostat dissection. The deep portion of the muscle is then slowly divided with electrocautery, exposing the supratrochlear nerves within the superficial aspects of this muscle. These nerve branches are preserved, and the remaining corrugator is completely divided from its underlying bony origins. Hypertrophy within the corrugator is then carefully feathered by further thinning the muscle until a flat, smooth glabellar contour is obtained.

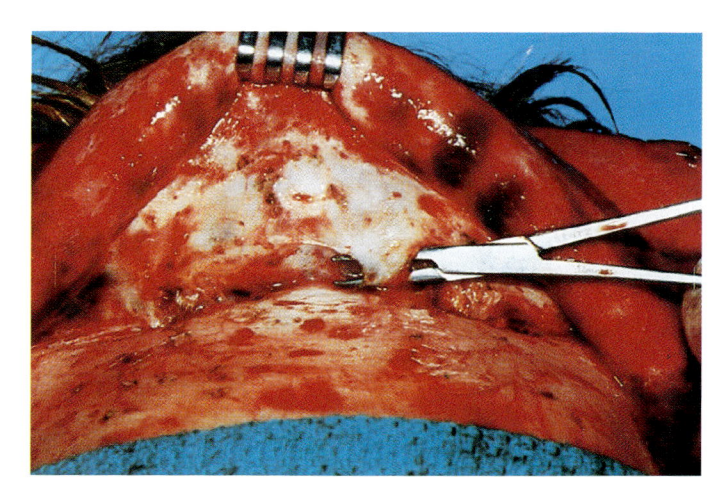

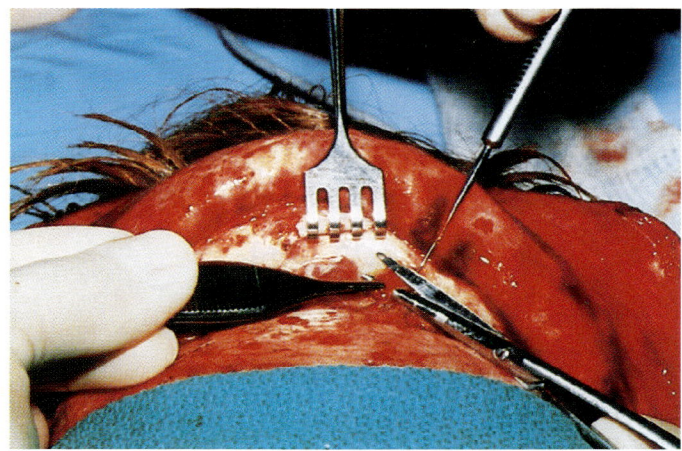

Corrugator muscular division. After the corrugator muscles are divided from their periosteal attachments, the hypertrophic muscle is then excised as far laterally as the supraorbital neurovascular bundle. Great care is used during this resection to preserve the supratrochlear nerve branches, which are commonly seen percolating along the superficial aspects of the corrugator muscle.

Attention is then turned to procerus muscle modification. This muscle is identified along the root of the nose. In most patients simple horizontal transection of the procerus is adequate as long as it is precisely performed. Usually the procerus is divided at a level between the eyelashes and the supratarsal fold.

If the patient has deep glabellar frown lines, these should be treated before flap redraping. These creases are formed from prolonged muscle action on the dermis, and freeing the skin from the underlying muscle and galea commonly produces significant improvement. The

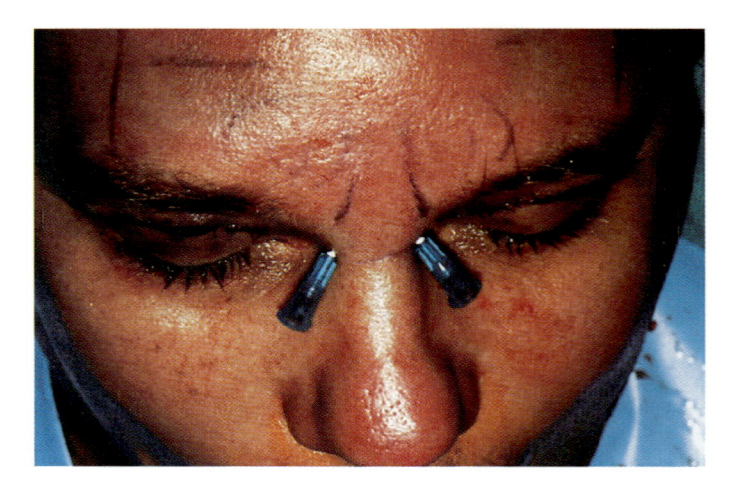

Procerus division is usually performed at the approximate level of the supratarsal fold. To ensure accuracy, the level of procerus division should be decided preoperatively, marked on the patient's skin, and transmitted to the galea via the use of needles.

glabellar frown lines are first marked along the interior of the scalp flap by passing needles through the skin and then marking the needles with methylene blue. After these lines are marked along the inside of

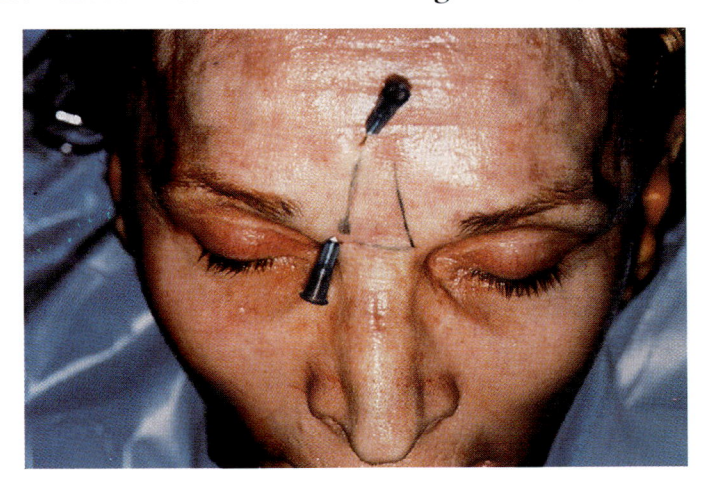

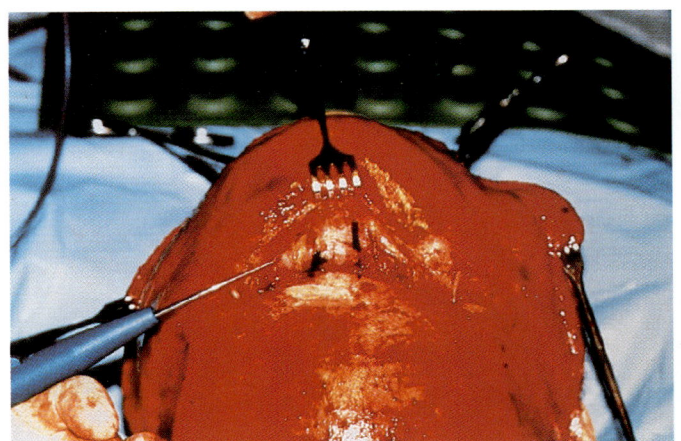

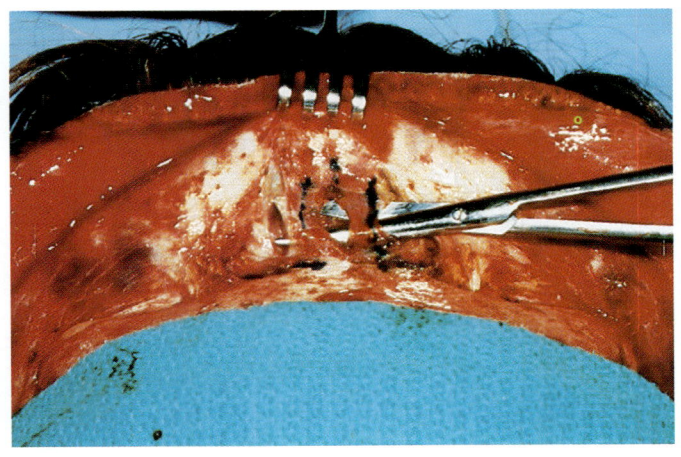

A, Marking of the glabellar creases with the use of needles inserted through the skin. B and C, Following the marking of the glabellar creases, the galea is incised approximately 7 mm lateral to both creases, as well as between the creases, followed by undermining of the glabella from the overlying subcutaneous tissue using blunt dissection. This effectively separates the galeal portion of the crease from the dermis, which tends to blunt these dermal rhytides postoperatively. It is important not to resect the galea in this region or it will produce a central forehead depression. Instead, in patients with very deep glabellar frown lines following galeal release, a graft of deep temporal fascia can be inserted between galea and dermis to add bulk to the central forehead region and prevent the readherence of dermis to the underlying galea. In most patients, adding this fascial graft is not necessary.

the flap, a relaxing incision is made both between the creases and laterally, approximately 7 to 10 mm on either side of the glabellar crease. The muscle and galea beneath the crease are then undermined in the subcutaneous plane between the relaxing incisions, separating dermis from muscle. The galea is not resected following this undermining because doing so would tend to produce postoperative contour depression in this region. The frontalis muscle should then be modified again according to the preoperative plan. This tends to improve forehead wrinkling. Whereas some authors discuss the removal of the galea or partial removal of the frontalis muscle to correct this problem, we have found that in some patients galea and muscle removal can produce forehead contour depression or uneven forehead animation following muscle modification. Alternatively, a common method of weakening the frontalis involves simply incising the galea and frontalis muscle horizontally, using three or four parallel incisions coursing between the supraorbital nerve bundles. In patients with very deep, coarse forehead

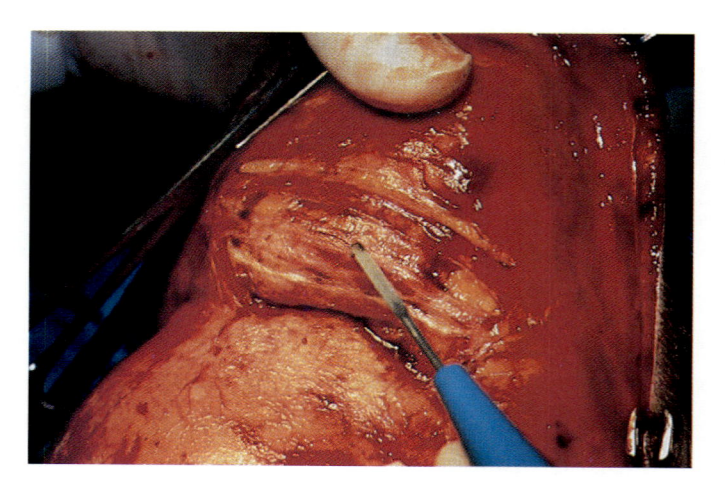

Treatment of forehead rhytides via horizontal scoring of the frontalis muscle between the medial to the supraorbital neurovascular bundles. In patients with deep forehead rhytides, a criss-cross "tic-tac-toe" pattern can be added to the scoring. As an alternative to this, partial resection of galea and frontalis muscle performed medial to the supraorbital bundles serves as an adequate treatment of frontalis hyperactivity in most patients.

wrinkles, vertical incisions in a "tic-tac-toe" type fashion will similarly weaken the frontalis muscle, helping to eliminate the grooves, but will not lead to an inanimate forehead.

If lateral forehead rhytides are especially prominent, relaxing incisions in the galea can be performed provided these incisions are made cephalad to the course of the frontal branch of the facial nerve.

CLOSURE

Before closing the incisions, the surgeon must make certain that the brow is mobilized and that it can be easily elevated. Following this, temporary tacking sutures are placed before trimming off the excess scalp. In redraping the coronal flap, it should be treated as an advancement flap rather than a rotation flap. Thus the predominant excision of scalp should occur directly cephalad to the lateral portion of the brow, since this is the portion of the flap that requires the greatest elevation. For this reason we draw a line from the lateral aspect of the brow (usually extending from the lateral canthus) superiorly into the hair; this marks where the first tacking sutures are placed. After the lateral brow is adequately elevated in a bilateral fashion, a similar key suture is placed in the midline to accommodate medial brow elevation. Over time it is very difficult to overelevate the lateral brow, although it is simple to overelevate the medial brow (because of the significant medial weakening of the corrugator, procerus, and frontalis muscle, combined with galeal scoring). These points should be kept in mind at the time of flap redraping.

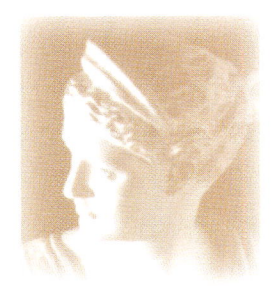

After the temporary tacking sutures are placed, the redundant scalp is excised with care to follow the direction of the hair follicles during scalp excision. In general, between 15 and 25 mm of scalp is removed laterally, although our average medial resection can vary between 5 and 15 mm. Because the scalp is closed as an advancement flap rather than a rotation flap, little scalp excision is required along the temporal aspects of the coronal incision. The closure is usually performed by placing deep buried galeal sutures and using metallic staples to close the skin. To improve lateral brow fixation, we will at times use deeply placed sutures, laterally fixating the lateral galea to the deep temporal fascia and galea posterior to the coronal incision.

Care must be taken to avoid excessive tension on the flap at the time of closure. The flap is stretched over a convex frontal bone, and necrosis and alopecia can result. The only tension points (tension should be kept to a minimum) should exist along the key sutures, and scalp excision between these key sutures should be performed with 2 to 3 mm of redundancy.

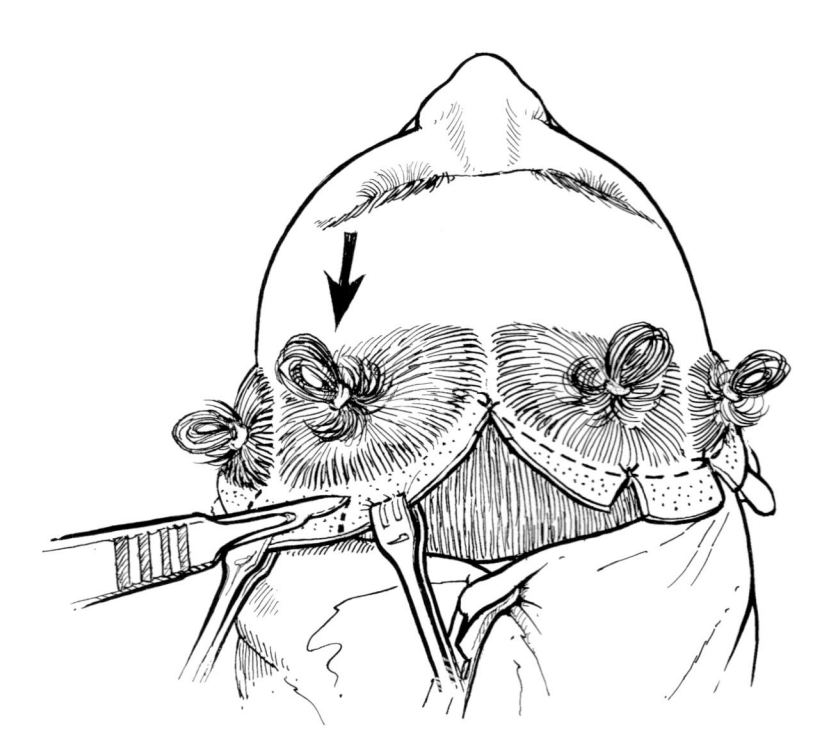

Scalp resection commonly performed in coronal browlifting. Note that the flap has been treated as an advancement flap, with the majority of the scalp resection performed directly above the lateral brow and little scalp resection performed along the midline. This crescent of scalp excision removed tapers into the central portion of the resection, as well as the lateral portion of the resection. Key sutures are placed first in the area directly superior to the lateral third of the brow bilaterally, followed by a similar key suture placed at the midline. Scalp excision between the key sutures is performed with 2 to 3 mm of redundancy.

ALTERNATIVE TO HAIRLINE INCISIONS IN PATIENTS WITH HIGH CENTRAL FOREHEADS

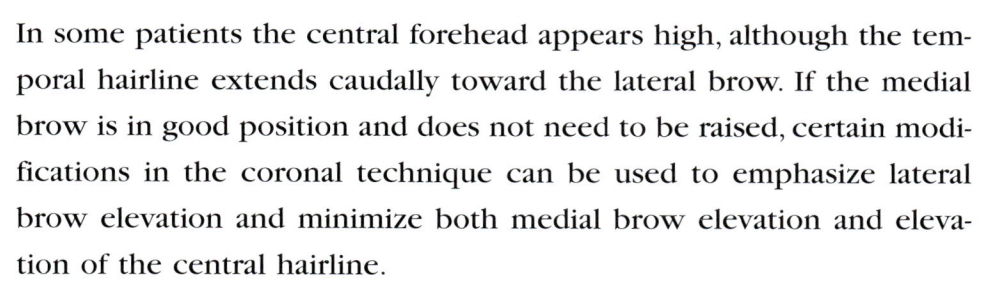

In some patients the central forehead appears high, although the temporal hairline extends caudally toward the lateral brow. If the medial brow is in good position and does not need to be raised, certain modifications in the coronal technique can be used to emphasize lateral brow elevation and minimize both medial brow elevation and elevation of the central hairline.

The surgeon must realize that much of medial brow elevation obtained in brow lifting has less to do with central scalp resection, but rather is secondary to extensive mobilization of the medial brow. The medial brow is fixated in position by firm attachments to the supraorbital rim which occur along the lateral nasal root. Anatomically, this junction of medial brow to periosteum occurs along the origin of the corrugator muscle along the nasal sidewall. If these attachments of the medial brow to the lateral nasal wall and most medial aspect of the supraorbital rim are left intact during dissection, then limited medial brow elevation will occur and with it little change in the central frontal hairline. Limiting dissection in this region of the glabella will still allow the surgeon adequate access to contouring the corrugator muscle in the region of the supratrochlear and supraorbital nerves, as well as will allow the division of the procerus muscle directly over the nasal bridge. In patients in which we do not desire medial brow elevation or a change in the central forehead, we will limit procerus division along its origins along the lateral nasal sidewall which similarly functions to prevent over-elevation of the medial brow.

Another adjustment we willl make in patients with high central forehead, to minimize central hairline elevation, is to vertically score the galea rather than horizontally incise it. We would point out that vertical incisions in the frontalis have less effect in terms of improvement of deep forehead wrinkles, and are perhaps most applicable when performing this procedure in the younger patient.

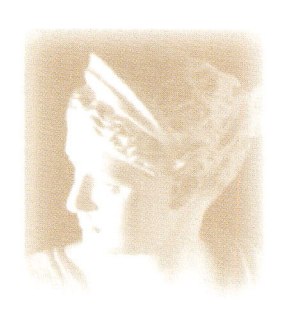

With these types of simple modifications, we are able to minimize central forehead elevation while maximizing elevation of the lateral eyebrow in the properly selected patient. We would stress that this type of modification is useful only in selected clinical situations, for patients who have both high central and lateral foreheads, a hairline incision is more appropriate.

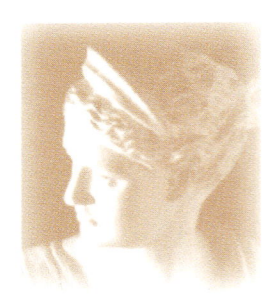

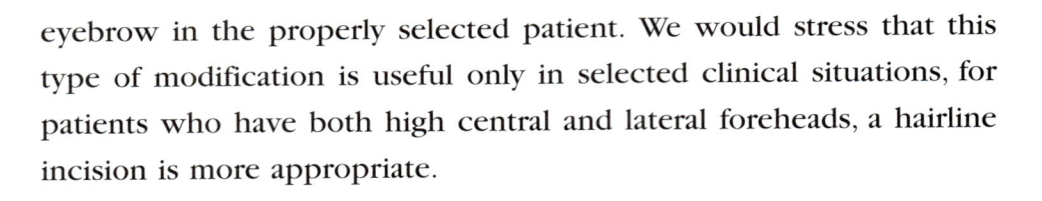

BLEPHAROPLASTY COMBINED WITH CORONAL BROWLIFT

If an upper lid blepharoplasty and coronal browlift are performed at the same time, a conservative approach should be adopted regarding the amount of upper lid skin to be removed. For the inexperienced surgeon it is probably best to perform the coronal browlift first, performing the upper lid blepharoplasty as the second portion of the operative procedure. Our experience has shown that either method can be successfully used.

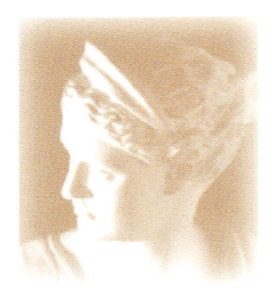

BROWPEXY

Occasionally the plastic surgeon will be confronted with a patient who requires lateral brow elevation and who refuses to undergo a coronal browlifting procedure. In these situations, we will occasionally offer a browpexy as an alternative method for brow elevation. This technique essentially involves elevating the lateral eyebrows through the upper blepharoplasty incision.

Technically, this procedure is quite simple to perform during blepharoplasty. The lateral and central portion of the brows are marked preoperatively for ideal suture placement. A routine upper blepharoplasty is then performed. Following removal of an appropriate degree of ROOF fat, blunt dissection is used directly deep to the orbicularis muscle (in the plane of the ROOF fat) to approximately 1 cm above the superior orbital rim. A permanent suture is then placed along the previously placed markings of the lateral brow, extending to the underlying periosteum superior to the supraorbital rim. Usually three to four sutures are placed; thus it is important to ensure proper preoperative marking to obtain symmetric results. Because of concomitant lateral brow elevation these patients usually require less upper lid skin resection to compensate for brow elevation.

Although the results in browpexy with upper lid blepharoplasty are more variable than those obtainable through a coronal browlifting approach, this method can somewhat improve brow position in patients who do not wish to undergo a more extensive procedure. The disadvantages of browpexy include less predictability in terms of postoperative brow descent.

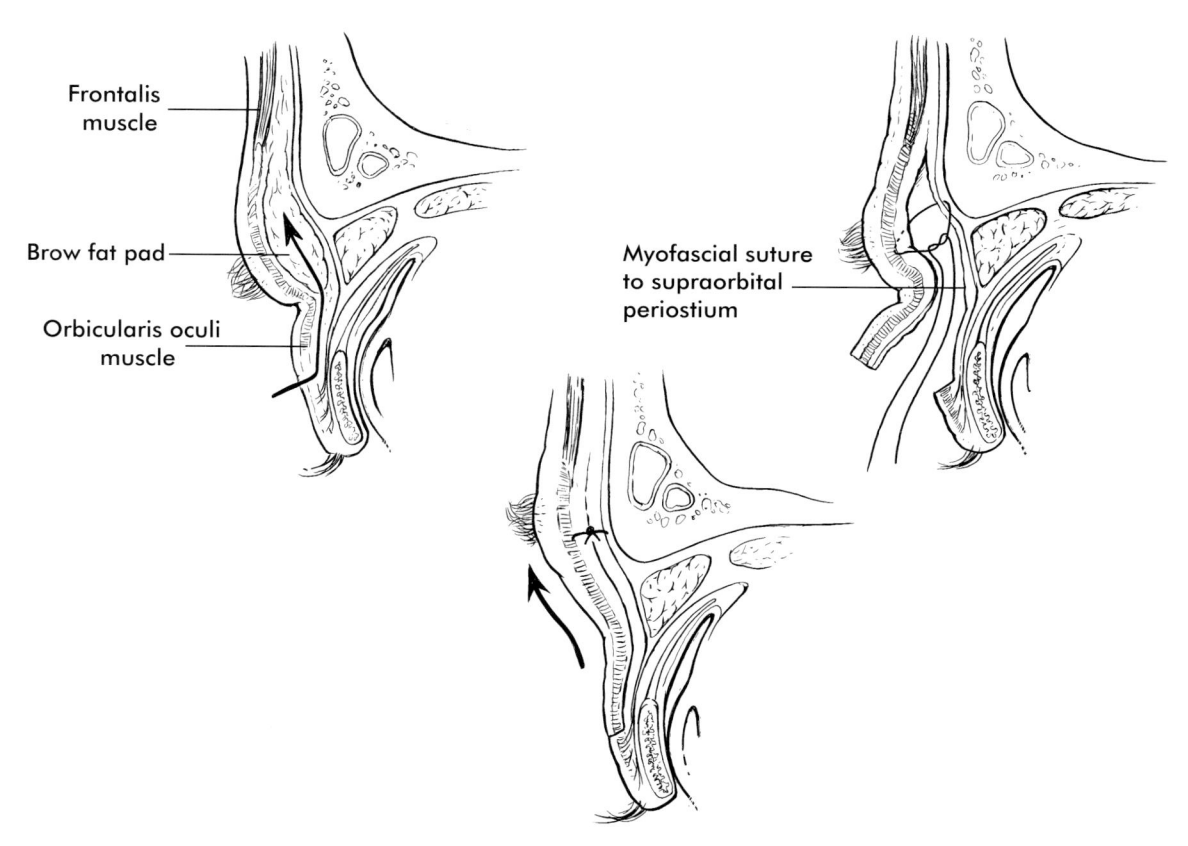

Browpexy procedure performed though an upper blepharoplasty incision. Following incision of the upper eyelid, dissection is continued in the retroarbicular plane (in the plane of the brow fat pad–ROOF fat) superior to the supraorbital rim. Tacking sutures are then placed between the brow pad and the underlying periosteum. Usually three to four permanent sutures (4-0 nylon) are placed with care to ensure proper elevation along preoperative markings. The blepharoplasty is then closed in a routine fashion. It is important to remove slightly less skin at the time of upper blepharoplasty if a browpexy procedure will be performed.

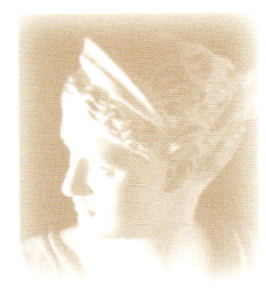

POSTOPERATIVE MANAGEMENT

Discomfort occurring as a result of the operative procedure can be controlled with mild pain medication. Narcotics are usually not necessary. Bandages are removed in 24 to 48 hours. The patient is instructed to wash his or her hair daily until the staples are removed, usually on the ninth or tenth postoperative day.

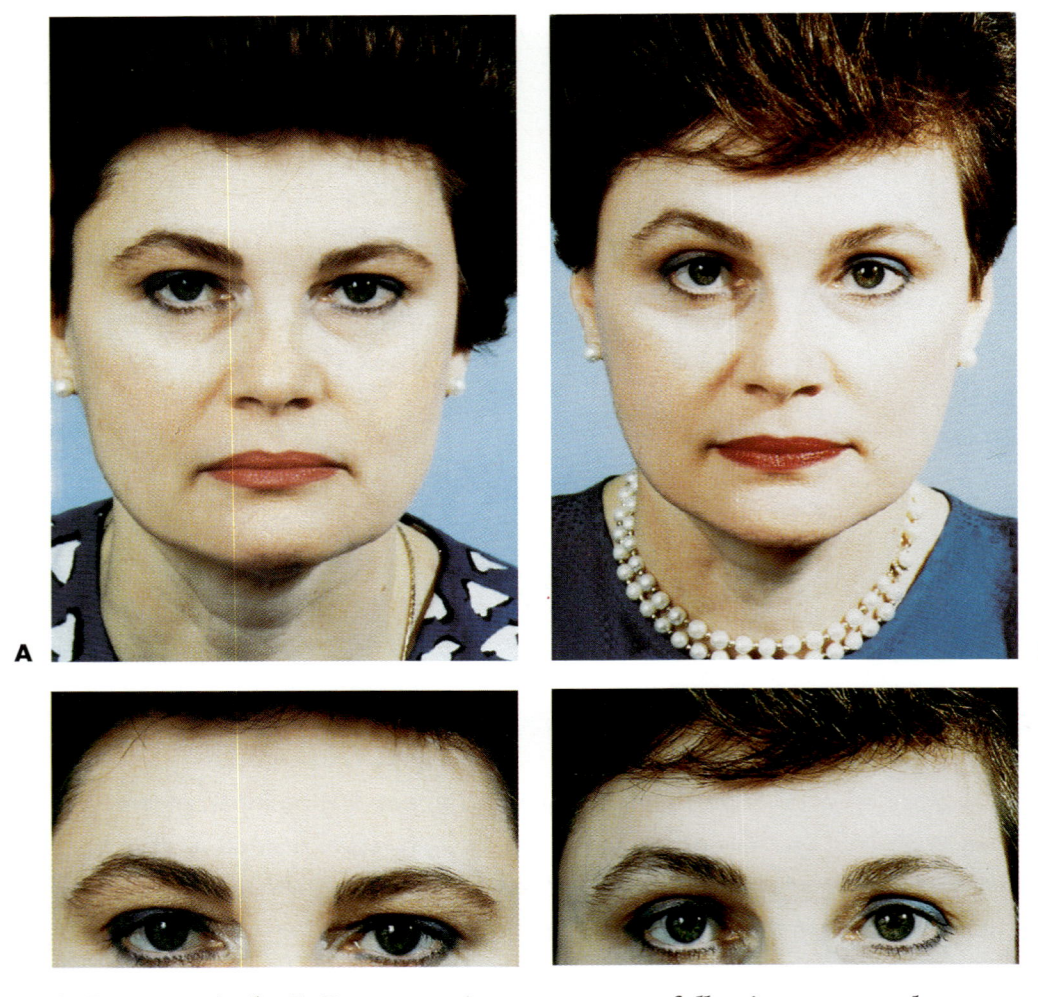

A, Preoperatively. B, Postoperative appearance following a coronal browlifting and rhytidectomy. No upper eyelid skin was resected during this procedure.

CORONAL BROWLIFTING

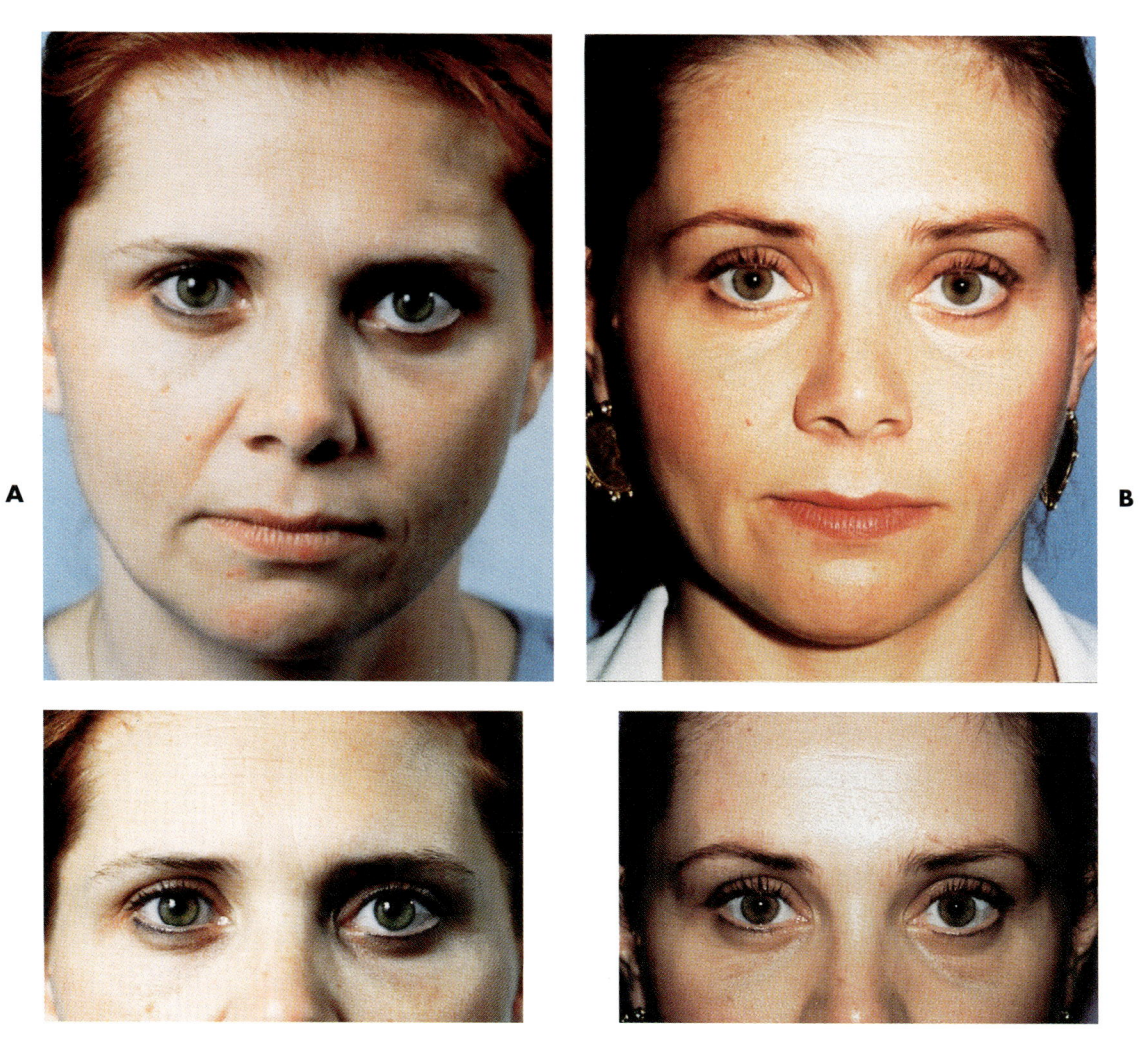

A, Preoperative appearance. B, Postoperative appearance following coronal browlifting. No upper lid skin was resected during this procedure. Of note, mobilization of the medial brow was limited, and the emphasis was placed on lateral brow elevation only. This enabled us to change a flat brow shape into an arched brow configuration postoperatively.

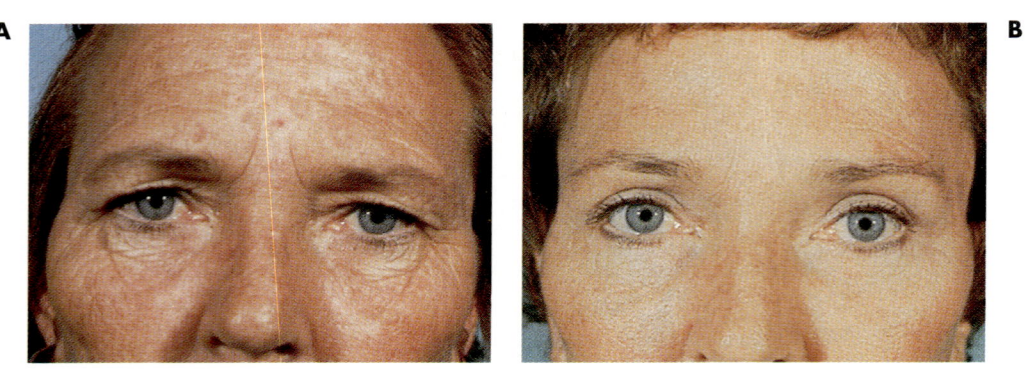

A, Preoperative appearance. B, Postoperative appearance following coronal browlifting with concomitant blepharoplasty.

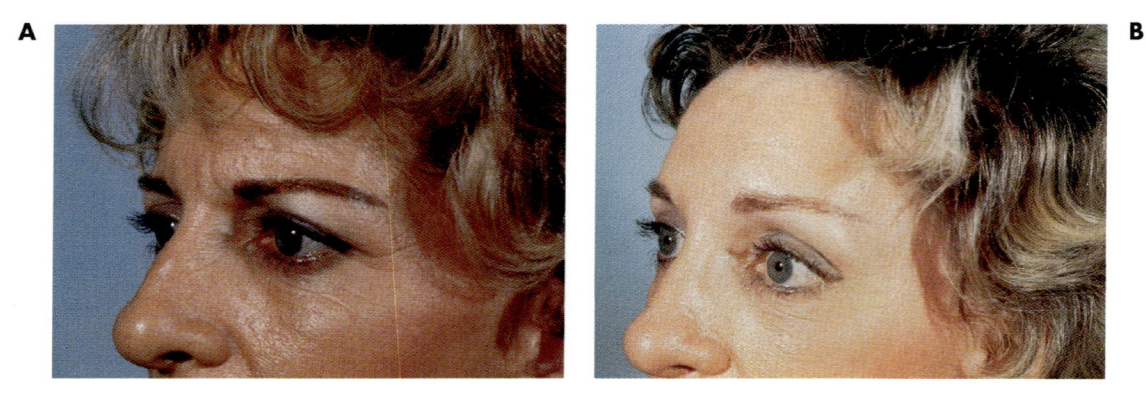

A, Preoperative appearance. B, Postoperative appearance following coronal browlifting. An upper blepharoplasty was not necessary in this patient.

COMPLICATIONS

◼ Frontal Nerve Injury

Injuries to the frontal nerve are rare. They can be minimized if the surgeon has a thorough knowledge of anatomy of the temporal branch of the facial nerve. If the plane of dissection is immediately external to the temporalis fascia, the nerve supply will be protected.

◼ Alopecia

Alopecia can be a problem, although it rarely occurs. It can be minimized by avoiding excessive tension on the scalp flap. Beveling the scalp incision along the direction of the hair follicles is an important technical point in minimizing this complication.

◼ Scarring

Unacceptable scarring can occur, but it is probably also caused by excessive tension on the line of closure. If the scars spread postoperatively, they can be revised in a few months to adequately correct the problem. Scars may also be located in undesirable areas.

The best way to avoid this is to place the incisions in inconspicuous locations so that the resulting scars will not be as visible. Hypertrophied or irregular scars at the hairline are difficult to correct.

◼ Infection

Infection is rare; we have never encountered this complication. If it occurred, the usual treatment would be to obtain a culture and administer appropriate antibiotics.

◼ Hematoma

Hematoma is also rare. We have encountered only two cases, both of which occurred in the immediate postoperative period. Treatment consists of opening the flap, exposing the operative site, and controlling the bleeding point(s). The bleeding vessel is usually found temporally from a branch of the superficial temporal artery.

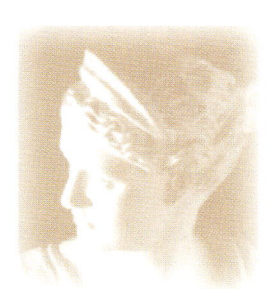

Itching

Itching can be a troublesome symptom in the first few weeks postoperatively; however, it is infrequent. The cause is probably associated with reinnervation of the scalp flap. Symptomatic treatment includes trimeprazine tartrate (Temaril) 2.5 or 5.0 mg every 6 hours. The patient should be reassured that the itching will eventually subside.

Numbness

Numbness is not truly a complication but instead is an anticipated sequela or by-product of the operation. It occurs in the area between the incisions and on the crown of the head. Sensation usually returns within 6 to 8 months, but in rare instances the numbness can be permanent.

Overcorrection—Lack of Harmony Between Medial and Lateral Brow

Over-correction can occur if the forehead flap advancement is extreme. The patient may have a surprised or startled look. It is important preoperatively to understand the amount of movement desired within each portion of the brow to obtain the desired aesthetic result.

Most problems with overcorrection occur because the medial brow is placed at a level equal to or higher than the lateral brow. Aesthetic overcorrection of the medial brow occurs because as the procerus and corrugator musculature are weakened during the brow lifting procedure, the muscular stress toward redescent of the medial brow is usually nonexistent. Thus the medial brow will remain where it is placed at the time of surgery. Unfortunately, this is not true of the lateral brow. The orbicularis oculi muscle remains the main depressor of the lateral eyebrow, and is unaffected by the surgery. In some patients the muscular closure of the orbicularis oculi can remain a powerful force, causing a redescent of the lateral brow in the postoperative period. It is sometimes difficult to overcome the dynamic stress of the orbicularis oculi through the static tension associated with brow mobilization and galeal closure.

CORONAL BROWLIFTING

It is important preoperatively to assess the degree of medial brow elevation which is required. There are only two methods available to the surgeon to prevent overelevation of the medial brow. First, as was previously discussed, limiting mobilization of the medial brow along

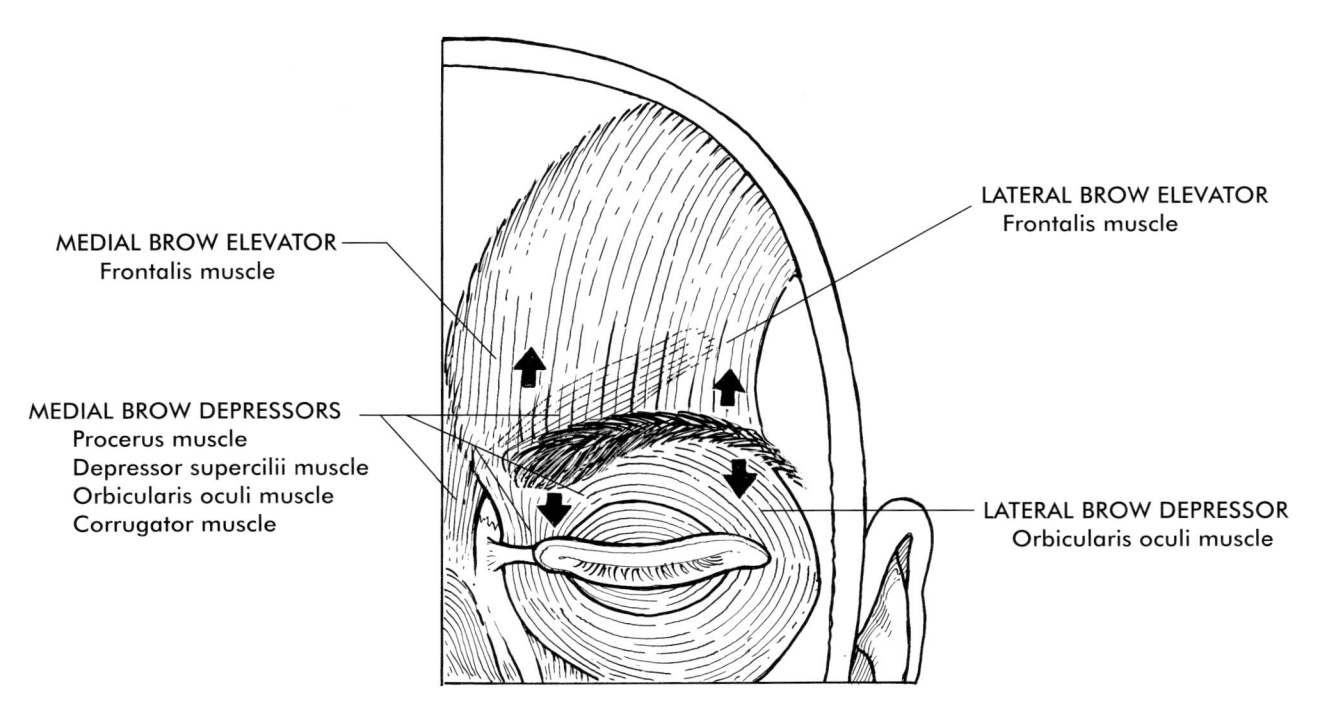

MEDIAL BROW ELEVATOR
Frontalis muscle

MEDIAL BROW DEPRESSORS
Procerus muscle
Depressor supercilii muscle
Orbicularis oculi muscle
Corrugator muscle

LATERAL BROW ELEVATOR
Frontalis muscle

LATERAL BROW DEPRESSOR
Orbicularis oculi muscle

It is important to understand that browlifting relies on the counterbalance between the dynamics of muscle pull versus the static elevation of the eyebrow through mobilization and fixation. The main problem in browlifting is that the medial brow tends to stay where the surgeon places it postoperatively because both the medial brow elevators (frontalis) and medial brow depressors (corrugator and procerus) are weakened during the procedure. Unfortunately, the major lateral brow depressor (orbicularis muscle) is not affected by browlifting procedures and remains active postoperatively. For this reason it is essentially impossible to overelevate the lateral brow via static tension through scalp excision, since the orbicularis muscle contraction postoperatively will tend to cause a redescent of the lateral brow. These factors must be gauged intraoperatively to account for the postoperative descent of the lateral brow so that the medial and lateral brow remain in harmony in the later postoperative period.

its attachments to the periosteum of the lateral nasal root will prevent a significant amount of medial brow elevation. This area should be mobilized only if medial brow elevation is required. Second, limiting the amount of central scalp resection will similarly help to prevent over

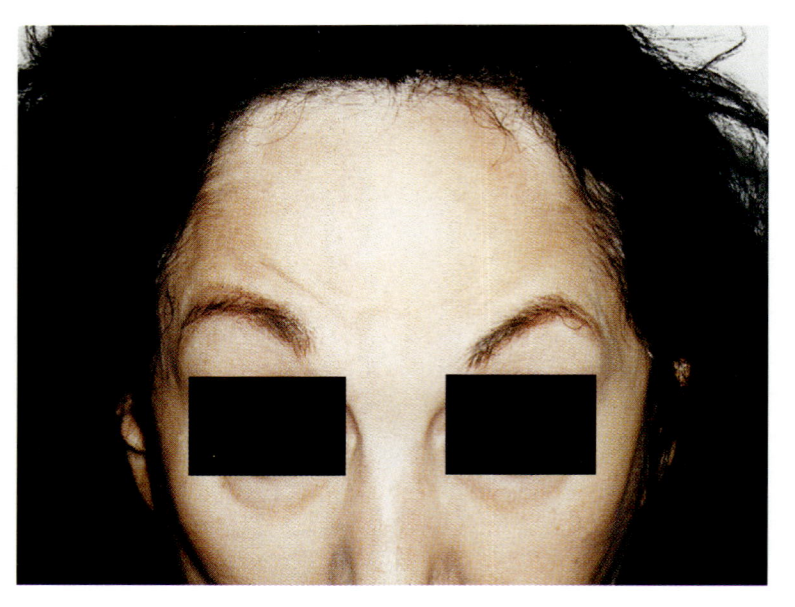

Overcorrection of the medial brows will produce an unnaturally startled or surprised look, the hallmark of surgical distortion. Note that this patient, besides the problems with medial brow positioning, also exhibits complete resection of the central aspect of the frontalis muscle, which over time has given an obvious contour deformity to the central aspect of her forehead. For this reason we prefer frontalis scoring rather than resection. Note also the central hairline displacement. In our opinion a hairline incision would have been preferable for this patient.

elevation of the medial brow. In our opinion, limiting dissection of the medial brow attachments is perhaps the more important factor in limiting medial brow elevation.

In summary, it is our feeling that it is perhaps best to undercorrect medial brow elevation while maximizing lateral brow elevation. Over time it is almost impossible to obtain overcorrection of the lateral brow and those forces which will improve lateral brow elevation, such as completely freeing the lateral brow from its lateral orbital attachments, mobilizing the lateral brow pad in a subperiosteal fashion down to the frontal zygomatic suture, and perhaps deeply placed sutures from galea to the deep temporal fascia, are methods to improve long term fixation of lateral brow position. Nonetheless, in some patients it is almost impossible to prevent some form of descent of the lateral brow over time, and this eventual descent should remain in harmony with medial brow position.

SUMMARY

The coronal browlift is technically a simple procedure. It is associated with few complications and produces a high degree of patient satisfaction. The results are usually as permanent as those produced by a routine rhytidectomy involving the lower two thirds of the face. There should be no hesitation in recommending surgical alterations of the upper third of the face because this often complements the procedures performed on the lower two thirds. Procedures performed on the lower part of the face may make forehead and brow deformities even more obvious if the coronal browlift is warranted but not performed.

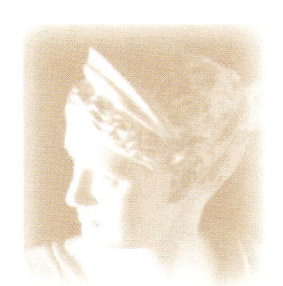

Q&A: FREQUENTLY ASKED QUESTIONS

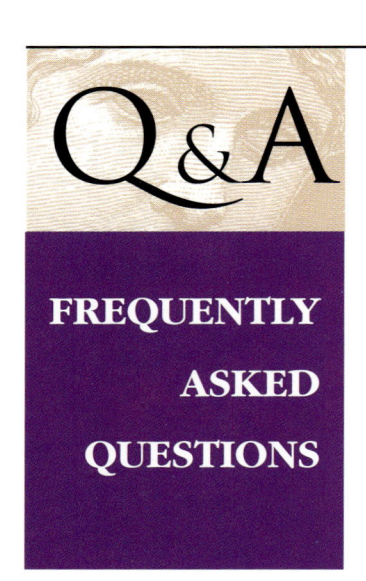

"Does it hurt more than other procedures?"
There is no pain associated with the actual operation. Some patients complain of headache or tightness of the forehead, but these are temporary symptoms.

"Does the incision show?"
The scar is usually placed within the hairline and therefore is not visible.

"Is the incision ever made in front of the hairline?"
In some cases this is done. If a patient has a high vertical dimension to the forehead, the incision may be placed at the hairline so as not to lengthen an already high hairline.

"Will I lose my hair?"
Hair loss is rare but could occur if tension were too great along the suture line or if other complications (hematoma or infection) occurred.

"Do I lose sensation in my forehead?"
There is some diminution of sensation immediately postoperatively. The sensation usually returns to normal within 6 to 9 months. The area most affected is the top of the head between the incision and the (occipital) crown.

"Will all of the lines in my forehead be removed?"
Probably not; however, they will be significantly improved for several years.

"Could I have my brows elevated without having the incision across the top of my head?"
Yes, but it would require another approach, most commonly an incision just above each eyebrow. A fine-line scar would result.

"Is it possible to have nerve damage to my muscles so that I would lose expression in the forehead?"
It is possible, but this is extremely rare. The nerve that supplies the area of the brows may be temporarily affected, but the damage is permanent in less than 1% of cases.

"Is there a chance of creating a 'wide-eyed' or 'surprised' look?"
Only if the correction were extreme. Even then there would be some relaxation over time, and the expression would eventually return to normal.

SUGGESTED READING

1. Abdul-Hassan HS, von Drasek Ascher G, Acland RD: Surgical anatomy and blood supply of the fascial layers of the temporal region, *Plast Reconstr Surg* 77:17, 1986.
2. Baker TJ: *The brow lift.* In Goulian D, Courtiss E, editors: *Symposium on surgery of the aging face, vol 19,* St Louis, 1978, Mosby, p 103.
3. Bames HO: Frown disfigurement and ptosis of eyebrows, *Plast Reconstr Surg* 19:337, 1957.
4. Connell BF, Manter TJ: The male foreheadplasty: recognizing and treating aging in the upper face, *Clin Plast Surg* 18:653, 1991.
5. Connell BF, Lambros VS, Neurohr GH: The forehead lift: techniques to avoid complications and produce optimal results, *Anesthetic Plast Surg* 19:217, 1989.
6. Connell BF: Eyebrow, face and neck lifts for males, *Clin Plast Surg* 5:15, 1978.
7. Castanares S: Forehead wrinkles, glabellar frown and ptosis of the eyebrows, *Plast Reconstr Surg* 34:406, 1964.
8. Furnas DW: Landmarks for the trunk and the temporofacial division of the facial nerve, *Plast Reconstr Surg* 52:694, 1965.
9. Gleason MC: Brow lifting through a temporal scalp approach, *Plast Reconstr Surg* 52:141, 1973.
10. Habal MB: The invisible frown plasty, *Anesthetic Plast Surg* 2:395, 1978.
11. Kaye BL: The forehead lift: a useful adjunct to face lift and blepharoplasty, *Plast Reconstr Surg* 60:161, 1977.

12. Le Roux P, Jones SH: Total permanent removal of wrinkles from the forehead, *Br J Plast Surg* 27:359, 1974.
13. Marino H: The forehead lift: some hints to secure better results, *Anesthetic Plast Surg* 1:251, 1977.
14. Noel A: *La chirurgie esthetique et sa role sociale,* Paris, 1926, Masson et Cie.
15. Ortiz-Monasterio F, Barrera G, Olmedo A: The coronal incision in rhytidectomy: the brow lift, *Clin Plast Surg* 5(1):167, 1978.
16. Pitanguy I, Silveira R: The frontal branch of the facial nerve: The importance of its variations in face lifting, *Plast Reconstr Surg* 38:352, 1966.
17. Pitanguy I: Section of the frontalis-procerus-corrugator aponeurosis in the correction of frontal and glabellar wrinkles, *Ann Plast Surg* 2:422, 1979.
18. Pitanguy I: Indications for and treatment of frontal and glabellar wrinkles in an analysis of 3404 consecutive cases of rhytidectomy, *Plast Reconstr Surg* 67:157, 1981.
19. Stuzin JM, Wagstrom L, Kawamoto HK, Wolfe SA: Anatomy of the frontal branch of the facial nerve: the significance of the temporal fat pad, *Plast Reconstr Surg* 83:265, 1989.
20. Tolhurst DE, Carsten SMH, Greco RJ, Hurwitz DJ: The surgical anatomy of the scalp, *Plast Reconstr Surg* 87:603, 1991.
21. Uchida J: A method of frontal rhytidectomy, *Plast Reconstr Surg* 35:218, 1965.
22. Vinas JC, Caviglia C, Cortinis JL: Forehead rhytidectomy and brow lifting, *Plast Reconstr Surg* 57:445, 1976.

CORRECTION OF PERIORAL WRINKLES

Approximately 50% of female patients requesting rhytidectomy also elect perioral wrinkle treatment. Most commonly we treat these patients with perioral dermabrasion, although on fair-complexioned patients who have deep rhytides, we will occasionally use a perioral phenol peel. The greatest advantage of dermabrasion in the treatment of perioral rhytides is that there is usually little change to the perioral color compared with that of the surrounding cheek skin. Although dermabrasion is not as effective as phenol peeling in the treatment of perioral rhytides, its improvement is usually significant enough to produce adequate patient satisfaction. Dermabrasion is much more effective in treating rhytides of the upper lip than those of the lower lip.

We rarely use trichloroacetic acid (TCA) peeling to improve perioral rhytides. Our experience with TCA in this area has been disappointing and not as predictable as treatment with either dermabrasion or phenol peeling (for the details of both dermabrasion and chemical peeling, see Chapter 3).

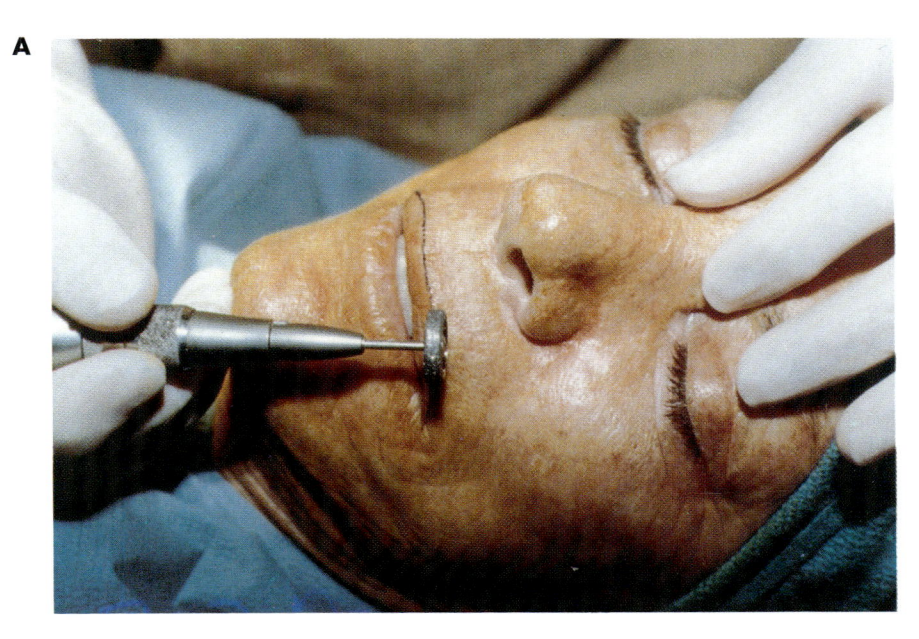

A, It is helpful to mark the vermilion-skin junction before beginning the dermabrasion. This aids in guiding the abrasive wheel along the border to eliminate the fine lines extending from the vermilion onto the skin.

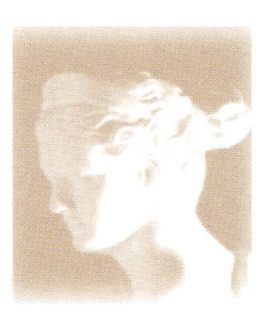

Continued.

SURGICAL REJUVENATION OF THE FACE

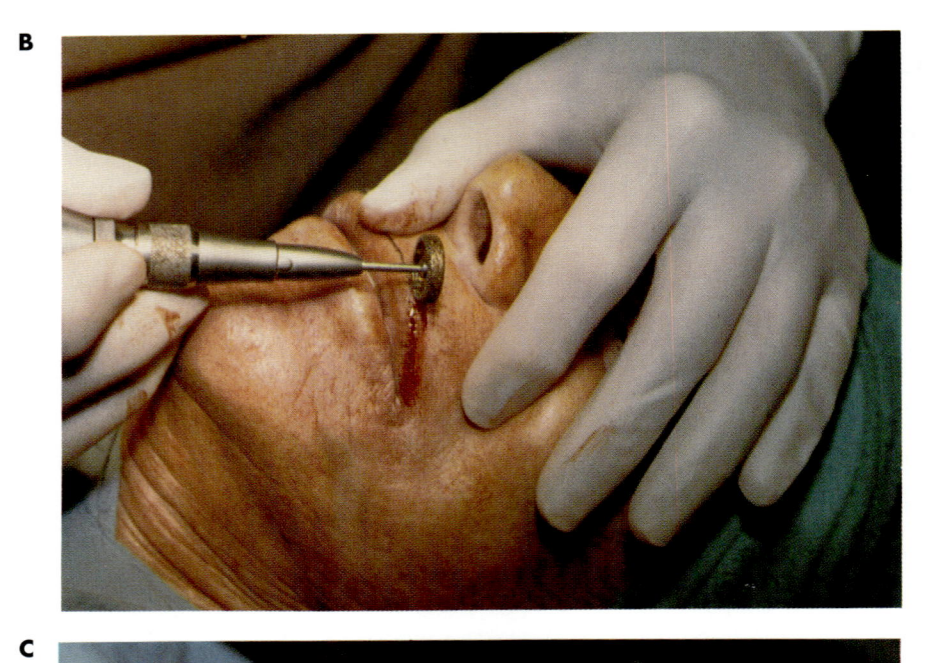

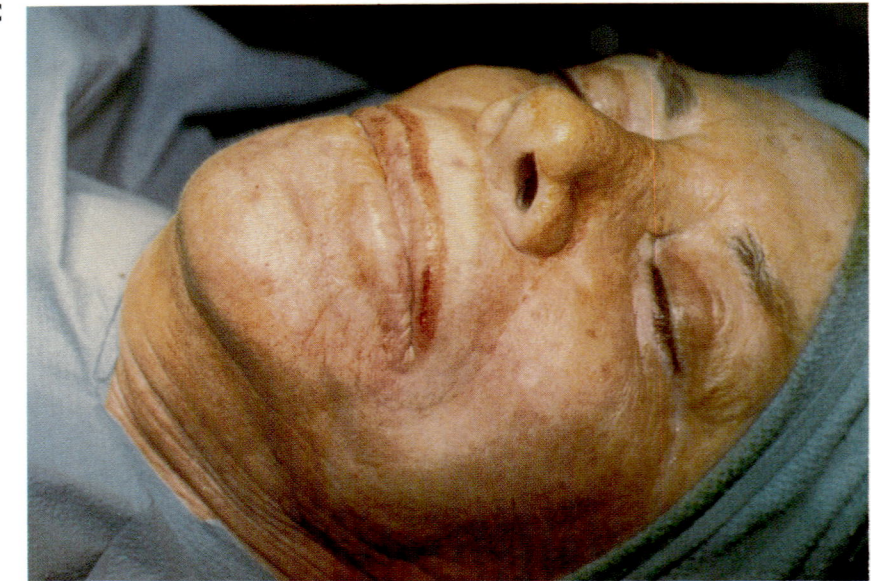

B, The vermilion-skin junction is abraded with a narrow fraise to outline the border. C, The skin adjacent to the vermillion border of the upper lip has not been abraded, and the procedure is carried out on the lower lip line.

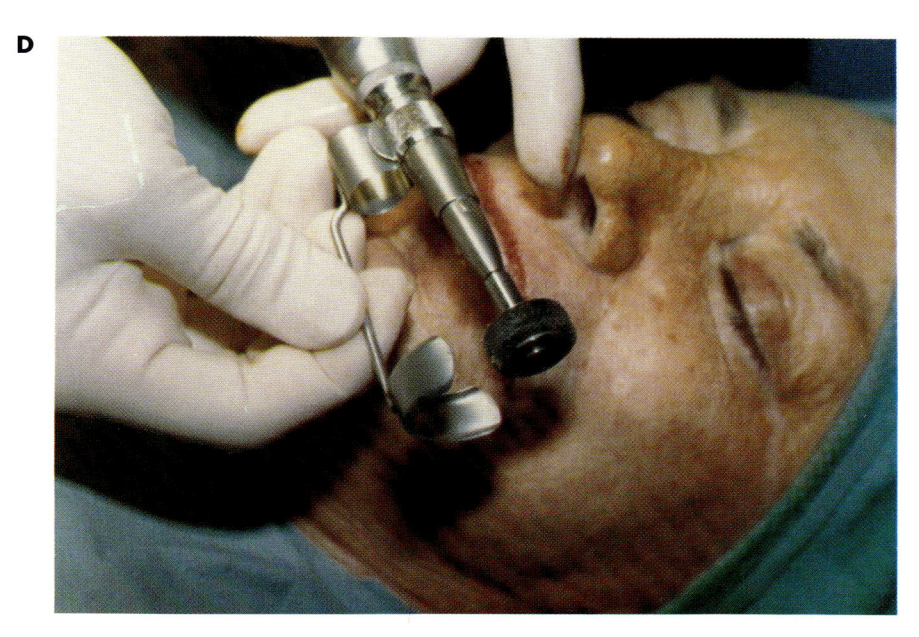

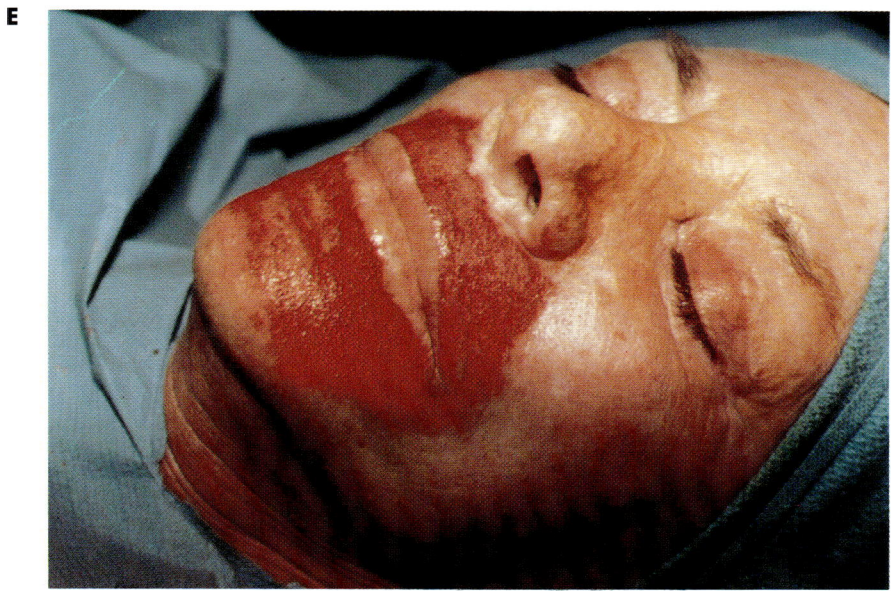

D, Using a large abrasive disc (in this case a wire brush and a guard), the surgeon performs the remainder of the perioral abrasion. E, The appearance of the perioral area when the dermabrasion has been completed. (From Baker TJ, Gordon HL: Surgical rejuvenation of the face, ed 1, St Louis, 1986, Mosby, pp 379-381.)

SURGICAL REJUVENATION OF THE FACE

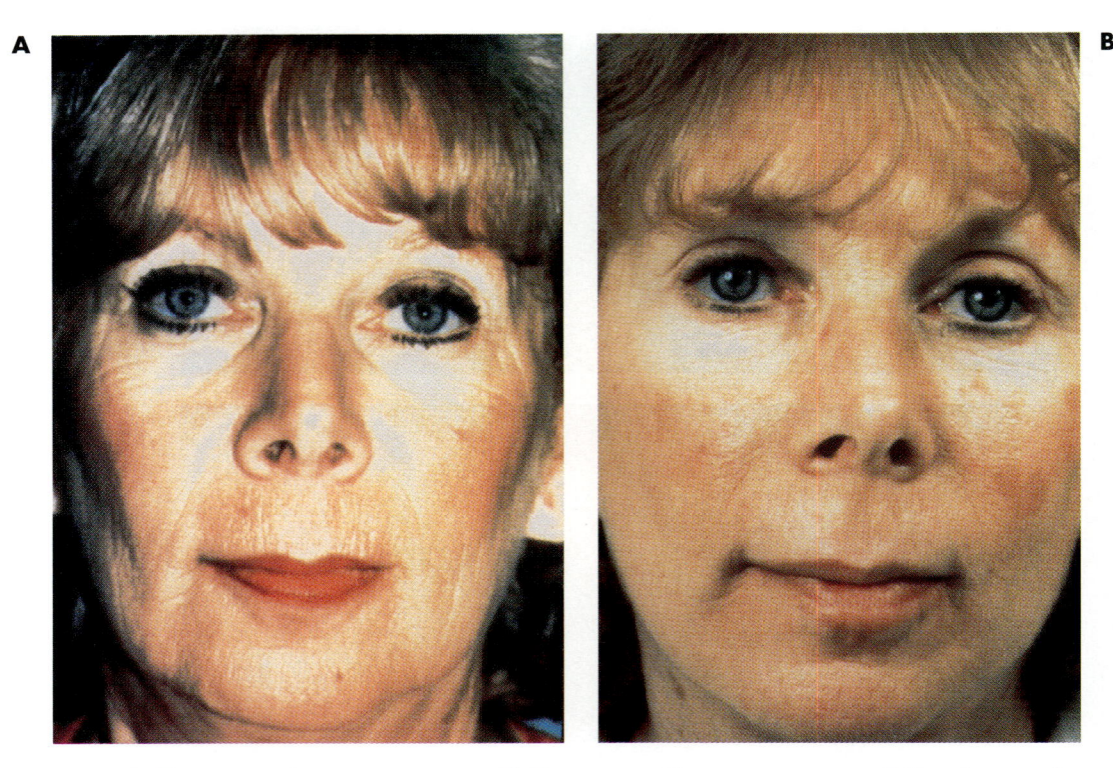

A, Preoperative appearance. *B,* Postoperative appearance following perioral dermabrasion. The primary advantage of dermabrasion as opposed to phenol peeling is the minimal change in perioral pigment. Although dermabrasion is an effective adjunct in removing perioral rhytides, its efficacy is slightly less than that obtained with phenol peeling.

DIRECT EXCISION OF NASOLABIAL FOLDS

Some individuals have laxity in the nasolabial folds but do not need a complete rhytidectomy. In these rare cases direct excision of the nasolabial folds occasionally is performed. The resulting scar in the nasolabial line is acceptable, particularly for male patients. The technique usually involves local anesthesia. The procedure is to excise an ellipse of skin that parallels the nasolabial fold, removing a sufficient amount of skin to eliminate the overhanging laxity from the cheek side of the nasolabial crease. No undermining is necessary, and the wound closes under minimal tension. To prevent cross-hatching, no sutures should be used if possible. By closing the wound in layers and reinforcing the skin closure with Steri-strips, the surgeon can achieve an acceptable scar.

In general we rarely use direct excision of the nasolabial folds, because we can often improve this area through contouring obtained using the extended SMAS dissection. Most of the patients on whom we have used direct excision have been males; our experience using this procedure on female patients has been limited. Although direct excision of the nasolabial fold can improve the contour in this region of the face, it has the obvious disadvantage of producing a cutaneous scar, as well as an abnormal flatness to the region of the nasolabial fold. Because of these problems this procedure is applicable only to very selected clinical situations.

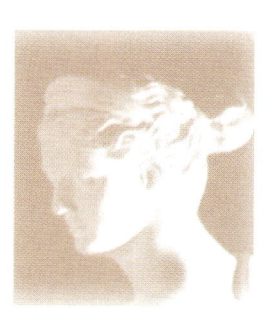

SURGICAL REJUVENATION OF THE FACE

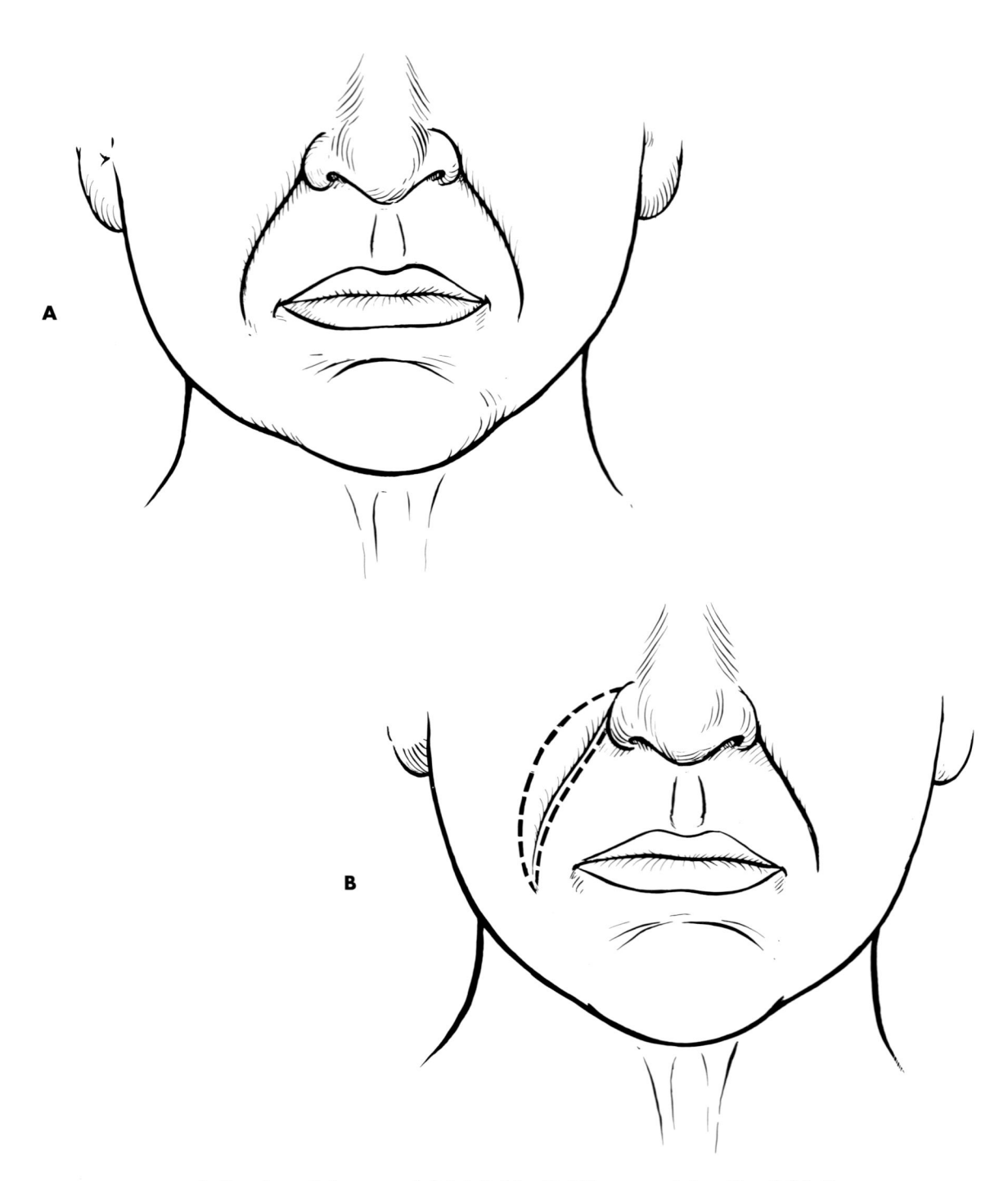

A, Laxity of the nasolabial folds. B, When excising the fold, the surgeon removes the major portion of the ellipse lateral to the nasolabial crease. The crease should be included in the excision.

ANCILLARY PROCEDURES

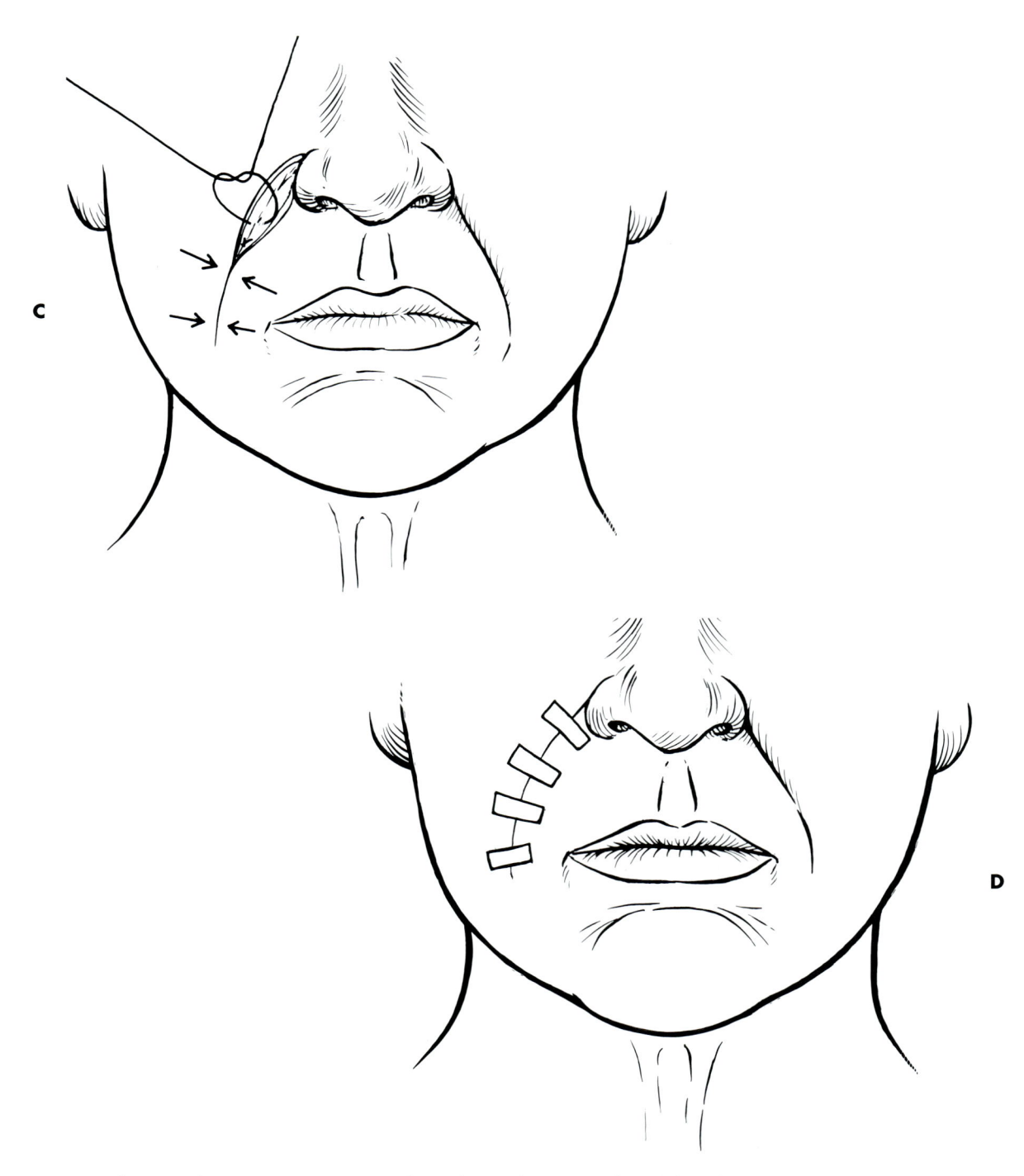

C, Subcuticular sutures are used to close the wound. D, The closure parallels the nasolabial crease. Steri-strips are used to reinforce the closure. (From Baker TJ, Gordon HL: Surgical rejuvenation of the face, *ed 1, St Louis, 1986, Mosby, pp 384-385.)*

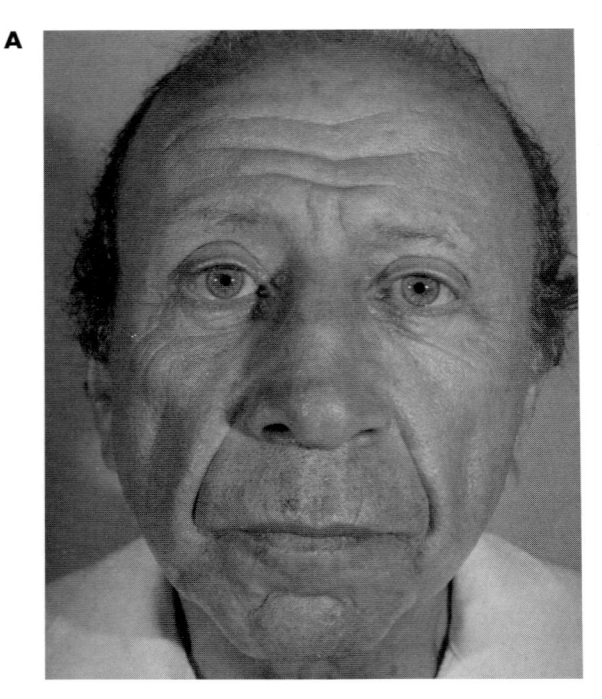

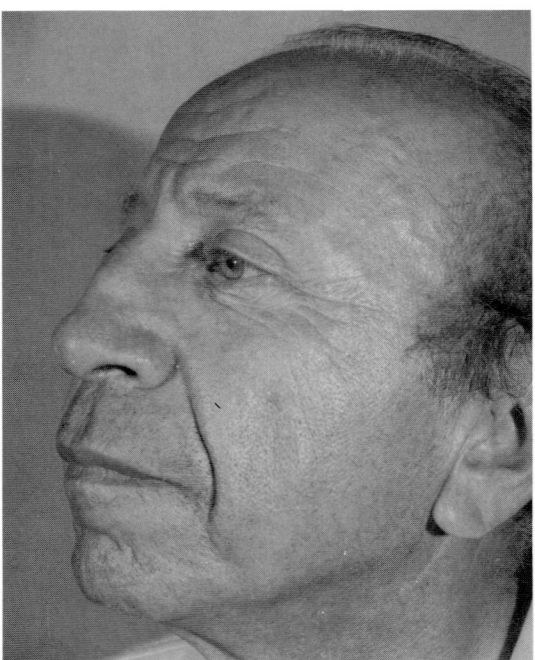

SURGICAL REJUVENATION OF THE FACE

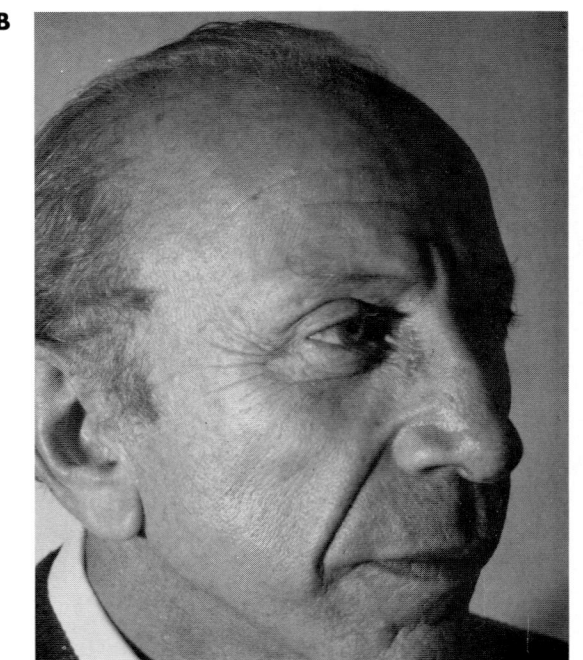

A, This patient has deep nasolabial folds. A standard face-lift will not appreciably correct his appearance. B and C, Note the deep nasolabial crease; it is actually a fold. Nasolabial folds of this depth respond well to direct excision.

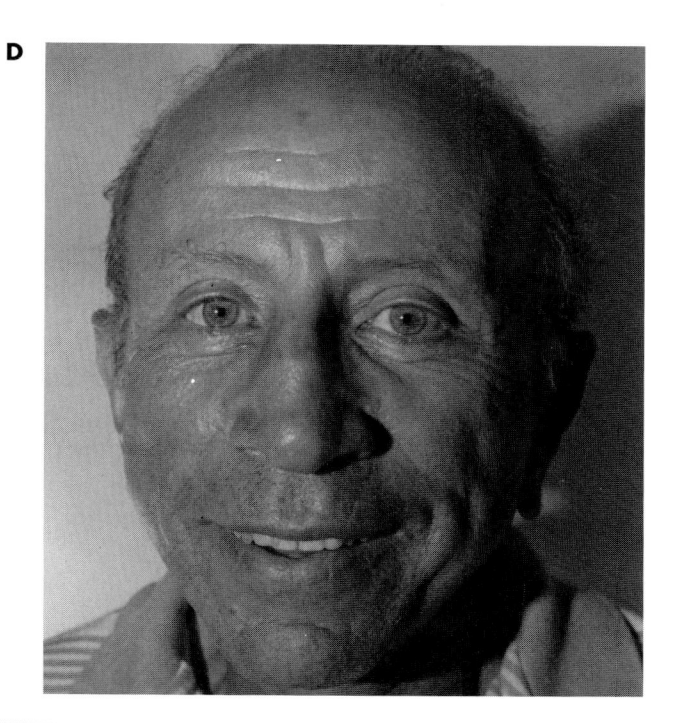

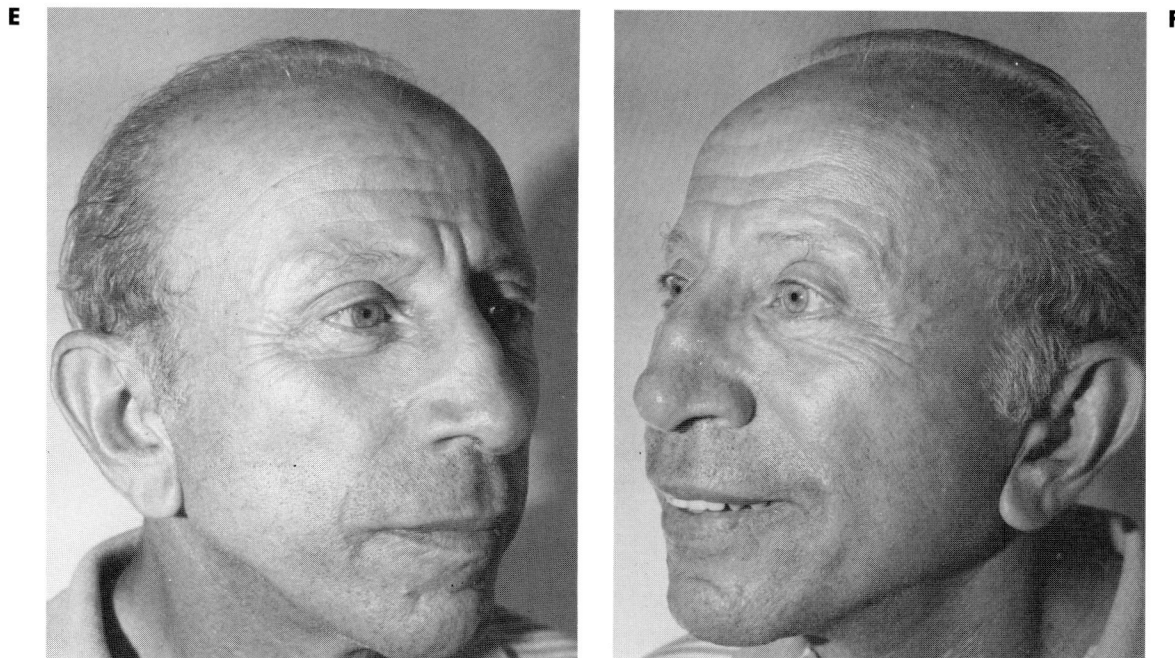

D, The nasolabial folds have been directly excised. The scar is well camouflaged. E and F, Patient's appearance after direct excision of the nasolabial fold. The scar is placed parallel to the nasolabial fold.

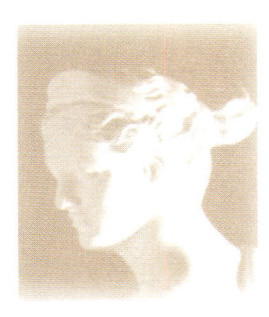

BUCCAL FAT EXCISION

Buccal fat excision is useful for the patient who has round, full cheeks and desires a tapering of facial contours and a highlighting of the malar eminences. Buccal fat excision is rarely indicated in facial rejuvenation surgery. As people age, they tend to lose fat within the face; buccal fat excision will tend to accentuate this gauntness. In the rare situation that buccal fat excision is indicated as a simultaneous procedure for patients undergoing rhytidectomy, we will usually remove the buccal fat by simply extending the subSMAS dissection anterior to the masseter muscle. The buccal fat pad is then identified within the buccal recess, lying just deep to the deep facial fascia.

With careful spreading through the deep fascia, buccal fat can be identified, brought superficially into the wound, and then carefully contoured. The buccal fat pad lies within the same plane as the facial nerve, and when we enter the buccal space through subSMAS dissection, we are careful to penetrate the deep fascia by spreading in the direction of the facial nerve branches. Similarly, we gently tease the buccal fat into the wound and then carefully contour it to prevent injury to the surrounding facial nerve branches.

Most patients undergoing buccal fat excision are young and either request buccal fat excision as an isolated procedure or in conjunction with such procedures as rhinoplasty or chin augmentation. In this situation it is quite simple to harvest buccal fat through an intraoral incision. In general this is a safer approach and has the advantage of an intraoral scar.

For buccal fat harvesting through an intraoral approach, we prefer to use an incision placed high in the maxillary vestibule, beginning above the second maxillary molar and extending posteriorly for 2 cm. The incision is made 5 mm above the attached gingiva of the second molar and extends through the mucosa and then the fibers of the buccinator muscle, exposing the maxillary periosteum.

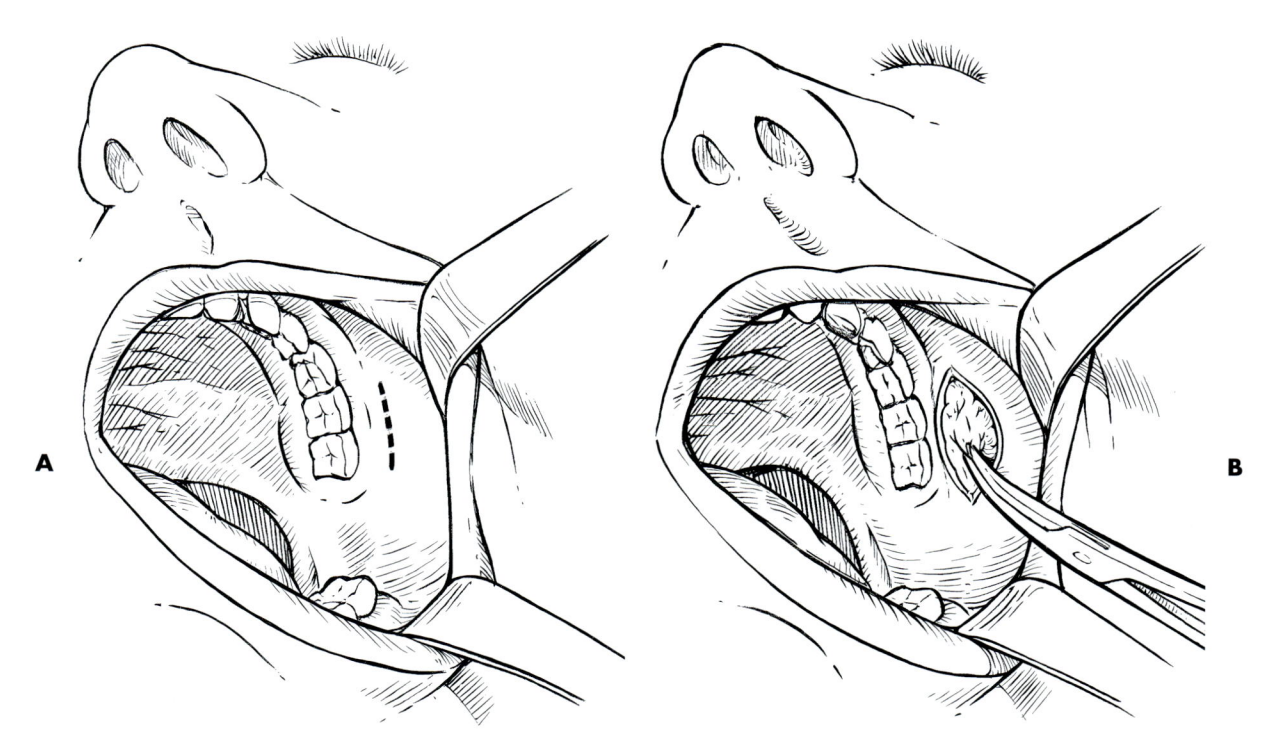

A, Buccal fat pad removal can be performed as an intraoral procedure. We prefer to make the incision above the second maxillary molar and extend posteriorly for 2 cm. The incision is made 5 mm above the attached gingiva, extending through the mucosa and the fibers of the buccinator muscle to expose the maxillary periosteum. B, Because the buccal fat pad is surrounded by a deep fascial envelope, this deep fascia must be incised before the masticatory space is entered. This procedure is similar to the opening of the orbital septum in blepharoplasty. After bluntly spreading through the deep fascia, the buccal fat pad will readily prolapse into the intraoral cavity. After being delivered into the mouth, the buccal fat pad can be carefully removed in incremental amounts, ensuring hemostasis.

Since the buccal fat is surrounded by a fascial envelope, this fascia must be incised before removal of the fat, similar to opening the orbital septum in blepharoplasty. We prefer to bluntly open this layer with a fine hemostat or a scissor and gently spread the fascia until the fat protrudes into the mouth. Because of the intimate association of the fat pad and the facial nerve, the fat should be teased into the mouth by gentle traction while external pressure is applied to the cheek. Deep dissection within the masticatory space should be limited. In general a conservative excision of buccal fat is indicated. We prefer to remove the buccal fat in increments to prevent overresection. Often it is necessary to remove only 1 to 2 grams of fat to obtain the desired aesthetic result. In the very full-cheeked individual, it may be necessary to remove as much as 5 grams of fat on each side. As the fat is removed, changes in cheek contour are obvious and should be appreciated. An overly aggressive initial resection can later lead to a hollowed-out look that is neither aesthetically pleasing nor simple to correct.

If the patient's cheek contour is symmetrical preoperatively, equal amounts of fat should be removed from both sides. If asymmetry exists before surgery, this can usually be improved by harvesting slightly more fat from the fuller cheek. Following excision, the wound is closed with interrupted chromic sutures. We usually give these patients perioperative antibiotics and advise them to apply iced compresses to the cheeks for 48 hours.

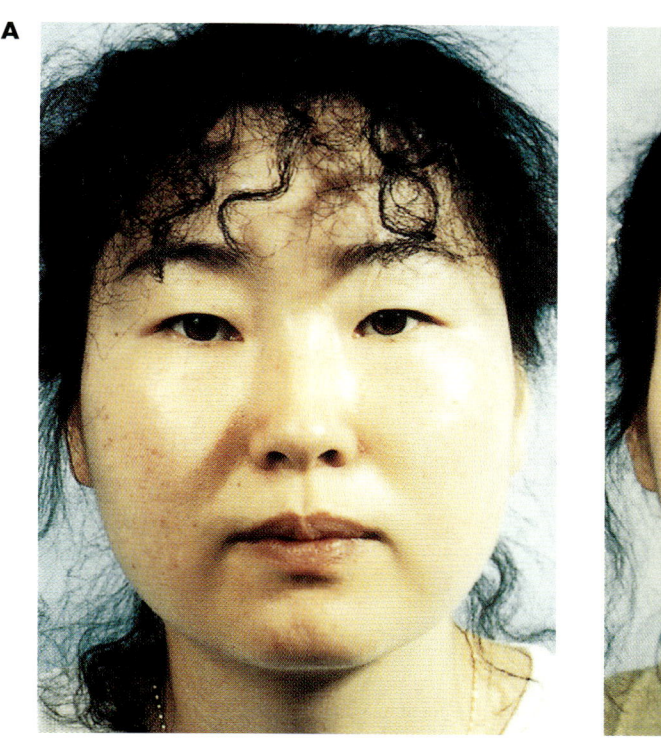

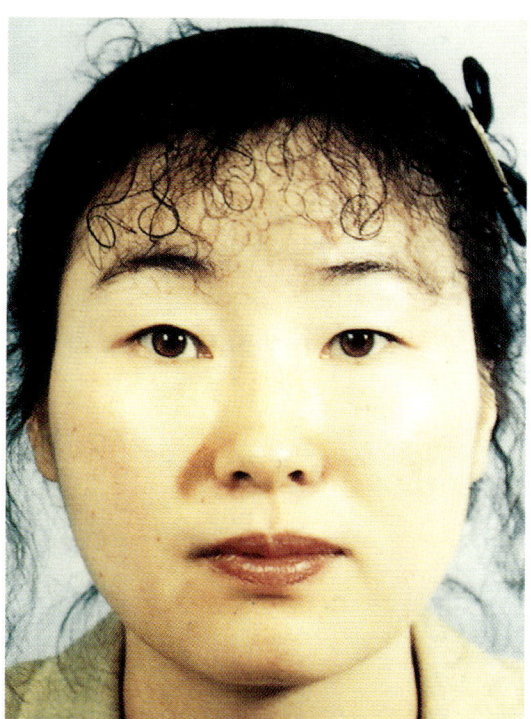

A, Preoperative appearance. *B*, Patient is seen following buccal fat removal performed in conjunction with closed suctioning of her facial jowls.

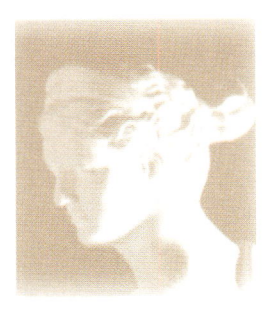

CHIN AUGMENTATION

If a patient requires chin augmentation at the time of rhytidectomy, we often place the chin implant through a submental approach since we will already be making a submental incision to help contour the neck. Placing a chin implant through a submental incision offers an advantage over intraoral placement because the chin implant can be fixated to the periosteum along the inferior border of the mandibular symphysis, which helps prevent postoperative displacement.

When a chin implant is placed through the submental approach, the dissection is continued cephalad toward the inferior border of the mandibular symphysis. The attachments of the platysma to the mandibular symphysis are divided, exposing the periosteum along the sym-

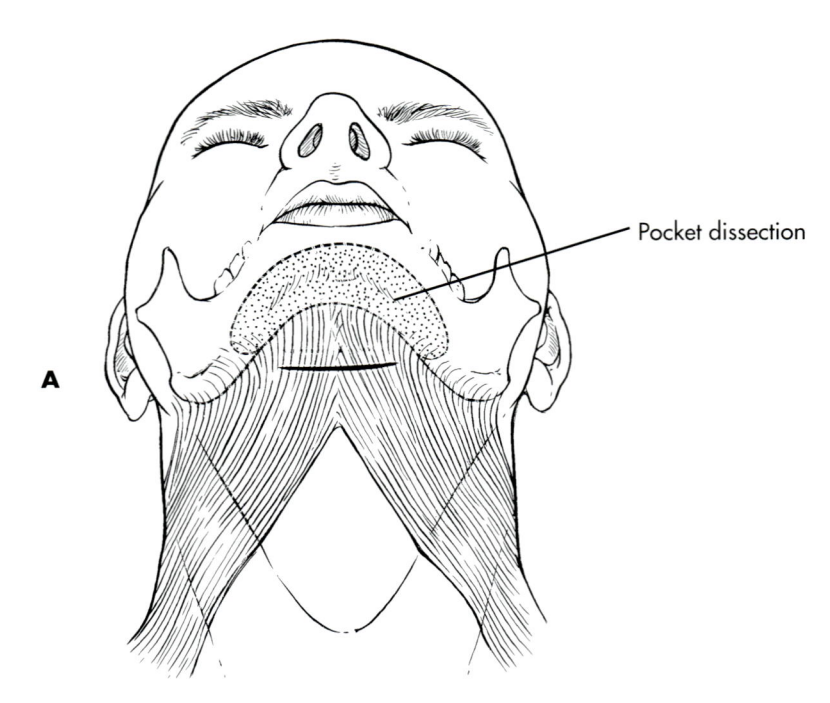

A, When placing a chin implant through a submental incision, it is preferable to make the incision approximately 5 mm caudal to the naturally occurring submental crease. Subcutaneous undermining is then performed in a cephalad fashion to free the crease from the underlying mandibular periosteum. Following this, the platysma is incised and the dissection is continued above the mandibular symphysis in the subperiosteal plane.

physis. The pocket is then made in a precise, symmetrical fashion, usually in the subperiosteal plane. The pocket is made so that the implant sits directly along the mandibular border and does not extend higher than the labial mental crease. It is important to leave some of the periosteum and muscular attachments along the lower lateral portion of the pocket intact so that the implant cannot slide caudally into the neck. After the implant is inserted, it is helpful to fixate it both in the midline and along its more lateral aspects by using interrupted sutures going from the implant into the periosteum and the fibers of the platysma. Following implant insertion, the submental fat and platysmal fascia are approximated with interrupted sutures so that the implant pocket is completely separated from the rest of the submental dissection.

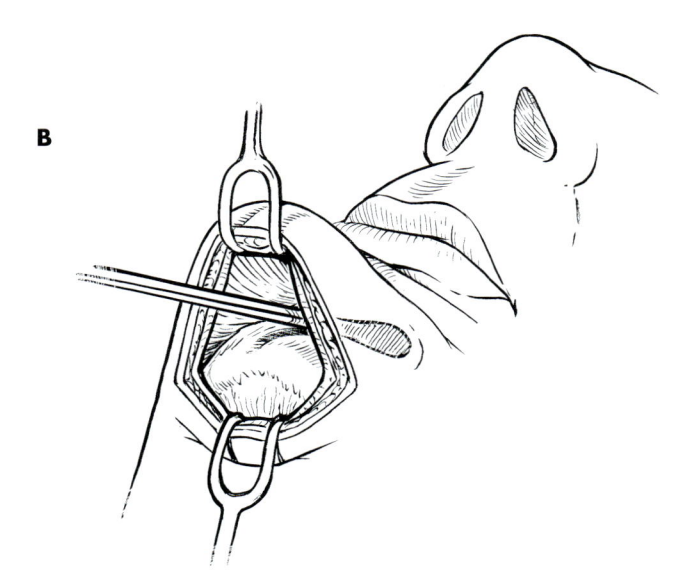

B, A pocket is then made directly overlying the mandibular symphysis, using blunt dissection. We prefer to make this pocket subperiosteal, although in reality there is little difference when the pocket is made either above or below the periosteum. The key to successful implant placement is precise pocket formation.

Continued.

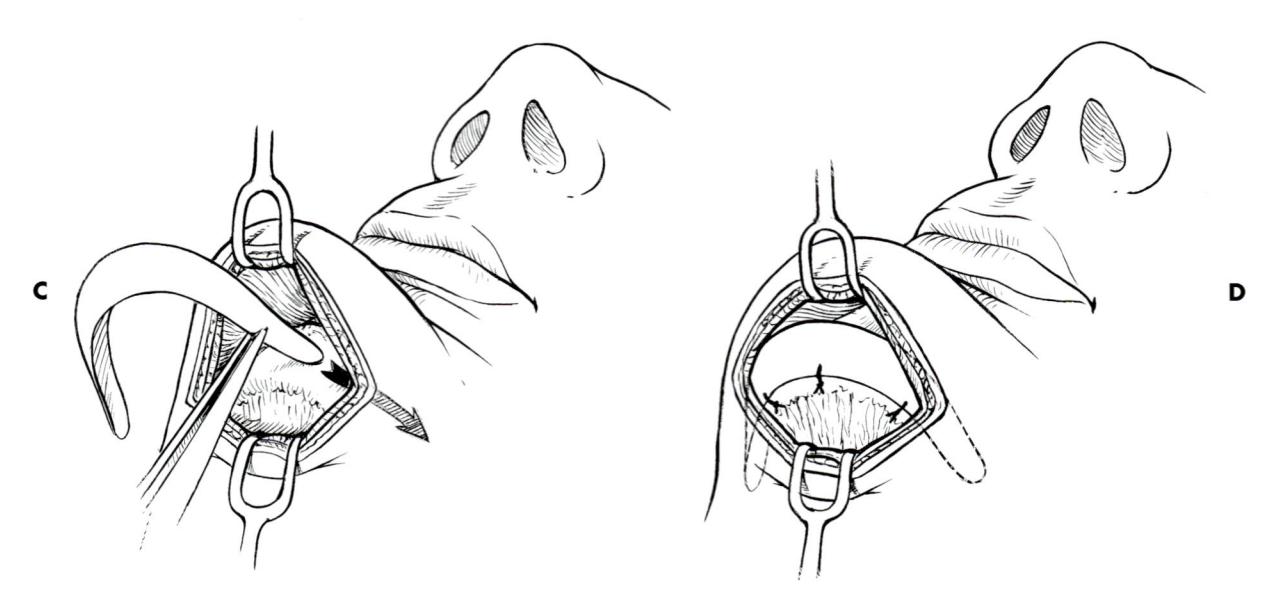

C, After the pocket is formed, the implant is positioned. D, After successful placement, we prefer to secure the implant to the inferior border of the mandible using several interrupted sutures.

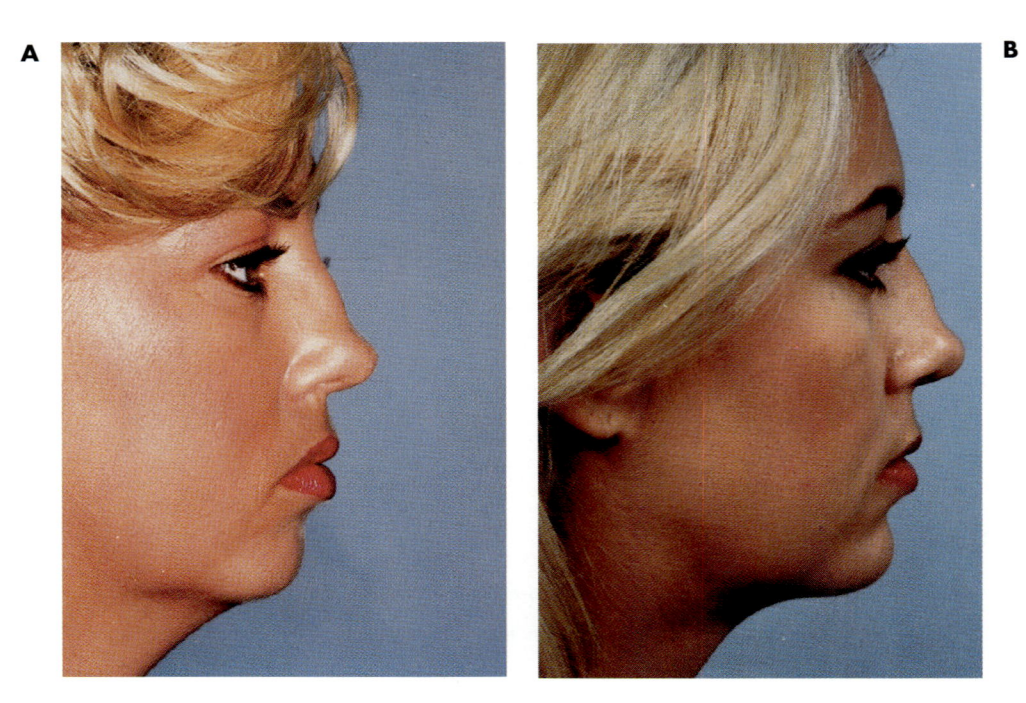

A, Preoperative appearance. B, Patient is seen 3 years after placement of chin implant and closed suction lipectomy of the submental and submandibular areas of her neck.

GENIOPLASTY

As an alternative to alloplastic chin augmentation, a horizontal osteotomy of the mandibular symphysis, also termed genioplasty, is a useful procedure. It is important when evaluating chin position in terms of facial aesthetics to determine the degree of horizontal discrepancy and understand the vertical relationships that exist within the face. Although perhaps oversimplified, an alloplastic chin augmentation is useful in patients who have a moderately retrusive chin and no vertical discrepancy in terms of facial length. In more difficult situations, as well as in patients who have had complications or failure of alloplastic chin augmentation, consideration should be given to the use of a horizontal osteotomy of the mandibular symphysis.

The greatest advantage of genioplasty over the use of alloplastic chin augmentation is the great versatility it offers the surgeon. Specifically, the osteotomized mandibular symphysis represents vascularized material that can be manipulated in different ways to either shorten or lengthen the chin, as well as add anterior projection. In our experience the possibility of controlling the osteotomized segment precisely and having this segment heal with bony union is a great advantage over alloplastic augmentation in the more difficult clinical situation. Proper analysis of the problem through patient examination and analysis of photographs and cephalometrograms is important in choosing an accurate operative plan.

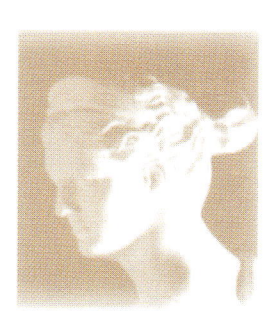

Technique

A genioplasty is performed through an intraoral approach. The oral mucosa is incised from canine to canine, 5 mm inferior to the attached gingiva, sparing the frenulum. A degloving of the mandibular symphysis is performed, extending lateral to the mental foramen. The soft tissue directly overlying the mental tubercle along the base of the mandibular symphysis is not underminded. The reason for not degloving the most inferior aspect of the mandibular symphysis is to leave intact the soft tissue attachments that exist between the periosteum of the symphysis and the base of the chin pad, which allows

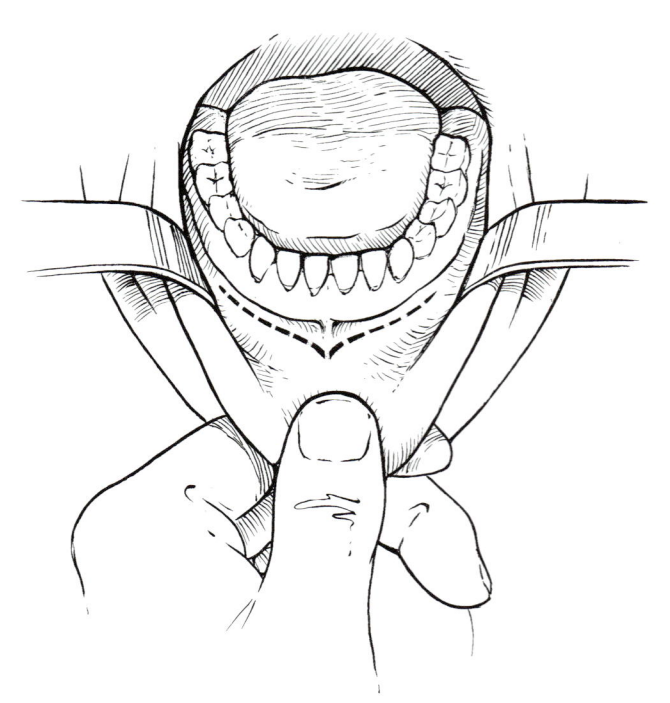

When performing genioplasty, we use an intraoral incision that extends from canine to canine, 5 mm inferior to the attached gingiva, taking care to spare the frenulum. Following this, careful degloving of the mandibular symphysis is performed, leaving intact some of the attachments between the mental tubercle and the overlying chin pad along the inferiomedial aspect of the dissection.

ANCILLARY PROCEDURES

the surgeon to control the movement of the chin pad once the bone is cut. This is especially applicable when shortening a long chin, in which case it is important that as the bone is shortened in the vertical dimension, the soft tissues of the chin pad similarly are elevated. Extensive degloving of the chin pad, when associated with a vertical reduction, has the possibility of producing a ptotic appearance to the chin (witch's chin deformity).

We prefer to perform the medial (or horizontal) portion of the osteotomy with an oscillating saw. In determining where to make this cut, it is important to first determine the location of the base

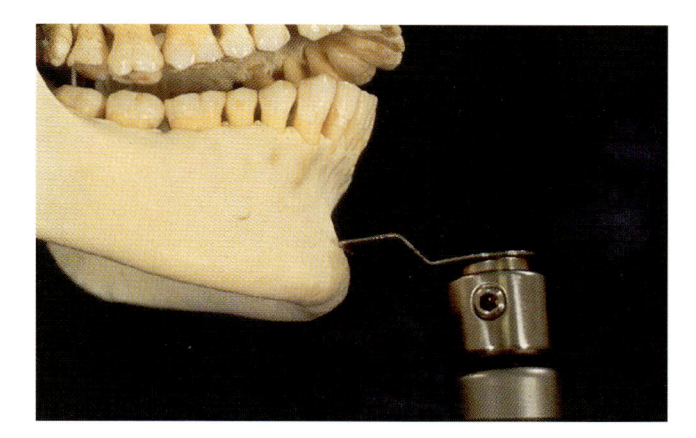

The horizontal medial portion of the osteotomy is performed with an oscillating saw after careful determination that the osteotomy will be performed below the root of the canine tooth. We generally make this horizontal cut between 1 and 2 cm superior to the inferior border of the mandibular symphysis.

of the root of the canine (which is the longest tooth root). Obviously, any cut through the mandibular symphysis should be well below the roots of the teeth. In general we make this horizontal cut between 1 and 2 cm superior to the inferior border of the mandibular symphysis. The lateral aspect of the genioplasty osteotomy is performed with the use of a reciprocating saw. This lateral cut must be at least 5 mm below the inferior alveolar foramen so that the mental nerve will not be jeopardized. The thickest bone encountered laterally during the osteotomy is along the inferior lingual aspect of the mandibular symphysis. To avoid comminution, great care should be used to ensure that this portion of the mandible has been divided during the osteotomy before any attempt at downfracture and advancement is made.

Once the osteotomy is complete, the suprahyoid musculature that remains attached to the inferior segment should be inspected. These muscle attachments vascularize the distal bony segment. Inspection of this area and meticulous hemostasis are important before advancement.

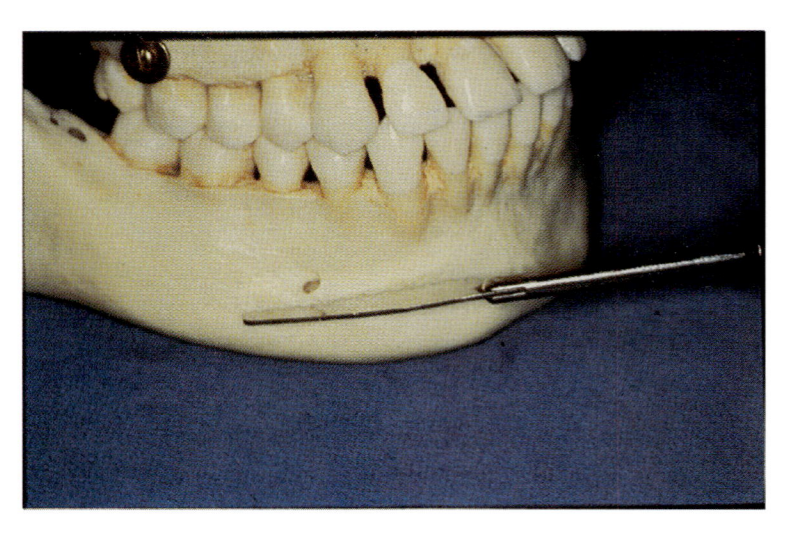

The lateral aspect of the osteotomy is performed with the use of a reciprocating saw. This lateral cut must be at least 5 mm below the inferior alveolar foramen so that the inferior alveolar nerve will not be injured during the osteotomy.

ANCILLARY PROCEDURES

Following osteotomy, several procedures can be performed on the inferior segment. Most commonly, the genioplasty segment is simply advanced, and as much as 10 mm of transverse augmentation can usually be obtained in an advancement genioplasty. If a vertical reduction is required, a second osteotomy must be performed and a wedge of bone removed from the mandibular symphysis. The degree of vertical reduction must be precisely determined by preoperative analysis.

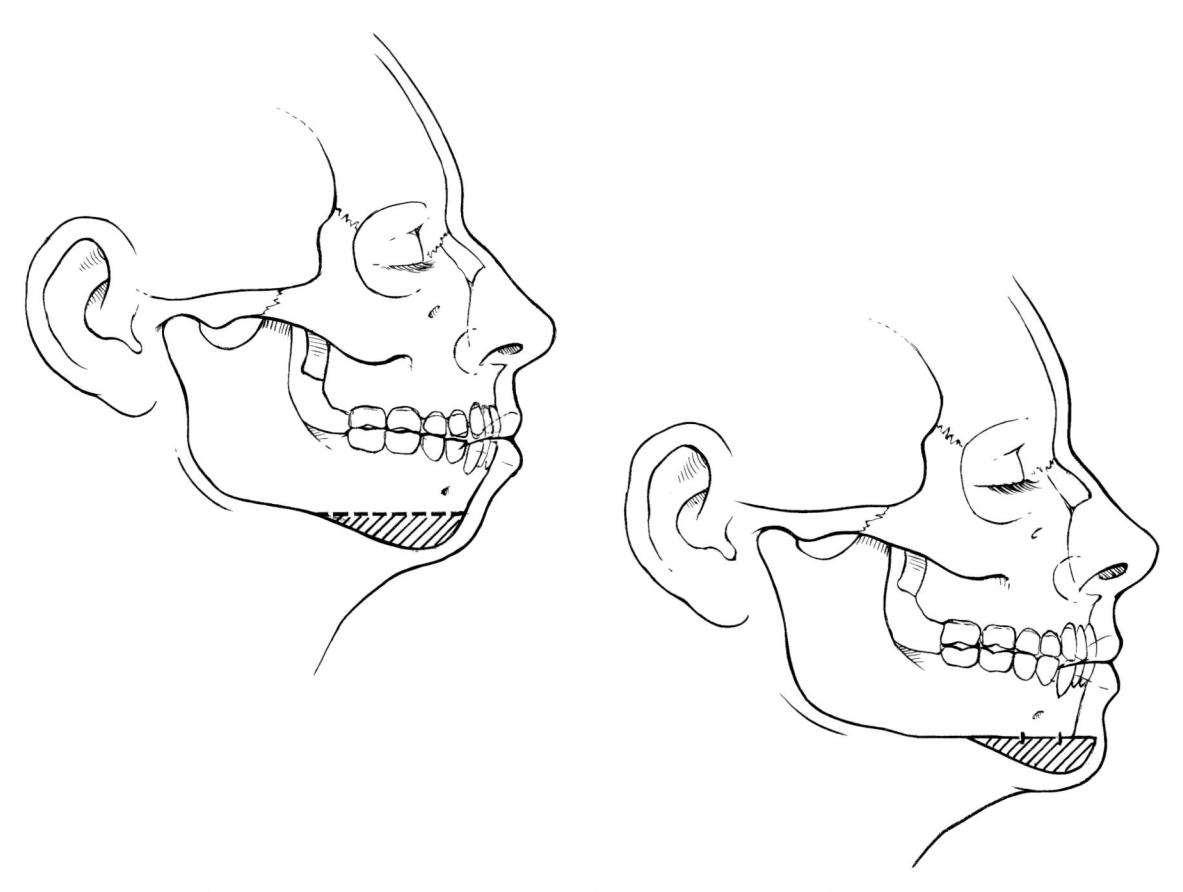

Once the osteotomy is complete, we commonly perform a simple advancement, which can gain approximately 10 mm of transverse chin augmentation. After advancement it is important to obtain secure fixation of the osteotomized segment by using either intraosseous wires or miniplates and screws.

SURGICAL REJUVENATION OF THE FACE

Following osteotomy and advancement, it is important to securely fixate the inferior segment to the mandibular symphysis. Rigid fixation with miniplates or interosseous wires adequately immobilizes the bone. Meticulous, watertight, intraoral closure is similarly important to prevent postoperative infection. All patients are given perioperative antibiotics.

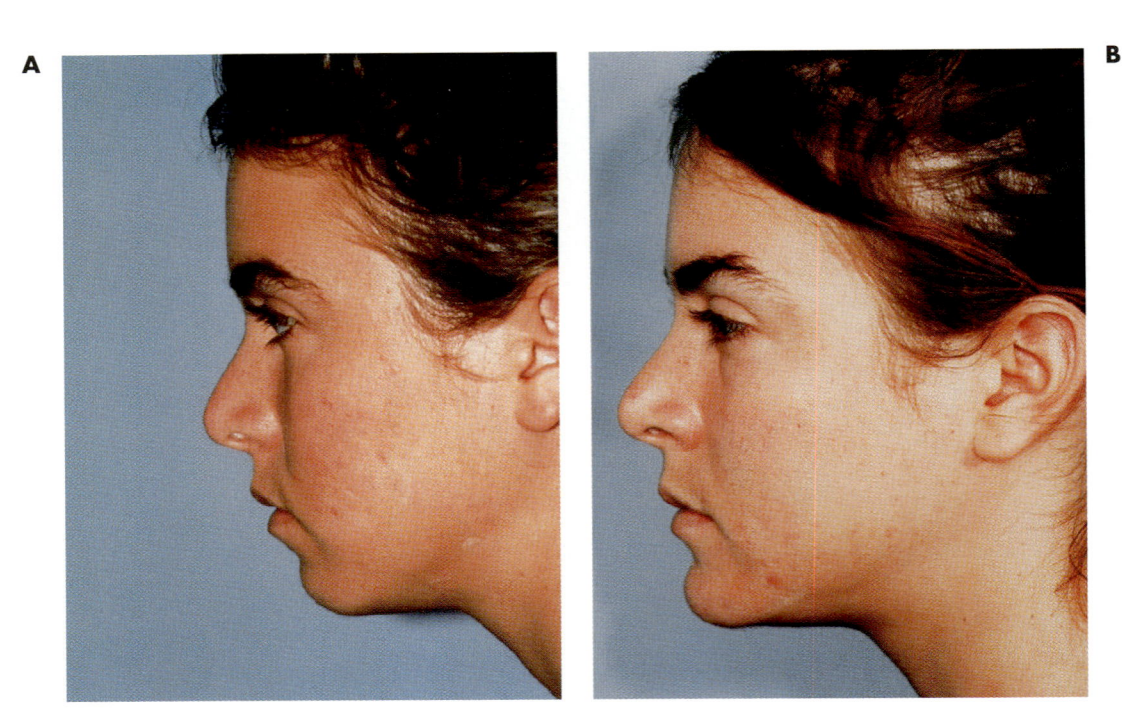

A, Preoperative appearance in a young patient with a recessive chin. B, Postoperative appearance 2½ years after advancement genioplasty.

ANCILLARY PROCEDURES

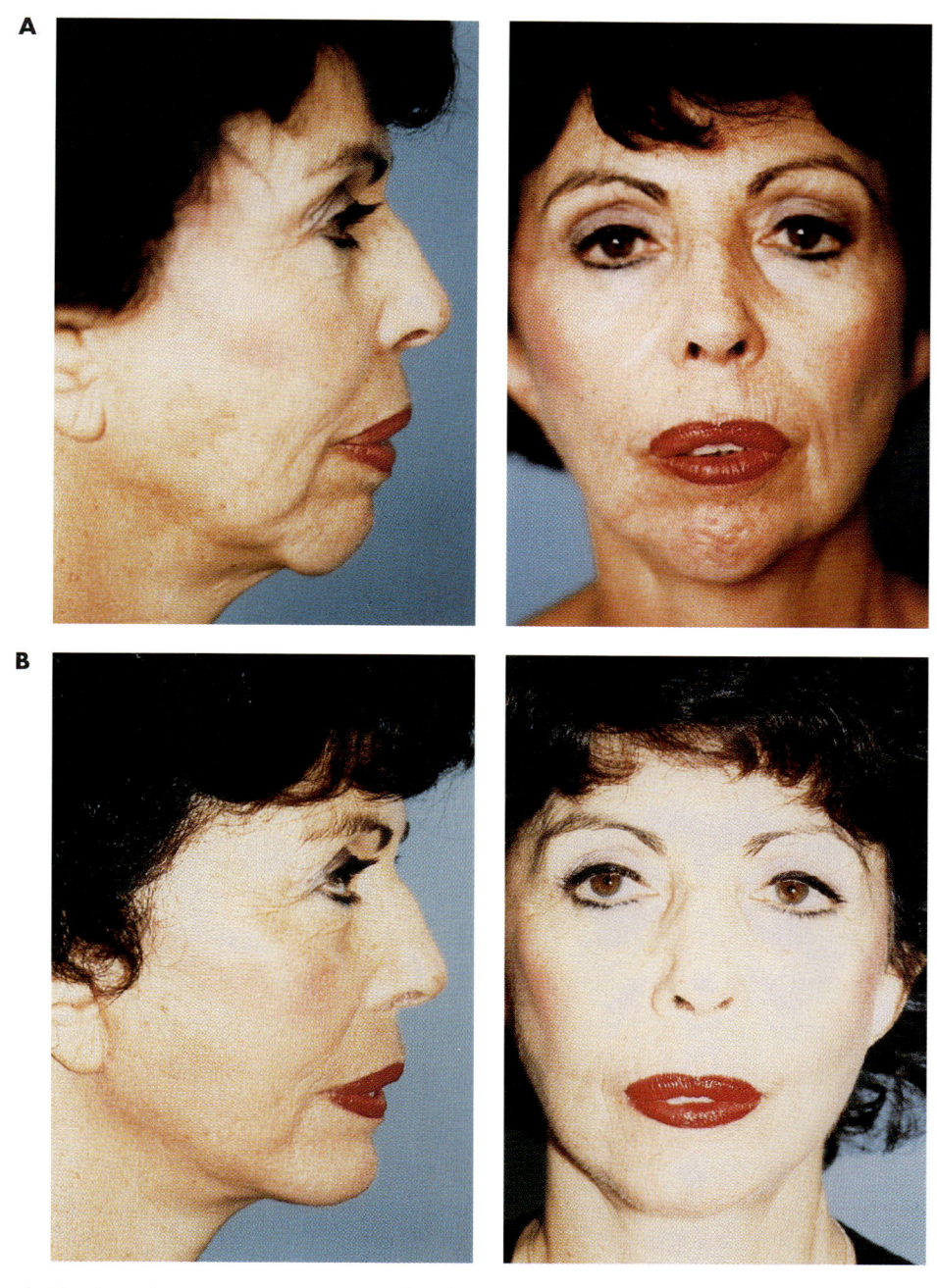

A, Patient is seen preoperatively; four previous attempts at chin implant placement have resulted in the implant slipping below the mandibular symphysis and producing a ptotic (witch's chin) appearance. B, Patient is seen following removal of her chin implant and performance of an advancement genioplasty and simultaneous rhytidectomy.

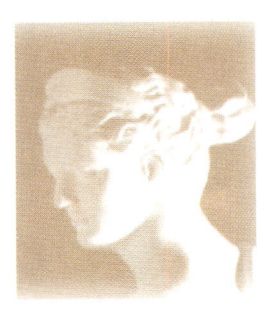

WITCH'S CHIN

A witch's chin, or ptotic chin pad, is commonly seen in the aging patient. What this problem represents is an attenuation of support from the numerous mandibular ligaments that hold the chin pad tightly to the underlying mandibular symphysis. As people age, they can lose the support of these retaining ligaments, which allows the chin pad to descend inferiorly. The patient who has a witch's chin usually has a chin pad that is significantly below the mandibular symphysis; is mobile; and is accentuated by the appearance of a deep, tight submental crease that marks the junction between the chin pad and submental skin.

Treatment of a witch's chin can be quite difficult. Efforts to relocate the chin pad superiorly and fix it to the mandibular symphysis are often frustrating. Thus most efforts are turned toward camouflaging the problem, with the possibility of slightly improving the ptosis of the chin pad.

■ Technique

The key to improvement of the ptotic chin pad is to improve the significant submental crease that demarcates the ptosis of the chin pad from the submental region. To improve this problem, an incision is made 5 mm caudal to the submental crease. Dissection is then performed very superficially, in the subdermal region cephalad past the submental crease, well up into the ptotic chin pad. From the original submental incision, the dissection is then carried deeply just beneath the cephalad margin of the platysma fibers in the submental region. Dissection is then continued cephalad toward the inferior border of the mandibular symphysis, essentially creating a flap that consists of platysma and submental fat. Following adequate mobilization, this flap of platysma and submental fat is brought caudally into the neck where it is sutured to the platysma fascia. Excess overhanging fat in the symphyseal region secondary to the ptosis of the chin pad is then removed to create a smooth contour from the submental region cephalad toward the mandibular border.

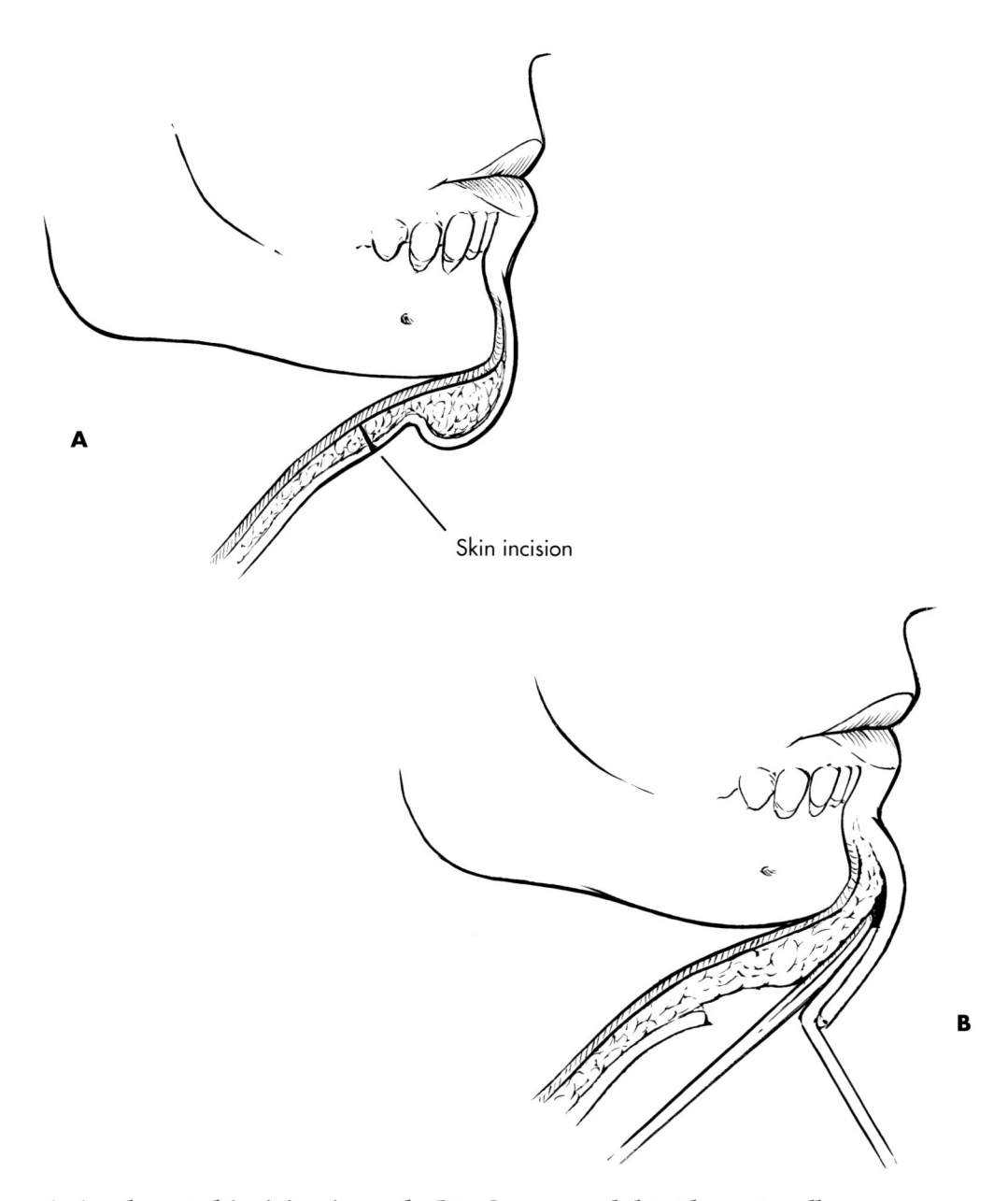

A, A submental incision is made 5 to 8 mm caudal to the naturally occurring submental crease. B, Dissection is then performed superficially in the subdermal plane cephalad to the submental crease to release the attachments of the crease to the mandibular symphysis.

Continued.

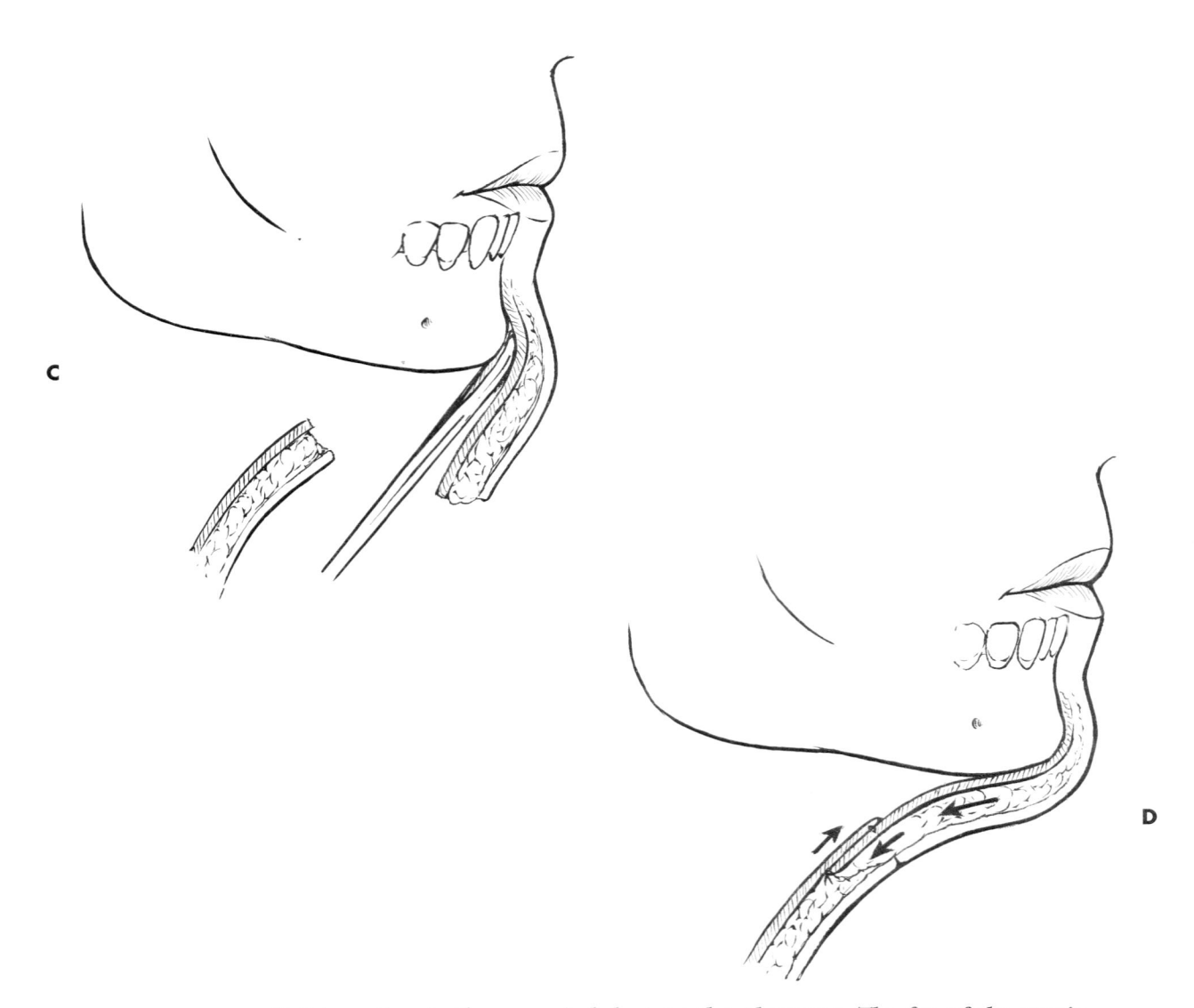

C, Dissection is then carried deep to the platysma. The fat of the ptotic chin pad, in continuity with the upper platysma fibers, is then mobilized to the inferior border of the symphysis. D, The fat-muscle flap is advanced caudally into the submental region and sutured to the platysma, filling the contour depression along the submental crease. After advancement, the subcutaneous fat cephalad and caudal to the submental incision is contoured so that there is an even blending of fat between the chin pad and neck.

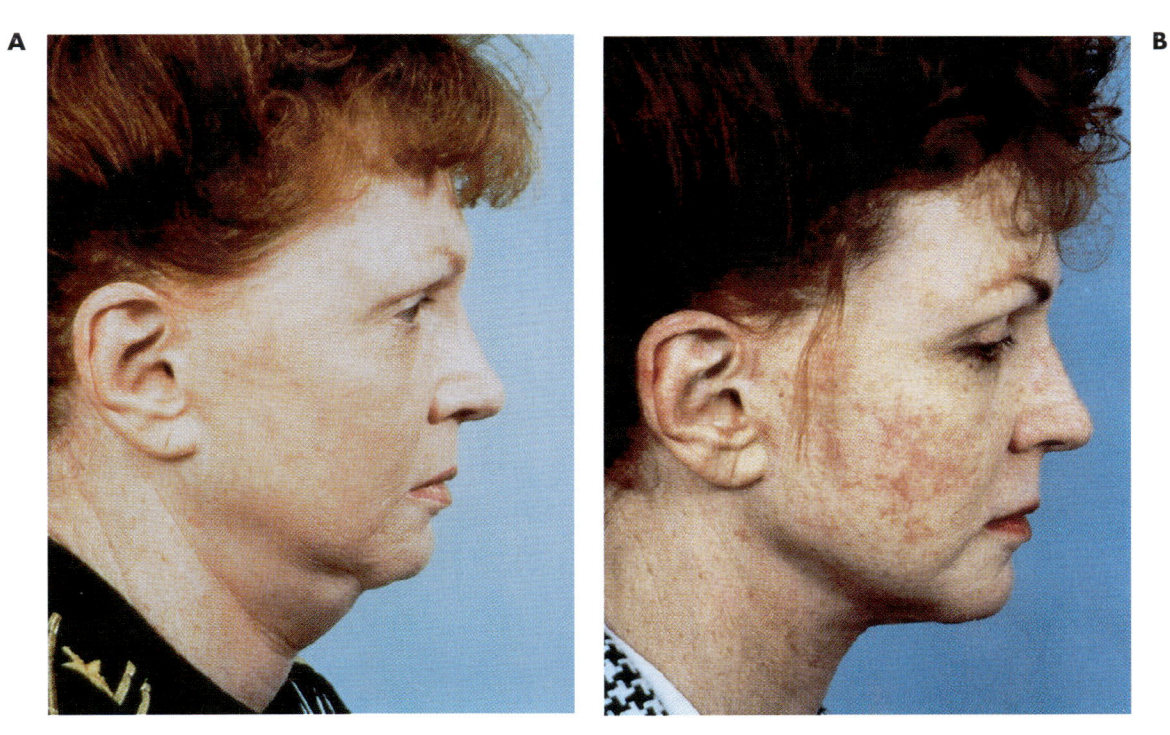

A, Preoperative appearance. B, Postoperative appearance after treatment of witch's chin through previously described technique. No chin implant was placed in this patient.

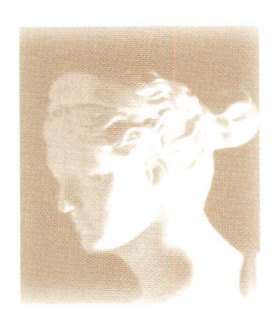

FAT INJECTION

In occasional clinical situations, autogenous fat injection has proven to be a simple filler for smoothing contour depressions and facial rhytides. We think of autologous fat injection as similar to collagen injection, though it offers the advantage of using the patient's tissue, thus decreasing the potential for allergic or host reaction following injection. In addition, it is easy to obtain large volumes of autologous fat, which allows the surgeon to treat significant depressions in a single session.

The largest problem with autologous fat injection is reabsorption, which is most likely caused by the inability of mature fat cells to survive the transplant. Rapid absorption often occurs within a few months of the procedure.

There seems to be a subgroup of patients who have longer-lasting results with fat injection. These usually are young patients, under the age of 40, who are healthy and not obese. We have seen long-lasting results in some of these patients, who usually have either significant contour depressions or heavy facial rhytides.

■ Technique

The procedure is usually performed with a slight amount of intravenous sedation. Alternatively, we ice the area (for 20 minutes) where the fat is to be harvested, which commonly provides enough anesthesia to minimize discomfort at the time of lidocaine infiltration. Similarly, ice is applied to the area where the fat will be injected, which is helpful in decreasing patient pain.

Any area can be used to harvest the fat. We commonly harvest the fat from the subcutaneous tissue of the abdomen, using an incision made within the umbilicus. Another favored donor site is the medial knee, where fat is obtained through a popliteal crease incision. After we make a small stab wound, a #13 Mercedes-type cannula is introduced and attached to a syringe. Several passes are made within the subcutaneous tissue, with the syringe on moderate vacuum. Usually within a few passes the syringe begins to fill with fatty material. After harvesting, the fat is centrifuged to remove aspirated serum.

We usually anesthetize only the area where the needle will be inserted along the recipient site, so that the effect on contour following the injection can be easily visualized. If a facial rhytide such as the nasolabial fold is to be injected, the fat is injected just beneath the rhytide line. If we are treating contour depressions, they are carefully marked preoperatively. The fat is then injected throughout the circumference of a contour depression. Overcorrection is usually recommended.

Following injection, the fat is carefully contoured by using pressure massage until it is evenly distributed throughout the area of injection, with no obvious bulges or nodules.

Most patients can wear cosmetics 24 hours after this procedure, although the area along the injection sites will be slightly swollen for up to 1 week.

The longevity of results following fat injection is unpredictable and can vary from a few weeks to several months. Before undergoing this procedure, the patient must understand that reinjection is frequently necessary within a few months.

SURGICAL REJUVENATION OF THE FACE

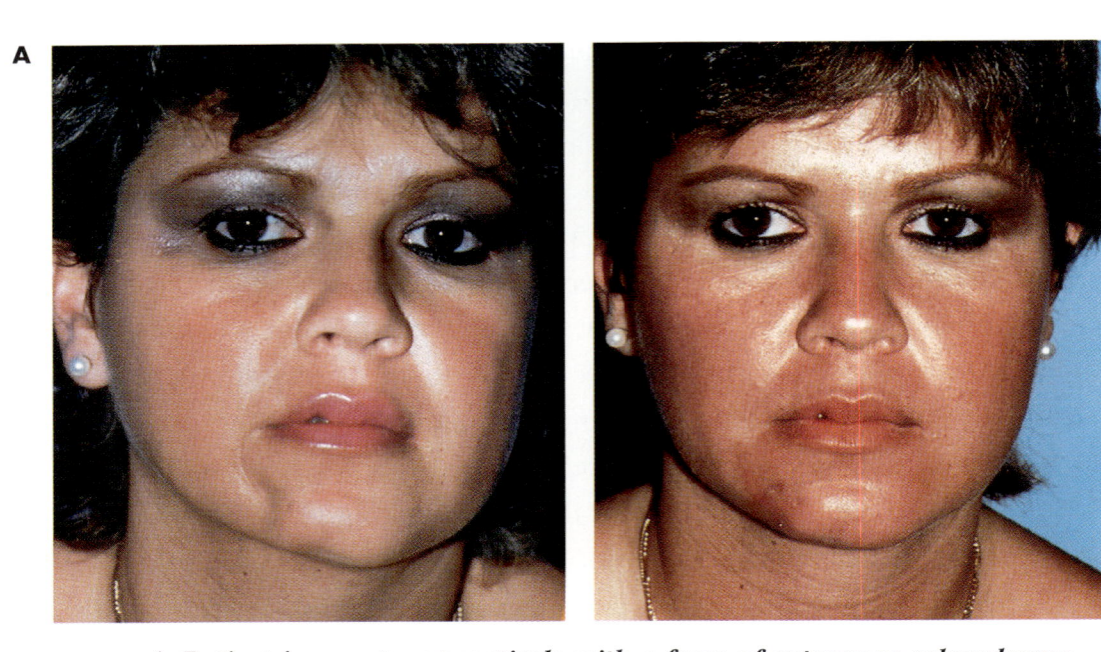

A, Patient is seen preoperatively with a form of cutaneous scleroderma. B, Postoperative appearance following the injection of 10 cc of fat into the depressed region. Although the patient has been seen several times over a 5-year period and has required reinjection, the injections have produced stable long-term results.

Autologous Collagen

Although a face-lift removes the laxity present within the face, facial rhytides usually remain if they were present preoperatively. We rarely use injectable bovine collagen in the treatment of these problems. However, we are currently evaluating the use of autologous collagen, which we feel is a preferable biomaterial because it represents autogenous grafting. This is performed by saving the skin removed during blepharoplasty, rhytidectomy, and browlifting procedures, processing the skin to extract the patient's collagen, and processing it into an injectable form (Autogenesis Tech Inc., Acton, Mass.). If the patient requests treatment of individual rhytides several months after the procedure, it is then quite simple to use their own collagen. Although the durability of these injections compared with bovine collagen injections remains untested at this time, we prefer to use autogenous material, rather than performing a xenograft, to avoid potential allergic hypersensitivity complications. (We have no financial interest in this product.)

SUGGESTED READING

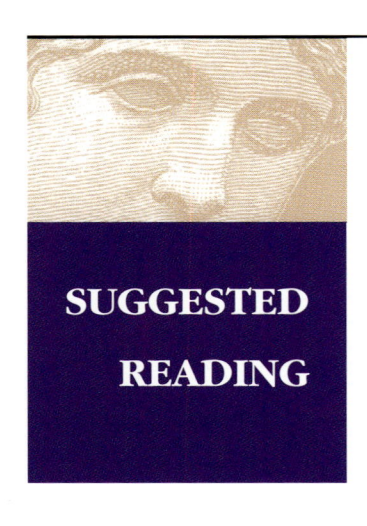

1. Baker TJ, editor: Symposium on the aging face, *Clin Plast Surg* 5(1):1-2, 1978.
2. Carlin GA, Gurdin MM: Ancillary procedures for the aging face and neck, *Surg Clin North Am* 51(2):371, 1971.
3. Converse JM, Woodsmith D: Horizontal osteotomy of the mandible, *Plast Reconstr Surg* 34:464, 1964.
4. Feldman JJ: The ptotic (witch's) chin deformity: an excisional approach, *Plast Reconstr Surg* 90:207, 1992.
5. Gonzalez-Ulloa M: Ptosis of the chin, *Plast Reconstr Surg* 50:54, 1972.
6. Hamra ST: *Composite rhytidectomy,* St Louis, 1993, Quality Medical, p 95.
7. Kawamoto HK, Jr: Reduction mentoplasty (discussion), *Plast Reconstr Surg* 70:151, 1982.
8. Marino H: Plastic correction of double chin, *Plast Reconstr Surg* 31:45, 1963.
9. Miller CC: The eradication by surgical mean of the nasolabial line, *Ther Gaz* 23:676, 1907c.
10. Pitanguy I: Ancillary procedures in face-lifting, *Clin Plast Surg* 5(1):51-69, 1978.
11. Snyder G: Chin disfigurement following removal of alloplastic chin implants (discussion), *Plast Reconstr Surg* 88:67, 1991.
12. Stuzin JM, Wagstrom L, Kawamoto HK Jr, Baker TJ, Wolfe SA: The anatomy and clinical applications of the buccal fat pad, *Plast Reconstr Surg* 85:29, 1990.
13. Stuzin JM, Kawamoto HK Jr: *Genioplasty.* In Gruber RP, Peck GC, editors: *Rhinoplasty: state of the art,* St Louis, 1993, Mosby, p 335.
14. Zide BM, McCarthy J: The mentalis muscle: an essential component of chin and lower lip position, *Plast Reconstr Surg* 83:413, 1989.

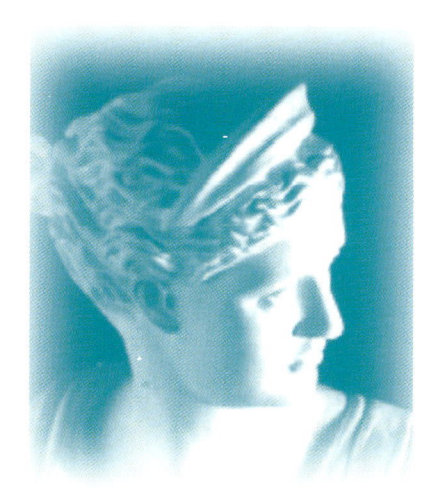

Index

A

Abrasive, 135-140
Absorption
  of drug, 18
  of phenol, 81-82
Accidental phenol spill, 113
Acne
  dermabrasion for, 136
  hyperpigmentation caused by, 74
Actinic keratosis
  histology of, 58
  phenol peeling and, 71
  subclinical, 59
  in unpeeled skin, 59
Adhesive tape masking, for chemical peel, 141
Adrenergic blocking agent, 29-30
Age, of rhytidectomy patient, 196
Aging
  anatomic changes with, 180-187
  stigmata of, 56, 192-193
Airway
  benzodiazepine overdose and, 25
  obstruction of, 38-39
Aliphatic drug, 27
Allergy, iodine, 141
Alloplastic chin augmentation
  genioplasty as alternative for, 595-601
  rhytidectomy and, 302
  technique for, 592-594
Alopecia, browlift causing, 565
Alpha-adrenergic agonist, 30-31
Alpha-adrenergic blocking agent, 30
Amide anesthetic, 18
Analgesic, types of, 21-22
Ancillary procedure, 575-611
  buccal fat excision as, 588-591
  chin augmentation as, 592-594
  fat injection as, 606-607
  genioplasty as, 595-601
  nasal alterations as, 577-578
  nasolabial fold excision as, 583-587
  perioral wrinkle correction as, 579-582
  witch's chin correction as, 602-605

INDEX

Anesthesia; *see also* Drug management
  for blepharoplasty, 439-440
  for browlift, 548
  dose-response curve for, 14
  maintenance of, 36-38
  for rhytidectomy, 216-218
Angle, cervicomental, obtuse, 211, 212-213
Antagonist, benzodiazepine, 26
Anticholinergic agent, 29
Antihistamine, 26
Aperture, eyelid, 389
Aponeurosis
  levator, 398, 400-401
  superficial muscular; *see* Superficial muscular aponeurosis
Arrhythmia
  cardiac, 40
  phenol causing, 81-82
Artery, supratrochlear, 533
Asymmetry, eyelid, 419
Atarax (hydroxyzine), 27
Atrial tachycardia, phenol causing, 82
Atrophy, steroid-induced, 492-493
Atropine, 29
Attenuation of soft tissue support; *see* Soft tissue, attenuation of
Augmentation, chin
  genioplasty as alternative for, 595-601
  rhytidectomy and, 302
  technique for, 592-594
Auricular nerve
  anatomy of, 178-179
  rhytidectomy and, 241
    injury caused by, 358-359
Autogenous fat injection, 606-608
Autologous collagen injection, 609

B

Band, platysma
  reoperative rhytidectomy and, 325-326
  rhytidectomy and, 203-213
Barbiturate, 22-23
Bell's palsy, 365
Benadryl (diphenhydramine), 26
Benzodiazepine, 24-26
Benzodiazepine antagonist, 26
Beta-adrenergic blocking agent, 30

Binding, protein, of drug, 15-16
Birth control pill, hyperpigmentation caused by, 73
Bleeding
  blepharoplasty and, 487, 492
  rhytidectomy and, 351-355
Blepharitis, 498
Blepharoplasty, 385-525
  anatomic considerations in
    lateral canthal tendon and, 397
    levator palpebrae and, 398-401
    lower eyelid fat pad and, 411-414
    lower eyelid retractors and, 404-407
    medial canthal tendon and, 395-396
    Muller's muscle and, 401
    orbicularis oculi muscle and, 392-393
    orbital fascia and, 401-403
    orbital fat and, 408-411
    orbital septum and, 394-395
    superficial eyelid and, 388-392
  anatomy and, 388-415
  brow ptosis and, 539
  browlift with, 559
  chemical peel after, 115
  complications of, 488-520
    bleeding as, 492
    blepharitis as, 498
    discoloration and, 490-491
    dry eye syndrome as, 488
    ectropion as, 514-517
    epiphora and chemosis as, 489
    fat pad overcorrection as, 495
    inability to close eyes as, 498
    infection as, 497
    inferior oblique muscle damage as, 497
    lateral canthopexy and, 510-513
    lower lid laxity and, 502-509
    paresis of lower lid as, 497
    persistent small wrinkles as, 495-496
    persisting malar pouches as, 500-501
    ptosis as, 495
    retrobulbar hematoma as, 494
    scars and keloids as, 488, 499

INDEX

Blepharoplasty—cont'd
 complications of—cont'd
  secondary blepharoplasty as, 498-499
  steroid-induced atrophy as, 492-493
  too much for skin remaining as, 499
  vision loss as, 494-495
  wound dehiscence as, 497
 goals of, 438-439
 operative technique for, 439-481
  anesthesia and, 439-440
  closure of upper lid and, 452
  incision placement for, 441-445
  of lower eyelid, 457-486
  muscle and fat resection in, 446-451
  supratarsal fixation in, 453-456
 patient selection for, 387-388
 postoperative care after, 487
 preoperative evaluation for, 423-438
  fat and, 428-431
  lower eyelid and, 432-437
  skin and, 423-427
 preoperative visit for, 415-423
 questions and answers about, 521-522
 secondary, 498-499
Blood pressure
 anesthesia management of, 39-40
 chlorpromazine affecting, 27-28
 clonidine and, 31
Blotchiness
 acne causing, 74
 chemical peel causing, 110
 chemical peel for
  phenol, 72-77
  trichloroacetic acid, 128
 oral contraceptives causing, 73
 in sun-damaged skin, 60
Brow, fat of, 410
Browlifting, 527-573
 blepharoplasty with, 559
 browpexy as alternative for, 560-561
 closure of, 557-558
 complications of, 565-568
 early approaches to, 530-531
 hairline incision for, 542, 543
 indications for, 539-541

Browlifting—cont'd
 preoperative planning for, 544-547
 results of, 562-564
 technique of, 548-557
 temporal region anatomy and, 531-538
Browpexy, 560-561
Bruising, 356-357
Buccal branch of facial nerve, 359-365
Buccal fat pad
 anatomy of, 176-178
 excision of, 588-591
Buccinator muscle, 156, 157
Bundle, neurovascular, 532
Bupivacaine, 19
Burn, 114
Burning sensation, 90, 98
Butyrophones, 28

C

Canthal tendon
 anatomy of, 395-397
 suture support to, 505-507
 tarsal strip procedure for, 510-513
Capsule, parotid, 162
Capsulopalpebral fascia, 406-407
Carbocaine (mepivacaine), 19
Cardiac arrhythmia
 management of, 40
 phenol causing, 81-82
Central nervous system
 drug toxicity to, 20
 midazolam and, 24
 propofol affecting, 33-34
Cervical fascia; *see also* Neck
 anatomy of, 154, 162
 superficial muscular aponeurosis and, 153
Cervical obliquity, 198
 platysma, 32-326
Cervicomental angle, obtuse, 211, 212-213
Cheek, dissection of SMAS and, 252
Chemical peel, 45-134; *see also other Chemical peel entries*
 examples of, 47-51
 questions and answers about, 141-143
Chemical peel, with phenol, 52-116
 histology of skin and peeled, 62-70

Chemical peel, with phenol—cont'd
　histology of skin and—cont'd
　　sun-damage and aging, 57-61
　history of, 52-57
　indications for, 72-81
　　for hyperpigmentation, 72-77
　　for wrinkling, 78-79
　patient education about, 87-88
　patient selection for, 82-85
　postpeel care in, 98-104
　preoperative visit for, 86-87
　procedure for, 88-98
　　application of phenol in, 89-92
　　ingredients in, 88-89
　　petroleum jelly dressing and, 94-98
　　waterproof mask and, 93
　regional, 104-107
　toxicology of, 81-82
　trichloroacetic acid peel and, 131
Chemical peel, with trichloroacetic acid, 117-134
　complications of, 132-133
　depth of, 119-122
　intermediate-depth, 126-131
　light, 123-125
　perioral wrinkles and, 579-581
　phenol versus, 134
　pretreatment for, 118-119
Chemosis, 489
Chin
　augmentation of
　　genioplasty as alternative for, 595-601
　　rhytidectomy and, 302
　　technique for, 592-594
　retrusive, platysma and, 209
　witch's, 602-605
Chlorpromazine
　characteristics of, 27-28
　for male rhytidectomy patient, 348
Citanest (prilocaine), 19
Cleansing of face, 89
Clonidine, 31
Collagen
　in peeled skin, 64, 66, 67
　in sun-damaged skin, 59
Collagen injection, 609
Commissure, 389
Compazine (prochlorperazine), 27

Complications
　of blepharoplasty, 488-520; *see also* Blepharoplasty, complications of
　of browlifting, 565-568
　of chemical peel, 107-116
　of nasal alteration procedure, 577-578
　of rhytidectomy, 350-379; *see also* Rhytidectomy, complications of
Consent, for blepharoplasty, 422
Contact lens, 521
Contour irregularity after rhytidectomy, 378
Contraceptive, hyperpigmentation caused by, 73
Contraction, premature ventricular, 40
Contracture, 373
Coronal browlifting, 527-573; *see also* Browlifting
Corrugator muscle
　anatomy of, 531
　division of, 552, 553
　hyperactivity of, 541
　hypertrophy of, 546-547
　overcorrection of browlift and, 567
Crease
　glabellar
　　as indication for browlift, 539-540
　　operative technique for, 554-557
　　preoperative evaluation of, 546, 547
　submental, 602
　supratarsal
　　anatomy of, 390-391
　　preoperative evaluation of, 426-427
Croton oil, 89, 141
Crow's feet, 416
Cutaneous scleroderma, 608

D

Deep fascia, 160-165
　superficial fascia in relation to, 164, 165
　temporal, 162, 163
Deep mimetic muscles, 155
Defatting, submandibular, 275
Deformity, 198-199

Dehiscence, wound, 497
Depigmentation, 107
Depression
  central nervous system, 33-34
  respiratory, 24-25
Dermabrasion, 135-140
  for perioral wrinkles, 580-582
Dermis, dermabrasion of, 135-140
Desquamation, 125
Detachment of earlobe, 227-232
Diazepam, 25-26, 32
Diphenhydramine, 26
Diprivan (propofol), 33
Discoloration, 490-491
Dissatisfaction with results, 8-10
Dissociative anesthetic agent, 31-32
Dose-response curve for drug, 14-15
Drain, 311
Dressing
  for chemical peel, 93-98
  for rhytidectomy, 311-312
Droperidol
  characteristics of, 28
  intraoperative, 32, 36
Drug management, 11-43
  adrenergic blocking agents and, 29-30
  alpha-adrenergic agonists and, 30-31
  analgesics and, 21-22
  anticholinergics and, 29
  antihistamines and, 26
  barbiturates and, 22-23
  basic principles of
    dose-response curve in, 14-15
    potency of drug and, 15
    therapeutic index in, 13-14
  benzodiazepine antagonist and, 26
  benzodiazepines and, 24-26
  butyrophenones and, 28
  chronic medication in, 17
  complications of, 38-41
  dissociative anesthetic agents and, 31-34
  drug interactions in, 16
  hydroxyzines and, 27
  local anesthetics and, 17-20
  pharmacokinetics in, 15-16
  phenothiazines and, 27-28
  postoperative, 42-43
  in recovery room and, 41-42
  technique of, 34-38

Drug reaction, hyperpigmentation from, 72
Dry eye syndrome, 488
Duct, parotid, 176
Duranest (etidocaine), 19

E
Earlobe, detachment of, 227-232
Ecchymosis, 356-357
Ectropion
  blepharoplasty and, 514-517
  chemical peel causing, 115
Edema
  blepharoplasty and, 487
  rhytidectomy and, 356
Education, patient
  about blepharoplasty, 415-423
  about chemical peel, 87-88
Elastic fiber, in peeled skin, 63, 67
Elastosis
  sun damage causing, 57-58
  in unpeeled skin, 65
Elevation of superficial muscular aponeurosis, 186-187
Eosinophilic grenz zone
  definition of, 59
  in unpeeled skin, 63
Epidermis
  dermabrasion of, 135-140
  of peeled skin, 69-70
  phenol peel affecting, 62
  in sun-damaged skin, 58, 59-61
Epinephrine, 216
Epiphora, 489
Epithelial lesion, 57
Epithelium, of peeled skin, 71
Erythema
  phenol, 108
  trichloroacetic acid, 124, 127
Ester anesthetic, 18
Etidocaine
  dosage of, 19
  lipid-solubility of, 19
Exophthalmos, 438
Expanding hematoma, 351-355
Expression, muscles of, 154-160
Extraocular muscle, 402
Eye
  chemical peel around, 106
    with phenol, 106

Eye—cont'd
  chemical peel around—cont'd
    with trichloroacetic acid, 128
  examination of, 420
Eyebrow, placement of, 545, 546
Eyelid; *see also* Blepharoplasty
  anatomy of, 388-392
  asymmetry of, 419
  chemical peel of, 87, 91
  cross-section of, 405
  ectropion of, 115
  fat of, 408, 409
  lower
    fat pad anatomy of, 411-414
    laxity of, 437
    orbital septum and, 395
    preoperative evaluation of, 432-437
    retractors of, 404-407

F

Facelift; *see* Rhytidectomy
Facial expression, muscles of, 154-160
Facial nerve
  anatomy of, 166-171
  buccal branches of, 177
    rhytidectomy causing injury to, 359, 362
  dissection of, 171
  forehead and, 534, 535-536
Fascia; *see also* Superficial muscular aponeurosis
  capsulopalpebral, 406-407
  deep, 160-165
  extraocular muscle and, 403
  of forehead, 536, 537
  messenteric, 162
  orbital, 401-403
  superficial versus deep, 164, 165
  Tenon's, 401-402
Fat; *see also* Fat pad
  browlifting and, 534, 538
  browpexy and, 560, 561
  of eyelids
    evaluation of, 428-431
    lower, 391, 435-436
    in lower blepharoplasty, 469-471
    resection of, 446-451
  injection of, 606-608
  orbital, 408-411
  ptotic chin pad and, 602-605

Fat; *see also* Fat pad—cont'd
  rhytidectomy and
    cervical lipectomy and, 274-283
    jowls formed by, 269, 270
    platysmal band and, 288-290
    removal of, 269
    reoperative, 322-323
    subcutaneous, 196-197
Fat pad
  blepharoplasty and, 446-451
    overcorrection of, 495
  buccal
    anatomy of, 176-178
    excision of, 588-591
  ROOF
    anatomy of, 538
    browpexy and, 560, 561
Fentanyl
  characteristics of, 21-22
  operative period and, 36-37
Fiber
  elastic
    chemical peel and, 63
    in peeled skin, 67
    platysmal band and, 288-289
Fibrous band, 175
Fine wrinkling; *see* Wrinkles
Fixation
  of superficial muscular aponeurosis, 262-263
  supratarsal, 453-456
Flap
  rotation of, 246-247
  superficial muscular aponeurosis; *see* Superficial muscular aponeurosis
Flumazenil, 26
Fluphenazine dihydrochloride, 27
Fold, nasolabial
  aging and, 180, 181
  direct excision of, 583-587
  rhytidectomy and, 201-202
Forehead; *see also* Browlifting
  nerves of, 532-534
  skin of, 531
Freckled skin, phenol peel of, 82-83
Frontal branch of facial nerve, 534, 535-536
  anatomy of, 166-169
  injury to, 565

Frontalis muscle
  anatomy of, 531
  frown line removal and, 556
  hyperactivity of, 540
  overcorrection of browlift and, 567-568
Frosting, in chemical peel, 120-122
Frown lines
  as indication for browlift, 539-540
  operative technique for, 554-557
  preoperative evaluation of, 546, 547

G

Galea, 153
  anatomy of, 154
Genioplasty, 595-601
Glabellar frown lines
  as indication for brow lift, 539-540
  operative technique for, 554-557
  preoperative evaluation of, 546, 547
Gland, lacrimal
  fat pad confused with, 412
  prolapsed, 518-520
Glasses, 521
Glaucoma, 421
Granule, melanin
  in peeled skin, 69
  in sun-damaged skin, 60
Great auricular nerve
  anatomy of, 178-179
  injury to, 358-359
  rhytidectomy and, 241
Grenz zone
  definition of, 59
  in unpeeled skin, 63
Ground substance
  in peeled skin, 65
  in unpeeled skin, 70

H

Hairline
  browlifting and, 542, 543
  rhytidectomy and, 224-226
    incisions in, 224-226
    in male patient, 341-343
    reoperative, 316-319
Half-life of drug, 21
Haloperidol, 28
Hematoma
  browlift and, 565

Hematoma—cont'd
  retrobulbar, 494
  rhytidectomy and, 351-355
Horn of levator palpebrae muscle, 398, 400
Hydroquinone, 118-119
Hydroxyzine, 27
Hyoid, platysma band and, 208, 209
Hyperpigmentation
  chemical peel for, 72-77
    trichloroacetic acid, 128
  drug reaction causing, 72
  oral contraceptives causing, 73
  phenol causing, 113
  sun causing, 75
Hypertension, 39-40; *see also* Blood pressure
Hypertrophic scar
  chemical peel causing, 111, 112, 131
    phenol, 108-112
  dermabrasion causing, 136-137
  rhytidectomy, 366-369
Hypertrophy
  of corrugator muscle, 541, 546
  of platysma, 210
Hypotension, 39-40

I

Implant, chin, 302
  technique for, 592-594
Incision
  for blepharoplasty, 441-445
    in lower eyelid, 457-461
    transconjunctival, 483-484
  for browlift, 542, 543, 548-550
  for rhytidectomy, 218-232
    earlobe detachment and, 227-232
    in male patient, 340-344
    postauricular, 223
    posterior neck, 224-226
    reoperative, 316-320
    tragal, 220-222
Index, therapeutic, 13-14
Infection
  blepharoplasty and, 497
  browlift and, 565
  chemical peel causing, 108
  rhytidectomy and, 378-379
    skin slough and, 371

INDEX

Inferior oblique muscle, 497
Inferior suspensory ligament of Lockwood, 402
Infiltrate, lymphocytic, 68
Injection, fat, 606-608
Injury, nerve
   browlift causing, 565
   rhytidectomy causing, 166, 358-365
Innervation; see Nerve
Interaction, drug, 16
Intermediate-depth chemical peel, 126-127
Intravenous sedation, 11-43; see also Drug management
Investing parotid fascia, 162
Iodine allergy, 141
Itching, from browlift, 566

J

Jawline, 197
Jowls
   fat removal from, 270
   rhytidectomy and, 200-201
   subcutaneous fat in, 240
   superficial muscular aponeurosis elevation for, 268

K

Keloid, 488
Keratocoagulation necrosis, 62
Keratosis, actinic, 59
Ketamine
   characteristics of, 31-33
   operative period and, 36, 37
   rhytidectomy and, 216

L

Lacrimal gland
   fat pad confused with, 412
   prolapsed, 518-520
Lateral canthal tendon, 397
   suture support to, 505-507
   tarsal strip procedure for, 510-513
Lateral canthopexy, 510-513
Lateral commissure, 389
Lateral horn of levator palpebrae muscle, 398
Lateral malar area, 170
Laxity
   of lower eyelid, 437, 502-508

Laxity—cont'd
   platysmal, 284-302
Lay clinic, chemical peeling by, 53
   burn caused by, 111, 114
LD_{50}, 13-14
Lentigo
   chemical peel of, 85
   solar, 61
Levator aponeurosis, 398, 400-401
Levator palpebrae muscle
   anatomy of, 398-401
   lateral extension of, 413
Lidocaine
   dosage of, 19
   properties of, 18-19
   rhytidectomy and, 216, 218
Ligament
   Lockwood's, 402
   masseteric cutaneous, 182, 183
   retaining, 172-176
   Whitnall's, 398
Light chemical peel, 123-125
Lipectomy, cervical, 274-283
   dissection for, 276-279
   suction lipoplasty for, 274-276
Lipid-solubility of drug, 19
Liver, drug metabolism in, 16
Local anesthetic; see also Anesthesia
   pharmacology of, 17-20
   for rhytidectomy, 216-218
Lockwood's inferior suspensory ligament, 402
Lower eyelid
   blepharoplasty of, 457-486
      crease and, 391
      fat pad anatomy and, 411-414
      fat removal in, 469-471
      goals of, 439
      incision placement in, 457-461
      laxity and, 437, 502-508
      preoperative evaluation and, 432-437
      skin excision in, 472-482
      skin flap for, 457-462
      skin-muscle flap for, 463-468
      transconjunctival, 483-486
   cross-section of, 405
   ectropion of, 514-517
      chemical peel and, 115
   laxity of, 502-509

INDEX

Lower eyelid—cont'd
　laxity of—cont'd
　　lateral cathopexy for, 510-513
　　orbital septum and, 395
　paresis of, 497
　retractors of, 404-407
Lymphocytic infiltrate, 68

M

Malar pouch, persisting, 500-501
Malar region
　implant removal in, 265
　muscles of, 155
　SMAS dissection in, 249-257
Malar soft tissue, 180, 181
Male patient
　chemical peel in, 85
　rhytidectomy for, 333-349
　　closure in, 348
　　evaluation of, 335-339
　　incisions in, 340-344
　　postoperative care for, 349
　　preoperative preparation of, 340
　　results of, 345-347
　　technical differences in, 334
Malignancy, chemical peel to prevent, 71, 80, 116
Mandibular ligament, 172-174
Mandibular nerve injury, 360-361
Marcaine (bupivacaine), 19
Marginal mandibular nerve, 170
　rhytidectomy causing injury to, 360-361
Mask, in chemical peel procedure, 93-98
　removal of, 99-100
　tape for, 141
Masseteric cutaneous ligament, 172, 173
　aging and, 182, 183
Masseteric muscle, 175-176
McGregor's patch, 239
Medial canthal tendon, 395-396
Medial horn of levator palpebrae muscle, 398, 400
Melanin
　in peeled skin, 69
　in sun-damaged skin, 60
Melanocyte
　in peeled skin, 69

Melanocyte—cont'd
　in sun-damaged skin, 60
Mentum, platysma band and, 208, 209
Meperidine, 22
Mepivacaine, 19
Mesotemporalis region, 237-238
Messenteric fascia, 162
Metabolism, of drug, 16
Methohexital, 23
Midazolam
　characteristics of, 24
　operative period and, 36
　rhytidectomy and, 216
Milia, 107-108
Mimetic muscle, 154-160
Monitoring, of analgesia, 34-35
Monoamine oxidase inhibitors, 16
Motor nerve injury, 359-365; *see also* Nerve
Mouth
　chemical peel with phenol and, 92, 105-106, 107
　dermabrasion around, 138-139
　wrinkle correction around, 579-582
Muller's muscle, 401
Muscle
　corrugator
　　anatomy of, 531
　　division of, 552, 553
　　of forehead and glabella, 532
　frontalis, 531
　　overcorrection of browlift and, 567-568
　inferior oblique, 497
　levator palpebrae, 398-401, 413
　Muller's, 401
　orbicularis oculi, 392-393
　platysma, 184, 185
　procerus, 554
　resection of, 446-451
Muscular aponeurosis, superficial; *see* Superficial muscular aponeurosis

N

Naloxone, 21
Narcotic analgesic, 21-22
Nasal alteration, 577-578
Nasolabial fold
　aging and, 180, 181

INDEX

Nasolabial fold—cont'd
  dissection of SMAS and, 254-255
    extended, 303
  excision of, 583-587
  rhytidectomy and, 201-202
Neck
  aging and, 184, 185
  cervical obliquity and, 198
  chemical peel of, 109, 110
  obtuse cervicomental angle and, 211, 212-213
  rhytidectomy and, 196-197
    cervical contouring in, 274-283
    dissection and, 242
    dissection of SMAS and, 252
    incisions in, 224-226
    male, 337-339
    redraping of skin flap and, 305-309
    scarring and, 369
    seroma in, 377
Necrosis
  keratocoagulation, phenol peeling causing, 62
  rhytidectomy and, 372
Nerve
  elevation of platysma and, 157
  facial, 166-171
  to forehead, 532-534
  great auricular
    anatomy of, 178-179
    rhytidectomy and, 241
  rhytidectomy causing injury to, 358-365
Nerve fiber, classification of, 17-18
Neuroleptic analgesia/anesthesia
  dose-response curve for, 14
  maintenance of, 36-38
  monitoring of, 34-35
Neuroleptic malignant syndrome, 41
Neurovascular bundle, 532
Nose, minor alterations to, 577-578
Novocain (procaine), 19
Numbness, browlift and, 566

O

Obstruction, airway, 38-39
Occlusive dressing, for chemical peel, 93-98
Oil, croton, 89, 141
Oozing of blood, 487
Oral contraceptive, hyperpigmentation from, 73
Orbicularis oculi muscle
  blepharoplasty and, 392-393
  overcorrection of browlift and, 567
Orbit, fascia of, 401-403
Orbital fat, 408-411
Orbital septum, 394-395
Osteotomy, in genioplasty, 598-599
Overcorrection of browlift, 566-568
Overdose, of midazolam, 24-25

P

Pad
  fat; see Fat entries
  ptotic chin, 602-605
Pain, postoperative, 41-42
  in male rhytidectomy patient, 348
Palsy, Bell's, 365
Parasympatholytic agent, 29
Paresis, 497
Parotid capsule, 162
Parotid cutaneous ligament, 172, 173
Parotid gland
  anatomy of, 176-178
  dissection of SMAS and, 252
Parotid-masseteric fascia, 160, 161
Patch, McGregor's, 239
Patient education
  about chemical peel, 87-88
  blepharoplasty and, 415-423
Patient-surgeon relationship, 3-10
Peel, chemical; see Chemical peel entries
Penrose drain, 311
Perioral region
  chemical peel of, 105, 106-107
  dermabrasion of, 136, 138-139
  wrinkle correction in, 579-582
Periorbital region, chemical peel of
  with phenol, 106
  with trichloroacetic acid, 128
Perivenular lymphocytic infiltrate, 68
Petroleum jelly dressing, 94-98
Pharmacokinetics, 15-16
Pharmacology, 11-43; see also Drug management
Phenergan (promethazine), 26

INDEX

Phenol
   accidental spill of, 113
   chemical peel with, 52-116; *see also* Chemical peel, with phenol
Phenol, *USP*, 88-89
Phenothiazine, 27-28
Phentolamine, 30
Pigment, in peeled skin, 103, 107
Piperazines, 27
Piperidines, 27
Plasma protein binding of drug, 15-16
Platysma band
   reoperative rhytidectomy and, 325-326
   rhytidectomy and, 203-213
Platysma muscle
   aging and, 184, 185
   anatomic variation in, 204-205, 208-209
   anatomy of, 155, 156
   anterior approach to, 242, 243
   deep fascia and, 163
   elevation of, 157
   in male patient, 344-346
   transection of, 293-303
Platysmal band, 284-302
Plication
   of platysma muscle, 291-293
   platysmal, in male patient, 345-346
Pontocaine (tetracaine), 19
Postauricular dissection, 242
Postauricular incision, 227-232
Postoperative period
   in chemical peel procedure
      with phenol, 98-104
      with trichloroacetic acid, 124-125, 127-131
   dermabrasion and, 140
   management during, 42-43
   pain in, 41-42
   reassurance during, 7
   for rhytidectomy, 313
      complications in, 350-379
      reoperative, 329
      superficial muscular aponeurosis and, 266-273
Potency of drug, 15
Pouch, malar, persisting, 500-501
Preauricular incisions for rhytidectomy, 221

Preauricular skin, redraping of, 306-307
Premalignant lesion, 57, 71, 80, 116
Premature ventricular contraction, 40
   phenol causing, 82
Preoperative care
   blepharoplasty and, 415-423; *see also* Blepharoplasty
   for chemical peel, 86-87
   rhytidectomy and, 192-213; *see also* Rhytidectomy
Preplatysmal fat
   preservation of, 278
   removal of, 277
Prilocaine, 19
Priscoline (tolazoline), 30
Procaine, 19
Procerus muscle, 554
Prochlorperazine, 27
Prolapse, lacrimal gland, 518-520
Prolixin (fluphenazine dihydrochloride), 27
Promazine, 27
Promethazine, 26
Prophylaxis for anesthetic toxicity, 20
Propofol, 33-34
Propranolol, 30
Protein binding of drug, 15-16
Psychotic side effects of ketamine, 32
Ptosis
   blepharoplasty for, 419
   brow, 539
   of brow, 423
Ptotic chin pad, 602-605

Q

Questionnaire, 5

R

Recovery room management, 41-42
Redraping, in rhytidectomy, 304-310
Regional peel
   with phenol, 104-107
   with trichloroacetic acid peel, 123, 126
Regitine (phentoaline), 30
Reoperative rhytidectomy, 314-332; *see also* Rhytidectomy, reoperative
Respiratory depression, 39
   midazolam causing, 24-25

INDEX

Retaining ligament
  aging and, 180
  anatomy of, 172-176
  rhytidectomy and, 197
Retractor, lower eyelid, 404-407
Retrobulbar hematoma, 494
Retrusive chin, platysma and, 209
Rhytidectomy, 147-383; *see also* Wrinkles
  anesthesia for, 216-218
  cervical contouring in, 274-283
  chemical peel and, 86-87
  closure of, 304-310
  collagen injection and, 609
  complications of
    contour irregularities as, 378
    ecchymosis as, 356-357
    edema as, 356
    hematoma as, 351-355
    infection as, 378-379
    nerve injury as, 358-365
    scarring as, 366-369
    seroma as, 376-377
    skin slough as, 370-375
  drains and, 311-312
  facial nerve injury from, 166
  incisions for, 218-232
    designing of, 219
    earlobe detachment and, 227-232
    postauricular, 223-226
    preauricular, 221
    tragal, 220, 222
  in male patient, 333-349
  patient education for, 214
  patient evaluation for, 188-189
  platysmal bands and, 284-302
  postoperative routine for, 313
  preoperative consultation for, 190-191
  preoperative evaluation for, 192-213
    attenuation of deep layer support and, 198-199
    jowls and, 200-201
    nasolabial fold and, 201-202
    patient's age and, 196
    platysma bands and, 203-213
    skin quality and, 194-195
    subcutaneous fat accumulation and, 196-197
  preoperative routine preceding, 215

Rhytidectomy—cont'd
  reoperative, 314-332
    attenuation of deep support and, 323-325
    fat accumulation and, 322-3231
    incisions for, 316-320
    patient evaluation for, 315-316
    platysmal bands and, 325-326
    postoperative care after, 329
    results of, 330-331
    skin laxity and, 321
    technique for, 326-329
  soft tissue anatomy and, 149-187; *see also* Soft tissue
  subcutaneous undermining in, 233-243
  redraping and, 244-247
  superficial muscular aponeurosis and, 248-261; *see also* Superficial muscular aponeurosis
ROOF fat
  browpexy and, 560, 561
  forehead anatomy and, 538
Root of tooth, in genioplasty, 598
Rotation of skin flap, 246-247

S

Scalp
  browlift incisions and, 548-550
  numbness of, 566
Scar
  blepharoplasty causing, 488, 499
  browlift and, 543, 565
  chemical peel causing
    phenol, 108-112
    trichloroacetic acid, 132-133
  dermabrasion and, 136-137
  rhytidectomy, 366-369
    contracture and, 373
    in male patient, 337
Scleroderma, 608
Scopolamine, 29
Secondary rhytidectomy; *see* Rhytidectomy, reoperative
Secretion, ketamine causing, 32-33
Sedation, 11-43; *see also* Drug management
Senile lentigo, 61
Sensitivity to sunlight, 108

INDEX

Sensory nerve; *see also* Nerve
  browlift and, 533
  rhytidectomy and, 358-359
Septum, orbital, 394-395
Seroma, 376-377
Shivering, 40-41
Skin
  anatomy of, 152
  blepharoplasty and, 499
  of eyelids
    anatomy of, 392
    lower blepharoplasty and, 472-482
    overresection of, 423-426
    preoperative evaluation of, 423-425
  forehead, 531
  rhytidectomy and, 194-195
    reoperative, 321
    sloughing of, 370-376
Skin cancer, 71, 80, 116
Skin flap
  redraping of, 304-310
  rotation of, 246-247
Skin graft, slough and, 376
Skin-muscle flap, 463-468
Sloughing of skin, 370-376
SMAS; *see* Superficial muscular aponeurosis
Soft tissue
  anatomy of, 149-187
    aging changes and, 180-187
    facial nerve and, 166-171
    great auricular nerve and, 178-179
    mimetic muscles and, 154-160
    parotid duct and buccal fat pad and, 176-178
    parotid-masseteric fascia and, 160-165
    retaining ligaments and, 172-176
    skin and, 151, 152
    subcutaneous layer, 152-153
    superficial muscular aponeurosis and, 153-154
  attenuation of
    deformities from, 198-199
    jowls and, 200-201
    nasolabial fold and, 201-202
    platysma band and, 206, 207
    reoperative rhytidectomy and, 323-325

Solar lentigo, 61
Spinal accessory nerve, 363
Spot chemical peel
  of face, 83, 84
  of hand, 85
Staphylococcal infection
  blepharoplasty and, 497
  rhytidectomy and, 378-379
Staple, 310
Steroid, for hypertrophic scar, 366
Steroid-induced atrophy, 492-493
Stigmata of aging, 56, 192-193
Subcutaneous fat
  in jowls, 240
  rhytidectomy and, 196-197
Subcutaneous layer, 152-153
Subcutaneous undermining, for rhytidectomy, 233-243
  age as factor in, 234-235
  ear and, 240-242
  mesotemporalis region and, 237, 349
  temporoparietal fascia and, 237, 238
Sublimaze (fentanyl)
  characteristics of, 21-22
  operative period and, 36-37
Submandibular fat, 275
Submental crease, 602
Submental incision, 242
Subplatysmal fat
  contouring of, 280-283
  rhytidectomy and, 196-197
Sub-SMAS fat, 534, 535-536
Suction drain, 311
Suction lipoplasty, submandibular, 275
Sun exposure
  blepharoplasty and, 521
  of peeled skin, 103
Sun-damaged skin
  chemical peeling for, 47, 50
  to dermis, 57-59
  hyperpigmentation in, 75
  lymphocytic infiltrate in, 68
  regional peeling in, 83-84
  rhytidectomy and, 194-195
Sunlight sensitivity, 108
Superficial fascia
  cervical, 154
  deep fascia in relation to, 164, 165
Superficial mimetic muscles, 155

INDEX

Superficial muscular aponeurosis
  anatomy of, 153-154
  brow fat and, 410
  browlifting and, 538
  deep fascia and, 163
  dissection of, 186-187
    attenuation of deep layer support and, 199
    extended, 254, 272-273
    reoperative, 327-329
  facial nerve injury and, 166, 168
  fibrous bands and, 175
  frontalis muscle and, 531
  jowls and, 200-201
  mimetic muscles in relation to, 158-160
  muscle anatomy and, 157
  operative technique for, 248-261
    closure of, 258
    fixation and, 262-263
    incisions in, 250-251
    in male patient, 344-346
    nasolabial fold and, 254-255
    parotid gland and, 252
    redraping and, 247, 259-261
  postoperative results of, 266-273
  reoperative rhytidectomy and, 324-325
  rhytidectomy and, 237
Superficial temporal artery, 169
Superior transverse ligament of Whitnall, 398
Supraorbital nerve, 532
Supratarsal crease
  anatomy of, 390-391
  evaluation of, 426-427
Supratarsal fixation, in blepharoplasty, 453-456
Supratrochlear artery, 533
Supratrochlear nerve, 533
Surgeon-patient relationship, 3-10
Surgery, chemical peel with, 141
Suture
  in browlift, 557-558
  browpexy, 561
  lateral canthal tendon and, 505-507
  rhytidectomy and, 304-310
    in male patient, 348
  superficial muscular aponeurosis and, 258

T

Tachycardia
  management of, 40
  phenol causing, 82
Tape mask in chemical peel
  procedure, 93, 141
  removal of, 99-102
Taping, for lower lid blepharoplasty, 507
Tarsal strip procedure, 510-513
Telangiectasia, in peeled skin, 65
Temporal artery, superficial, 169
Temporal branch of facial nerve, 361
Temporal fascia, 162, 163
Temporal region
  anatomy of, 531-538
  cross-section of, 537
  facial nerve in, 166, 168
Temporoparietal fascia, 153; *see also* Superficial muscular aponeurosis
  anatomy of, 154
  rhytidectomy and, 237, 238
  superficial muscular aponeurosis, 239
Tendon, canthal
  anatomy of, 395-397
  suture support to, 505-507
Tenon's fascia, 401-402
Tertiary rhytidectomy; *see* Rhytidectomy, reoperative
Tetracaine, 19
Therapeutic index, 13-14
Thorazine (chlorpromazine), 27
Thymol iodide powder, 141
Tolazoline, 30
Tooth, in genioplasty, 598
Toxicity, of local anesthetic, 19-20
Toxicology, of phenol chemical peel, 81-82
Tragal incision for rhytidectomy, 223
  in male patient, 340-341
  reoperative, 316
Transconjunctival blepharoplasty, 406-407
  lower eyelid, 483-486
Transection, of platysma muscle, 293-303
Trapezius muscle, nerve injury and, 363-365

INDEX

Trauma, to nerve
  browlift causing, 565
  rhytidectomy causing, 166, 358-365
Tretinoin, 118
Trichloroacetic acid peel, 117-134; see also Chemical peel, with trichloroacetic acid
Triflupromazine, 27
Trigeminal nerve, branches of, 533
Turgor, 122
Turkey gobbler neck, 338

U

Upper eyelid; see also Blepharoplasty; Eyelid
  crease of, 390
  cross-section of, 405
  fat of, 408, 409

V

Vaseline dressing, 94-98
Ventilation, in anesthetic toxicity, 20
Ventricular contraction, premature, 40
Vermilion
  dermabrasion around, 138
  perioral wrinkle correction and, 580
Versed; see Midazolam
Vesprin (triflupromazine), 27
Vessel
  in peeled skin, 65
  in sun-damaged skin, 58

Visual loss, 494-495

W

Waterproof mask, 93
Whitnall's ligament, 398
Witch's chin, 602-605
Wound, 497
Wrinkles
  blepharoplasty and, 416, 495-496
  browlift for, 539-540
  chemical peel for, 78-80; see Chemical peel *entries*
    examples of, 47-51
    trichloroacetic acid, 130
  dermabrasion for, 136
  phenol peeling for, 72
  reoperative rhytidectomy for, 321
  rhytidectomy for; see Rhytidectomy

X

Xylocaine; see Lidocaine

Z

Zygomatic ligament
  aging and, 180, 181
  anatomy of, 172
  dissection of SMAS and, 255
Zygomaticus muscles
  anatomy of, 155, 156
  dissection of SMAS and, 254